CHILDREN'S LITERATURE FOR HEALTH AWARENESS

by
Anthony L. Manna
and
Cynthia Wolford Symons

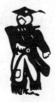

The Scarecrow Press, Inc.
Metuchen, N.J., & London
1992

British Library Cataloguing-in-Publication data available

Library of Congress Cataloging-in-Publication Data

Manna, Anthony L.
    Children's literature for health awareness / by Anthony L. Manna
and Cynthia Wolford Symons.
        p.   cm.
    Includes bibliographical references and index.
    ISBN 0-8108-2582-1 (acid-free paper)
    1. Health—Study and teaching (Elementary) 2. Health—Study
and teaching (Elementary)—Bibliography. 3. Children's
literature—Bibliography. I. Wolford Symons, Cynthia, 1953– .
II. Title.
    LB1587.A3M36   1992
    372.3'7—dc20   92-29737

Contents

Foreword, by Diane DeMuth Allensworth vii
Acknowledgments xi
Preface xiii

1. INTRODUCTION 1
 Chapter Notes 20
 Children's Books Cited 22

2. THE COMPREHENSIVE SCHOOL HEALTH
 PROGRAM: A MEANS TO IMPROVING
 CHILD HEALTH 23
 Chapter Notes 58

3. EVALUATING AND SELECTING
 LITERATURE FOR CHILDREN 61
 • Folktales: Health Issues Across Time and
  Cultures 68
 • Fantasy Literature: Health Issues in "Another
  Kind of Real" 78
 • Realistic Fiction: Health Issues Here and Now 97
 • Historical Fiction: Health Issues in Past Times
  and Places 115
 • Poetry: Health Issues in Sound and Motion 129
 • Informational Books: Humanizing the Facts and
  Figures of Health 162
 • Biography: Health Issues in the Lives of Real
  People 183
 • Plays: Health Issues on Stage 192
 • Book Selection 210
 • Chapter Notes 227
 • Children's Books Cited 230

4. INTEGRATING LITERATURE WITH THE
   SCHOOL HEALTH PROGRAM   242
   • Book Selection and Children's Development   246
   • Correlating Literature and Health Issues   255
   • Growing Healthy: Health Education Curricular
     Progression Chart   259
   • Chapter Notes   301

5. EXPERIENCING LITERATURE WITH
   CHILDREN   303
   • Commercialized Reading Instruction   304
   • Current Attempts at Reform   311
   • Extending Children's Encounters with Literature 332
   • Addressing Controversial Health Topics in the
     Elementary Classroom   353
   • Chapter Notes   359
   • Children's Books Cited   361

6. ANNOTATED BIBLIOGRAPHY OF
   CHILDREN'S LITERATURE FOR
   HEALTH AWARENESS   365
   A. Growth and Development   365
   B. Emotional and Mental Health   372
   C. Personal Health   411
   D. Family Life and Health   420
   E. Nutrition   466
   F. Disease Prevention and Control   481
   G. Safety and First Aid   489
   H. Consumer Health   494
   I. Drug Use and Abuse   497
   J. Community Health Management   500
   K. Careers in the Health Field   512
   L. Miscellaneous Issues   513
      • Persons with Handicaps   513
      • Death and Dying   523
      • Abuse   531
      • Suicide   535

APPENDIX I: HEALTH-RELATED MATERIAL
AND RESOURCES   539
  A. Growth and Development   539
  B. Mental/Emotional Health   542
  C. Personal Health   545
  D. Family Life   551
  E. Nutritional Health   557
  F. Prevention and Control of Diseases and
    Disorders   563
  G. Safety and Accident Prevention   568
  H. Consumer Health   571
  I. Substance Use and Abuse   571
  J. Community Health   586
  K. General Resources for Health Educators   587
  L. Miscellaneous Issues   592

APPENDIX II: CHILDREN'S LITERATURE
RESOURCES   603
  • Booklists and Bibliographies   603
  • Indexes   606
  • Resources on Special Topics   607
  • Periodicals   609

Subject Index   611
Author and Illustrator Index   623
Title Index   635

About the Authors   660

Foreword

> We have met the enemy and he is us.—*Pogo*

Medical scientists have concluded that the major cause of premature death and illness is the lifestyle an individual chooses. Often this lifestyle has its origin in one's childhood. Many of the health decisions that one makes as an adult are based upon the habits adopted as a child. Further, if a child establishes health-enhancing attitudes and behaviors, it is most likely that these will continue throughout a lifetime. Although the primary responsibility for the transference of knowledge and attitudes which lead to the adoption of a healthy lifestyle lies with the family, the school must also share in this responsibility because a child whose psychological, sociological, or physical health is impaired is a child who is at risk for failing in school.

> What is very clear is that education and health for children are inextricably intertwined. A student who is not healthy, or suffers from an undetected vision or hearing deficit, or who is hungry, or who is impaired by drugs or alcohol, is not a student who will profit optimally from the educational process. Likewise, an individual who has not been provided assistance in the shaping of health attitudes, beliefs, and habits early in life will be more likely to suffer the consequences of reduced productivity in later years. [J. M. McGinnis, Director, Office of Disease Prevention and Health Promotion, US Public Health Service]

Two concepts are involved: ensuring children are healthy so that they are capable of learning, and providing learning experiences that will facilitate the adoption of a health-enhancing lifestyle which will allow the individual to most effectively and efficiently utilize the knowledge gained during the schooling experience.

Although the professionals within the school who have some responsibility to provide health instruction include the teacher, nurse, physical educator, guidance counselor, and food service director, it is the teacher who has the most significant role to play. The daily contact of the teacher with the student provides an opportunity to structure the learning experiences necessary for the development of intelligent and self-directed choices leading to health-enhancing behaviors, as well as to teach by example as a role model.

A course of study in health education is fundamental to the curriculum. However, even when students are provided with a sequential kindergarten-through-high-school course in health education, it is often difficult to ensure that students spend sufficient time on tasks to master the health-content concepts. The School Health Education Evaluation study noted that it took forty to fifty hours of instruction in health education for significant changes in behavior to be realized. In order to attain or exceed this minimum, it is recommended that the teacher consider utilizing the concept of correlation in order to maximize the amount of time that students study health. While any number of subjects, such as mathematics, art, science, social studies, and physical education can be used in the elementary school, the language arts and reading are particularly useful for this endeavor because they can be used by the teacher in direct instruction, by the student in a self-directed learning activity, or by parents who can supplement the lessons at school.

Children's Literature for Health Awareness provides the elementary teacher with a long-needed resource detailing how health can be taught through correlation with language arts. Children's literature can serve as a valuable tool to convey health concepts by capturing the child's imagination and intellect. To assist the teacher to plan appropriate learning experiences, this book provides annotated entries of fiction and nonfiction for all ten content areas of a comprehensive health education course. Literature opens new horizons and engages the child in a holistic way, making learning incidental to a pleasurable activity.

> Literature is my Utopia. Here I am not disenfranchised. No barrier of the senses from the sweet, gracious discourse of my book friends. They talk to me without embarrassment or awkwardness. [Helen Keller]

The authors use one of the most popular elementary health education curriculums, Growing Healthy, as an organizational focus. To further assist the teacher, the books mentioned are also organized according to the developmental needs of children. Exciting and innovative learning strategies using literature are provided. *Children's Literature for Health Awareness* promises to be a most valuable resource for all elementary teachers.

The need for children to receive an abundance of health messages in the formal curriculum is critical. Their current and future health depends upon it. *Children's Literature for Health Awareness* will make it easier for the school to respond to that need.

DIANE DEMUTH ALLENSWORTH,
PH.D., R.N.
Associate Executive Director
for Programs and Past President
American School Health Association

Acknowledgments

This book came into being with the gracious support and helpful advice of many people. A research fellowship in 1987 at the Alden B. Dow Creativity Center in Midland, Michigan, helped to launch the project by allowing me a summer of study and the type of discussion that provides meaningful direction. Many thanks to Carol Coppage, Executive Director, and Liz Drake, Assistant Director, for their indefatigable attention to detail and their constant care and concern. A fellowship during the 1988–89 academic year at the Institute for Humanities and Medicine—sponsored by Hiram College and the Northeastern Ohio Universities College of Medicine with a grant from the National Endowment for the Humanities—put me in touch with a special group of humanities specialists and clinical professionals from various medical fields whose efforts to integrate the humanities with the health-care professions provided an invaluable source of inspiration and new ways of thinking about the ties that bind art and science.

I am grateful to Carol Donley and Marty Kohn, Institute codirectors, for believing that we musn't forget to include the children. I am also indebted to Joanne Rand Whitmore, Dean of the College of Education at Kent State University, for granting me a leave to finish this book; Dona Greene Bolton, of the Child Development Center at Kent State University, for giving me so many opportunities to witness a gifted teacher in action; my students over the years who have allowed me into their classrooms by graciously sharing their work with me; Ellen King and Cheryl Levy, children's librarians, Grace A. Dow Memorial Library, Midland Michigan, for helping with the initial search; Darwin Henderson, University of Cincinnati, for the strength of his convictions; Arlene Lawson, Center for Peaceful Change at Kent State

University, for her remarkable editorial expertise and her extraordinary friendship; and, finally, my son Serge, for liking the idea and knowing when it was time to call me out of my study.

A.L.M.

I would like to thank Dr. Diane Allensworth for introducing me to this project and Dr. Charles F. Kegley for his suppport and consistent direction. I hope that this book serves children like Jessica, Laura, Kyle, Vanessa, and Christopher.

C.W.S.

Preface

This book has been written for anyone committed to promoting the holistic health of all children. In the following chapters, parents, librarians, elementary school teachers, and allied health practitioners, such as the school nurse, the pediatric nurse, and community health agents, will find descriptions of many examples of children's books that address health topics. All of the books discussed in the text and included in the supplementary lists were selected on the basis of their proven or potential appeal to children in the elementary school grades as well as their usefulness for reinforcing children's understanding of health-related topics and issues and for helping them clarify important personal concerns that affect their health. We have presented examples of classics as well as examples of more recent books.

In our attempt to demonstrate that fiction as well as nonfiction can be used by health educators, we have described many different types of literature, including poetry, the realistic novel, fantasy, biography, folktales, and plays that contain topics which correspond with those discussed in health education classrooms. We hope that with so many appealing selections from which to choose, our readers will find a variety of books that match the specific interests, needs, and ability levels of the children with whom they come into contact each day. Throughout the book, we have suggested activities for facilitating and managing individualized and large-group reading and for stimulating active involvement in the reading and learning processes through structured discussion as well as through art, dramatics, writing, and other activities that can enrich students' experiences with literature.

According to the *1985 School Health Education Survey,* 66 percent of the nation's kindergarten teachers and 76 percent of those teaching in grades one through six received inservice training in some aspect of health education during 1985.* Workshop leaders who want to offer experienced teachers a practical and substantial way to correlate health education and language arts instruction should find the ideas in this book helpful. We speak from experience. On many occasions we have integrated the materials and methods described in this book into inservice workshops. It is important to remember that many of these teachers work with various populations of children, the gifted and talented, the physically and mentally challenged, and the economically disadvantaged. As we point out in the following chapters, both research and experience demonstrate that health education and children's literature are equally vital to the well-being of these children.

Finally, we believe that school and public librarians will find this book helpful. Over the years, we have discovered that librarians are just as eager as classroom teachers to have access to specialized bibliographies and other materials that can help children develop and that can assist teachers in their efforts to reach their students. As many teachers and students know, libraries and librarians are important links to valuable information. Librarians are often called upon to help students who seek information about health matters for personal reasons and for class reports. School librarians in particular frequently work with teachers in order to make students aware of what a library contains and how to use its resources. We hope this book will foster the kind of collaboration between teachers and librarians which stems from a genuine concern for the well-being of children.

The lists of children's books will allow librarians to recommend books about specific health questions and concerns, and the professional resources described at the end of the book should prove particularly helpful to teachers seeking further information about children's literature, health education, and tried-and-true instructional practices for involving children in both of these areas.

---

*1985 *School Health Education Survey* (New York: Metropolitan Life Foundation, 1985), p. 3.

Wishing to make the book useful to as wide an audience as possible, we used the Growing Healthy Curriculum as our guide for recommending various children's books and for suggesting appropriate learning activities. Developed as a combination of the Primary Grades Health Curriculum Project and the School Health Curriculum Project, two standard and respected curricular models in the health education field, the Growing Healthy Curriculum offers elementary school teachers a comprehensive model for students in kindergarten through grade seven. Since this curriculum covers such a wide range of essential health-related information and skills, the topics outlined in the Growing Healthy Curriculum guide, as well as the lifestyle goals and learning objectives listed on the Growing Healthy Curricular Progression Chart, provided some direction for insuring a thorough treatment of the topics encountered in a typical elementary school health education program at a given grade level.

Overview of the Chapters

The organization of this book closely parallels the format we have used in our workshops and classes on correlating health education and children's literature. By following this format, we have been able to focus on the topics and issues that actually concern educators, librarians, parents, and others who are committed to promoting the health of children with the aid of meaningful trade books.

In Chapter 1, we define and elaborate on the nature of the relationship between children's literature and health education. The case for using literature to develop health awareness is put forward by contrasting the standard approach to health education, through textbooks, with the much broader potential offered by the creative use of good children's literature, both fiction and nonfiction.

In Chapter 2, we provide a rationale for comprehensive health programming within the context of each elementary school grade. Specific characteristics of an exemplary health program are provided through a detailed description of the topics and objectives contained in the Growing Healthy

Curriculum. This inclusive model is the basic framework for describing the knowledge, skills, and attitudes that health educators attempt to inculcate in children as they progress through each level of a comprehensive health curriculum.

Chapter 3 contains a guide to evaluating and selecting specific types of children's books. Along with general evaluative criteria that can be applied to both the language and illustrations in children's books, specific questions are provided for assessing books that deal with health-related topics, concepts, and themes. For the purpose of selecting books that correspond to the needs and interests of children at various stages in their growth, we highlight specific developmental characteristics that have implications for selecting books for children's private as well as shared experiences with literature. A framework for book selection based on research in the development of children's reading interests is also discussed.

In Chapter 4 we describe specific children's books that reflect the lifestyle goals and health topics contained in the Growing Healthy curriculum. The supplementary lists of annotated books found in Chapter 6 contain many other examples of books that can be used to enhance the topics, issues, and themes that comprise a comprehensive health education program.

Chapter 5 is a methodology chapter. We discuss some of the ways to share literature with children. The focus here is on creating a supportive, child-centered classroom environment, and the emphasis is on promoting children's active responses to literature that depicts health-related content. We offer a theoretical model for integrating reading, writing, speaking, and listening through literature and we describe specific activities for enhancing children's experiences with books. In Chapter 5 we also summarize the benefits and objectives of making children aware of health topics and concerns with children's literature.

Chapter 6 provides an extensive annotated bibliography of children's books that can be used for health education. It is organized by topics in the Growing Healthy Curriculum and further subdivided by grade/reading level and specific subjects.

Two appendixes have been included: Appendix I contains an annotated list of nonbook health-related materials and resources. Appendix II contains an annotated list of various selection aids for children's literature. Three indexes complete the book.

1. Introduction

> Science offers so few clues that we
> need to draw on all the humanities to
> understand human behavior.—*Margaret Walker*, M.D., Harvard Medical
> School[1]

Children's Literature for Health Awareness has evolved out of
our growing perception that the topics and issues found in
many selections of children's literature closely parallel the
health-related topics and issues dealt with each day in a typical
elementary school classroom. In fact, the main goal of this
book is to demonstrate that there are literally hundreds of
appropriate children's books which can enhance and reinforce
children's knowledge and understanding of skills and attitudes that affect personal and public health. Throughout this
book we also demonstrate that just as children's discussions of
the subjects and themes found in many provocative children's
books can stimulate them to think about health-related issues,
their discussions of health-related topics will become much
more meaningful and personalized when they see these topics
come alive in carefully selected children's books that reflect
various aspects of the human condition.

The idea for writing this book began when we started to
communicate across two seemingly different curriculum areas, health education and children's literature. We soon
discovered that we were exploring similar issues and concerns
with the teachers and parents who took our classes and
workshops. We began to realize that we shared a deep
concern for the welfare of children and a similar professional
commitment to improving the quality of children's lives.
Based on our own experiences in elementary and secondary
schools and our ongoing work with many dedicated and

1

sensitive teachers, parents, and librarians, we knew, for example, that it is possible to create safe and nurturing places for children to grow and learn and flourish. We both believe that, with the right kind of information and adult support, children can learn to take control and ownership of their physical and emotional well-being in order to live their lives to the fullest.

In becoming aware of the degree to which health-related issues and the content of many types of children's literature are interrelated, we realized that each of our fields deals directly with essential life skills and attitudes that can have a profound and lasting impact on children, not only during their formative years but throughout the course of their lives. While some of this development can be enhanced by children's acquisition of skills that are immediately observable and measurable, much of it is less concrete but no less vital to their well-being. For example, through their exposure to all types of literature and through their involvement in a comprehensive health education program, children can develop positive feelings about themselves. At the same time, they can learn about and practice effective ways of living with and relating to others. Further, the topics they discuss in response to good books and the issues that capture their attention in a health education classroom can make them aware of their responsibility for helping to create and maintain healthful environments.

The Range of Children's Books

To recognize the extent to which the topics and themes in children's books deal with personal and public health issues, one needs only to spend some time in the children's room of a public library or the children's section of a good bookstore. Of the 40,000 children's books now in print, to which approximately 3,000 books are added annually, hundreds speak directly, honestly, and accurately to both children and adults about specific and universal questions, concerns, and problems that are functions of children's health. Such concepts are revealed in an impressive array of books, including many different versions of ancient folktales, realistic novels that reflect contemporary life, and provocative informational books that satisfy children's natural curiosity about the world and the people who inhabit it. With remarkable insight, the best authors and illustrators of children's books focus on children and adults of every race and every cultural and socioeconomic background who confront and cope with issues of social and personal change.

Within this wide range of books the entire gamut of moods and emotions, as well as the positive and negative consequences of human experiences, are depicted for children. Many children's books not only reflect typical experiences associated with preventive health maintenance and healthy lifestyles, including visits to a dentist or physician and the need for physical fitness and judicious dietary practices, but these books also examine, through fact as well as fiction, such abstractions as the relationship between the physical, mental, social, and emotional aspects of health, the importance of satisfying our basic physical and psychological needs, and the value of weighing consequences before choosing one action over another.

At the same time, other authors and illustrators are critically conscious of the fact that many of today's children are exposed to the harsher realities of life through their own personal experiences and through various media. These authors and illustrators depict more disturbing and alarming experiences that are inevitable and unavoidable facts of life which can intensely affect children. Opening its doors wide to these unsettling events and circumstances, the children's book market contains many types of literature—including fantasy, poetry, plays, and nonfiction—about death and dying, prejudice, the debilitating effects of drug abuse and addiction, children's confrontations with abusive adults, the threat and potential effects of nuclear war, patterns of human sexuality, the rise of suicide rates among young people, and the repercussions of an unwanted or unintended pregnancy.

Like literature for adults, children's literature both reflects and interprets the concerns and issues that characterize the age in which it is written. As more and more studies of childhood and child development provide specific and pertinent information about how children grow and develop, what they are capable of learning and understanding, and the ways quality literature can enhance even the youngest child's cognitive, emotional, and social development, books written for children continue to demonstrate increasing and remarkable sophistication. This is evident in the topics explored in children's books and in the range and quality of their language style, their illustrations, and their overall design. Far from depicting only a sunny, one-sided view of the world, the literature available to today's children continues to explore all facets of life—the poignant as well as the pleasant, the disturbing as well as the happy. These books can have a significant impact on a child's life because they have the potential to offer the help and guidance children need in order to survive the best and worst of times.

Teachers and parents often ask us, "Is it really necessary to expose children to the darker side of life and to life's problems? Won't there be plenty of time for that once they grow up and experience some of these problems firsthand?" We believe, as does child psychologist Bruno Bettelheim, that to pretend that there are no disturbing circumstances in life and that people always act from a perspective of kindness and goodness does children a disservice. Such a protectionist attitude insulates and incapacitates children in areas to which they are already exposed and about which they have many questions. Based on his use of fairy tales to help children develop personal awareness and to find meaning in life, Bettelheim argues that "the child needs most particularly to be given suggestions in symbolic form about how he may deal with these issues and grow safely into maturity."[2] According to Bettelheim, "when children are young, it is literature that carries such information best."[3] This is the case because much good literature shows children effective ways to cope with life's problems and predicaments through their imaginative and sympathetic participation in the experiences of the characters they meet in the books they read or the ones read to them. In this sense, literature can be both an important part of a child's rehearsal for adult life and, at the same time, an aid for helping him or her to deal with immediate concerns and experiences.

Echoing the sentiments and practices of many contemporary writers, illustrators, and publishers of children's books, award-winning author and illustrator Maurice Sendak has said:

> You must tell the truth about the subject to the child as well as you are able without any mitigating of the truth. You must allow that children are small, courageous people who have to deal everyday with a multitude of problems, just as we adults do, and that they are unprepared for most things, and what they most yearn for is a bit of truth somewhere.[4]

While escape and entertainment are often the rewards of reading, literature can offer children much more than an escape from life's circumstances and far more than mere entertainment. A good poem or story, or a good informational book that augments understanding and offers accurate and current factual knowledge, can stimulate children as well as the adults who share books with them to think about what it means to be human. Like all effective art, a well-written work of literature provides insights into human existence and shows us not only how life is lived but also how it might be lived. Children's literature is no exception.

There are of course many children's books that are poorly written and others that are poorly designed and illustrated. These books were produced as though their authors and illustrators were oblivious to the fact that just as children need and long for quality and sustenance in all aspects of their lives, from their diet to their relationships, they also need the kind of nourishment good books supply in such abundance. At the same time, there are just as many books that ring true because they contain honest accounts of how people act and interact in positive and negative ways and what they value and believe. The books that endure and continue to offer children insights into what it means to grow up are the ones that show respect for children's rapidly developing intelligence and for the intensity of their feelings and discoveries.

The good book, whether fiction or nonfiction, answers basic but important questions children ask about the world and the people who inhabit it. As Charlotte Huck has explained, "Literature helps a child understand what it means to become fully human."[5] This is possible because good literature is by and about real people in the midst of living and learning, sometimes bumbling through or celebrating their relationships, and at other times wondering about or desperately trying to survive disruptive experiences that cause them to change, to form new values, to gain a deeper sense of themselves, and to grow in compassion for others. "Literature enhances children's knowledge of the world," writes Dorothy Strickland, a well-known reading expert. "It allows children to tap a wide range of human emotions and experiences, and it stimulates curiosity and reflective thought."[6]

The Role of School Health Education

This same concern for all facets of the physical, mental, social, emotional, and spiritual development of children and other members of society should be at the heart of every comprehensive health education program. This is what the Oxford English Dictionary implies when it defines health not only as a "soundness of body," but as a "spiritual, moral and mental soundness" as well. The current and growing concern among health professionals is for comprehensive educational programs that emphasize prevention and attitudinal changes toward health practices. This concern is based on increasing evidence that risks to longevity, such as heart disease, cancer, stress, and accidental injury, are very closely related to lifestyle factors.[7] In 1976, for example, medical scientists concluded that perhaps as much as 50 percent of mortality could be attributed to unhealthy behaviors or lifestyles and that most incidences of unhealthy conditions found among adults and children can be reduced in severity, if not prevented, through avoidance of risk factors by lifestyle modifications.

It is vital to note that the personal health habits and behaviors to which most serious health problems can be attributed do not appear overnight; they are dependent on habit patterns learned and integrated in childhood. One study suggests that as many as 40 percent of children exhibit one or more of the risk factors associated with heart disease, including hypertension, high cholesterol levels, and lack of exercise.[8] A further review of child and adolescent health statistics reinforces the fact that health risk behaviors are pervasive among the following populations:

- Nearly one-half of all deaths to children aged one to fourteen are due to unintentional injuries. About one-half of injuries to children in this age group result from being passengers in cars involved in motor vehicle crashes. Although all 50 states now require safety restraints for very young children, there is great variation in these mandates for children over the age of three.
- About one-fourth of high school seniors who have ever smoked report having smoked their first cigarette by grade six, over one-half by grades seven or eight, and three-fourths by grade nine. Although cigarette smoking is declining for all age groups, those who do smoke are starting at younger ages.
- The three leading causes of death among American youth aged fifteen to twenty-four, in descending order, are unintentional injuries, homicide, and suicide. Importantly, three-fourths of the injury deaths to youth in this age cohort involve motor vehicles, and more than one-half of the related motor vehicle crashes involve alcohol.[9]
- Teenage girls are the most likely victims of sexual abuse.
- More than one-half of all committed juvenile offenders used alcohol or other drugs regularly before being imprisoned.[10]

While this list—however brief—is alarming, it strongly implies just how critical it is to empower children, while they are in the stages of habit formation, with knowledge, skills, and attitudes that will have lasting effects on enhancing the quality of their lives. What better place for them to examine and learn about such vital lifestyle issues than in a health education classroom where, with the facilitation of a concerned and qualified adult, they can gain a sense of responsibility for their lives that can lead to the integration of a health-promotion attitude and lifestyle into their personal development. Health promotion and the wellness movement that emphasizes the interdependence of community and individual measures for ensuring a state of well-being are concepts whose time has come.[11]

Comprehensive school health programming has limitless potential to address the holistic health concerns of children, youth, and the culture at large. Recognizing the compulsory nature of schooling in the United States, the American Public Health Association asserts, "no other community setting even approximates the magnitude of the grades K–12 school education enterprise, with an enrollment . . . of 45.5 million students in nearly 17,000 school districts comprising more than 115,000 schools with some 2.1 million teachers."[12] In *Health Education and Youth: A Review of Research and Development,* Lloyd Kolbe is even more specific about the role health educators can play in health promotion when he points out that quality health instruction should be "designed to help students recognize how their personal behavior affects their health, learn to make responsible health-related decisions, acquire health-related knowledge, develop positive attitudes and habits, and learn to influence factors in the home and community that affect health."[13]

By promoting a student's health and the adoption of a healthier lifestyle, schools can protect, maintain, and foster holistic health not only during the student's years in school, but also into adulthood. Further, in a time such as ours when schools in the United States are called upon to be accountable for what children learn and how they develop, it is important to remember that healthy children are more likely to participate in and benefit from learning experiences.[14]

Within the health field it has been unequivocally demonstrated that school health education is not only an effective means of improving health knowledge and attitudes but can also decrease the likelihood that children will adopt behaviors that are hazardous to health.[15] In light of the School Health Education Evaluation Survey, schools can no longer be responsible for merely disseminating information about a variety of health matters but must extend their concern for enhancing their students' well-being into a comprehensive quality health promotion role. The American Medical Association notes, "Any future advances in improving the nation's health will not result from spectacular biomedical breakthroughs. Rather, advances will result from personally initiated actions that are directly influenced by the individual's health-related attitudes, beliefs, and knowledge. School health education can make a valuable contribution in areas such as these. . . ."[16]

The Role of the Textbook in Health Education

Although the standard textbooks used in health education classrooms may be helpful for introducing elementary school children to basic facts and concepts about personal and community health, health educators cannot expect these texts to convey to children all the dimensions of well-being. This is particularly true when well-being is viewed holistically as "an expression of each person functioning as an integrated whole, a totality of body, mind and spirit."[17] Even the exceptional textbook, which can justifiably serve as a starting point for a heterogeneous class, must naturally limit its content to basic understandings about health. It simply cannot cover all the pertinent health matters children will encounter in specific situations.

Textbooks are limited in other ways as well. Several recent studies of texts commonly used in American elementary and secondary schools revealed that textbook writers often impede rather than facilitate the reader's comprehension of the information the text is responsible for communicating. One major problem found by schoolbook researchers is referred to as "mentioning," a term used to describe the superficial treatment topics routinely receive in textbooks. Although mentioning has been found in texts used to teach nearly every subject at every grade level, it is most prevalent in textbooks dealing with social studies, history, and science.[18]

Mentioning causes a number of difficulties for readers. When textbook writers move quickly from one idea or fact to another as though they were compiling a list, they frequently fail to indicate which ideas are the most important. As a result, they do not give enough attention to the most significant information. David Elliott, codirector of Educational Media Associates, believes that such "thinness of detail" often makes schoolbooks inaccurate, misleading, and uninteresting.[19]

In a study conducted at the University of Illinois' Center for the Study of Reading, researchers found other problems with textbooks. For example, a large sample of social studies and science texts contained deficient transitions and connectives between ideas, no clear cause-effect relationships, insufficient and irrelevant information, and a faulty structure that affected the overall logic and coherence of the writer's presentation.[20] Many of these problems were a direct result of the writers' reliance on short, simple sentences which, instead of aiding understanding and basic comprehension, obscured meaning and forced readers to grope for meaning relationships. In contrast, other studies have shown that children read faster and have better comprehension when they have access to a more sophisticated and complex writing style rather than the primer-type style that writers of textbooks and other curriculum materials often use.[21] Since students spend 75 percent of classroom time and 90 percent of homework time using texts, many reading experts recommend exposing children to texts whose styles reflect the complexity of natural language usage, particularly if understanding rather than mere recall and regurgitation of facts is the goal of instruction.[22]

Trade Books as an Alternative

Well-written children's books employ a distinctive, even a fresh and memorable, language style that is appropriate to the author's purpose and content. The best ones capture the expressive rhythms, patterns, and diversity of authentic language, thus offering children language models that can enhance their oral and written language development. In fact, it is not uncommon for authors themselves to point out that although their books are intended for children, they in no way feel obligated to restrict their topics or themes, or to limit their vocabulary or language style. For example, Cynthia Rylant, an award-winning children's author, feels that she writes *up* rather than *down* to her readers. Rylant says,

> I'm not out to instruct children and I don't think I restrict myself in any way because children will be among the readers of my books. Actually, within the world of children's literature I feel extremely free to share the things I observe and feel so deeply because I believe children are interested in anything that has to do with living. My challenge is to find that beauty and to see if I can capture it in words—regardless of the age of my readers.[23]

When used as a viable and stimulating alternative to a constant diet of textbook language and, even more important, to the often questionable way textbook writers convey information, good children's books can benefit both teachers and students of health education. While many health education texts do provide important information about healthful ways of living, what is frequently missing from these texts is the human element that trade books provide in such abundance and with such variety because they are rooted in all kinds of genuine and identifiable human experiences. This is particularly true of authors of informational trade books, whose purpose and challenge are to make the facts and figures about a subject come alive by providing information in the form of absorbing characters and incidents that highlight personal attitudes and understandings, while at the same time heightening the reader's knowledge. *No Measles, No Mumps for Me* by Paul Showers, for example, explains to children in the primary grades the reasons why they need shots and how antibodies fight germs. A sensitively written informational book, *No Measles, No Mumps for Me* offers accurate information through an inventive and lively story narrated by a young person with whom children can identify. The colorful illustrations and detailed diagrams that complement the factual information teach as much as they entertain and sustain the interest of young readers.

While a textbook must limit the coverage and depth of its information due to constraints of space, a trade book, which is usually written on one specialized topic, can provide much more detail and a more thorough treatment of a subject. The range and depth of a subject can also be increased for children who read trade books because so many different writers and illustrators have focused on, and continue to treat, the same subjects. This can not only demonstrate to children how one topic can be explored from several equally legitimate and defensible points of view, but it can also provide young learners opportunities to compare and contrast attitudes and opinions about a subject. In this way, they can develop the kinds of critical thinking skills that are essential for all true learning to take place and for a firm grasp of specific content.

The variety trade books offer also means that different

students can find books on the same subject that complement
their interests, abilities, and reading levels. As numerous
researchers have shown, when children's interest in what they
read is high, they enjoy reading and they also tend to move
beyond the basic comprehension and recall levels in their
reading responses, demonstrating, for example, an ability to
interpret and evaluate a text.[24]

Given opportunities to choose freely from a collection of
appropriate trade books that match their interests, tastes, and
abilities and extend the materials treated in their textbook,
students will also be more inclined to discuss what they read.
They will feel they have something valuable and unique to
contribute to class discussions since each trade book contains
a distinctive approach to a topic. Such discussions are important for learning. When students work together and talk to
one another about ideas that interest and excite them, greater
clarification of concepts is made possible through reinforcement, through the need to verify and support ideas, and
through opportunities to make choices and decisions based
on their knowledge and understanding of various perspectives and interpretations of basic facts and attitudes.

The type of student interaction and involvement that trade
books encourage, and the informative and lively debate trade
books can stimulate, make learning purposeful, functional,
and enjoyable. Jerome Bruner believes that such involvement
can have a lasting impact on how children see themselves as
learners and how they approach future learning tasks. He
says, "To the degree that one is able to approach learning as a
task of discovering something rather than 'learning about' it,
to that degree will there be a tendency for the child to carry
out his own learning activities with the autonomy of self-
reward."[25] How different this is from the picture painted by
Julie Chan of California State University when she describes
what often happens when textbooks control instruction: ". . .
when students all read from the same textbook, the same
chapter, the same page and perhaps the same section, they
have the same information. It is difficult to listen to others tell
about something which is common knowledge to the entire
class."[26]

Nathan Perry, former president of Harvard University,

reflects these same sentiments when he suggests: "The close observer soon discovers that the teacher's task is not to implant facts but to place the subject to be learned in front of the learner and, through sympathy, emotion, imagination, and patience, to awaken in the learner the restless drive for answers and insights which enlarge the personal life and give it meaning."[27] By making a wide selection of relevant children's books an integral part of the entire health education curriculum, teachers can practice the type of sensitive student-centered instruction Nathan Perry endorses.

Literature, then, can help to promote health awareness in the following ways:

- Provides opportunities to make abstract information about health concrete, relevant, and personal.
- Provides opportunities for students to explore health-related attitudes, values, options, choices, and coping strategies from a human perspective.
- Provides access to various points of view, behaviors, and lifestyles of people from various backgrounds and cultures.
- Reinforces the concept that health is a continuously evolving process which involves constant decision-making and lifestyle choices which can promote or hinder wellness.
- Helps young people see that they are not alone regarding their emotions, problems, concerns, and questions as well as their triumphs and successes concerning life and living.
- Stimulates young people to discuss and perhaps find solutions to health problems and concerns they might not otherwise talk about openly or even acknowledge.
- Reinforces language skills and reading skills within the context of health-related topics and issues.
- Introduces young people to a wide variety of literature which can enhance various aspects of their personal and social development while they learn health-related content.

Benefits for Teachers

Students are not the only ones who can benefit from an exposure to children's books. There are just as many rewards for elementary school teachers and other health professionals who use trade books to reinforce, enrich, and enliven health-related content and concepts. By having access to a wide and relevant selection of children's literature, health educators can choose materials that match the different concerns, abilities, and learning styles of their students. Many of the teachers we know claim that this type of freedom, and the trust in their professional judgment implied by it, is all too rare in today's schools. In many cases, the selection of textbooks and other types of instructional aids is done by a district-wide committee, often without adequate input from the teachers who will be asked to use the materials and without careful consideration of the kinds of students who are supposed to learn from them. As a result, textbooks more often become a burden than an aid for motivating students to learn and for sustaining their enthusiasm about a topic. Because the same textbook is frequently too difficult for some students and too easy for others, students often become frustrated or bored when a textbook is used as the primary learning tool, not to mention the effect these attitudes can have on a teacher's attempt to keep students interested.

We have found that when teachers learn about the enormous variety that characterizes the contemporary children's book market, they soon realize that by using appropriate trade books to supplement textbook lessons they can have greater control over what goes on in their classrooms and greater autonomy regarding the countless instructional decisions they need to make each day. In this case, control should not be confused with manipulation or the misuse of a teacher's authority. Rather, it refers to an essential professional privilege that allows teachers to accomplish an important professional objective: to give every type of learner many opportunities to experience the joy and satisfaction that are associated with successful learning.

Because teachers spend so much time with their students, they get to know them as individuals with specific emotional, social, and cognitive needs. They should therefore be trusted as knowledgeable and sensitive professionals who know how to create productive classroom environments, to design meaningful learning tasks, and to select the kinds of materials that can best enhance their students' development. In this book, we suggest that by using children's literature in their classrooms and by engaging their students in imaginative activities which can promote learning and awareness through literature, health educators can become empowered to exercise their rights as qualified and concerned professionals.

The teachers in our classes and workshops tell us that it is very tempting to become wholly dependent on textbooks and the student workbooks and drill sheets that are intended to insure students' mastery of textbook material. This dependence is not surprising. Elementary school teachers are busy people. They are held accountable for teaching many subjects and for teaching them efficiently and on a prescribed schedule. Since instructional resources such as textbooks and worksheets contain a built-in management system and a planned sequence of observable skills that can be quickly measured, they can naturally become a type of cookbook to be relied upon for immediate proof of instructional success. But what are the costs of such a heavy, and often exclusive, dependence on predominately cognitive resources of this sort? In the first place, these types of materials tend to restrict teachers as much as they restrict their students. Too often, standard textbook lessons and the instructional techniques outlined in a teacher's manual imply that teaching is merely a matter of communicating and testing basic facts about a subject and that true learning is simply factual recall. However, teaching and learning are both complex processes that are not quite as uniform and orderly as producers of textbooks would have teachers and students believe.

The assign-read-test approach that frequently characterizes a textbook-dominated classroom is a far cry from the spontaneous discoveries and happy accidents that distinguish true learning and sustain us as teachers. As anyone who has ever stepped inside a dynamic classroom knows, the task a teacher faces each day is not merely to provide a viable structure for learning tasks, but also to make a subject meaningful and functional for students so that what they learn has some personal significance in their lives. A teacher's challenge is to make the content come alive, consequently helping students recognize the relationship between the concepts and skills they are learning and how these concepts and skills impact on their lives.

Even an exceptionally written textbook can provide only the most basic ingredients that go into the dynamic process and sensitive, humane interaction that characterize the art of effective teaching. On the other hand, a memorable work of literature paired with an effective informational book more closely reflects and approximates this process, because the fundamental concern of all writers of literature is to promote significant human experiences. As aware and close observers of life and living, writers of literature can be included among our most impressive and impressionable teachers because they have the potential to make such a deep and enduring impact on our beliefs, attitudes, and knowledge as well as on how we see ourselves fitting into the world. Graham Greene, the well-known novelist, has observed that writers whose works appeal to young people are no exception:

> . . . in childhood all books are books of divination, telling us about the future, and like the fortune-teller who sees a long journey in the cards or death by water, they influence the future. I suppose that is why books excite us so much. What do we ever get nowadays from reading to equal the excitement and revelation of those first fourteen years?[28]

This notion of the writer as teacher has important implications for health educators. Considering the impact quality literature of all types can have on children, it is not surprising that teachers who are responsible for health education often point out that they gain a great deal of practical information from the techniques writers and illustrators of children's books use to communicate to their readers and to hold their attention. This is due in part to the honest and authentic ways good books characterize children and depict childhood. Just as the best writers and illustrators of children's books do not talk down to their readers, they also present accurate depictions of different types of children and different aspects and conditions of childhood. Similarly, they need to have a firm understanding of how children learn and develop.

A writer or illustrator who is aware of the experiences and circumstances of childhood can therefore remind adults of what it is like to be a child, of how children relate to those around them, and, particularly in the case of a worthwhile informational book, how they perceive, integrate, and use newly acquired information and concepts. The approaches to life and learning contained in many first-rate children's books offer adults positive models to follow in their own teaching and in the ways they relate to the children with whom they come into contact.

Children's books can also serve teachers in other practical ways. For example, a knowledge of appropriate trade books can help teachers plan curriculum sequences that span various grade levels. This type of planning is possible because many different books that treat the same general topic are available for readers of all ages and abilities. Thus, trade books with similar content can be used at each grade level to reinforce attitudes, knowledge, and skills learned in previous and subsequent grades.

Consider, for example, the issue of smoking. When the topic is first introduced in the primary grades, teachers could read aloud and perhaps have their students dramatize *Where Does All That Smoke Come From?* by the Sandbergs, a clever, though serious, fantasy with vivid illustrations that depicts how two young children learn about the dangers of cigarette smoking when they meet a chain-smoking dragon who is a victim of cigarette advertising. In the same elementary school, students in the upper grades could read and discuss Wrenn and Schwarzrock's *Facts and Fantasies About Smoking,* one of the many informational books in the "Coping With" series published by American Guidance Service.

Following the format of other books in this timely series which emphasizes decision making about important health matters, *Facts and Fantasies About Smoking* focuses on a younger adolescent who, after being introduced to the consequences of cigarette smoking, must decide if the pleasure of smoking is greater than the risks which, in this case, are appropriate to the target audience for whom the book is written. Role playing and an informal class debate would be natural follow-up activities for any of the "Coping With" books.

As we will demonstrate throughout this book, this same

type of sequential curriculum planning with trade books is possible for any of the topics covered in a comprehensive elementary school health education program. Teachers can choose from literally hundreds of trade books, ranging from simple to complex selections of fiction and nonfiction, about safety and first aid, nutrition, the protection of environmental resources, human reproduction, and many other pertinent topics that comprise a comprehensive knowledge of personal and public health issues.

By using appropriate selections of children's literature, health educators can also correlate several of the subject areas they are responsible for teaching. An efficient and effective way to combine instruction in several subject areas, correlation is based on the premise that there are many basic similarities among the various content areas of an academic curriculum. In practice, correlation occurs when the content of two academic disciplines is taught concurrently for the sake of fostering divergent thinking among students. For example, elementary school teachers who follow the suggestions described in this book will plan and present lessons that relate the concepts, skills, and activities usually covered in a health program to the ones traditionally dealt with in reading or language arts instruction.

While many curriculum guides imply that each subject area should be given its own time slot and specified attention during the school day, there is much to be said for a correlated approach to curriculum planning. Classrooms of students are heterogeneous in nature. Even when students are grouped according to the skills they can demonstrate, they still have different backgrounds, learning styles, and health statuses. While direct teaching done in separate strands with a uniform text may serve as a starting point for such an eclectic group, children do not live in isolation from one another, nor do events in their lives occur in isolation. Through correlated approaches to classroom instruction, children are encouraged to explore the degree and nature of the relationships between thoughts, events, and phenomena, and develop skills to deal with the interrelated nature of life's events. Opening children to this concept in the safety of a nurturing classroom environment serves significantly more important ends than closing or categorizing their minds into time or content slots. Several studies have demonstrated the positive effects of a correlated curriculum on the development of skills. In one of these studies, a fourth-grade textbook science unit on oceanography was supplemented with a selection of relevant trade books and related extension activities. After the entire class completed the textbook unit, one-half of the students read trade books on the topic of oceanography and participated in enrichment activities that integrated writing, speaking, reading, and listening.[29] While the other students had access to several literary selections, their involvement ·in follow-up activities was restricted to a panel discussion on the conservation of ocean ecology. In contrast to the experimental group whose involvement was extensive, these students did not participate in activities that were intended to reinforce the information and concepts acquired through both the textbook and the trade books. As might be expected, students in the experimental group not only scored higher on tests of factual recall, but also demonstrated better interpretive skills.[30] While the study underscored the value of using both fiction and nonfiction in a science unit, it also demonstrated the effectiveness of planning activities that correlate science and the language arts.

Correlation is an instructional practice which seems particularly useful to classroom teachers who are responsible for planning and implementing a health education program. According to a survey conducted by the Metropolitan Life Foundation in 1985, more than 81 percent of the teachers in grades one through six across the country are regular classroom teachers who, because of mandates or insight, or issues of conscience, become responsible for the health education of their students.[31] Few elementary educators in this country have specialized degrees that qualify them to teach health education. It is not surprising, then, that most of the elementary school teachers in our classes and workshops feel they need all the help they can get for dealing with the critical health incidents that arise daily in their classrooms, for teaching health education effectively, and for motivating their students to become personally involved in learning health-related content. Because our approach to health education demonstrates an effective and practical way to correlate two areas of the elementary school curriculum, health education and the language arts, teachers accept it as a viable model for developing their students' skills in health and language arts concurrently. They like the idea of combining instruction in reading, writing, speaking, and listening with instruction in various facets of health, since this type of correlation not only provides them a "way into" health topics and issues, but also offers them a practical solution to the problem of having to fit health education into an already overcrowded curriculum.

NOTES

1. "Medical Summit Sees Need for New Social Contract," *Brain/Mind Bulletin* 12, 9 (June 1987):5.
2. Bruno Bettelheim, *The Uses of Enchantment* (New York: Knopf, 1976), p. 8.
3. Ibid., p. 4.
4. Walter Lorraine, "An Interview With Maurice Sendak" in *Wilson Library Bulletin* 52 (October 1977) :157.
5. Charlotte S. Huck, *Children's Literature in the Elementary School,* 3d ed. (New York: Holt, Rinehart and Winston, 1976), p. 704.
6. Dorothy Strickland, "Foreword" in Eileen M. Burke, *Early Childhood Literature* (Boston: Allyn and Bacon, 1986), p. xiii.
7. Harold J. Cornaccia, et al., *Health in Elementary Schools* (St. Louis: Times Mirror/Mosby, 1984).
8. Marian B. Pollock and Kathleen Middleton, *Elementary School Health Instruction* (St. Louis: Times Mirror/Mosby, 1984), p. ix.
9. U.S. Department of Health and Human Services (Public Health Service), *Healthy People 2000: National Health Promotion and Disease Prevention Objectives,* DHHS Publication No. (PHS) 91-50212 (Washington: U.S. Government Printing Office, 1991), pp. 13–16.
10. Janet Simons, Belva Finlay, and Alice Yang, *The Adolescent and Young Adult Fact Book* (Washington: Children's Defense Fund, 1991), pp. ix–x.
11. Concerning the concept of health promotion, see U.S. Department of Health, Education, and Welfare, *Healthy People: The Surgeon General's Report on Health Promotion and Disease Prevention* (Washington: U.S. Government Printing Office, 1979).
12. "Education for Health in the Community Setting," *American Journal of Public Health* 56 (1975) :65.
13. Lloyd J. Kolbe, "Improving the Health of Children and Youth:

Frameworks for Behavioral Research and Development," in *Health Education and Youth*, ed. George Campbell (London: The Falmer Press, 1984), p. 11.

14. Steven Nelson, *How Healthy Is Your School?* (New York: National Council of Health Education, 1986), p. 12.
15. David B. Connell, et al., "Summary Findings of the School Health Education Evaluation: Health Promotion Effectiveness, Implementation, and Costs," *Journal of School Health* 55 (October 1985) :316–23.
16. *A Guide to Curriculum Planning in Health Education* (Madison: Wisconsin Department of Public Instruction, 1985), p. 5.
17. Dianne E. Cmich, "Theoretical Perspectives of Holistic Health," *Journal of School Health* 54 (January 1984):3.
18. "Schoolbooks Skim Surface, Fail as Tools," *The Cleveland Plain Dealer*, 7 September 1986, p. 25A.
19. Ibid., p. 25A.
20. These findings were reported in *Learning to Read in America: Basal Readers and Content Texts*, eds. Richard C. Anderson, et al. (Hillsdale: Lawrence Erlbaum Associates, 1984). In this volume see, in particular, "Content Area Textbooks " by Thomas H. Anderson and Bonnie B. Armbruster, pp. 193–226; "The Problem of 'Inconsiderate Text' " by Bonnie B. Armbruster, pp. 202–17; and "A Synthesis of Research on the Use of Instructional Texts: Some Implications for the Educational Publishing Industry in Reading" by Richard J. Tierney, pp. 287–96.
21. Armbruster, "The Problem of 'Inconsiderate Text,' " p. 209.
22. Ibid., p. 207.
23. Anthony L. Manna, "Profile: Cynthia Rylant," *The Bulletin* 10 (Winter 1984):14.
24. Studies of response to literature are numerous. For some of the most pertinent, see *Hooked on Books* by Daniel Fader and Elton B. McNeil (New York: Berkeley, 1966); *Literature Education in Ten Countries* by Alan C. Purves (New York: Wiley, 1973); and *Literature and the Reader: Research in Response to Literature, Reading Interests, and the Teaching of Literature* by Alan C. Purves and Richard Beach (Urbana: National Council of Teachers of English, 1972).
25. Jerome Bruner, "The Act of Discovery," in *Concepts in Art and Education*, ed. George Pappas (New York: Macmillan, 1970), p. 96.
26. Julie M. T. Chan, "Trade Books: Uses and Benefits for Content Area Teaching," ERIC Document 189 578 (Arlington: ERIC Document Reproduction Service), p. 7.
27. Quoted in *The Read-Aloud Handbook* by Jim Trelease (New York: Penguin Books, 1982), pp. 36–37.
28. Ibid., p. 21.
29. Betty Anderson, "Books Make Social Studies and Science Come Alive," ERIC Document 240 604 (Arlington: ERIC Document Reproduction Service), pp. 9–11.
30. Ibid., p. 11.
31. *1985 School Health Education Survey* (New York: Metropolitan Life Foundation, 1985), p. 2.

CHILDREN'S BOOKS CITED IN CHAPTER 1

Sandberg, Inger, and Sandberg, Lasse. *Where Does All That Smoke Come From?* trans. Merloyd Lawrence. Delacorte, 1972.
Showers, Paul. *No Measles, No Mumps for Me.* Illus. Byron Barton. Crowell, 1980.
Wrenn, C. Gilbert, and Schwarzrock, Shirley. *Facts and Fantasies About Smoking.* Illus. Dick Gravender. American Guidance Service, 1970.

2. The Comprehensive School Health Program: A Means to Improving Child Health

> Any future advances in improving the nation's health will not result from spectacular biomedical break-throughs. Rather, advances will result from personally initiated actions that are directly influenced by the individual's health-related attitudes, beliefs, and knowledge. School health education can make a valuable contribution in areas such as these. . . .—*American Medical Association*[1]

There is a game commonly played with young children called "What's wrong with this picture?" in which a caregiver shows the child a depiction of a situation and the child is asked to figure out what is portrayed incorrectly or illogically. This same notion can be applied by adults as a very effective way to quickly evaluate the logic or congruence of activities that go on in educational environments. Consider the frequency with which the intentional or formal instructional program of a school is undermined by much more powerfully reinforced contradicting messages. This often occurs when school policies or procedures are not evaluated carefully to discern exactly what lessons they are unintentionally reinforcing. Imagine, for example, the confusion in the mind of a fifth grader, whose formal health instruction for several days has focused on nutrition concepts. The lessons have included developmentally appropriate cognitive information, strategies to enable students to evaluate feelings and beliefs about foods, and practice in food choice skills. Coincidentally, however, it is also time for the kick-off of the annual

23

schoolwide fundraiser, which has traditionally been a candy sale. At the end of the school day, the closure activities include distribution of the candy bars for sale by each child, and an inspirational announcement by the chief school administrator reminding the children of the prizes to be won by those individuals selling the most candy bars. This kind of situation begs the question, "What's wrong with this picture?"

This should not be interpreted as an indictment of school fundraisers. Rather, parents, teachers, and administrators are urged to evaluate a variety of situations in the school program where policy or practice is contradictory or inconsistent with intentional health education. Other common examples include school district policies that support the celebration of special occasions with caries-producing and high-fat foods, but require that nutrition education be a featured unit in the curriculum; policies that establish smoke-free environments for students, but provide designated smoking areas for faculty and staff who may have power with students as role models; and those that fail to require the installation of seat belts in school buses, particularly in states that mandate child restraints and seat belt use in passenger cars. Such contradictions render the best health instruction program ineffective in the context of having an impact on student health behaviors. It is, therefore, the intention of this chapter to visit the school health program, examine the current status of the health of young children, and provide a model for teachers, parents, administrators, and concerned others to improve the health status of the school community and the constituent students.

Current Health Issues of Americans

With the 1979 publication of *Healthy People: The Surgeon General's Report on Health Promotion and Disease Prevention,* it was confirmed that due to the conquest of infectious disease, changes in public health policy, and pharmacologic discoveries, Americans are living longer and healthier lives.[2] Since 1900, there has been a twenty-year increase in our life span.[3]

While many of our ancestors died when plagues of infectious diseases swept through their communities, an examination of our current ten leading causes of death reveals that approximately 50 percent are the result of unhealthy lifestyle and behavior patterns pursued by the individual. An additional 20 percent of our most common causes of death result from hereditary or biological factors, 20 percent from exposure to environmental toxins or pollutants, and the remaining 10 percent is due to inadequacies in access to quality health care.[4] While it is true that financial constraints prohibit many individuals from receiving appropriate health care, for others who live in more rural areas where population is less dense it is more a matter of access.

When we compare the primary health concerns of previous generations with those of today's Americans, we can better understand that our philosophy of health and health care has made a dramatic shift. When the leading causes of death were a result of infectious disease, it was quite reasonable for us to put the care of our health in the hands of trained medical practitioners. This medical model or disease orientation, however, is no longer appropriate, as a majority of us now die prematurely as a result of conditions or diseases that are related to and influenced by our personal lifestyles. We need, instead, to adopt a philosophy that shifts us toward health promotion. In *Healthy People,* the Surgeon General defined promotion as any effort which begins ". . . with people who are basically healthy, and seeks the development of community and individual measures which can help them develop lifestyles that can maintain and enhance the state of well being."[5] This health promotion orientation asserts that each individual must have knowledge, attitudes, and skills necessary to assume a much larger role than previous generations of Americans in controlling or at least influencing the destiny of personal health status.

In light of this discussion of health promotion, it is interesting that the citizens of the world are currently confronted with the disease AIDS and HIV infection which, until a cure is found, usually result in premature death. As a result of this disease, some individuals are tempted to again place the fate of their health in the hands of the medical community. In the case of AIDS, perhaps we feel for the first time in years how our ancestors must have felt in attempting to respond to epidemics of smallpox, tuberculosis, or polio. There is, however, a significant difference when the nature of AIDS and HIV infections are closely examined. Although AIDS does fall into the category of a viral infectious disease, for most of its sufferers, the modes of transmission are very closely linked to lifestyle-related behaviors. Excluding those congenital cases passed from infected women to their children, and those that resulted from exposure to tainted blood supply prior to adequate testing regimens, individuals who practice sharing needles and less-than-safe sexual behaviors are at greatest risk for contracting HIV/AIDS. Consequently, we are faced with the fundamental understanding that we as Americans will die as a result of how we live our daily lives. If we fail to manage personal stress levels and don't exercise regularly, if we use tobacco products, eat a high salt and cholesterol and low fiber diet, and if we fail to wear our seatbelts, or participate in risky drug and alcohol consumption, we can fairly accurately predict our personal causes of death. With this in mind, *Healthy People* concluded:

> Beginning in early childhood and throughout life, each of us makes decisions affecting our health. They are made, for the most part, without regard to, or contact with, the health care system. Yet their cumulative impact has a greater effect on the length and quality of life than all the efforts of medical care combined.[6]

The concept of health promotion as it has been defined by the Surgeon General in *Healthy People* has particular implications for educators. According to this document, no group ". . . is more able than school teachers to provide information and instruction that can help young people make decisions to promote good health."[7] Given the universal and compulsory nature of schooling, it is not surprising that schools have been singled out as primary, if not *the* primary vehicle through which school-aged children and youth should be informed about those factors which will influence their health.[8]

The American Public Health Association suggests, "The school, as a social structure, provides an educational setting in which the total health of the child during impressionable years is a priority concern."[9] Further, we must remember that in addition to the issue of convenient access to large numbers of children, there is growing evidence that the habits and behaviors most closely related to a variety of serious health problems do not appear overnight. Rather, these conditions are influenced by habits and behavior patterns developed during childhood. For example, Pollock and Middleton assert that as many as 40 percent of American children exhibit one or more of the risk factors commonly associated with heart disease, including hypertension, high cholesterol levels, and lack of exercise.[10]

The Comprehensive School Health Program

An examination of the health issues facing us today, and the impact of these concerns on the quality of life of our children, suggests that it is appropriate for us to evaluate how our children have traditionally been educated about their health and explore avenues for improving this process. Children entering school bring with them strongly held beliefs and perceptions about health that reflect their culture and upbringing. These concepts and values have been intentionally, and in many cases not so intentionally, taught to them by the media and significant others in their lives.

From the time they are born, children receive very powerful messages that strongly reinforce very specific values about exercise and fitness, nutrition, drug use, the importance of preventive medical care, family styles, patterns of expressing love and concern for others, self-management and decision-making skills, etc. It is therefore important for school based educators who are responsible for formalizing health education in the classroom and throughout the school program to recognize that children bring their world with them when they come to school. Consequently, to be effective, classroom teaching strategies and the school environment as a whole must be sensitive to the diversity of the health education "upbringing" that children bring with them. It is equally necessary for school programmers to recognize that the cultural shift from a traditional disease model or approach, to the health promotion model previously discussed, dictates that the kind of school health education that may have been appropriate in the past is no longer going to serve the needs of children well. Rather, school health practitioners must understand the impact of lifestyle behaviors on health status, and plan programs that will enable and empower children to establish or reinforce those habits and behavior patterns that will enhance their short- and long-term well-being.

Historically, experts in the field of health education have asserted that the schools could best accomplish this by establishing comprehensive health programs for children that focused on: (1) a formalized classroom health instructional component, (2) health related services, and (3) a healthful school environment.[11] Although we have evolved to a health promotion orientation, this comprehensive approach still serves as the fundamental base of quality school health education. Following is a closer look at these three critical programs:

- *Health Instruction.* Those involved in health instruction are usually the classroom teacher for elementary children, or science, physical education, or health specialists for secondary students. The instructional program consists of those planned, sequential, and intentionally structured learning activities designed to help students acquire knowledge, examine attitudes, and develop skills necessary to enhance personal health.[12] In 1977, the Secretary of Health Education and Welfare stated, "Effective health education early in life can help prevent the major disease of adulthood. . . as children grow older, we must teach them how to become responsible, informed consumers of health care."[13]
- *Health Related Services.* The delivery of school health services is usually coordinated by a registered nurse, school nurse practitioner, or physician. These individuals assess the health status of students, screen for specific problems, develop nursing care plans, and manage health problems to restore health, prevent illness, and facilitate rehabilitation.[14] To this end, "the school nurse should be the case manager of the student with health

needs. Basing practice on (a conceptual) framework that emphasizes 'prevention' and 'health promotion,' the school nurse is in a unique position to facilitate the attainment of high level wellness by the children, families, and school personnel whom she serves."[15]

• *Healthful School Environment.* Finally, the third portion of the traditional comprehensive health program focuses on those energies directed toward maintenance of a healthful school environment. While the tone for the school environment is set by administrative policies,[16] healthful school living ". . . embraces all efforts to provide at school physical, emotional, and social conditions that are beneficial to the health and safety of pupils. It includes the provision of a safe and healthful physical environment, the organization of a healthful school day, and the establishment of inter-personal relationships favorable to mental health."[17]

Health educators have long agreed that a quality school health program should include developmentally appropriate instruction, timely services, and a safe and nurturing schoolwide environment at its core. The health issues facing today's school-age children and youth and the culture in which they have been raised, however, are of such a degree of complexity that our definition of "quality" as it pertains to school health programs must be reevaluated. This is a time when the three leading causes of death of American adolescents are not diseases, but accidents,[18] homicide,[19] and suicide.[20] Such issues have their causes rooted in multifactorial social, cultural, and developmental phenomena. We can no longer afford to turn to only a few people within the school in a crisis intervention or reactive fashion. Rather, it is much more appropriate to expand our definition of quality comprehensive health programming as a means to incorporate all resources at our disposal in both the school and community. To deal with the complex issues facing today's children and youth, support must be mobilized from many sources to send proactive consistent messages about health and health issues through multiple and diverse channels.

To this end, Lloyd Kolbe of the Centers for Disease Control has asserted that physical educators, school counselors, and food service practitioners should coordinate their health-related efforts as active participants in the comprehensive school health program.[21] Further, school/community task forces comprised of such concerned individuals as parents, clergy, civic leaders, law enforcement professionals, agency representatives, and business persons need to become critical agents for making sure that there is consistency between the school and community efforts. This is not only an effective educational concept, but can also reduce costs and duplication of services, and result in more diverse and effective programs that reinforce clearly articulated messages offered at multiple sites.[22] Finally, many school districts are developing school-site health promotion programs for the faculty and staff. In addition to reducing absenteeism and decreasing healthcare costs to the taxpayers of that district, healthy teachers provide better quality and continuity of instruction. Healthier faculty and staff members also reinforce a consistent commitment to the notion of the individual taking responsibility for engaging in health-enhancing behaviors through providing a more appropriate and consistent role model. Because this is a relatively new concept at the school site, we provide the following resources to help districts considering such a program:[23]

- Ruth Behrens. *Work Site Health Promotion: Some questions and answers to help you get started.* Office of Disease Prevention and Health Promotion, Public Health Service, U.S. Dept. of Health and Human Services, Washington, DC, 1983;
- Health Insurance Association of America. *Wellness at the School Work Site: A manual.* Health Insurance Association of America, 1850 K St., NW, Washington, DC 20006–2288;
- Wolford, C. A., Wolford, M. R., Allensworth, D. D., "A Wellness Program for Your Staff Sets a Health Example for Students." *The American School Board Journal* 175, 5 (May 1988).

This Kolbe model of comprehensive school health programs includes the critical foundation of:

- health instruction
- school health services
- healthful school environment

but goes further to also include:

- the physical education program
- the school counseling and psychology program
- the school food service program
- integrated school/community task forces
- school-site health promotion programs for faculty and staff.[24]

Interestingly, such a configuration does not require any school district or community to spend additional money, but rather takes advantage of pre-existing programs that by their nature have a critical role in sending powerful messages that reinforce some aspect of child health. Implied in this diverse conceptualization of the comprehensive school health program, therefore, there is a role for everyone who comes in contact with children, including bus drivers, custodians, secretaries, playground monitors, and other support persons to serve as child health advocates.

Further, it is not sufficient for schools to be satisfied with health-enhancing programs reinforced by committed resource persons serving as advocates for child health. School administrative personnel must also adopt policies that reinforce, rather than sabotage, the health-enhancing messages intentionally delivered through these planned activities and programs. It is very destructive when policies or precedent sanction school-based activities that send the message suggesting that expediency or dollar issues are more important than health. For example, when school fundraising or a tobacco policy conflicts with the intentional health education program, children are quick to infer that health is something that goes on in a classroom, not a part of daily behavior. In summary, by coordinating personnel, programs, and policies, schools and communities can join forces to maximize resources most effectively while reinforcing health-enhancing behaviors. This philosophy of sending consistent messages through multiple channels is not only educationally sound but is also a cost-effective way to respond to both the short- and long-term health education needs of children.

Critical Health Issues of Children

Parents, teachers, librarians, and other caregivers often believe that childhood is an idyllic and stress-free time. For a variety of reasons, American children today face a unique and complex set of issues. The Children's Defense Fund has clarified some very important characteristics of those children who will be members of the graduating class of the year 2000. This is where these children stand on the following critical indicators:

- More than one in five is poor. Poverty rates are even higher among minority children: four of nine black six-year-olds, and two of every five Hispanic six-year-olds are poor.
- One of every four does not live with both parents. Most children in single-parent families live with their mothers. Of children living with their mothers, 40 percent have mothers who have never married and 30 percent have mothers who are divorced.
- More than one of every two has a mother in the workforce. Sixty percent of all American six-year-olds have working mothers, yet only a minority of these youngsters are in safe, affordable, quality child care.
- More than one in five is without health insurance. Of all age groups in America, children are most likely to lack health insurance. This problem has been increasing in recent years as a result of high rates of child poverty, cutbacks in government help for the poor, and reductions in employer-provided health coverage.
- At least one in three has never seen a dentist. Few low-income families can afford to pay for their children's medical expenses out of pocket. The result: children often go without essential care.[25]

Rather than focusing our interpretation of this information on a scathing indictment of American culture, it would be much more appropriate to direct our energies toward the needs of our children and the issues and circumstances that they must be prepared to face. Because "the good old days" are never coming back, parents and educators must recognize that education in general, and health education in particular, must be contemporary and effective as a means to empower children to cope with the set of cultural circumstances that will face them. An educational philosophy that is grounded only in cognitive teaching methods delivered by a health teacher in a formal classroom setting is not likely to reach a majority of our children. As the culture has evolved, so have the needs of children, and educational strategies that may have been effective with "Wally and the Beaver" or the children of "Father Knows Best" are essentially ineffective with the children who grew up on "Sesame Street." Anspaugh, Ezell, and Goodman (1987) assert that, "Presenting factual information alone—the cognitive aspect of health education—is not enough. Knowledge alone does not lead to changes in behavior. The failure of so many cognitive drug education programs in the past is evidence of this. The knowledge must become personalized—the affective aspect of health education."[26] Only when effective classroom practice in the cognitive, affective, and psychomotor domains takes on a fundamental role as part of a comprehensive health education program, can a school district and the constituent community hope to get the best learning experience for children and the greatest return for its investment.

Quality Classroom Instruction: A Powerful Foundation

The School Health Education Evaluation (SHEE) study unequivocally demonstrated that the classroom instructional component of a comprehensive school health education program is an effective means of helping children improve health knowledge and develop positive attitudes about health. Further, this study proved that classes in health education content can decrease the likelihood that children will adopt behaviors such as cigarette smoking that are hazards to their health.[27] In a Louis Harris study conducted for the Metropolitan Life Foundation, data gathered between January and May 1988 revealed the following positive impacts of comprehensive health instruction:

- Whereas 43 percent of students with one year of health education have a drink sometimes or more often, that proportion decreases to 33 percent for students who have had health education for three years.

- Twenty percent of students with one year of health education smoke a cigarette sometimes or more often, as opposed to 14 percent among those having had health education for three years.
- In contrast to 13 percent of students having received health education for one year who have taken drugs a few times or more, only 6 percent of those with three years of health education have done so.
- The proportion of those who have ridden with a driver who has been drinking decreases from 70 percent for students with one year of health education to 63 percent for students with three years of health education.[28]

Careful scrutiny of such data reveals that there is no distinction made between the behavior of children who completed one year of health instruction and children who participated in no health instruction. Rather, the evidence of behavior change demonstrated by the Harris Associates for the Metropolitan Life Foundation occurred when comparisons were made between students who had completed one and three years of health instruction.[29] The impact of this information is astounding, for while there is an abundance of evidence that demonstrates that health instruction has an impact on health knowledge and attitudes, there is very little documentation that demonstrates the existence of a relationship between limited classroom time invested in health-related content and actual student behavior. Both the SHEE study and the Harris study for the Metropolitan Life Foundation provide evidence that a significant amount of time must be invested in health instruction if the desired outcome is to have an impact on student health behavior. Justification is, therefore, provided for increasing the commitment of time typically afforded to health instruction in the school day.

When we consider the impact of lifestyle behaviors and personal health status, the demonstrated link between the amount of time invested in classroom health instruction and the actual behavioral risks in which students engage, we are provided with a rationale for a shift in perception about health instruction in elementary school classrooms. Traditionally, health becomes a rainy-day alternative for outdoor recess, or a substitute for a broken science film. Given current evidence, however, school programmers must be willing to provide sufficient time for developmentally appropriate health instruction and consistent reinforcement throughout the school day. To this end, health must become a philosophy—not a specific class that is graded. Like reading skill development, which requires consistent reinforcement across all content areas, health education must take place across disciplines throughout the school program if we want children to apply health knowledge, attitudes, and skills in their daily lives.

While we certainly recognize that time is a most limited and precious commodity in the elementary school day, an investment in developing a strong philosophical commitment to health will not only have an impact on children's health behaviors, but will positively influence their general academic success as well. Kolbe and his colleagues have demonstrated a strong and positive relationship between the health status of children and their academic performance. These researchers conclude that health factors such as dietary patterns influence short-term memory, attention span, analytical abilities, and social and emotional functioning.[30] In 1987, the Deputy Assistant U.S. Secretary for Health, J. Michael McGinnis, asserted, "Unless a child is alert, healthy, well-fed, and fit, you cannot teach that child those subjects traditionally called basics."[31] Allanson has, therefore, concluded that no school can choose either to maintain or not maintain a school health program; it can choose only to have an adequate or inadequate one.[32]

As we focus our attention on the classroom instructional component of the comprehensive school health program, it is appropriate to turn to the National Education Association for a definition of health education. Interestingly, the NEA definition of health education is very closely related to the previously discussed concept of health promotion, and the broad-based conceptualization of the comprehensive school health program endorsed by contemporary health educators. According to the NEA, health education is "the process of providing learning experiences which favorably influence understanding, attitudes, and conduct relating to individual and community health."[33]

Specific criteria to help educators evaluate the quality of school health instruction has been outlined by the American Medical Association. The AMA maintains that there are four critical elements in effective school health instructional programs:

- *Sequential,* wherein concepts are covered in all grades, K–12, at developmentally appropriate times, with lessons from one year building on what has been learned in previous years;
- *Planned,* with clearly stated objectives, activities, and evaluation criteria, taught at scheduled times within the total curriculum;
- *Comprehensive,* covering the complete diversity of health content and issues facing children, and showing how these issues are interrelated and have an impact on the quality of life;
- *Taught by qualified teachers,* who have the ability to create learning experiences that relate in realistic and current ways to the lives of students.[34]

These characteristics, however, are a far cry from actual practice in most school districts. In a 1989 analysis of comprehensive school health programs entitled *School Health in America,* it was revealed that:

- Only thirty-two states (64%) require that health education be taught sometime during grades K–12.
- Only nineteen states (38%) require that health education be taught sometime during grades 1 through 6.
- Only twenty-two states (44%) require that health education be taught sometime during grades 7 and 8.
- Only twenty-five states (50%) require a course in health education for high school graduation.[35]

Consequently, it is estimated that American students are required to participate in an average of only 13.87 hours of health instruction annually throughout their K–12 schooling experience.[36] While there is diversity in the amount of instructional time afforded to health education across school districts, we can only conclude that the current practice of placing health instruction on such a low priority sends a tacit message to students that health issues are simply not that pressing a priority. Although they are told that their health is very important and that certain critical issues are worthy of conversation, the verbal messages are not reinforced in practice.

From the perspective of the taxpaying public and parents, health education doesn't fare much better. In a recent Phi Delta Kappa/Gallup Poll which evaluated the attitudes of the public toward the public schools, those questioned ranked health education ninth in importance among thirteen required core courses required for college-bound students, and ninth again among eleven course requirements for students not planning to attend college. Ironically, that same public rated the use of drugs as the biggest problem the schools must now face.[37]

This low priority may be due in part to the lack of adequately trained health teachers, particularly in the elementary school environment. Currently, in the U.S. there is only one certified health teacher for every 21,500 students, or about one for every fifty schools.[38] Because most elementary schools don't hire health education specialists, classroom teachers have direct responsibility for health instruction. These individuals, therefore, need adequate preparation for this task.[39] This is far from actual practice. Only twenty-six states (52%), however, currently require that elementary teachers have some coursework in health education to qualify them for an elementary teaching certificate.[40] The fifth edition of *School Health in America* also clarifies the nature of the coursework that states require preservice elementary teachers to take. The following breakdown reinforces the general lack of preparation of preservice elementary teachers to deal with health issues of children:

- Only nine states (18%) require preservice teachers to take a methods and materials of teaching health course.
- Only nine states (18%) require these individuals to take both a personal health and teaching methods course.
- Only seven states (14%) require only a personal health concepts class to be taken.
- Only five states (10%) require a health *or* physical education class be taken to meet certification requirements.

- Five states (10%) permit elementary teachers-in-training to meet this competency with some other set of stated requirements.[41]

Without proper training, how can teachers be alerted to the importance of health education? Without the requisite skills, how can they build and implement viable health education programs? Without adequate background, how can teachers, regardless of their content area specialty, be expected to interact in any meaningful way with students who, on a daily basis, may face such critical health issues as child abuse, drug use, alcohol consumption, and developmental sexual concerns?

A massive nationwide certification effort in health education for elementary teachers is unlikely. It is also unlikely that teachers will gladly welcome health instruction as yet another subject to be added to a curriculum that already suffers from a surfeit of content. Further, it is unrealistic to assume that the hiring of trained health-content specialists will become the rule rather than the exception in elementary schools, even though this is often the case with the content areas of art, music, and physical education.[42]

Effective Alternative Strategies for Elementary School Personnel

Given the limitations on classroom instructional time and preservice elementary teacher training, even concerned teachers who are fortunate enough to work with a comprehensive team of supportive administrators, colleagues, and parents find health instruction frustrating to plan and deliver to students. Rather than "reinventing the wheel," many school districts have chosen to adopt a previously developed course of study or series of curriculum materials. There are a variety of such curriculums available from various health agencies, state departments of education, textbook publishers, and curriculum developers. One that is held in very high esteem among many health education professionals is "Growing Healthy." "Based on a long term goal of emphasizing active participation in the process of achieving and maintaining health for themselves and their communities, the generation of children who have experienced *Growing Healthy* may be able to help contain health care costs and improve the quality of their own lives."[43] Growing Healthy is a K–7 curriculum model that evolved from the companion projects, the *School Health Curriculum Project* for grades 4–7 and the *Primary Grades Health Curriculum Project* for grades K–3. The development of this project began in 1969, and was funded by the U.S. Public Health Services, the Department Health and Human Services, the Centers for Disease Control, and the American Health and American Lung Association.[44] This comprehensive instructional model incorporates a variety of experiential methods, including a wide range of resources and multimedia techniques that link the school and community as a means not to only increase cognitive knowledge, but also to build self-confidence and self-esteem among children in grades K–7. The Growing Healthy Curriculum receives high marks from teachers, as particular strengths of this program lie in its self-contained structure, the inclusion of a teacher-training component, and its potential adaptability to meet local needs and circumstances.[45] On pages 40–54 is the "Curricular Progression Chart" that serves as the basic organizer of the Growing Healthy model.

More than thirty professional evaluators have demonstrated that Growing Healthy has a significant and positive effect on health knowledge and attitudes.[46] Further, it is one of the only health education curriculum models in existence that has been validated by the National Diffusion Network of the U.S. Department of Education. The National Diffusion Network recognizes exemplary programs and helps local school districts to adopt the programs it recognizes.[47] School districts that are interested in receiving more information about the Growing Healthy Curriculum are encouraged to direct questions to their local chapter of the American Lung Association or the National Center for Health Education, 30 East 29th Street, New York, N.Y. 10016.

Because of the diverse and comprehensive nature of topics included in the Growing Healthy Curriculum, its widespread

(continued on page 55)

GROWING HEALTHY
HEALTH EDUCATION
CURRICULAR PROGRESSION
CHART

	A	B
	GROWTH AND DEVELOPMENT	**MENTAL/EMOTIONAL HEALTH**
	Structure and function of the systems of the body; their interdependence and contribution to the healthy functioning of the body as a whole; reciprocal relationships between growth and development.	Ability to handle stress appropriately; to apply problem-solving skills to the resolution of individual and family concerns; achievement of a positive self-concept that respects the right of others to be different; and acceptance of responsibility for his/her own health as well as for that of others.
	Lifestyle Goals The individual: • Appreciates the contribution of each of the body systems to the survival and health of the total system; • Views growth and development as a lifelong process fostered by responsible behavior.	**Lifestyle Goals** The individual: • Exhibits a positive self concept; • Expresses emotions comfortably and appropriately; • Weighs potential benefits against possible consequences before choosing one action over another; • Communicates and cooperates effectively with others; • Develops and maintains interpersonal relationships.

From Growing Healthy Health Education Curricular Progression Chart, 1985.
Used by permission of the National Center for Health Education.

(continued)

Grade	A Curriculum Level Objectives The student:	B Curriculum Level Objectives The student:
K	1. Describes the growth and development of healthy teeth and gums. 2. Explains the structure and function of teeth.	1. Names ways in which people are the same as and different from other people. 2. Describes the relationship between feelings and senses. 3. Defines the meaning of friendship.
1	1. Names major body parts. 2. Describes the kinds of information provided by each of the senses.	1. Explains ways people are unique. 2. Describes positive qualities of self and others. 3. Differentiates between acceptable and unacceptable behavior.
2	1. Describes the structure and function of the eye and ear.	1. Differentiates between pleasant and unpleasant emotions. 2. Compares responsible with irresponsible expressions of emotions. 3. Illustrates ways emotions are revealed through physical reactions.
3	1. Lists characteristics common to all living things. 2. Describes the balanced relationships among body systems. 3. Illustrates ways the skeletal and muscular systems work together.	1. Describes how one person's behavior can help or harm others. 2. Illustrates similarities and differences among people. 3. Describes personal health responsibilities.
4	1. Describes the functions of body cells in the production of energy. 2. Explains how growth and development occurs at the level of the cell. 3. Describes the structure and function of the digestive system.	1. Illustrates the importance of physical and psychological need satisfaction. 2. Explains the relationship between physical well-being and mental/emotional health.

(continued)

Grade	A	B
5	1. Explains the physiological needs of a cell. 2. Describes interdependence among body systems. 3. Describes the structure and function of the respiratory system.	1. Describes positive personality traits. 2. Explains the influence of peer pressure on behavior.
6	1. Differentiates among kinds and functions of body cells. 2. Explains how body systems are interrelated in their functioning. 3. Identifies the role of blood in meeting cell needs for nourishment and excretion. 4. Describes the structure and function of the circulatory system.	1. Analyzes the influence of peer pressure on health choices. 2. Identifies positive and negative effects of stress. 3. Describes constructive ways to help reduce stress. 4. Explains the significance of the problem-solving process in making health-related choices.
7	1. Compares the functions of the cell to the functions of the total organism. 2. Explains the function of the nervous system in controlling and coordinating body systems. 3. Explains the function of hormones in regulating body systems. 4. Describes the basic structure and function of the nervous system.	1. Analyzes the interrelationship among physical, mental/emotional and social well-being. 2. Describes the function of emotions in producing and relieving tension. 3. Describes the importance of setting realistic personal goals.

(continued)

C   D

PERSONAL HEALTH	FAMILY LIFE AND HEALTH
Development of positive health care habits; includes grooming, physical fitness, and other personal health practices that help maintain the body and promote overall wellness.	Exploration of the roles and interactions of individuals within the family life cycle: responsibilities and privileges experienced by each family member; physical, mental and social changes anticipated for each person from birth to death; the family's responsibility for the healthy maturation and socialization of children.
Lifestyle Goals The individual: • Adheres to a lifestyle that promotes personal well-being; • Pursues leisure time activities that promote physical fitness and relieve mental and emotional tension; • Follows health care practices that prevent illness and maintain health.	**Lifestyle Goals** The individual: • Respects the rights and privileges of every family member; • Adjusts appropriately to changing physical, mental and social roles, responsibilities and privileges as they occur throughout the life cycle; • Deals comfortably and appropriately with the demands of his or her own gender; • Communicates effectively as a member of a family or society; • Supports the belief that the health of all children is an individual, family, and community responsibility.

(continued)

Grade	**C** Curriculum Level Objectives The student:	**D** Curriculum Level Objectives The student:
K	1. Defines the meaning of personal health practices. 2. Describes ways that health care practices promote physical, mental, and social health.	1. Describes things that parents do to promote the health of the family.
1	1. Identifies personal health practices that can protect the health of self and others. 2. Explains the importance of regular visits to health advisors.	1. Explains the function of a family. 2. Describes various kinds of families. 3. Explains ways each family member can help the family work together as a unit.
2	1. Explains benefits of personal health care practices. 2. Lists reasons for regular visits to the dentist. 3. Describes ways to protect the eyes, ears, gums, and teeth.	1. Explains why family members should be considerate of each other. 2. Explains ways family membership changes. 3. Describes ways friends help each other.
3	1. Explains individual needs for exercise, relaxation, and sleep. 2. Describes physical, mental, and social implications of cleanliness. 3. Defines the meaning of personal fitness. 4. Identifies characteristics of good posture.	1. Explains the responsibilities and privileges of each family member. 2. Identifies unique social and physical characteristics of girls and boys. 3. Describes different kinds of friendships.
4	1. Illustrates correct dental health practices. 2. Analyzes the relationship between fitness and diet.	1. Describes the growth spurt that occurs during adolescence.

(continued)

Grade

	C	D
5	1. Explains how personal health behavior is influenced by that of peers and family members. 2. Describes physical advantages of good posture and regular exercise.	1. Explains the function of the reproductive system. 2. Describes the progression of the individual through the cycle of life.
6	1. Describes physical, social and emotional benefits of regular exercise and fitness. 2. Compares immediate and long-range effects of personal health care choices.	1. Describes changes in physical, social, and mental/emotional characteristics that occur during adolescence.
7	1. Identifies areas in which personal patterns of health care may need improvement or change. 2. Synthesizes a plan combining regular physical activity with personal health habits that promote and maintain total health.	1. Describes the reproductive processes. 2. Explains why some adolescents begin the growth spurt earlier than others. 3. Analyzes the effect of the mother's health on prenatal development and birth of her child. 4. Identifies ways to cope with family conflicts common during adolescence. 5. Identifies social and cultural forces in the development of responsible health behavior.

(continued)

	E	**F**
	NUTRITION	**DISEASE PREVENTION AND CONTROL**
	Sources of the principal nutrients; functions of food in meeting body needs; essential components of a balanced diet; significance of eating a wide range of foods; potential influence of food fads and fallacies on nutrition.	Factors contributing to the development of chronic, degenerative, and communicable diseases and disorders; methods for the detection, prevention, and/or control of cardiovascular disease, digestive and respiratory disorders, sexually transmitted diseases, cancer, and other such health problems.
	Lifestyle Goals The individual: • Eats a daily diet that provides adequate nutrients for the maintenance of health; • Selects food representative of a wide range of food stuffs; • Balances calorie intake with energy needs; • Avoids dependence upon food fads as the sole criterion for diet choices or meal planning.	**Lifestyle Goals** The individual: • Adheres to a lifestyle that promotes well-being and minimizes exposure to known risk factors; • Maintains immunizations of self and family at recommended levels of effectiveness; • Seeks preventive measures such as examinations at specified intervals.

(continued)

E   F

Grade	**Curriculum Level Objectives** The student:	**Curriculum Level Objectives** The student:
K	1. Names foods that contribute to strong bones and teeth. 2. Lists many kinds of foods.	1. Describes germs. 2. Names ways to avoid germs.
1	1. Lists sources of commonly eaten foods. 2. Explains the role of breakast in providing energy for work and play. 3. Identifies appropriate foods for healthful snacks.	1. Explains the difference between illness and wellness. 2. Names ways to break the communicable disease cycle.
2	1. Describes individual and ethnic variations in food choices. 2. Describes sources of different kinds of foods. 3. Explains how certain foods can be harmful to oral health.	1. Names diseases and disorders of the eyes, ears, gums, and mouth. 2. Explains the functions of mechanical aids for vision, hearing, and dental health. 3. Explains ways sound health habits help prevent disease.
3	1. Classifies foods according to their principal nutrients. 2. Illustrates food combinations that provide a balanced daily diet. 3. Explains why certain foods have limited nutritional value.	1. Differentiates between communicable diseases and chronic—degenerative diseases. 2. Describes preventive measures for injuries to bone and muscle tissue.
4	1. Names energy sources common to all living things. 2. Describes the functions of the major nutrients. 3. Identifies factors that influence personal food choices. 4. Analyzes the nutritional worth of food choices for meals and snacks.	1. Identifies problems and diseases that may interfere with the functioning of the digestive system. 2. Explains the importance of good dental practices in the prevention of problems of the mouth, teeth, and gums. 3. Explains ways digestive upsets and diseases may be avoided.

(continued)

Grade	**E**	**F**
5	1. Explains why a variety of foods is needed every day. 2. Explains how diet choices based upon food fads may provide inadequate nourishment.	1. Describes ways to prevent diseases of and injuries to the respiratory system. 2. Explains how lifestyle choices help reduce the risk of cancer.
6	1. Explains why nutrition requirements vary from person to person. 2. Illustrates the function of nutrients in building strong bodies. 3. Interprets physical and mental consequences of a poorly balanced diet.	1. Describes disorders and diseases that may harm the circulatory system. 2. Analyzes the relationship of certain risk factors to the occurrence of heart disease. 3. Explains how lifestyle choices help reduce the risk of heart disease.
7	1. Evaluates individual diets according to nutritional requirements of adolescents. 2. Explains the relationship between calorie intake and level of activity to body weight. 3. Analyzes implications of dependence of food fads and fallacies in selecting a diet. 4. Describes ways to lose weight safely.	1. Describes measures for the prevention and control of chronic and neurological disorders. 2. Explains the function of immunization in preventing disease. 3. Describes ways to prevent or control sexually transmitted diseases.

(continued)

G   H

SAFETY AND FIRST AID	CONSUMER HEALTH
Methods for the identification and elimination of hazardous conditions or situations; rules and procedures for safe living in the home, school, and community; patterns of behavior promoting accident prevention; techniques for first aid and emergency care.	Forces influencing an individual in the selection of health information, products, and services; delineation of criteria for those selections; evaluation of commercial appeals motivating the sale and purchase of health-related products and services.
Lifestyle Goals The individual: • Takes steps to correct hazardous conditions when possible; • Follows rules and procedures recommended for safe living; • Avoids unnecessary risk-taking behavior; • Applies correct emergency treatment when appropriate.	**Lifestyle Goals** The individual: • Chooses health products and services on the basis of valid criteria; • Accepts only that health information provided by recognized health authorities; • Utilizes services of qualified health advisors in the maintenance and promotion of his/her own health.

(continued)

Grade	**G** Curriculum Level Objectives	**H** Curriculum Level Objectives
	The student:	The student:
K	1. Identifies safety hazards at home, at school, and in between. 2. Names places and people who can provide help if needed.	1. Lists health products people commonly purchase. 2. Names people whose job it is to help keep us well.
1	1. Explains the importance of having playground safety rules. 2. Describes how the senses help protect us from accidents and injury. 3. Explains how to obtain help in an emergency.	1. Explains ways TV advertising influences choices of foods and other products.
2	1. Explains how to prevent accidental eye, mouth, and ear injuries. 2. Differentiates between hazards and accidents. 3. Describes basic first-aid treatment of eye, mouth, and ear injuries.	1. Describes the many kinds of health advisors.
3	1. Explains the need for obeying safety rules at home, school, work, and play. 2. Describes personal responsibility for reducing hazards and avoiding accidents. 3. Explains accepted procedures of safe bicycle travel.	1. Identifies advertising methods used to promote the sale of health-related products. 2. Analyzes reasons for choosing health products commonly used.
4	1. Describes ways to handle and store foods in a sanitary manner. 2. Explains reasons for appropriate fire safety measures.	1. Interprets the meaning of nutritional information provided on food labels. 2. Explains how information contained on a label can be used in selecting health products.

(continued)

Grade	G	H
5	1. Demonstrates the ability to provide rescue breathing. 2. Describes procedures for saving a choking victim. 3. Explains the importance of playing safely in and around water.	1. Analyzes methods used to sell health products and services. 2. Differentiates between health quackery and sound medical practice.
6	1. Describes the importance of following appropriate first-aid measures for bleeding and shock.	1. Explains why prescriptions for medications and other professional advice must be carefully followed. 2. Identifies sources of reliable health information and services. 3. Identifies sales appeals used in media promotion of health-related products.
7	1. Lists, in order, the first-aid steps to be taken when accidents occur. 2. Explains the relationship between unnecessary risk taking and accidents.	1. Describes the role and function of official consumer protection agencies. 2. Identifies criteria for the selection of an appropriate health advisor. 3. Interprets data provided on prescription and over-the-counter drug labels.

(continued)

I   J

DRUG USE AND ABUSE	COMMUNITY HEALTH MANAGEMENT
Beneficial and appropriate versus harmful and inappropriate uses of mood modifiers such as opiates, cannabis, amphetamines, barbiturates, hallucinogens, tranquilizers, tobacco, alcohol, and volatile substances, including those medications commonly sold over the counter either with or without a prescription.	Ways the individual can effectively contribute to the solution of community-wide health problems such as: environmental pollution, spread of disease, and waste disposal; protection of environmental resources; functions of voluntary, official, professional and other health organizations; community health care opportunities.
Lifestyle Goals The individual: • Adheres to medical recommendations in the use of drugs and medications; • Refrains from the abuse of potentially harmful drugs; • Obeys laws and regulations regarding the use of controlled substances.	**Lifestyle Goals** The individual: • Obeys laws and regulations designed to protect the health of the community; • Contributes to community programs designed to promote community health; • Accepts responsibility as a citizen in supporting the activities and programs of community health workers; • Avoids any personal action that might contribute to the deterioration of the environment.

(continued)

Grade

	I Curriculum Level Objectives The student:	**J** Curriculum Level Objectives The student:
K	1. Names hazardous substances that people use or abuse. 2. Explains reasons for consulting adults before using an unknown substance.	1. Defines *pollution*. 2. Names sources of air pollution. 3. Explains how people can work together to solve problems.
1	1. Describes correct uses of medicine. 2. Explains how use of unknown substances can be hazardous. 3. Names methods of identifying potentially hazardous substances.	1. Describes characteristics of a healthy community. 2. Names groups who help maintain and promote community health. 3. Describes ways the senses can be protected from air pollution.
2	1. Defines the term *drug*. 2. Explains why people choose to avoid certain mood modifiers such as tobacco.	1. Differentiates among kinds and sources of environmental pollution. 2. Describes ways to avoid hearing loss due to noise pollution.
3	1. Explains the difference between use and abuse of drugs. 2. Predicts the effect of certain drugs on physical, mental, and social functioning.	1. Identifies ways health agencies help in protecting health and the environment. 2. Describes ways individuals can help keep a healthy school environment. 3. Identifies ways to help health agencies in the promotion of health.
4	1. Describes effects of drugs on organs of the body. 2. Identifies similarities and differences between drugs and foods. 3. Explains the relationship between drug use and nutritional status.	1. Identifies causes of water pollution. 2. Describes community facilities and procedures that ensure safe water supplies and sanitary trash and sewage disposal.

(continued)

Grade	I	J
5	1. Analyzes the effects of drugs on the functioning of body systems. 2. Describes effects of the use of drugs that may be inhaled. 3. Explains the necessity of sound decisions concerning the use of any drug.	1. Describes methods used to control environmental pollution. 2. Identifies individual and community responsibilities in the control of environmental problems.
6	1. Describes hazards associated with the use of any drug. 2. Describes reasons why some people abuse drugs.	1. Explains the role of community health agencies in protecting and promoting the heatlh and safety of community members. 2. Describes ways in which improving the environment can enhance physical, mental, and social health.
7	1. Analyzes physical, mental, and social effects of drug abuse. 2. Identifies variables that modify the effect of a given drug dose. 3. Explains reasons for laws regulating drug use (including OTC, prescription, alcohol, tobacco, as well as illicit drugs). 4. Describes alternatives to the use of mood modifiers as a means to solving problems and imitating good feelings.	1. Describes community efforts in preventing and controlling disease. 2. Describes the importance of individual participation in community health activities. 3. Identifies career opportunities in the health field.

adoption in many of the Nation's elementary schools, and its familiarity and credibility among many educators, we have chosen to use its "Curricular Progression Chart" as the basis for linking the correlation of children's literature and critical health issues.

Another strength of the Growing Healthy Curriculum is found in the many opportunities for teachers to review content or issues that are introduced in a previous grade level or during the study of a different content area. The impact of such planned repetition shouldn't be overlooked. To this end, Table 1 clarifies places from the "Curriculum Progression Chart" where issues or concepts are introduced and reinforced across the content areas and grade levels.

Table 1

Introduction and Reinforcement of Health Issues by Content Area and Grade Level in the *Growing Healthy Curricular Progression Chart*

Health Issue or Topic	Chart Content Area & Grade Level Where Topic Is Introduced	Chart Area & Grade Levels of Reinforcement
Dental Health	Growth & Development—K	Personal Health—2,4 Nutrition—2 Disease Prevention & Control—2 Consumer Health—2
Vision & Hearing	Growth & Development—2	Personal Health—2 Disease Prevention & Control—2
Digestive System	Growth & Development—4	Personal Health—4 Nutrition—All Grades Disease Prevention & Control—4
Respiratory System	Growth & Development—5	Disease Prevention & Control—5 Drug Use & Abuse—5

Source: Adapted from *Growing Healthy Health Education Curricular Progression Chart,* 1985. Used by permission of the National Center for Health Education.

Health Issue or Topic	Chart Content Area & Grade Level Where Topic Is Introduced	Chart Area & Grade Levels of Reinforcement
Circulatory System	Growth & Development—6	Disease Prevention & Control—6
Nervous System	Growth & Development—7	Mental/Emotional Health—7
Friendship	Mental/Emotional Health—K	Family Life & Health—2
Impact of behavior on health of others	Mental/Emotional Health—3	Disease Prevention & Control—1 Community Health Management—K, 5
Health Advisors	Personal Health—1	Consumer Health—K,2
Influence of Family	Personal Health—5	Family Life & Health—K,1,2,3
Nutrients	Nutrition—3	Nutrition—4,6
Communicable Disease	Disease Prevention & Control—1	Disease Prevention & Control—3,7
Sensory Health	Safety and First Aid—1	Growth & Development—1
Sanitary Food Storage	Safety & First Aid—4	Nutrition—4,5,6,7
Television Advertising Effect on Food Choices	Consumer Health—1	Nutrition—5,7
Hazardous Substances	Drug Use & Abuse—K,1	Consumer Health—3,7
Drug Use & Nutritional Status	Drug Use & Abuse—4	Nutrition—6,7

Health Issue or Topic	Chart Content Area & Grade Level Where Topic Is Introduced	Chart Area & Grade Levels of Reinforcement
People Cooperating to Solve Problems	Community Health Management—K	Mental/Emotional Health— 3,6

Summary

Recently, the federal government sponsored a report on the health of America's youth entitled *The National Adolescent Student Health Survey*. The results of the study have provided much needed data on the knowledge, behaviors, and attitudes of eighth and tenth grade students with regard to such critical health issues as: injury prevention, suicide, AIDS, violence, nutrition, tobacco, drugs, and alcohol. Among the recommendations of the study are the following, which have particular impact on elementary classroom teachers and administrators:

- Health must have a higher priority in the total school curriculum.
- Educational programs and interventions must go beyond simply providing information to students.
- Planned sequential health instruction (K–12), supported by other school health promotion components, such as food service, counseling, and physical education, is essential. The need for comprehensive school health programs is supported by this survey.
- More attention to health instruction in the elementary grades is needed because that is the time when many health behaviors are developing. In particular, the survey results support beginning alcohol and drug education at the elementary school level.
- Elementary school classroom teachers in particular need special preparation to teach health education. . . . Early childhood curricula in colleges and universities need to include preparation for teaching health education at the elementary school level.

• In-service education of teachers is needed to provide better preparation for teaching health at the elementary and secondary levels.[48]

Given the health issues facing the contemporary child, and because schooling is universal and compulsory, it behooves curriculum developers, librarians, and teachers to create learning environments that are not only safe, but are also enriching and empowering. Only in this way will children have the knowledge and skills necessary to live full and healthy lives. This book provides a model based on the correlation of critical health issues with the language arts. It is not the intent of the authors that this book take the place of a comprehensive instructional program, but rather that it serve as a timely and useful supplement for teachers, librarians, and parents. Through correlating health issues with language arts skills with which most elementary educators and librarians are more familiar and comfortable, it is our hope that today's children will be better served.

The third chapter of this book provides a review of various types of children's literature and suggests ways that they can be used effectively to explore child health issues. It is our hope that readers will find the organizational style of this book "user-friendly."

NOTES

1. *A Guide to Curriculum Planning in Health Education* (Madison, WI: Department of Public Instruction, 1985), p. 5.
2. Diane DeMuth Allensworth and Cynthia A. Wolford, *Achieving the 1990 Health Objectives for the Nation: Agenda for the Nation's Schools* (Kent, OH: American School Health Association, 1988), p. 19.
3. S. M. Weiss, "Foreword: The Case for Work Site Health Promotion," in *Occupational Health Promotion,* ed. G. Everly and R. Feldman (New York: John Wiley and Sons, 1985), pp. 9–18.
4. U.S. Department of Health, Education, and Welfare, Public Health Service, *Healthy People: The Surgeon General's Report on Health Promotion and Disease Prevention* (Washington, DC: U.S. Government Printing Office, 1979), p. 9.
5. Ibid., p. 119.
6. Ibid., p. 119.

7. Ibid., p. 143.
8. Donald Iverson and Lloyd J. Kolbe, "Evaluation of the National Disease Prevention and Health Promotion Strategy: Establishing a Role for the Schools," *Journal of School Health* 53 (1983) :294–302.
9. American Public Health Association, "Education for Health in the Community Setting," *American Journal of Public Health* (1975): 65.
10. Marion Pollock and Kathleen Middleton, *Elementary School Health Instruction* (St. Louis, MO: Times Mirror/Mosby, 1984), p. IX.
11. Allensworth and Wolford, *Achieving the 1990 . . .*, p. 23.
12. Ibid., p. 24.
13. Joseph Califano, "School Health Message," *Journal of School Health* 47, 7 (1977) :395–96.
14. Allensworth and Wolford, *Achieving the 1990 . . .*, p. 24.
15. S. Wold and N. Dagg, "School Nursing: A Framework for Practice," *Journal of School Health* 48, 2 (1978) :111–14.
16. Allensworth and Wolford, *Achieving the 1990 . . .*, p. 24.
17. H. Cornacchia, Larry K. Olsen, and C. Nickerson, *Health in the Elementary Schools,* 6th ed. (St. Louis, MO: Times Mirror/Mosby, 1984), p. 45.
18. U.S. Department of Health and Human Services, *Healthy People 2000: National Health Promotion and Disease Prevention Objectives* (Washington, DC: U.S. Government Printing Office, 1991), p. 16.
19. Ibid., p. 16.
20. Ibid., p. 16.
21. Lloyd Kolbe, *Indicators for Planning and Monitoring School Health Programs* (Los Angeles: University of California Symposium on Indicators of Health Promotion Behavior, 1985).
22. Allensworth and Wolford, *Achieving the 1990 . . .*, p. 27.
23. Ibid., p. 26.
24. Kolbe, *Indicators for Planning.*
25. *CDF Reports* (Washington, DC: Children's Defense Fund, September, 1988), p. 3.
26. David Anspaugh, Gene Ezell, and Karen N. Goodman, *Teaching Today's Health.* 2d ed. (Columbus: Merrill, 1987), p. 9.
27. James O. Mason and J. Michael McGinnis, "The Role of School Health," *Journal of School Health* 55, 8 (1985) :299.
28. Louis Harris and Associates, *Health You've Got to be Taught: An Evaluation of Comprehensive Health Education in American Public Schools* (New York: Metropolitan Life Foundation, 1988), p. 5.
29. Ibid., p. 5.
30. Lloyd Kolbe, Lawrence Green, et al., "Appropriate Functions of Health Education in Schools: Improving Health and Cognitive Performance" in *Child Health Behavior: A Behavioral Pediatrics Perspective,* ed. N. Kraisuegor, J. Arastele, and M. Cataldo (New York: John Wiley and Sons, 1986) pp. 178–84.
31. J. Michael McGinnis, *Why School Health* (Arlington: American Association of School Administrators, 1987) p. 1.
32. J. Allanson, "School Nursing Services: Some Current Justifications

and Cost Benefit Implications," *Journal of School Health* 48, 10 (1978):603–607.

33. C. Wilson, ed., *School Health Services* (Washington, DC: National Education Association, 1971) p. 2.

34. *Why Health Education in Your School?* (Chicago: American Medical Association, 1982).

35. Diane Allensworth, Christine Lovato, et al. *School Health in America,* 5th ed. (Kent, OH: American School Health Association, 1989) p. 11–14.

36. Lloyd Kolbe, Diane Allensworth, et al. *School Health in America: An Assessment of State Policies to Protect and Improve the Health of Students,* 4th ed., (Kent, OH: American School Health Association, n.d.) pp. 5–6.

37. A. M. Gallup and D. L. Clark, "The 19th Annual Gallup Poll of the Public's Attitudes Toward the Public Schools," *Phi Delta Kappan,* 69, 1 (1987) :22, 28.

38. National Center for Educational Statistics, *The Condition of Education,* NCES Pub. No. 84–401 (Washington, DC: U.S. Government Printing Office, 1984).

39. D. Oberteuffer and Mary K. Beyer, *School Health Education,* 4th ed. (New York: Harper and Row, 1966).

40. Allensworth, Lovato, et al., *School Health,* p. 11.

41. Ibid., p. 11.

42. Anthony Manna and Cynthia Wolford Symons, "A Case for Promoting Student Health Through Children's Literature," *Educational Horizons,* fall 1990.

43. *Growing Healthy: Comprehensive Education—for Health* (New York: National Center for Health Education, 1985).

44. Ibid.

45. Ibid.

46. Ibid.

47. Ibid.

48. American School Health Association, Association for the Advancement of Health Education, and Society for Public Health Education, Inc. *The National Adolescent Student Health Survey: A Report on the Health of America's Youth* (Oakland, CA: Third Party Publishing Company, 1989) pp. 132–35.

3. Evaluating and Selecting Literature for Children

> Children deserve the best you give
> people you care for.—*Betsy Hearne,*
> **Choosing Books for Children**[1]

Parents, teachers, and health professionals who are committed to enabling children to take responsibility for their health and to clarifying children's health-related questions and concerns are well served by a wide variety of relevant children's books that can lead children to valuable insights into all aspects of personal, family, and community health. In this chapter, we discuss some criteria for evaluating different types of children's books, and we consider some things to keep in mind when selecting the right book for the right reader, or group of readers, at the right time. We first examine the characteristics of a number of health-related children's books in order to demonstrate how the evaluative criteria apply to specific types of literature. We then show how what we know about children's reading interests at various stages in their development can serve as a guide for selecting books for individual children or for large-group reading experiences. Along the way, we describe some useful professional resources for selecting literature on many topics and themes that can help to foster children's understanding of personal and public health issues.

The Adult As Critic

Whether you are an experienced health educator, a future teacher, an allied health professional, or a parent concerned about your child's well-being, it is important for you to be able to distinguish the exceptional book from the kind of book that our students call "kiddie lit." Well-written and beautifully illustrated books are the ones both child and adult will return to again and again. There is so much honesty and truth in such books that they can stand up under the pressure of repeated readings. The artless children's book, with its pointless plot, unbelievable characters, and sentimental point of view toward children and childhood, provides little nourishment for the heart, soul, or mind. Years ago, Paul Hazard, the French critic and child advocate, summed up the worst features of dull, poorly written and poorly illustrated books for children when he pointed out that these books contained "...disguised sermons, hypocritical lessons, irreproachable little boys and girls who behave with more docility than their dolls."[2]

Like good nutrition, good relationships, and good role models, good books make a lasting impression on children. Just as children form positive attitudes toward health based on their early experiences, they can be hooked by books and reading from a very early age. Many studies of children's reading habits and development have shown that the child who is tuned in and turned on to books from infancy onward not only has a positive attitude toward reading, but is also a more skilled reader, is more comfortable with language in general, and may even be more emotionally and socially well adjusted than the child who has not started life with this advantage.[3]

Children rely on us a lot. They model our convictions and values when they sense that we are honest, sincere, and concerned for their welfare. They depend on us for their basic needs, and even though they may rebel against our beliefs in order to test their own, they basically trust our direction and counsel. Regarding such vital health issues as personal identity, control over one's existence, and a feeling of connection with others in the world, what truly matters to children is what mattered to us as children: not merely the things parents, teachers, and other significant adults *say,* but rather what they *do* and how they *act.*

The same thing is true for the type of sustenance literature offers to children. Our obvious enthusiasm and excitement about the value of reading good, timeless literature, combined with our awareness of how literature can help children to make sense of the world and their place in it, will demonstrate to children in a clear and concrete way the reasons why worthwhile literature is—and has been since the first stories were told—both an endless source of enjoyment and information and a direct route to the most significant questions, problems, dilemmas, and discoveries that have always concerned people in every culture.

Children's literature can be a sturdy bridge that connects child to adult and adult to child—the common ground being the human condition, human experience, and the human spirit. Jim Trelease, in *The Read-Aloud Handbook,* says "Literature brings us closest to the human heart. . . .[It] arouses [children's] imaginations, emotions, and sympathies. It awakens their desire to read, enlarges their lives, and provides a sense of purpose and identity."[4] Because of the personal, intellectual, and social enrichment literature can provide, Trelease feels we should "count among the needs of the world those special people who help children discover the meaning behind those strange marks that add up to an alphabet, who thankfully let children know there is more to reading than workbook pages."[5]

When parents and teachers begin to see the value of using literature to help children understand the information, attitudes, and habits which can influence their health, the first things they want to know about are the kinds of children's books available for this purpose and what they should be thinking about when evaluating and selecting books for children. When it comes to choosing children's books, they usually ask questions like these:

- How do I tell a good book from a bad book?
- How important are illustrations, and what should I be looking for when I pick up an illustrated book?
- How do I know if a book is the right one for the child or children with whom I intend to share it?
- How do I know if a book will be too difficult or too easy for children?

- Is there some way to tell which books to recommend for individualized reading and which ones to select for an entire group of students?
- Which books work best with reluctant readers and students with reading problems?

There are no easy answers to any of these questions, nor are there hard-and-fast rules to follow for every book and every child all of the time. It does help, though, to be aware of the characteristics of good literature, to have an understanding of children, and to be able to use a great deal of common sense. These can lead the way to sensible choices and judgments about books that children will enjoy and that have the potential to stimulate rich responses and genuine discussion among children and among children and adults.

How to Evaluate Children's Literature

Because a children's book is meant to be enjoyed by children, the tendency sometimes is to judge its worth solely on the basis of guesswork about whether or not it will attract the attention of children—before we look closely at the book's characteristics as literature and even before we read it to children or have them read it on their own. Parents and teachers frequently make judgments like these—particularly about books that contain controversial topics or behaviors like the eavesdropping incidents in *Pippi Longstocking* by Astrid Lindgren, or the homosexual incident in *I'll Get There, It Better Be Worth the Trip* by John Donovan. It is not uncommon for adults to dismiss a book such as *Outside Over There* by Maurice Sendak because "it's too weird for kids." In the same way, many adults feel that *Hiroshima No Pika* by Toshi Maruki, which depicts the physical and emotional effects of the dropping of an atomic bomb, is "too frightening to share with children."

Although subjective judgments like these are understandable and only natural, there are several problems with this approach to deciding which books will matter to children and which books will not. In the first place, a book may be well written, beautifully illustrated, and carefully designed, but our notions of children and childhood and our prejudices concerning children's capabilities prevent us from seeing this, and so we put the book aside. As Sutherland and Arbuthnot point out in *Children and Books,* "If an author's attitude toward parent-child relationships, sex mores, civil rights, or any other issue is in agreement with ours, we may tend to approve of the book as a whole, but if the values and assumptions are at variance with our own, we tend to dismiss it, regardless of its other qualities."[6]

Sometimes this happens because we have had bad experiences with certain types of literature such as poetry, or because we let our own preferences or interests determine what a child will like or dislike. In each case, we sacrifice evaluation to a type of censorship, perhaps missing an opportunity to forge an important and powerful connection between a child and a book. Imagine how many of the nearly forty thousand children's books now in print would remain on library shelves if every adult in this country were allowed to remove a book that didn't agree with his or her beliefs or dealt with subjects that adults regard as inappropriate for children. Because children need access to a wide selection of good books, wider in range than most of us can even imagine from our adult perspectives, parents, teachers, and librarians—anyone, that is, who is concerned with the intellectual and emotional welfare of young people—should know how to look at books objectively and to evaluate them according to how well they satisfy standards of excellence. The critic Lillian Smith tells us why this is so important: "A poor book sets a child back, a mediocre one leaves children where they are, but a good book moves children on to growth and pleasure, to new understandings and discoveries."[7]

It isn't necessary to have a college degree in children's literature to distinguish talented writers and illustrators from writers who have little sense of language and life and illustrators who seem to use a paint-by-numbers kit to do their illustrations. What it does take to tell the difference between superior, mediocre, and uninspired children's books is a willingness to read lots of children's books with an open mind and an attention to detail. There is simply no way around this need to sample a large selection of books in order to get to know the field of children's literature and to discover the best authors and illustrators. Like other types of art, literature is supposed to grab and hold our attention by involving both our senses and our minds. Good children's books are no exception. They are meant to be pored over and savored in the way that a good painting, a good movie, or a good play makes us slow down and look at familiar things in a different way, or lures us into an experience we ourselves may never have had or even thought about.

Because the best children's books reflect the special brand of curiosity and exuberant attentiveness that children bring to each situation, the search for worthwhile children's books can be a refreshing and enlightening experience for adults. For example, in *Dawn* by Uri Shulevitz, both children and adults rediscover the hushed sights and sounds of an early morning in the woods through luminous pictures and simple, poetic language that together depict the gradual awakening of a new day. In *Return to Bitter Creek,* a realistic novel by Doris Buchanan Smith for children in the intermediate and upper grades, we live through a year of personal changes with twelve-year-old Lacey as she adjusts to life in the conservative rural town where her mother grew up and where she has recently moved with her mother and her mother's boyfriend. Because her grandparents don't approve of their daughter's lifestyle, Lacey watches and wonders and learns as her mother struggles to gain her family's acceptance without forfeiting her integrity.

In two informational books for ten- to twelve-year-old readers by author/photographer Jill Krementz, *How It Feels When Parents Divorce* and *How It Feels When a Parent Dies,* young people themselves talk candidly about their first experiences with separation and loss, reminding us of the resiliency of the human spirit. In *Heartbeats* by the Silversteins, we share the child's fascination with discovering how the heart works, how it functions to keep us alive, and why so vital an organ must be kept fit. Powerful books such as these are more the rule than the exception among a rich and varied body of literature created by some of the best writers and artists in America.

Parents and teachers are often overwhelmed by the staggering number of children's books. It is not surprising that they sometimes resort to giving children the classics they themselves enjoyed as children, or that they simply keep using the same books year after year because those are the ones that held children's attention in the past. Although both of these approaches to book selection can reap some pleasurable moments with literature, most parents and teachers need to vary what they read and recommend to children—for their own sake as well as children's. To paraphrase an old saying, variety is the spice of a child's reading life.

One quick and efficient way for busy parents and teachers to find some new books to share with children is to use the book selection guides that we introduce throughout this chapter. These guides describe a variety of books on a variety of topics that interest children of all ages. Most of these selection aids, such as *Appraisal: Science Books for Young People* and *Health, Illness and Disability: A Guide to Books for Children and Young Adults,* contain annotations that both describe and evaluate a book. Although these resources are useful, it is important to remember that they reflect the opinions and tastes of others. They should not be viewed as a substitute for the real thing, but rather as a kind of map that can lead to some interesting areas in the territory of children's literature. As any seasoned traveler knows, a map can never reveal the excitement of experiencing a place firsthand or the satisfaction of discovering pleasant surprises on the way to one's destination.

This is certainly the case when one's goal is to find good children's books that address personal and social health issues. In spirited folktales and thoughtful fantasy stories that contain timeless themes, in sensitive realistic stories that depict the problems and concerns of contemporary children, in lively Mother Goose rhymes and provocative poems, in attractive informational books and other types of literature, children of all ages, abilities, and backgrounds have access to an enormous range of vivid experiences and accurate information that elevate health concepts to a human issue. There is truly something here for every child's tastes and needs and for every adult who believes it is necessary to make health a relevant and personal issue for children. Quality literature paired with meaningful activities that genuinely involve children in the process of reading can make health concepts come alive. And the better the literature, the better the opportunity to capture children's attention with accurate information and honest situations that demonstrate how good or poor health habits affect the lives of all types of people.

In the pages ahead, we survey numerous selections of children's literature that relate health issues and concerns to the human experience. The selections have been organized into eight sections that represent the eight standard types of literature. In the first section, we examine **folktales** and other types of literature that originally were communicated by oral storytellers all over the world. The other sections describe examples of **fantasy and science fiction**, **realistic fiction**, **historical fiction**, **poetry**, **informational books**, **biography and autobiography**, and, finally, **plays**. Within each section, we discuss selections of literature for children of various ages that depict the experiences of people from a number of cultural, racial, ethnic, and socioeconomic groups. In order to provide an extensive examination of an immediate and common health concern, special attention is given in most of the sections to literature that deals with nutrition, although readers will also find references to literature on many other health topics.

FOLKTALES: HEALTH ISSUES ACROSS TIME AND CULTURES

"To count the themes of folklore," writes Betsy Hearne in *Choosing Books for Children,*

> is to count the heartbeat of the human race. . . . Folktales are time frozen, the epitome of ageless literature. Created, told, and retold to mixed groups of children and adults, they still wear well on every level. They are the bare bones of story. Each archetypal character represents a part of humanity, each action a part of life, each setting a part of existence.[8]

The territory of traditional literature is vast, for it contains a multitude of zesty Mother Goose rhymes, clever fables, intriguing myths that are filled to the brim with adventure and suspense, epics and legends in praise of invincible heroes, and a worldwide collection of serious and humorous folktales that explore humanity's basic needs, desires, motives, and emotions, and provide answers to humanity's timeless questions about every conceivable aspect of life and living. Born of the imaginations of oral storytellers, this literature represents a hearty tradition that has survived the best and worst of times throughout history. Even in a fast-paced technological world, this limitless body of literature continues to entertain children and adults alike and to remind them that people in every culture used stories to explain their origins and to preserve the values, virtues, and moral beliefs they espoused.

Considering how folk literature reflects humanity's fundamental concerns and needs, it is not surprising that food and eating play a significant role in many traditional stories. This is especially true of folktales, the type of traditional literature we will discuss here. While folktales do not overtly teach children specific facts about the science of nutrition, these stories show children that food plays an important role in every culture. More specifically, folktales reveal habits, customs, and beliefs related to food and eating in various parts of the world, and they provide information about the types of foods found in various cultures. Because food is such a human concern in folktales, these appealing stories can enliven and make concrete the facts and advice adults try to convey to children about nutrition. The following list details some of the ways storytellers have incorporated food and eating into their tales. Information about the folktales mentioned in the list can be found at the end of this chapter.

- A human or animal character's survival depends on certain types of foods—"**Rapunzel**" (Germany); "**The Corn in the Rock**" (Maya); "**Hansel and Gretel**" (Germany).
- Food causes or leads to conflict—"**Tom Tit Tot**" (England); "**Rumpelstiltskin**" (Germany); "**The Talking Fish**" (Armenia); "**Little Red Riding Hood**" (Germany); "**The Three**

Wishes" (England); "The Pancake" (Norway); "The Bun" (Russia); "The Three Little Pigs" (England); "The Funny Little Woman" (Japan); "The Marvelous Pear Seed" (China).
* Food helps to unite people or animals—"The Three Wishes" (England); "Beauty and the Beast" (France); "Snow White" (Germany); "The Pancake" (Norway); "The Lad Who Went to the North Wind" (Norway); "The Enormous Genie" (Armenia).
* Food causes comical and outrageous predicaments—"How the Peasant Helped His Horse" (Russia); "Hans in Luck" (Germany); "The Wee Bannock" (Scotland); "The Pancake" (Norway); "The Ash Lad Who Had an Eating Match With the Troll" (Norway).
* The consequences of greed for food—"Being Greedy Chokes Anansi" (Jamaica); "The Magic Pear Tree" (China); "The Crane Wife" (Japan).
* A human or animal is considered food by his or her enemy—"The King of Ireland's Son" (Ireland); "Jack and the Beanstalk" (Appalachia); "The Wolf and the Seven Little Kids" (Germany); "Little Red Riding Hood" (Germany).

The Characteristics of Folktales

Whether a folktale is retold by an oral storyteller or by a writer, the most memorable retellings capture the distinctive elements that give folktales their special flavor. The characteristics of folktales such as plot, character, and theme are the elements which an adult needs to consider when searching for the best of the lot. Consider, for example, the typical folktale plot, which includes what happens in the story as well as when and where it happens. The plot develops swiftly and directly, and descriptions are brief and to the point. At once, time, place, character, and conflict are established with minimal detail so that the action can get underway. Immediately, we are caught up in the conflict and carried along by it, wondering if things will work out for better or worse. A fast pace, a very obvious conflict or problem, lots of action in contrast to lengthy descriptions and extended side trips into the characters' thoughts—these are the ingredients that make the folktale a compact, abbreviated story with more going on between the words and lines than first meets the eye.

Barbara Rogasky's faithful retelling of "**Rapunzel**" is a good example of how quickly and economically a folktale gets to the heart of the matter. In this classic tale from Germany which tells of the terrible consequences of a woman's obsession with an ordinary garden vegetable, it takes just a little over two hundred words to introduce all the basic details. No sooner do we learn about the poor couple who long for a child when the wife becomes pregnant and reveals her intense desire for the lettuce that grows in a nearby garden belonging to a much-feared witch. The wife believes she will surely die unless her husband can fulfill this need. Given a very brief description of the characters, a sketchy setting ("in the woods"), a typical folktale time frame ("once upon a time"), and the makings of a tense conflict, our attention is caught and we are interested and involved in the story's development and the fate of its characters. In the same concise way, "**Rapunzel**" reveals how the witch claims the couple's daughter for her own in retribution for the husband's theft of the lettuce, and how, when the child turns twelve, the witch locks her in a tower to isolate her from the world. Later, when Rapunzel falls in love with a prince, the witch banishes her, and the prince, blinded in his fall from the tower, is forced to wander helplessly through the countryside. Finally, Rapunzel, the twins she gives birth to, and the prince are reunited, Rapunzel's tears serving as the cure for the prince's blindness.

Behind the simple, terse, and straightforward manner of a folktale like "**Rapunzel**," there is a wealth of possible insights into human nature. This helps to explain why the same folktale can mean so many different things to different readers, depending on their ages and experiences. It also explains why both children and adults can find new meanings in the same folktale each time they read or listen to it. Responding to one of the many versions of "**Rapunzel**," for example, younger children tune into the suspense and fear the story evokes. Intrigued by the woman's attraction to the lettuce, they like to talk about their own attraction to any kind of food they can never seem to get enough of. They often imagine themselves as the baby and wonder how the parents felt when she was taken from them. Responding to the parents' dilemma, a seven-year-old boy with whom we have worked wondered why the parents "don't just beat up the witch and take Rapunzel back."

Even though "**Rapunzel**" has a "happily ever after" ending, which is typical of most folktales, younger children are frequently disappointed with the way "**Rapunzel**" ends because the witch doesn't die, as she does in many of the folktales they know. Younger children have a very clearcut sense of justice and a clearly defined notion of right and wrong. Perceiving acts as totally right or totally wrong, they like to see evildoers of any kind—the cunning witch, the mighty giant, the vile stepmother—punished, just as they like to see good characters win out in the end. The psychologist Bruno Bettelheim believes that the "crime doesn't pay" attitude revealed in many folktales, along with the opportunity to identify with virtuous characters who struggle to the bitter end, can help to enhance children's moral development.[9]

Like many folktales, "**Rapunzel**" can be just as provocative for older readers. They, too, wonder about the woman's obsession with the lettuce, and they are appalled when Rapunzel, at age twelve, is put into the witch's tower and loses her freedom. Older readers also try to imagine what it would be like not to have anyone to talk to and, even worse, to be without one's friends. What especially appeals to older readers, though, is the love that unites Rapunzel and the prince and how their relationship is the most important thing in their lives. When these children learn that Rapunzel gives birth to twins, they are more concerned with the separation the couple has to endure than the fact that there is no mention of their ever having been married.

When illustrations accompany a folktale, the pleasure and understanding the story offers can be even greater. As in all illustrated books for children, the pictures in an illustrated version of a folktale should provide much more than a pleasant visual backdrop. Just as musicians need to study a written musical score before they can adequately interpret a piece of music in performance, illustrators need to spend a great deal of time studying the language in a text before they can do justice to the sensations and thoughts the text evokes in them or to the information the text contains. Relying on the clues they find in the writing, the best illustrators use an artistic medium, such as watercolors, pastels, or woodcuts, and an artistic style—such as realism, impressionism, or surrealism—to capture the spirit of the writer's words. In a worthwhile illustrated book, the words and pictures work together, one medium supporting and illuminating the other to communicate the book's meaning.

Trina Schart Hyman's full-bodied watercolor illustrations for Rogasky's retelling of "**Rapunzel**" are a case in point. They extend the details in the text by placing the characters and the action in distinctive and appropriate settings—a dark, somewhat eerie forest and rustic interiors. They highlight key scenes and dramatize the tension and conflict, and, through Hyman's subtle use of subdued light and carefully placed shading, they enhance mood, atmosphere, and feeling. Like explorers who are discovering a new territory, children of all ages pore over the details in enticing illustrations such as these, for illustrations help them to make sense out of what they read or what is read to them.

Something to Do

Find an illustrated version of a folktale in the children's section of your library or local bookstore. Examine the book by following these steps:

1. Look at the cover or book jacket. Is it inviting? Does it make you curious about the story? Based on the details and design of the cover, what do you think the story will be about?
2. Page through the book. How are the illustrations arranged? Do the illustrations interest you? What is your general impression of the illustrations and the layout of the book? Is the quality of the paper good or bad? What kind of type is used for the text? How and where are the words arranged on the page? Are the words easy or difficult to read? Does the style of the print seem to fit the overall mood and style of the book?
3. Randomly choose a few sections of the story to read. Does the writing have a distinct style that keeps you interested and involved? Does the writer talk down to the reader? Does the

dialogue sound natural? Are the descriptions vivid? Do you
get a clear sense of character, conflict, and action from the
writing?
4. Reexamine the illustrations. Does their placement in the text
correspond with the written text? Do the details and style of
the illustrations fit the details and style of the written text?
How do the illustrations work with the text?

Food and Nutrition in Folktales

There seems to be no limit to the problems, conflicts, and
predicaments that food causes in folktales. For example, a
family's lack of food sets the story of "**Hansel and Gretel**"
into motion, and the hunger of the two abandoned children
leads to their struggle with a thoroughly malicious witch who
would have them for dinner. "**Hansel and Gretel**" wastes no
time in getting to the hard, cold facts of a pretty gruesome
situation. As the result of a famine, the already impoverished
family of four may die from starvation. With the intensity and
cunning of someone bewitched by her own needs, the wife
finally convinces her husband that unless their children are
left in the woods to fend for themselves none of them will
survive. What a relief it is for children when Hansel and
Gretel's resourcefulness and perseverance prove more powerful than the witch's terrifying deviousness and their
mother's wretched deceit! Children spend no time grieving
over the witch's violent demise or the death of Hansel and
Gretel's mother. It is life and living and survival that matter
here. That Hansel and Gretel end their family's poverty
forever with the jewels they take from the dead witch's cache
makes these two courageous children that much more heroic
in children's eyes. Hansel and Gretel appeal because they
take control of their destiny; they are brave, they never lose
hope, and they are deeply concerned for one another. These
are values and virtues which need to be a big part of every
child's heritage.

Many translations, retellings, and illustrated versions of
"**Hansel and Gretel**" and other folktales fill the children's

book market. As a rule of thumb, avoid the ones that talk down to the reader, that underestimate children's abilities and feelings, that cloud the succinct style of folktales with excessive description, and that contain illustrations which play down the emotional intensity of the story by sentimentalizing the characters' problems. Instead, find retellings—and there are plenty of them—with strong, distinctive illustrations that stretch the imagination and deserve to be looked at again and again. Share the ones that have a fresh, vivid language style which captures the rhythm and vitality of a story meant to be told or read aloud—again and again.

Checklist for Evaluating Folktales

1. Does the language style capture the characteristics of oral language, or does it sound more like a writer's words? Does the dialogue between characters sound natural and authentic, or stiff and wooden?
2. Is there a simple and direct movement to the plot, and a quick development of episodes that leads to an obvious climax and a brief ending?
3. Are time, setting, and other story elements briefly sketched, rather than described elaborately?
4. Are the characters' traits, qualities, and shortcomings briefly outlined? Is it clear which aspect of human nature each character represents?
5. Does the reteller allow the reader's imagination to work, or does he/she too often attempt to fill in the missing details, the connections between incidents, and the characters' motives?
6. Is there a theme in the story, and is it revealed naturally through the character's actions, thoughts, and conflicts?

Humorous folktales about food and eating can also transport children to cultures around the world. From England comes "**The Three Wishes.**" In this popular tale, a woodcutter and his wife rescue an imp who returns the favor by promising to fulfill three of their wishes. As poor and humble as these folks are, it is not surprising that they first imagine themselves owning all sorts of treasures. Because they are so unfamiliar with such good fortune, however, the husband, forgetting the power he now has, wishes for a simple dinner of sausages. When the steaming dinner magically appears, the angry wife, forgetting *her* power, wishes that the sausages were hanging from her husband's nose. After they use the final wish to remove the sausages, the husband and wife are content to settle down at last to an appetizing dinner! In Paul Galdone's picturebook version of this much-told tale, the rough-hewn pictures are a good fit with the foolish couple's homespun language style. By comparing Galdone's version of the story with Margot Zemach's more subdued retelling, children can discuss specific reasons why they favor one story over the other. At the same time, they discover why two different interpretations of the same folktale can be success-ful. This, in turn, can be an effective rehearsal for their own written or dictated retellings of "**The Three Wishes**," done individually, in small groups, or as a large-group collaborative story experience. Later, the children could add interpretive illustrations.

The magic cooking pot is a popular motif in a number of humorous folktales. The magic pot takes center stage in Tomie dePaola's *Strega Nona*. Set in a small town in Italy, the story features a benign and amiable witch (the title means "grandma witch"), a typical noodlehead or dumbkin character found in stories around the world, and the traditional magic pot which gets out of hand. Big Anthony, who works for Strega Nona and who has a habit of not paying attention, is headed for big trouble when he decides to impress the people who live in the town by cooking pasta for all of them with Strega Nona's magic pot. Because he doesn't know the secret words that cause the pot to stop cooking—and because he doesn't pay attention to Strega Nona's warning not to use the pot in her absence—the town is nearly destroyed by a deluge of pasta. When Strega Nona returns, she saves the day by stopping the pot from cooking, but she makes Anthony eat every last string of pasta in order to teach him a lesson he will never forget. DePaola's larger-than-life, cartoon-style illus-trations are a perfect complement to this zany drama which children enjoy acting out.

The magic pot also appears in folktales from Germany (*The Magic Porridge Pot*), India (*The Magic Cooking Pot*), Japan (*The Funny Little Woman*), and other places. Since the food the pot cooks is different in each of these distinct tales, teachers can use the stories to spice up nutrition units in the primary and intermediate grades by introducing children to foods that are indigenous to each of the cultures depicted in the stories, possibly before or after the children sample the foods which are the center of attraction.

Teachers and parents can develop similar experiences with different versions of the story about food that escapes from its startled cook and sets off on a breakneck chase, usually with the cook in hot pursuit. These runaway food tales are cumulative and repetitive; incidents and details are added on in a logical, straightforward, and rhythmic fashion. They also contain short verses that are used throughout to keep the story moving and to hold the incidents together. Some cultural variations of this tale include "**The Gingerbread Boy**" (America), "**The Pancake**" (Norway), "**The Bun**" (Russia), and "**The Wee Bannock**" (Scotland).

Share these cumulative stories with younger children and they immediately join in, predicting what will happen next and reciting or singing the infectious rhyme right along with the storyteller or story reader. Besides the enjoyment and pleasure cumulative tales offer children, they are suitable for young readers or listeners for several reasons. First, because the cumulative tale moves in a straightforward, linear fashion, it can help young children remember basic story incidents and story sequence when they are first getting accustomed to how stories work. Second, children soon learn to use the cumulative pattern of events found in this type of story to predict what will happen next, a skill that fosters comprehension and increases children's confidence with print. Finally, cumulative tales with repetitive rhymes provide opportunities for oral interpretations of manageable stories through choral reading and dramatization. Oral interpretation of literature not only makes literature come alive, but, by stimulating children to read between the lines, it also facilitates comprehension by actively involving them with language.

Summary

When children are learning important concepts and information which, it is hoped, will lead to good nutritional habits, folktales can add a human perspective to the topic. The best of these stories not only entertain children; they also invite them to witness the value of food in all cultures as well as the origins of food customs, rituals, and traditions. From folktales they can gain some understanding of attitudes toward food and eating, not as an abstract concept but as a real-life issue that genuinely concerns people—even humanlike animals—of all ages, cultures, and backgrounds. An awareness of values, attitudes, and behaviors concerning nutrition is, after all, the main reason why we ask children to consider what and why they eat. As the authors of *Teaching Today's Health* point out, "Too often nutrition is taught as a grim and dry subject, divorced from the human perspective. No wonder that children often emerge from health education with scorn for nutritional principles; they associate nutrition with the imagined somber atmosphere of a health food store." How to work against this problem? "Avoid a rigid, by-the-rules approach," this team advises, "and do not reduce nutrition to a set of rules." Instead, "Your job in teaching is to make that concept more concrete and real to your students by presenting learning opportunities that relate nutritional information to daily life."[10] Folktales can help toward this effort because they provide children with situations that root nutrition in genuine human experience.

FANTASY LITERATURE: HEALTH ISSUES IN "ANOTHER KIND OF REAL"

Mention fantasy literature to some people and they immediately think of cherry-cheeked sugarplum fairies prancing through a Disney type of Never-Never Land where it is forever spring, or they picture a smiling heroine who always makes wishes come true with a sprinkling of magical dust. Mention it to parents and educators, and many wonder about the value of having children read any type of literature—or engage in any type of activity for that matter—which seems to remove them from the here-and-now. "Doesn't fantasy encourage children to avoid their real concerns and problems?" they sometimes ask. "Doesn't it distract children from the need to get on with their lives and to learn how to function in society?" Convinced that fantasy literature will give children a false sense of life and their place and role in the world, some adults even launch into a sermon like the one delivered in the London *Times Literary Supplement* by a critic who felt that fairy tales, which contain some of the basic ingredients of modern fantasy literature, "ultimately contribute to a more general alienation, a preference for living wholly in dreams and an inability to face reality."[11]

Many people have similar reservations about science fiction. Without having read much science fiction themselves, they assume that it deals only with farfetched situations and outlandish characters. These people tend to associate science fiction with stereotypical images, such as weird and hostile aliens who arrive in high-tech spaceships to conquer and control the universe, or superintelligent robots who eventually rebel against their master, or a strange scientist who is so preoccupied with inventing devious creatures that he (and it is more than likely a male) simply can't be bothered with the everyday world and the concerns of "normal" people. Although these skeptics sometimes believe that science fiction can involve young readers in an exciting though bizarre adventure story, they often see little worth in this type of literature beyond the immediate enjoyment it can provide.

Attitudes like these reflect a common misconception about the nature and function of fantasy stories and science fiction. The basic assumption is that this type of literature is primarily a vehicle for escaping from the problems and pressures of daily living. This implies that a child or adult who reads fantasy and science fiction enters into the world created by the writer in order to avoid life rather than to face it. With its vision focused on extraordinary happenings, with its manipulation of time and place as we know them, and with its frequent use of magic and dreamlike sensations, fantasy literature is seen as a diversion that helps to lessen the stress of having to live through the trials of ordinary, everyday life.

Take this type of reasoning to its extreme, and it is easy to see why writers of fantasy literature are often accused of catering to whimsy and encouraging daydreaming, wish-fulfillment, and all sorts of impractical thinking that lead the way to inattentiveness, negligence, and procrastination.

Characteristics of Fantasy Literature

Far from distorting or misrepresenting life, the topics and themes which the best writers of fantasy and science fiction explore in their stories actually focus on many important aspects of human nature and the human condition. Although these writers invite children to venture into other worlds or into a familiar world where the unusual becomes familiar and the extraoidinary takes on the characteristics of the ordinary, escapism for its own sake is not the reward that children gain from such reading. Rather, well-written fantasy and science fiction, like all good literature, can lead children to some valuable insights into themselves and others. Pointing out the fantasist's ability to carry children out of themselves and away from their ordinary world only to make them more aware of personal and social issues, the critic Sheila Egoff has observed:

> Fantasy is a literature of paradox. It is the discovery of the real within the unreal, the credible within the incredible, the believable within the unbelievable. . . .
> The creators of fantasy may use the most fantastic, weird and bizarre images and happenings but their basic concern is with the wholesomeness of the human soul, or to use a more contemporary term, the integrity of self. . . . The tenet of the fantasist is "there is another kind of real," one that is truer to the human spirit, demanding a pilgrim's progress to find it.[12]

Think of writers of fantasy and science fiction as highly imaginative individuals who are experts at devising and acting out situations in what could be an imaginary game called "What If?" Here are several "What If" scenarios based on a few well-known examples of fantasy and science fiction stories for children:

- *Where the Wild Things Are* by Maurice Sendak. What if a little boy who was having a bad day were sent to his room without any supper? Once he got there, what if he dreamed of a place where he met and controlled some undisciplined creatures who acted somewhat like himself?
- *Charlotte's Web* by E. B. White. What if a group of barnyard animals were given the power of speech? What would they say? How would they interact? With what would they be concerned?
- *Z for Zachariah* by Robert C. O'Brien. What if in the near future a nuclear war devastated the earth and killed all but two of its inhabitants? What if one of the survivors were a tyrant? How would the other survivor, a teenage girl, defend herself against such a person, in light of all else she must face while trying to stay alive?

As with all worthwhile stories, the best fantasy and science fiction stories contain well-defined, multifaceted characters, whether they are personified animals or human beings. To be believable, these characters must have distinct personalities and distinctive ways of talking, thinking, acting, and interacting. If they are genuine individuals, both the child and the adult will think, "I know someone like that!" or "This character is like (or not like) me." Having lived through the characters' experiences right along with them, we should respond, "Yes, this is the way things are" or "That's how I would have done it" or "I hope I never act this way." These are the kinds of "Ah ha!" recognitions that draw us into meaningful selections of fantasy or science fiction and give us something valuable to take away.

With the child beside us, we watch Max tame the Wild Things and realize that a healthy fantasy is a legitimate way for both children and adults to come to terms with their emotions. Reading *Charlotte's Web* to a group of second graders, we watch young Wilbur mature from an egocentric pig into an altruistic one, with Charlotte's support and guidance, and we celebrate the value of true friendship given with no strings attached. In a private conference with a seventh grader, we talk about Ann Burden's dilemma in *Z for Zachariah* and try to imagine the horror of such a terrible war, wondering how we would act if all of our familiar relationships and other securities suddenly vanished. The point is that with *good* fantasy literature, readers never doubt the existence of the characters and circumstances created by the writer because both are so well drawn and so convincingly portrayed that they seem possible.

Jane Yolen, the author of many fine works of fantasy and science fiction for children and adolescents, believes that "speculative fiction" is the label which best captures the hypothetical situations and plausible hunches that fantasists pursue. "Fantasy," she says, "is fiction that speculates on the possibilities that this and other worlds hold, limitless possibilities. . . . It is up to the author of speculative fiction to give us windows that open onto all those possible worlds."[13]

Surely, it is the pleasure of living through a vicarious experience that entices children and adults into the "possible worlds" which writers of fantasy create. But, like every other type of worthwhile literature, fantasy and science fiction should provide something more. In addition to a believable plot, credible characters, realistic dialogue, a plausible setting, and a fresh and engaging language style—the ingredients of all effective stories—fantasy and science fiction should lead to some type of significant discovery about people and society. In fact, one of the ways to single out the best fantasy literature is to ask whether the story contains an important theme. In any type of fiction, from the folktale to the realistic story of contemporary life and living, theme is the universal truth or idea that holds the story together and draws the reader's attention to some aspect of human nature or some characteristic of the human condition.

Perhaps the element of theme seems too abstract for children's books and too difficult for children to grasp. Theme is certainly one of the ingredients in literature that causes more problems for readers than is necessary. In a recent study of college students' perceptions of their reading development, the majority of these students reported that they were raised on the notion that theme is the "hidden" or "deep" meaning which readers are required to find whenever they read a poem, story, or play.[14] These students often characterized the search for theme as a kind of game they played with teachers, whether they were in elementary school or graduate school. In order to win this game, they had to correctly guess what the teacher or college instructor considered the author's "message" or the "intended meaning" of the piece. It is not surprising that these students learned at an early age to distrust their thoughts, feelings, and reactions to the literature they read in school because they soon realized that their ideas didn't matter. Thus, some became "literature drop-outs" who developed an aversion to reading altogether, while the ones who continued to read simply accepted the fact that their personal connections to literature would have to be reserved for the reading they did outside the classroom.

Theme is actually no more "hidden" than plot, character, setting, or any of the other elements which writers use to shape a story. Rebecca Lukens hits the mark when she suggests that theme is "a discovery of some kind."[15] It may be related to some abstract concept like love, hope, or fear, but it is always revealed in concrete ways through the tangible actions, thoughts, and feelings of lifelike characters who are involved in a situation that unfolds before us and, one hopes, involves us. For example, when Max returns from the land of the Wild Things, theme is the focus as you and the child think and talk about how good it feels to have a parent who loves you so much that even when you are having a rough day, you know you will still be cared for and accepted.

Theme is also the focus of a discussion of *Charlotte's Web* when a third grader realizes that "It's neat how Charlotte saves Wilbur, but I like how she lets him know that he will do all right on his own, too." The same is true when an eighth grader is talking to his teacher about *Z for Zachariah* and comments, "Ann knows that even a war can't make somebody give up. She's *got* to do everything she can to stay alive, even if it means leaving her family's farm." It is important for teachers and parents to remember that every good piece of literature can lead to different discoveries for different readers. Part of the excitement and satisfaction of reading literature, whether you are six, sixteen, or sixty-six, is making these personal discoveries and perhaps being changed because of them. This is what keeps readers reading.

Something to Do

Read one of the selections of fantasy or science fiction mentioned at the end of this chapter. List the major ideas the selection makes you think about. Take note of the ones that change as you continue to read and the ones that remain the same. Ask a child or a group of children to volunteer to do the same thing with the same story. In what ways are your ideas similar to and different from the child's or children's? What do the items on the lists reveal about readers of fantasy and science fiction?

Fantasy and Science Fiction on Health Issues

Writers of fantasy and science fiction have dealt with a wide range of personal and social issues that can complement children's understanding of the issues they explore in a comprehensive school health program. The best of these writers, as well as the illustrators who interpret their stories visually, have focused on all sorts of emotions and values: family and social relationships, the search for self identity, the nature and purpose of government, the causes and effects of war, and humanity's respect for and misuse of the natural environment. These topics can be found in classics that have proved to be perennial favorites with younger children, such as *The Ugly Duckling* by Hans Christian Andersen, *The Tale of Peter Rabbit* by Beatrix Potter, *The Wind in the Willows* by Kenneth Grahame, and *The Cricket in Times Square* by George Selden. All these stories depict the adventures and the troubles of personified animals and creatures who have problems, faults, and moods; who learn about responsibility to self, others, and the community at large; who survive difficult times and rejoice in easy ones; and who grow, change, and develop in positive ways much as we hope children will. *The Little House* by Virginia Burton, winner of the Caldecott Medal in 1943 for illustration, introduces young children to some of the negative effects of progress as the attractive house, formerly set in a peaceful rural environment, suffers through the confusion of increasing urbanization and the pollutants caused by modern technology. Through *The Velveteen Rabbit* by Margery Williams, a continual bestseller on college campuses, children can become aware, along with an endearing toy rabbit, of what it means to be real and how love and affection can help to sustain life and influence the attainment of personal identity.

Fantasy literature can be just as provocative for readers in the intermediate grades. In *Mrs. Frisby and the Rats of NIMH* by Robert C. O'Brien, they not only find an intriguing story of survival and a struggle for freedom, but they also learn about some aspects of the nature of scientific research and receive a great deal of information about modern medical concepts, discoveries, and issues. In an attempt to save her family's home from a spring plowing so that her son can recuperate from pneumonia, Mrs. Frisby, a widowed mouse, realizes that she must seek the help of a group of rats. Gradually, she learns the details of their remarkable experiences. The rats, along with her late husband, had been used in an experiment in which they were given DNA and steroids to develop their intelligence and extend their life spans. Having escaped from the laboratory, they now plan to develop a farming community where they can survive without being forced to steal. Later, Mrs. Frisby helps to save all but two of the rats by alerting the group to the arrival of government exterminators who have come to destroy them with cyanide gas. Among other things, this Newbery Award-winning novel deals with courage and determination, the value of cooperation, the repercussions of scientific investigation, and each individual's responsibility to defend and protect the rights of others.

Of course, not all fantasy literature is as intense as O'Brien's story. Just as many children like to think about and discuss the themes revealed in serious fantasies, they also welcome the special brand of zany comedy which characterizes humorous fantasy stories. When it comes to humor, Dr. Seuss's unique plots and characters are among younger children's favorites—from bewildered Bartholomew in *The Five Hundred Hats of Bartholomew Cubbins* to the quarrelsome Yooks and Zooks in *The Butter Battle Book,* where an increasingly ludicrous argument over how to butter bread threatens to end with a terribly destructive war. Because Seuss is a master at winding his way into children's hearts and minds with contagious rhythms and rhymes, they frequently memorize his stories. Still, they need the guidance of a sensitive adult to alert them to Seuss's observations of human nature that always raise his stories from entertaining language play to perceptive social commentary.

A number of humorous fantasy stories that feature eccentric characters and preposterous situations appeal to readers in the intermediate grades. *Freaky Friday* and *Summer Switch,* both by Mary Rodgers, can stimulate some very lively discussions about family relationships. In the first book, a daughter finds that she has been turned into her mother, while in the second, a son finds that he has been turned into his father. Needless to say, the situations make both the children and their parents more understanding and considerate of each other's responsibilities, roles, and needs.

The needs as well as the rights of others are central issues in *The Pushcart War* by Jean Merrill. Here, a group of New York City street vendors band together to protect themselves and their businesses from being destroyed by ruthless truck drivers. The story is written from the point of view of a historian in 1996 who, in describing the famous Pushcart War of 1986, explores why wars start and how we can prevent them. True, stories like these are outlandish and often bizarre, but by upending whatever is ordinary and familiar, they can make us and the children with whom we work pause long enough to reconsider, often from an entirely new perspective, the possibilities and choices all of us must deal with in the process of living through real-life experiences. From the child's point of view, part of the humor comes from witnessing the vulnerability of what seems to be a predictable adult world. For children, this makes the world a little more manageable.

Older students also have access to a variety of challenging fantasy literature, much of which complements their increasing sensitivity to social and political issues and their developing awareness of who they are and how they might fit into society. In the novels that comprise Patricia Wrightson's trilogy, *The Ice Is Coming, The Dark Bright Water,* and *Journey Behind the Wind,* Wirrun, an Aborigine, accepts the responsibility to save his people and their land from coming under the control of mysterious spirits from the past. Because of Wrightson's emphasis on humanity's need to respect and protect the natural environment, the trilogy can be particularly relevant in upper-grade units on environmental issues. Several challenging science fiction novels by H. M. Hoover and Sylvia Engdahl also deal with the environment. Set in a future world where the atmosphere is so unsafe that most people live in domed underground cities, *This Time of Darkness* by Hoover depicts the adventures and struggles of two young friends who decide to escape to the uncertain world outside their crowded, squalid environment. In *The Far Side of Evil* by Engdahl, also set in the future, Elana, a recent graduate of the Anthropological Service Academy, is given the task of working on the planet Toris, where the misuse of nuclear power may destroy an entire civilization.

Just as the themes that children discover in fantasy and science fiction can help them gain fresh insights into personal, social, and political issues, the believability of these stories is the element that sustains their interest and makes them receptive to the ideas and truths the stories contain. Believability may seem a strange characteristic in literature that is filled with extraordinary happenings and unusual characters, but unless the characters and incidents ring true, we will fail to take them seriously. The key to making fantasy and science fiction plausible begins with the writer's own belief in the world he or she creates. Writers of fantasy and science fiction must be as familiar with this imagined world as they are with their own environments. They must know every detail of the setting, from the lay and the look of the land to its climate, exact location, and resources, and they must know intimately each one of their characters. Jane Yolen advises the aspiring fantasist to ". . . write out a travelogue of your world. Take yourself for a trip to its most famous points of interest. Or pretend you are writing an article for an encyclopedia that will include customs, laws, historical background, flora and fauna, and the Gross National Product."[16]

Nutrition in Fantasy and Science Fiction

Included among the essential details in many fine selections of fantasy and science fiction are references to food, eating, and other nutritional matters. A case in point is *The Tale of Peter Rabbit* by Beatrix Potter, the animal fantasy cherished by generations of very young children. A good story to read aloud to children who are first learning about nutritious types of food, the tale tells of Peter's sortie into Mr. McGregor's lush vegetable garden, despite his mother's warning that in that very spot Peter's father lost his life. Stuffed to his ears with fresh lettuce, beans, and radishes, incorrigible Peter manages to make it back home, but only after a wild chase with furious Mr. McGregor in hot pursuit! Potter's tiny pictures are little cameos of setting, mood, character, and action, and the affectionate but firm way Peter's mother deals with her disobedient child is a model of patience for harried parents. Without losing sight of the instincts of the animals (and humans) she depicts, Potter adds another dimension to the notion that "kids will be kids." She also proves that a simple story does not have to be simplistic and condescending.

Whereas Peter Rabbit's physical agility saves him from Mr. McGregor's wrath, the lost mouse in Emily Arnold McCully's *Picnic* survives because she keeps her wits about her and forages for edible foods. A good example of a wordless picturebook in which the illustrations alone supply all the details of the story, *Picnic* shows how a mouse family's outing on a delightful summer day turns into a frantic search for one of its missed and missing children. On the way down an isolated country road, one of the children is accidentally thrown from her family's pick-up truck. Off the family goes before she can get their attention. Clutching a toy animal, she survives the frightening ordeal by eating the raspberries she finds in the woods, until she is discovered by her distraught family and they all settle down to a well-balanced picnic that includes the major food groups.

This closely knit family also appears in *First Snow,* a wordless sequel to *Picnic.* This time the same child takes her first solo sled ride down a steep hill with the support and encouragement of her family. Used to their best advantage, wordless books give children opportunities to "read" the pictures and to find in them story sequence, details, and characteristics. They have to infer from the pictures what is happening in each scene, what the characters might be saying and thinking, and even the appropriate sound effects that can be made to make the scenes come alive. A good follow-up activity is to have the children write or dictate their own captions to the pictures or to create a series of related pictures for their own wordless books that provide a sequel to the book they have just "read."

Eating problems and problem eaters appear in a number of inventive fantasy stories for younger readers. Finicky eaters easily relate to the young child's obsession with one kind of food in *Bread and Jam for Frances,* one of the selections in a series of picture storybooks by Russell Hoban that focus on the everyday situations and ordeals of an engaging family of badgers. When Frances refuses to eat anything but bread and jam, her parents use reverse psychology and allow their inflexible child to overindulge while they continue to enjoy a variety of foods including breaded veal cutlets, string beans, baked potatoes, and spaghetti and meatballs. Add to this the scrumptious lunches her friend brings to school each day, and Frances soon realizes that having too much of one thing can simply get boring. Typical of the succinct, compressed style of the picturebook form, *Bread and Jam for Frances* and the other timeless books in this popular series cover a lot of ground in a brief space and therefore make the reading experience a good fit for the young child's often-short concentration span. Children who ask for other books about Frances are pleased to find out that Frances's escapades are continued in *A Birthday for Frances*—where jealousy prompts her to eat most of the present she prepares for her baby sister—as well as *Bedtime for Frances, A Bargain for Frances,* and *A Baby Sister for Frances.*

In James Marshall's *Yummers!* and its sequel, *Yummers Too,* the problem is rotund Emily Pig's insatiable appetite for the oddest assortment of any kind of food—much of it the wrong kind. No matter how she worries about her weight, Emily's willpower always weakens at the sight of a popsicle, a scone with butter and jam, an eclair, or the other delectable treats that have an almost hypnotic power over her, as she moves from one enticing edible to another, accompanied by her faithful friend, Eugene Turtle, whose restraint is a sharp contrast to Emily's lack of self-control. Even when she is forced to work at Healthy Harriet's Health Food Store in *Yummers Too,* she manages to overindulge in honey-dipped papaya, ginseng soda, frozen yogurt, and carob candy bars. Because Emily is so oblivious to the negative effects of her compulsive eating habits, children enjoy the opportunity to become the experts who give an "adult" some sound advice about nutrition as they suggest ways to improve her diet, to lose weight, and to curb her craving for junk food. Marshall's brightly colored, cartoon-style illustrations add just the right touch of exaggeration to Emily's disproportionate desires.

A lack of willpower is also the problem two close friends face in "Cookies," one of the five stories found in Arnold Lobel's *Frog and Toad Together.* Because it is so hard to resist eating the entire batch of cookies Toad has just baked, Frog and Toad decide to keep the temptation out of sight by putting the remaining cookies in a box on a high shelf. Realizing that what is out of sight is not necessarily out of mind, they feed the cookies to the birds. Anyone who has ever weakened will surely recognize the extremes one sometimes engages in to subdue an overzealous appetite. The books in the Frog and Toad series are good examples of "easy readers." Created specifically for children who are just beginning to read on their own, easy readers feature a limited vocabulary, some repetition of key words, and fewer pictures than are found in a typical picture storybook. Lobel is a master of the form because he successfully meets the challenge that writers of easy readers must face: to simplify without being simplistic. In addition to the understated, almost dry manner in which he tells these tales, a great part of Lobel's success comes from the fresh and natural language style which he uses to shape Frog and Toad's very human problems and experiences, as in this conversation from "Cookies":

"Will Power is trying hard
not to do something
that you really want to do,"
said Frog.
"You mean like trying *not*
to eat all of these cookies?"
asked Toad.
"Right," said Frog.*

The Frog and Toad series abounds with authentic feelings and a genuine understanding of typical human predicaments. These are believable stories about how all creatures behave when they deal with the surprises, disappointments, and understanding they gain as they risk relating to others in open and honest ways. For other examples of easy-to-read stories with just as much good-natured humor and good feelings shared by friends and family members, see the Little Bear series written by Else Minarik and illustrated by Maurice Sendak.

Food looms large in a number of fantasies and science fiction stories for readers in the intermediate grades, although many of these stories can be read aloud to younger children whose listening comprehension usually exceeds their independent reading ability. The various Warton and Morton books by Russell E. Erickson are a case in point. In each of these novel-length stories, Warton and his brother Morton, a pair of down-to-earth toads, get involved in action-packed, danger-filled adventures whenever they leave their safe underground home. In contrast to Warton, a born adventurer, timid Morton prefers to stay put and prepare good meals. In *Warton and the Castaways,* Warton lures his brother into the wiles of the woods when Morton discovers that he is out of honey. There they are pursued by a crafty raccoon until they find a short-term refuge in the home of two eccentric old tree frogs. It is food at every turn here: the toad brothers' incessant hunger, the tree frogs' initial selfish concern for satisfying their own appetites, and the raccoon's frustration with being so near, yet so far, from a tasty meal of four healthy

---

*Excerpt from "Cookies" from FROG AND TOAD TOGETHER by Arnold Lobel. Copyright © 1971, 1972 by Arnold Lobel. Reprinted by permission.

creatures. In fact, it is the sharing of food which brings these creatures together in the end and helps to solve the conflict to everyone's satisfaction.

Children who have enjoyed following Warton and Morton on their many ventures into the dangerous bog that surrounds their peaceful home could move on to a more challenging story with similar characters, settings, and situations, such as *The Wind in the Willows* by Kenneth Grahame. In Grahame's classic story, a host of distinctive male animals live a content and peaceful life in the woods until the vicious creatures of the Wild Wood and the values and pressures found in the Wide World interfere with their orderly existence, which includes established rules of etiquette, loyalty to friends, a tolerance for frailties, and the sharing of food.

Psychologist Nicholas Tucker makes a number of interesting points about children's attraction to fantasies like *The Wind in the Willows* that depict a close-knit community of personified animals. Tucker believes:

- Because children, like animals, can be small and vulnerable, they can identify with and be sympathetic to animal characters' lifestyles and problems in a world dominated by "adults."
- Animal fantasies which portray how well a community works can give children clues to how they might adapt socially and live successfully in the world.
- In many animal fantasies, the animals survive without "adult" supervision; this contributes to the child's growing desire to survive independently without adult control.[17]

Also, the personified animals and objects which children meet in fantasy stories are compatible with the way children think and experience the world. In *The Uses of Enchantment,* Bruno Bettelheim explains that animistic thinking provides a clue to how children come to grips with their basic questions about who they are and how they fit into the world. He says:

> To the child, there is no clear line separating objects from living things; and whatever has life has life very much like our own. If we do not understand what rocks and trees and animals have to tell us, the reason is that we are not sufficiently attuned to them. To the child

> trying to understand the world, it seems reasonable to
> expect answers from those objects which arouse his
> curiosity. And since the child is self-centered, he ex-
> pects the animal to talk about the things which are really
> significant to him, as animals do in fairy tales, and as the
> child himself talks to his real or toy animals. A child is
> convinced that the animal understands and feels with
> him, even though it does not show it openly.[18]

The important thing for adults to keep in mind is that
children's tendency to personify animals and objects helps
them come to grips with their basic questions about life and
living—"Who am I? Where did I come from? How did the
world come into being? Who created man and all the animals?
What is the purpose of life?"—in concrete terms that make
sense to children in light of their mental and emotional
development.[19]

Humorous fantasies are also popular with many intermediate
grade readers. At the top of their list of favorites are Daniel
Pinkwater's offbeat science fiction stories which center around
nutrition. Parodying the lofty, serious tone of the traditional
science fiction novel, Pinkwater has created a gallery of
eccentric characters who become involved in bizarre situations
that provide some credible observations about contemporary
society. *Fat Men From Space* involves a worldwide junk food
takeover by hordes of overweight spacemen from the planet
Spiegel who invade Earth in streamlined spaceburgers. People
have become so attached to unhealthy foods that they panic and
nearly start a war as they watch these aliens confiscate such
staples as Twinkies and fast-food dinners.

Pinkwater continues this slapstick indictment of humanity's
inordinate attachment to bad foods in his Magic Moscow
trilogy which includes *The Magic Moscow, Attila the Pun,* and,
most recently, *Slaves of Spiegel.* In this latest story, the
spacemen from Spiegel are on a mission to search the
universe for the makers of "the greasiest, heaviest, and
most fattening cooking" who will then compete in an inter-
galactic cooking contest. Among the three top contest-
ants transported to Spiegel in the spaceship "Cholestrol" are
Steve and his assistant Norman, who own the famous Magic

Moscow gourmet restaurant, where customers can find a mixture of ice cream, vegetable, and fish delights such as The Day of Wrath and The Nuclear Meltdown. Using broad humor, exaggeration, and puns, Pinkwater instills new life into the need to raise children's consciousness about the differences between nutritional and unhealthy foods. Because of their own adeptness at creating humorous stories, intermediate graders like to model their writing after Pinkwater's to create sequels to the Magic Moscow trilogy. This is a good way to reinforce information students are learning about nutrients, a well-balanced diet, and the ill effects of junk food. Incorporating this information into inventive stories makes it less abstract for students and less distant from real-life experience. At the same time, story writing gives students opportunities to practice writing and thinking skills.

In the same way, selections of fantasy and science fiction can enhance the nutritional information, attitudes, and behaviors that teachers and parents strive to instill in children in the upper elementary grades. As their reading tastes develop, older children seek fantasy stories that satisfy their distinctive interests, concerns, and needs. Many of these stories are serious in tone and intent and contain the complexity of plot, character, and theme that complement the older elementary school student's search for answers to complex moral, political, and social questions.

In some of the more demanding selections of fantasy literature, nutritional concerns and issues help to reveal the characters' values and attitudes, uncover themes, and advance the action of the plot. In *The Voyage Begun,* Nancy Bond transports her readers to the not-so-distant future in the United States where many natural sources of food and energy are in short supply, due to shifts in the climate and rampant environmental problems such as toxic waste, oil spills, and radiation leaks. Unlike his scientist father who avoids the problems by putting all of his trust in new technological developments, Paul is horrified when he explores the once thriving coastal colonies that surround the area to which his family has recently moved and begins to understand the long-term effects of the devastating environmental conditions.

From a local conservationist, Paul learns that more and more people are being forced to hunt for the few remaining species of wild game and that what is left of edible foods from the sea is no longer safe to eat. Though Bond's portrait of the future is bleak, it is not hopeless. Without offering an easy and contrived solution to the disturbing problems that, according to Bond, could plague America in the twenty-first century, she reveals how a group of concerned citizens band together and try to save a crumbling environment. This is the kind of book that can transform classroom lessons on environmental awareness into crucial, close-to-home issues that should concern every citizen, since Bond shows that we are all affected by how well we care for our natural environments and how well we respect the resources they provide us. With the right direction on the part of the teacher, students could finish *The Voyage Begun* wondering what they themselves can do to help control environmental problems and why the maintenance of a safe and healthful community is each individual's moral responsibility. Bond implies that the continuation of life as we know it will surely depend on the development of attitudes like these.

Life as we know it has been altered irrevocably by a nuclear war in Robert C. O'Brien's disturbing futuristic novel *Z for Zachariah*. For sixteen-year-old Ann Burden, who thinks she may be the only person left on earth, survival is tenuous at best. But, when a crazed tyrant enters the scene with his selfish motives and deep suspicions, Ann becomes involved in a fierce struggle to maintain her rights and dignity. With Mr. Loomis serving as an increasing threat, Ann attempts to reestablish her family's farm so that she will have a lasting supply of wholesome provisions. Written in the form of a diary Ann keeps, this tense story is like a vivid documentary that describes the terrifying effects of a totally destructive war as seen from the perspective of a resourceful and sensitive teenager. In the end, Ann decides that even if it means she will have to abandon the farm she cherishes and the new crops which will surely keep her alive, she must leave Mr. Loomis in order to preserve her self-respect. As much as older children are intrigued by Ann's relationship with evil Mr. Loomis, they are just as eager to discuss the ways a nuclear war might affect humanity's basic human needs, from the need for love and companionship to the need for food and shelter. O'Brien's speculations can stimulate children to wonder about the things people value and the reasons why they would choose political ideals over love.

Summary

All of the most effective writers of fantasy and science fiction have in common their exploration of human behavior, human values and beliefs, and human needs. These should be crucial concerns and issues in a comprehensive school health program that views the attainment of well-being as a constant, lifelong process which involves critical thinking about choice, behavior, and personal responsibility. As in all good literature, such issues are not presented as abstract principles and prescriptions but as concrete experiences lived through by individuals who are seen in the act of making choices that either enhance or inhibit their well-being. By talking and writing about these characters and their experiences, by dramatizing their conflicts, problems, and successes, by reshaping their attitudes and behaviors into art and movement, students of health can be led to think about their own lives and the decisions and choices they make concerning their own health in the largest, most comprehensive meaning of that word. Through literature children can learn that human change is constant and that we do, in fact, have the power and right to influence the courses our lives take and even the course of the world.

Checklist for Evaluating Fantasy and Science Fiction

1. Does the writer tell a gripping story? Are the story and characters believable? Are the characters distinct individuals rather than stereotypes? Does the action develop logically and consistently within the fabricated world created by the writer,

or do things just seem to happen? As you are reading, can you say, "Yes, I can really see how this might happen" or do you disbelieve?

2. Does the story make you consider some important ideas about life and living in the past, the present, or the future?

3. Is the setting so vividly detailed that you can see, hear, and feel the place where the action unfolds and the characters develop? Do you have a clear sense of the time and era in which the story takes place?

4. Does the language style fit the characters? Does the dialogue sound natural, given the world fashioned by the writer?

5. If there are illustrations, do they work integrally with the language and ideas revealed in the text?

REALISTIC FICTION: HEALTH ISSUES HERE AND NOW

When we read well-written fantasy or science fiction, we willingly put our disbelief on hold and, for the time being, accept hypothetical incidents and situations. We never doubt the existence of the characters, no matter how extraordinary or unusual they may seem at first. When writers of fantasy and science fiction have control of the situations and characters, they also have control of our imaginations and so we believe. Realistic stories, on the other hand, place readers in more familiar territory right from the start. In realistic stories the characters must, from the beginning, have all the trappings of real people, and it must seem as though their experiences could actually take place in the world as we know it. It is as though the writer of realistic fiction has the power to remove a curtain that, once opened, reveals the lives and circumstances of real people—people both like and unlike ourselves—those we would like to emulate as well as those we would be glad to avoid. It is as though the writer invites us to eavesdrop on the private lives of all types of people who could very well live next door or down the street. Once there, we are allowed to become fully acquainted with these people and perhaps to learn something from them as they live through their experiences.

Characteristics of Realistic Fiction

The characters that readers meet in well-written realistic fiction as well as the problems, conflicts, and circumstances they face must seem so authentic that we can't help but wonder if they really do exist. It is not surprising, then, that writers of realistic fiction are frequently asked if they have written about people they actually know, places they have really lived in or visited, and situations they themselves have really experienced. That is how in touch these writers should be with every detail of their characters' lives, including their strengths and weaknesses, their appearances, and how they talk, feel, think, and behave. The same is true for the environments in which the characters live and interact, the difficulties and struggles they face, and the discoveries they make. Jane Yolen tells writers of realistic fiction to know all they can about their characters:

> Before you do anything else, you must make your characters real to yourself. Catalogue their looks, their likes, their dislikes. Fill in a family history. Think of small anecdotes about their childhood—or infanthood, if they are still children. If you have a tape recorder and are a frustrated actor, speak your characters' dialogue into the tape to see if it sounds realistic.[20]

The payoff for writers who know all of these details and weave them into their stories is a convinced and involved reader, for what we look for in realistic fiction is an accurate picture of life unfolding in a possible time and place. "A realistic story," Sutherland and Arbuthnot contend, "is a tale that is convincingly true to life."[21] If the story is a good one, readers of all ages should be able to say, "This is exactly how it is or how it could be. This is how people act. This is what they wonder about and contend with. These are the compromises and mistakes they make. These are the problems they experience and the understandings they gain."

The writer's attempt to be true to life influences every detail in realistic fiction. The characters' style of speaking and thinking should capture the variety, freshness, and rhythm of the language of real people. The themes discovered in realistic fiction should reflect and shed light on all types of significant concerns, problems, and conflicts that genuinely occupy children and adults who are living through the best and worst of times. The most effective writers allow these ideas to emerge naturally and honestly from what their characters do, say, think, and feel in the same way that truths emerge in real life from the concrete experiences of everyday living. Ultimately, what attracts readers of all ages to realistic fiction is first and foremost the pleasure of getting caught up in an exciting, thoughtful plot that has lots of unexpected twists and surprises and interesting characters. Like adults, children read to find out what happens next, to whom it happens, why it happens, and who makes it happen.

Whether it is a humorous picturebook about coping with the stresses of a bad day, such as *Alexander and the Terrible, Horrible, No Good, Very Bad Day* by Judith Viorst, or a novel that explores the psychology of overeating, such as *Fat* by Barbara Wersba, an effective realistic story is always about some beliefs, values, and attitudes which lead to a "main idea or central meaning" that readers of all ages take away with them at the story's ending in much the same way that any meaningful real-life experience has the potential to make us think about personal, social, and moral issues.[22] It is the writer's challenge—and a sign of his or her skill as an artist and his or her sensitivity to the way life works—to make the theme or themes an integral part of the fabric of a story that includes credible characters and plausible actions and experiences. Revealed in this way, the theme of a story is less a moral or lesson to be taught and learned than an underlying meaning or insight which readers discover as they follow along and put together the pieces of evidence and information the writer shows through the characters and their actions. Sutherland and Arbuthnot draw attention to the types of discoveries children can make through realistic fiction:

> If these books center on children's basic needs; if they give them increased insight into their own personal problems and social relationships; if they show that people are more alike than different, more akin to each

other than alien; if they convince young readers that
they can do something about their lives—have fun and
adventure and get things done without any magic other
than their own earnest efforts—then they are worthwhile books.[23]

Checklist for Evaluating Realistic Fiction

1. Are experiences, situations, and circumstances of everyday
   life and living revealed accurately and authentically?
2. Do the tempo and pace of the plot fit the situation? Does what
   happens in the story hold your interest? Do solutions evolve
   naturally and realistically with plausible and reasonable out-
   comes?
3. Are the characters believable? Are they multidimensional
   individuals who speak, act, interact, and feel in distinctive
   ways? Are their experiences, problems, conflicts, and awarenesses true to life? Do the characters provide us a better
   understanding of life and living?
4. Is the setting possible and recognizable? Are time and place
   fully described?
5. Are the discoveries and awarenesses about human experience
   worthy of attention? Do they develop naturally from the
   characters' experiences?
6. Is the language style appropriate to the characters and
   situations? Is there variation in the texture and rhythm of the
   language?
7. If the book is illustrated, do the illustrations complement the
   mood and language style of the story? Do they help to tell the
   story? Do they extend it?

The realistic writer's ability to accurately portray human
experience is the main reason that well-written realistic
stories are so valuable when it comes to shedding light on the
issues and problems which concern children. These stories
demonstrate what happens when children and adults alike
take charge of their lives and when they don't. They demonstrate that each of us has the power to make the right or wrong
choices regarding our happiness and, ultimately, our health.
In realistic fiction for children, the dominant point of view is
that genuine well-being cannot be reached or maintained

apart from considerations of mind, environment, and spirit, just as many contemporary medical and health professionals envision health as an integrated network of physical, emotional, mental, social, and spiritual factors.[24] Realistic stories translate these concepts into personal issues that children can recognize and to which they can relate as they read about and think about people their own age who meet the challenges of life head on and grow and learn from their experiences.

In the past twenty years or so, realistic fiction for children has come of age. There are few topics and issues about the realities of life that have gone unnoticed by contemporary writers of realistic fiction for children. These writers not only focus on the ordinary experiences and typical problems of people from every racial, ethnic, and socioeconomic group, but they also depict the harsher and more traumatic events and crises in life which deeply affect many children personally and which most children wonder about at some time.

Realistic Stories About Families

Many writers of realistic fiction have explored living in a family. A number have dealt with the many facets of sibling rivalry. Younger children who long to be accepted by an older, unsympathetic sibling will appreciate how young Tim, in *Timothy Too!* by Charlotte Zolotow, sticks by his older brother like a shadow until he makes friends with the new boy on his block and can begin to be his own person. Complemented by Ruth Robbins' compassionate illustrations, this little gem of a book for primary grade children is filled with warmth and understanding. It depicts a problem that many children need to talk about in order to work through their feelings and to recognize that their reactions are normal.

With the same sensitivity to the way children think and feel, Beverly Cleary uses a great deal of gentle humor in *Ramona and Her Mother* to reveal why seven-year-old Ramona believes that her mother loves her less than she loves Ramona's older sister. This is one of several short novels by Cleary that explores the ups and downs of a typical middle class American family as seen through the eyes of Ramona, a spunky, irresistible, and many-faceted little girl who has proved popular with both primary and intermediate grade readers.

The birth of a sibling can be a disruptive time for children. It is only natural for them to wonder if the new arrival will receive all of the family's attention and affection to their exclusion. Stories about the birth of a sibling can reassure youngsters that other children have had similar feelings and that they survived the ordeal and even began to feel excited about having someone new in their family. The title of *When the New Baby Comes, I'm Moving Out* sums up Oliver's initial attitude toward the impending birth of a brother or sister. With a number of perceptive family stories to her credit, author and illustrator Martha Alexander has Oliver describe the reasons why he thinks a new baby will usurp his special place in a very special family. Oliver may not be totally convinced that things will work out in his favor, but at least he has had a chance to voice his worries. Oliver can also be found in *Nobody Asked Me If I Wanted a Baby Sister,* where he decides that the best thing to do is to give his new baby sister away. He changes his mind when he discovers how indispensable he is to his sister because he has the power to make her stop crying.

In *She Come Bringing Me That Little Baby Girl* by Eloise Greenfield, which focuses on the experiences of a black family, Kevin resents all of the attention the new baby is receiving—especially because the baby is a girl. When his uncle explains how he used to take care of his baby sister, who is now Kevin's mother, Kevin gladly accepts his responsibility and invites his friends to see the new baby. Lois Lowry's *Anastasia Krupnik,* a feisty fourth grader who lives in a secure family, is downright appalled when she learns that her mother is pregnant. She begins to accept the inevitable, however, when her grandmother's death convinces her of the importance of a closely knit family. Intermediate grade readers can follow Anastasia's development in a series of fast-paced, humorous novels that tell of her growing affection for her baby brother and depict a variety of crises centered around family life and the little dramas and perplexing dilemmas that are an inevitable part of the process of growing up.

Realistic stories also show children that families can have their share of painful and tragic experiences. In *Nadia the Willful* by Sue Alexander and *My Twin Sister Erika* by Ilse-Margaret Vogel, both picturebooks for younger children, young people grieve over the death of a sibling. Lois Lowry presents older readers with a similar situation in *A Summer to Die*. Here, the jealousy Meg feels for Mollie, her attractive and vivacious older sister, eventually turns into guilt and then into heart-felt compassion as Meg watches Mollie succumb to leukemia. Without detracting from the intense sorrow that Meg and her parents feel, Lowry draws attention to the natural cycle of life and death by incorporating seasonal changes into the story and by making the birth of a neighbor's baby a central incident. This in no way lessens the intensity of Mollie's death or the fact that she will be missed, but it does show children how death is an integral part of the flow of life's changes.

Other realistic stories tell of children struggling through severe family situations that test their endurance and their ability to cope. This is certainly the case for fourteen-year-old Jeff Duncan in *CF in His Corner* by Gail Radley. Jeff has to contend with his divorced mother, who believes it is best to protect her sons from the truth by pretending that her younger son, Scotty, is afflicted with asthma rather than cystic fibrosis and that their modest trailer is really a fancy home. Jeff's determination to make his family face the harsh facts of their life is the catalyst for bringing the family together, but only after the three of them are forced to deal with some hidden emotions and genuine doubts. Because information about cystic fibrosis is woven naturally into the plot, readers can also learn how debilitating disease affects the body.

A search for the truth is also Babe's challenge in *Reasons to Stay* by Margaret Froelich. As if coping with the responsibility of caring for her brother and sister, her dying mother, and her alcoholic father isn't enough, Babe learns a terrible secret about her mother which leads to some painful discoveries. She also learns a gradual acceptance of the love of a new family and an awareness of how much her brother and sister mean to her. In this book for older readers, Babe's strength and resilience help her to survive intact as she begins to recognize her worth and to satisfy her basic needs without avoiding her responsibilities to others. She is a model of a young person who refuses to let life's difficulties defeat her because she relies on her inner strengths and convictions to see her through.

The theme that life's turmoils and tragedies can result in lasting personal change is also depicted in *The Solitary,* by Lynn Hall. After her mother killed her abusive father, Jane Cahill lived for years with resentful relatives who considered her a burden. At the age of seventeen, Jane returns to her deserted family home, where she intends to make an independent life for herself even though she is socially inept and terribly insecure. With the help of some sensitive neighbors, she slowly becomes aware of her courage and talents and is finally able to put the past behind her in order to take responsibility for the direction of her present and future life.

Nutrition in Realistic Fiction

Realistic stories that focus on nutrition include a similar range of feelings, moods, and themes. In many realistic picture books and in longer, more complex novels, nutritional issues are an integral part of personal, social, and cultural experiences that reflect life and living in today's world. The characters and situations found in these stories add a human and personal dimension to the facts and advice that parents and teachers give to children about nutrition to make them aware of the immediate and long-range effects of both a healthy and unhealthy diet on all aspects of a person's life. Just as a list of rules and prescriptions can be threatening and overwhelming to adults who want to change their habits and behaviors, children, too, need more than factual information to make the right decisions about nutrition. In the best realistic stories for children that deal with some aspect of nutrition, the topic is transformed into a human condition that both influences and is influenced by a young person's lifestyle.

Food serves a number of important functions in a variety of illustrated books. Many highlight the pleasures of sharing food with friends and family members. For example, one of the most memorable things about the summer *The Relatives Came* from Virginia for an extended visit is the home-cooked meals they prepare and eat with their country hosts. Stephen Gammell's lively colored pencil sketches for this good-natured and heartwarming story by Cynthia Rylant depict the homespun, folksy feelings that fill this lively book from start to finish. There is also an abundance of good feelings in *The Great Giant Watermelon Birthday* by author/illustrator Vera B. Williams. To celebrate the birth of their great grandchild, the owners of the Fortuna Fruit Market give away watermelons to anyone who wants to participate in the celebration. One hundred children and their relatives meet in a local park to have a wonderful party, complete with candles in the watermelons.

Food is also an important part of a more subdued type of celebration for young David in *Breakfast With My Father,* by Ron Roy. At first David wonders if he will ever see his father again after his father moves out of the house, but now David lives for Saturday morning, when he and his dad have breakfast at a nearby diner. Then, one Saturday morning David finds his father sitting at their own kitchen table. He has returned, but he makes no false promises about staying. The stark black-and-white illustrations for this story are as understated as the writing style, and both writer and illustrator are equally true to the tensions and insecurities that a troubled marriage typically causes for every member of a family.

Children will become sensitive to the feelings and motivations of others when they hear or read a story like David's and observe and interpret the body language and facial expressions the illustrations reveal. Following their exposure to the book, they might talk about, write about, and dramatize the thoughts, emotions, and reactions of both the young character and his parents. Since children often believe that they are the cause of their parents' troubles, a discussion of their responses to the book could culminate in making a large class chart on which the students contrast the characteristics of David's view of the situation with his parents' view, including the possible motivations for their separation. The word "possible" is the key here, since the characters' motivations and feelings are implied rather than stated outright in the story. To make sense of what the characters are thinking and feeling, readers of any age will need to read between the lines and fill in the gaps by inferring emotions and thoughts from the clues found in the illustrations and the brief text. During a large-group writing session, children can also explore character relationships, intentions, and feelings by contributing to a sequel to the story which tells of the family's situation in the future. This will involve them in problem solving and decision making while they learn more about story sequence, characterization, and other story elements.

Activities such as these not only encourage children's active involvement in literature and enhance their reading and language skills; they also help them develop important social skills as they move out of the egocentric stage that characterizes early childhood and toward a greater awareness of the needs, feelings, and motivations of others. In addition, when children participate in focused, meaningful discussions of literature, they will learn to listen to the opinions of others and, perhaps, gain new understandings and insights from them, especially when these opinions and reactions differ from their own. This ability to listen to others and respect the opinions of others is a valuable skill and habit—for reading and for getting along in life. Like life itself, reading is an active process that requires anyone at any age to "build" personal meaning based on the experiences one brings to the text as well as on clues and ingredients the author—and illustrator—supply.

In order for children to develop into confident and competent readers who turn to books for answers, insight, and information, they need to be assured that the feelings and thoughts and questions they have while reading are legitimate. They also need to see how others, including adults, actually work through worthwhile selections of literature as though they were putting together the pieces of a puzzle—tentative and unsure at first about what the experience means, until they gradually become aware of how things fit and relate and how all the elements add up to significant ideas and issues about people and life. In a classroom where risk taking is the norm for both students and teacher, this constructive, mean-ing-making process can be further enhanced and nurtured when collaboration is provided for and encouraged through a variety of activities. What a far cry this approach to reading is from limiting children's responses to literature to skill sheets and fill-in-the-blank exercises!

Something to Do

Choose a selection of realistic fiction from among the illustrated books listed at the end of this chapter. Consider the title and examine the illustration on the cover to deter-mine the possible subject of the story. Do the same with the title page. When you begin to read the book and look at the illustrations, note your initial reactions. Which types of questions do you have about the story at this point? Make note of the things you do not understand and the details you will need to help you answer these questions and give you a better understanding of the story. How do the illustrations help you as you read? At what points do you begin to make better sense of the story? When do you understand the themes and other "big" ideas which the author and illustrator are addressing? When you finished reading the book, what were you still wondering about and did you still have questions about?

Share the same book with a child or a group of children. How does the young reader's process of reading the book differ from your own? Show them some of the things you did and thought about as you read the book. Compare and contrast.

Children's ability to relate to and understand others can also be developed through their experiences with books that depict people from cultures different from their own. A number of realistic picture books reveal customs and tradi-tions pertaining to food and eating in a variety of cultures. These books can stimulate worthwhile discussions about the similarities and differences among the lifestyles and eating habits of people of various ethnic, cultural, and religious

backgrounds, the objective being children's increased respect
for all types of people. Children see behaviors and attitudes
modeled in these stories, and the attractive illustrations
reinforce, in tangible ways, the issues and concerns the writer
is addressing. Both writer and illustrator can help to dispel
myths and stereotypes about particular groups of people
because they reveal a culture from a human perspective.
These stories focus on feelings and needs that cut across
cultural differences. The underlying attitude is that people
throughout the world have more in common than any of us
might at first think. This is an important observation to share
with children, since studies of their perceptions of foreign
peoples have shown that young children in particular tend to
emphasize the differences rather than the similarities among
people and that they have a tendency to withhold affection
from foreigners.[25]

In their responses to good books that depict the experiences of people from other countries, children should be
encouraged to express both their positive and negative
feelings for people from various national backgrounds. When
children expose their perceptions and attitudes concerning
any person unlike themselves, a teacher or parent can help
them to compare impressions that stereotype people with
ones that take into consideration the unique traits of the
members of a particular social group as well as the basic
human needs, drives, and other characteristics that concern
individuals the world over and thus unite humanity. Consider,
too, the ways that effective selections of realistic fiction
dealing with cultural experiences can be included in a social
studies unit which focuses on life among foreign peoples.

How My Parents Learned to Eat by Ina Friedman is a realistic
picturebook that strikes a balance between cultural differences and the similarities among people. In this story, a young
girl explains why it is natural for her family to alternate
between a Japanese eating style on some days and an
American style on others. She describes how her American
father and Japanese mother secretly learned the other's way
of eating when they were courting in Japan so they could
finally eat together and thus continue to date. The child-
narrator implies that she is fortunate because now the family

knows two distinct ways to eat. Allen Say's full-color pictures reveal the amusing details of the parents' unique courtship and show how they learned about one another's culture partly through each other's food customs. Their daughter's pride in being part of the two cultures is felt in each episode.

A feeling of pride for cultural differences is the farthest thing from young Joey's mind when he and his friend Eugene pay a visit to Joey's Italian grandmother in *Watch Out For the Chicken Feet in Your Soup* by Tomie dePaola. In fact, Joey is embarrassed by what he believes to be his grandmother's strange behavior, the strange foods she prepares, and the even stranger way she speaks English. No need for Joey to worry. The visit turns into a fascinating experience for his friend, who not only finds the various foods delicious but is completely won over by Joey's endearing and gracious grandmother, especially when she invites the boys to make bread dolls for which DePaola supplies an easy-to-follow recipe. Without preaching, the author offers Joey and the readers of the book a simple lesson in respect.

The mood is much more serious in *Very Last First Time* by Jan Andrews, which tells of a Canadian Inuit girl's close encounter with death as she gathers mussels for the family dinner below the thick sea ice when the sea is at low tide. In the remote village where Eva lives, it is the custom for people who want to eat mussels in the winter to search for them along the bottom of the seabed. In the past, Eva has always gathered the mussels with her mother, but this is the first time she is allowed to make the search alone. Eva is thrilled as her mother lowers her through a hole in the ice, terrified when her candle goes out and she hears the tide beginning to flood, relieved when she safely rejoins her mother, and very proud as she sits at the kitchen table eating the food she has gathered—for the "very last *first* time" alone.

Children can follow Eva's experience by carefully viewing and interpreting the startling illustrations which use yellows and purples to contrast the safe above-ice world with the eerie under-ice world into which Eva journeys. Putting themselves in Eva's place, they can see how her feelings mirror their own and vice versa. A teacher might integrate this book into the language arts area of the curriculum by having the students discuss, write about, and act out their own significant first experiences, with the teacher's own writing serving as a model of the writing process. Also, Eva's story could serve as an introduction to a social studies unit on Canada that examines the Inuit people. *People of the Ice,* an informational book by Heather Smith Siska with illustrations by Ian Bateson, describes many aspects of Inuit life.

With approximately one out of every four school-aged children suffering from obesity, it is not surprising that many writers of realistic fiction have dealt with the personal and social problems which extremely overweight and obese children frequently face.[26] Because most of these authors probe the psychological and emotional causes of an inordinate dependency on food, by reading and discussing these stories children can begin to understand the reasons that mental attitudes affect physical and emotional conditions and how harmful dependencies of any sort can be overcome only when a person makes a commitment to modify his or her behavior or lifestyle. In most cases, the writers portray likable young people on the brink of making a deep-seated personal change as they begin to see their weight problems in the context of their confusion about self-identity and self-acceptance.

In the best of these stories, the characters are so believable and their problems so authentic that they evoke empathy and compassion, just as they would if we actually knew them. They draw us into their lives and we want them to change because we see even more than they do that they have the ability to live full and satisfying lives. This concern for the well-being of story characters is another way for children to explore the consequences of personal choice and personal change—to look for various solutions to personal problems, and to learn how to support and help others in need. Again, through their exposure to literature children can learn and practice important social and personal skills and attitudes that can influence their health and the health of others in the broadest, most concrete, and most practical sense of that word.

Among the many characters with weight problems in contemporary realistic stories for children, several are particularly memorable and believable for the way they develop into more self-assured individuals, partly through the help they receive from others, but mostly through a specific incident that puts them in touch with their qualities and worth. Harold V. Coleman, the endearing but lethargic central character in *After the Goat Man* by Betsy Byars, is a good example. Just on the brink of adolescence, grossly overweight Harold is experiencing a terrible summer, between dieting and having nothing to do except play Monopoly with Ada, his closest friend. He begins to gain the strength and insight he needs to get his life in order when he helps Figgy, his and Ada's new friend, search for Figgy's eccentric grandfather who is known as the Goat Man. By helping someone else, Harold realizes that he has the potential to help himself.

The process of growing up is just as complicated for Elsie Edwards, who thinks she has plenty of reason to believe that *Nothing's Fair in Fifth Grade.* An obese, temperamental, and stubborn child, Elsie steals lunch money to keep a well stocked supply of food, but she eventually takes charge of her unhappy condition and starts to slim down by the end of fifth grade. Several years later, in *How Do You Lose Those Ninth Grade Blues?,* she is still feeling unloved and unlovable as she struggles to overcome the earlier scars of rejection. Barthe DeClements's skill at juxtaposing humorous situations and emotionally poignant episodes, her thoroughly authentic characters who alternate between wit, wisdom, and confusion, and her use of lifelike contemporary dialogue give depth to these popular stories that lay out erratic and rocky journeys toward self-discovery.

For older children moving into adolescence, the process of maturing and developing a concept of self can be a remarkably stormy time. For older children with weight problems, the process becomes even more unsettling because the repulsion they often have for their bodies causes low self-esteem. Realistic fiction includes a range of stories that portray overweight adolescents in the midst of changing from self-conscious and often embarrassed individuals into assertive and confident young adults equipped with a clearer sense of who they are and what they hope to become. *One Fat Summer,* by Robert Lipsyte, chronicles this kind of personal turning point for fourteen-year-old Bobby Marks, who weighs more than two hundred pounds. Through a grueling summer landscaping job, he slowly and painfully comes to recognize his physical strength as well as the inner resources he needs to survive. At last, he finds the courage to stand up for himself against the vicious thugs who have been humiliating him the entire summer. The first-person telling of this story adds to its immediacy and contemporary sound and enables Lipsyte to get inside the mind and emotions of an alert and often funny young man who can now begin to live his life on his own terms.

Undernourished emotions are often the cause of an overzealous appetite. This is certainly the case for Dinky Hocker, another fourteen-year-old, who seems to eat everything in sight because she really craves her mother's attention and respect. Consumed by her mission to cure drug addicts, Mrs. Hocker has little time for her daughter's needs, until Dinky gets her mother's attention by inscribing "Dinky Hocker Shoots Smack" on the sidewalks, curbstones, and buildings in the neighborhood on the very night her mother is to receive the Good Samaritan Award for social service. Thus begins the task of rebuilding a strained relationship. M. E. Kerr, the author of this novel and many others which are always bestsellers with scores of adolescents, writes convincing, frank, and honest stories about the genuine needs and real problems of young people making their way in the contemporary world.

Barbara Wersba, another writer with a knack for evoking the emotional and psychological experiences of adolescence, has created a gallery of unconventional teenage characters. Most of these characters are intensely sensitive young people who are set apart from the norm because of their interests, their unwillingness to live by the rules and expectations prescribed for people their age, and the way they perceive the world. Alienated from their peers and parents, they are usually emotionally and physically insecure. In most cases, it is their relationship with an older person, who is as much an eccentric loner as they are, which helps them to develop a sense of self and an appreciation of their individuality. With sympathetic humor and a fluent writing style, Wersba lays out this route to identity for feisty, overweight Rita Formica in *Fat, A Love Story* and *Love Is the Crooked Thing.* In the first novel, sixteen-year-old Rita uses food as a crutch to cope with her loneliness and to compensate for feeling unloved and unlovable. Then she meets and eventually falls in love with Arnold Bromberg, an affectionate teddy bear of a man who is twice Rita's age. Arnold may be a penniless dreamer, but his true rewards come from reciting poetry, playing the organ, and writing a book on Johann Sebastian Bach. Through her love affair with Arnold, Rita begins to sort through her emotions and her weight problem and to celebrate her ability to love and be loved in return.

In *Love Is the Crooked Thing,* which takes place one year later, Rita's life is not turning out as she had hoped it would. She tells of how her parents forced her to break up with Arnold and how he moved to Switzerland, apparently to make things easier for her. Rita's true and most lasting personal change occurs when she tracks Arnold down in Zurich and realizes that he is unwilling to make a commitment to her, not because of her age or her parents' disapproval, but because of his fear of the responsibility that a relationship entails. Realizing that she deserves more than Arnold is capable of giving her, Rita can now take responsibility for her life because she no longer believes that her happiness and value as a human being depend on another person.

Few contemporary writers of realistic fiction for young people have penetrated the experiences of black children and adolescents with such sensitivity, depth of characterization, and poignant themes as Virginia Hamilton. Hamilton, who has won a number of prestigious awards that are given to writers of books for young people, is known for her ability to create unique and demanding stories that explore racial issues within the context of universal human issues that concern all peoples. In *A Little Love,* Hamilton tells a convincing, multi-layered story of an overweight and emotionally intense teenager's struggle to overcome her insecurities and fears. Sheema, a black high school student who is preparing for a career in the culinary arts, is consumed by her fear of the Bomb that could destroy the entire world, her sense of her inadequacies, and a negative physical image. Having been raised by her concerned and caring grandparents since her mother died and her father disappeared, Sheema convinces herself that if she could only establish a relationship with her estranged father, she would then experience the kind of reassuring love that would surely make her feel more secure and more accepting of herself.

Accompanied by her boyfriend Forrest, Sheema sets out to find her father who, as it turns out, is unwilling to accept the responsibility for his daughter. Through this disappointment, Sheema discovers the source of her strength and courage, and she recognizes the power of the commitment which Forrest and her grandparents have made to her. She now knows that it is not a little love which these people show her; it is a selfless, enriching kind of love that will help her to survive.

Summary

Since well-written realistic stories present children with true-to-life characters involved in authentic situations that reflect both commonplace and traumatic human experiences, realistic fiction can help enhance health-related knowledge, attitudes, and behaviors. In a health program that emphasizes promotion, prevention, and awareness, realistic stories allow children to read about and think about people their own age who deal with a wide range of vital health-related issues. It can be reassuring for children to see how others have faced and survived all sorts of problems and conflicts. These stories suggest to children that, though there may be no easy answers and solutions to life's dilemmas and difficulties, all of us can develop the ability and awareness to take hold of our lives, to make the right kinds of decisions, and to live life in healthy and satisfying ways.

By looking closely at the experiences of story characters, children can also weigh the choices, decisions, and options of others and explore alternative behaviors, attitudes, and solutions. This personal engagement with story characters can help children to develop empathy for others. A concern for the welfare of others is an important social skill that has many positive implications for the ways children relate to others and for the growth of their respect for the rights of different kinds of people. Through their exposure to realistic stories, children may also discover the types of personal and social concerns and problems that affect all types of people from every type of cultural and socioeconomic background. As Charlotte Huck and her colleagues have pointed out, "Realistic fiction serves children in the process of understanding and coming to terms with themselves as they acquire 'humanness.' "[27]

HISTORICAL FICTION: HEALTH ISSUES IN PAST TIMES AND PLACES

Just as some writers of fiction try to illuminate life as it is lived in the here-and-now, other writers of fiction set out to give their readers an accurate picture of life in the past. We should expect writers of realistic fiction to be in touch with the details of daily life and the concerns and issues which affect all types of people in the world about which they are writing. In the same way, writers who attempt to transport us to a time in the past need to be thoroughly familiar with all aspects of life and living in the era in which they set their stories. This is no less true of illustrators, who have a responsibility to communicate a genuine visual sense of what life and people must have been like in former times and places. Writers and illustrators of historical stories face quite a challenge, if they are to meet the requirements of a type of literature that should not only tell an interesting story but must also contain a true and factually correct picture of a specific period of history.

How do both of these artists learn about the period of history that will become an integral part of their stories? In order to acquire a full understanding of and, even more important, a feeling for the people and events they want to bring to life, these artists should be alert and perceptive researchers who delve into the past like sleuths who need to examine a wide range of resources—books, newspapers, private letters, journals, speeches, photographs, forms of entertainment, and types of art, to name a few—for possible clues about life and living in former times. To capture and sustain a reader's attention and interest with a believable story, writers—and illustrators—of historical fiction must have a complete knowledge of the beliefs, values, and mores which characterized the period they are depicting. They also need to become familiar with all of the details of daily life, such as how people dressed, what they ate, how and where they lived, what they did for entertainment, and how they related to one another. For the sake of creating authentic dialogue and description, they also need to know something about the language of the time, including the idioms and language styles used by different social classes and groups of people. At the same time, they must be aware of the social, economic, political, and religious ideals, issues and problems that influenced the thinking of the time and affected people's lifestyles in positive and negative ways.

Geoffrey Trease, author of many historical novels, sums up the challenge a historical novelist faces when he says that the true historical novel not only strives for an "authenticity of fact but—as far as is humanly possible—a faithful re-creation of minds and motives."[28] This emphasis on depicting the human element behind movements and trends in history aligns historical fiction with the human issues and concerns that should underlie every topic included in a comprehensive health education program.

When the goal of an imaginative writer is to resurrect the past, every detail is significant and relevant to creating a true slice of life. Geoffrey Trease tells an interesting story of how even the smallest detail can contribute to the believability of historical fiction. In *Mist Over Athelney,* Trease's historical novel about the Danish invasion of England, he has a group of young adventurers share a campfire meal of rabbit stew with a hermit they meet on one of their journeys. Although many professionals reviewed the book, it was an eleven-year-old reader who informed the author that his characters couldn't possibly be eating rabbit stew because there were no rabbits in England before the Norman Conquest, an event which occurred after the events Trease described in his novel.[29]

Of course, the typical child will rarely have a refined

knowledge of such specific historical details. In fact, children will usually have little or no knowledge of the life and times the writer is depicting. Since children must rely on the accuracy of the historical novelist's account and interpretation of the past, it is important for writers of historical fiction to have much more than a superficial understanding of the eras around which they build their stories. True, historical stories are fictional, but they are stories shaped out of facts and a knowledge of specific human issues and conditions that were an integral part of the fabric of life in a former time and place. As with all types of fiction, readers of historical fiction want an interesting story with interesting characters, a gripping conflict, and significant themes. But they should also gain an understanding of the spirit of a former time. By examining life and living in the past, they can perhaps gain a better understanding of the problems and issues of their own time.

Types of Historical Fiction

Today, children of all ages can choose from a large selection of stories that introduce different historical periods from nearly every culture in every part of the world. In general, there are three basic types of historical stories for children. In the first type, the writer weaves actual persons, events, or settings from the past into a fictionalized story which also contains imaginary characters, incidents, and places. Although writers of this carefully researched type of historical fiction may have little or no knowledge of the exact details of the things real people of the past said and did or what a particular locale in the past actually looked like, they use their research on the period to make educated guesses about each element they include in the story. This is what James and Christopher Collier did when they wrote *My Brother Sam Is Dead,* a Newbery-medal novel which focuses on the divided political loyalties within a family and an entire society during the Revolutionary War period in this country.

At the center of this tense and often brutal story is Tim Meeker, a youngster who is torn between his father's belief in the Tory cause and his brother Sam's determination to fight for the freedoms sanctioned by the Patriots. In a note at the end of the book, the authors explain that many of the characters in the story, including most of the military men and the majority of the townspeople, are based on real persons. Using the basic facts about these people they had discovered while researching the period, the authors set out to create multifaceted characters whose conflicts and experiences reflect the political situation in this country at the time of the Revolutionary War.

In *Johnny Tremain,* Esther Forbes also blends fact and fiction to dramatize the ideals and conflicts that caused the American Revolution. Johnny, her central character, may be fictional, but his job as a dispatch rider for the Committee of Public Safety puts him in touch with Paul Revere, John Hancock, Sam Adams, and several other famous freedom fighters whom we come to know as complex individuals having a full range of human feelings and concerns. Around Johnny's gradual transformation from an obnoxiously self-centered boy to a courageous and politically astute young man, Forbes has woven a classic tale that captures the very essence of the words freedom and loyalty in terms that older children can relate to and appreciate.

After they have read fictional stories that examine the American Revolution from a human perspective, children in the upper grades can learn a great deal about this turbulent period from Milton Meltzer's *The American Revolutionaries,* which contains the firsthand accounts of people who actually lived during that time. Using letters, diaries, journals, interviews, newspaper articles, pamphlets, speeches, and other sources, Meltzer has reconstructed the contagious fervor and arresting experiences of ordinary people, many of them youngsters, who helped build the modern world's first democracy.

Writers of the second type of historical fiction fill their stories with completely imagined characters and incidents that nevertheless capture the spirit of a known historical happening. These writers must also use their knowledge of the past to present—"as far as is humanly possible"—a true picture of the circumstances that characterized a period of

history and the ways real people lived, behaved, and interacted in the past.

Immigrant Girl by Brett Harvey, with illustrations by
Deborah Kogan Ray, fits this category. This is ten-year-old
Becky Moscowitz's first-person account of the conditions she
and her family had to face when they emigrated from a quiet
town in Russia to a crowded New York City neighborhood at
the turn of this century to escape a massacre of the Jews.
While the illustrator's black-and-white pictures are like candid snapshots of significant moments in the immigrant experience, the author's awareness of turn-of-the-century social and
economic history filters into every informative incident. By
zeroing in on an imaginary little girl whose perceptions and
reactions are intended to represent the experiences of many
immigrant children and their families, both the author and the
illustrator reveal a historical phenomenon that raises many
questions about the assimilation of different types of people
into a new culture. This is the kind of book that makes history
a living and dynamic chronicle because it shows how people,
especially young people, were affected by the conditions and
values that shaped a specific incident in history.

In *Prairie Songs,* Pam Conrad also creates imagined people
and incidents to highlight a well-documented period of
American history. Set on the Nebraska prairie at the turn of
this century, the novel depicts the experiences of an established pioneer family while telling of a young girl's first
startling encounter with the complexities of human nature.
Surrounded by vast miles of wild, flat grasslands and open
sky, young Louisa spends her days caring for her terribly shy
younger brother and helping her mother and father with the
endless chores that typify pioneer life. Then, when the new
doctor and his beautiful wife, Emmaline, arrive from New
York City to live nearby, Louisa's secure and simple existence
is changed irrevocably as she develops a relationship with
Emmaline and eventually watches her slip into a perplexing
state of madness and despair. Through the experiences and
relationships of a small group of people, the author reveals
the characteristics of a particular era and, in the process,
identifies a range of universal problems, conflicts, and needs

that are certainly not restricted to one place or an isolated time period.

The third type of historical fiction is the "remembered" story. In this type, the author presents a somewhat fictionalized version of either actual experiences from his or her own life or the experiences lived through and perhaps recorded by one of the author's relatives. Among the most well-known examples in this category are the Little House books by Laura Ingalls Wilder, which portray pioneer life in several locales of the American frontier. Each of these popular books is based on the actual experiences of the author or her husband.

A more recent selection that fits this category of historical fiction is Brett Harvey's *My Prairie Year*. To portray the joys and sorrows of pioneer life, the author used the details her grandmother remembered about her own experiences as a child in a homesteading family which moved from Maine to the Dakota Territory in 1889. Accompanied by dramatic black-and-white impressionistic illustrations which fill each page, this picturebook captures a wide range of authentic facts and feelings about the way homesteaders survived on the American frontier.

For any writer who weaves past events, ideologies, and beliefs into a story, the past is not only a record of remarkable facts, famous incidents, and the deeds of larger-than-life historical figures. Rather, writers of historical fiction view history as an ongoing process which involves all types of people—young, old, ordinary, famous, and infamous people—who had a part in shaping the past and whose experiences can cause readers of any age to think about the present. The best writers of historical fiction make the past relevant, real, and vivid for children. They prove to children that to become truly aware of the past, a person needs to become immersed in the lives of people because the choices and commitments that every individual makes, for better or worse, do in fact have an effect on the way history takes its course. The best of these writers see each era as another chapter in what historian Arthur Schlesinger refers to as "our common continuing humanity."[30]

The study of history doesn't have to be a lackluster

experience for children. Imaginative, enthusiastic teaching can help motivate children to examine both past and current events and the people behind them the way explorers examine an unfamiliar territory. Carrie Goddard, a fourth grade teacher in Hartville, Ohio, uses appropriate selections of literature to generate excitement about history in order to inspire her students to study and interpret a variety of historical events. She frequently enlivens social studies lessons with poems that dramatize incidents in history. In one of her history lessons, her students read and discussed "The Midnight Ride of Paul Revere" before they looked closely at the techniques Longfellow used to mold this legendary incident into a story poem. Equipped with this awareness of how a poet uses language, her students researched past and contemporary events to write poems of their own. After the students revised their poems and shared them with their peers, they set up a classroom publishing "company" called Goddard's Kids, Inc., and collaborated to organize the poems into a bound book which they called "History in Poetry." Among the subjects included in the book are the dropping of the atomic bomb on Hiroshima, the sinking of the "U.S.S. Arizona," the first flight to the moon, and the invention of the light bulb. One of the most popular topics was the explosion of the space shuttle "Challenger." Here is one ten-year-old's reaction to the incident:

The Challenger
At 11:38 on a cold clear January day
All spirits were high for the first teacher in space.
And so near the end of the countdown the crowd
    cheered
For they had never gotten this far before.
In the final seconds of the countdown, engines started.
Then liftoff, the crowd roared as the Shuttle
Soared high above them.

The Shuttle flight only 74 seconds old, the
Mighty Challenger explodes
And with it go the hopes and dreams of seven souls.
So remember these names:
Francis Scobee, Michael Smith, Christa McAuliffe,

Gregory Jarvis, Judith Resnick,
Ellison Onizuka, and Ronald McNair.

Jason Vestfals

Children can develop a wide range of skills from an
assignment like this. In addition to learning that all sorts of
interesting and personal topics can be appropriate material for
poetry, they can learn how to brainstorm for their own topics
which can insure ownership on their part as they work
through the writing process. Their need to find information
about their topics will motivate them to become researchers
who gather, choose, and organize a variety of facts and
impressions about their topic from the library as well as
community resources. Also, while writing and revising their
poems for the sake of "going public" with them, they can
learn some important language skills within the context of
real writing for real purposes and real audiences, from how to
effectively organize and communicate their thoughts to how
to use correct punctuation.

At the conclusion of the unit in Carrie Goddard's classroom, Kasi Olson, a student who wrote about the flight of the
space shuttle "Columbia," reflected on the value of her
involvement in the project. "It's been fun to learn about
history," she said. "You can write it and say how you feel."

Something to Do

Recall your personal experiences as a history student. What
are some of your best memories? What made these experiences positive? What are some of your worst memories?
What made these experiences negative? Recall your most
effective teachers of history. Why were these teachers effective? Recall your least effective teachers of history. What do
you remember about the way they taught? After you have
thought about these experiences, read a selection of historical
fiction from among the books listed at the end of this chapter.
How do the author's and/or illustrator's methods of presenting history compare with your positive and negative experiences with the study of history? What did you learn about the

period of history the author or illustrator is depicting? What might children gain from reading this book?

Nutrition in Historical Stories

When writers attempt to capture the spirit and conditions of a period of history in their stories, it is only natural for many of them to make the past that much more complete and human by showing what and how people ate in former times and places. In many carefully researched illustrated books and longer, more complex historical novels for children, food and eating are important concerns and needs that help to delineate a way of life. These stories introduce children to former habits and traditions pertaining to food and nutrition, and they reveal how some sources of nutrients have replaced others over the course of time while others have remained the same in each era. They also provide a timeline for people's tastes and preferences for certain types of foods. In some cases, they describe the debilitating effects of hunger and other nutritional problems, and in others they emphasize the fact that a proper supply of food will always be necessary for human survival.

A number of delightful picturebooks integrate factual information about food customs into entertaining stories that contain accurate details about specific societies. The painstaking energy and skill needed to prepare *A Medieval Feast* for the king and queen of England is the subject of Aliki's meticulously detailed story set in the early fifteenth century. In addition to describing with both words and illustrations a wide range of foods such as a cockatrice, wild boar, meats preserved in salt (there was no refrigeration back then, Aliki reminds her readers), and a variety of delectable desserts like a marzipan sculpture decorated with natural food colors, the author/illustrator focuses on accepted styles of eating and serving food, table manners, and forms of entertainment that accompanied an attractive, longlasting meal, showing why medieval feasting was considered an art. An interesting companion to Aliki's book is James Cross Giblin's *From Hand to Mouth,* a lively information book that documents the history of eating utensils and table manners of various cultures from the Stone Age to the present day. Subtitled "Or, How We Invented Knives, Forks, Spoons, & Chopsticks, & the Table Manners To Go With Them," the book is illustrated with photographs, prints, and drawings from a number of collections found in museums around the world.

Also set in medieval times, *Merry Ever After*, written and illustrated by Joe Lasker, compares a wedding for members of the nobility with a peasant wedding. Like Aliki, Lasker incorporates information about the social and economic conditions of the period into details of people at work and play through large watercolor illustrations and a simple, but never simplistic, text. Among many other things, readers learn that wine, beer, and cider would have been abundant at the wedding feasts, since tea and coffee did not yet exist and water was considered unsafe to drink. The manner of eating in those days could spark some lively discussion about present-day etiquette.

Considering how family life influences children, it is not surprising that stories about families in the past interest them. Some of the most memorable incidents in these historical stories that depict family experiences center around caring for, cultivating, and sharing a variety of basic foods. The *Ox-Cart Man*, by Donald Hall, with illustrations by Barbara Cooney, reveals the simple day-to-day life of an early nineteenth-century farming family. Throughout the seasons, the parents and their two young children work hard on their tidy farm nestled among the rambling hills of a New England countryside. Together they grow and harvest a crop of vegetables, pick apples, prepare maple sugar from sap, and make a variety of household goods, much of which is sold at a city market in the autumn. Even the feathers that the children collect from the barnyard geese are treasured in this clear and vivid portrait of an industrious family that actually practices the old saying "to waste not is to want not." Accustomed to prepared, packaged, and fast foods, contemporary children are fascinated by a family that literally lives off the land and survives with the help of a truly natural foods diet.

In *My Prairie Year,* a picturebook for intermediate grade

readers, Brett Harvey has taken actual experiences and impressions from a diary kept by her own grandmother when she settled with her family in the Dakota Territory. The author has shaped these facts into a dramatic story of pioneer life as seen through the eyes of an eager child who leads us through the days of the week and the seasons. While tornadoes, blizzards, and fires threaten the fragile life the members of this closeknit family build on the plains, the hearty crops they grow and the foods they share with fellow homesteaders help to sustain their energy as well as their spirit. The charcoal and pencil illustrations in a variety of muted tones help to bring to life the constant dramas that a hardworking and determined group of people must face in order to eke out a meager but rewarding existence.

Few books have presented as graphic a picture of the hardships and triumphs of a midwest pioneer family as the Little House books by Laura Ingalls Wilder. Beginning with *Little House in the Big Woods,* which is set in the Wisconsin woods in the late nineteenth century, Wilder combines fact and fiction in the chronicle of her family's experiences as settlers in the wilds of Kansas (*Little House on the Prairie*), Minnesota (*On the Banks of Plum Creek*), the Dakota Territory (*By the Shores of Silver Lake*), and other regions. Sustained by a great deal of love and security, this remarkable family survives floods, droughts, and near starvation as they create a life together. Since the series follows the Ingalls children as they move from early childhood into adulthood, children can grow along with Laura and her sisters. Many children in grades three or four who first get hooked by *Little House in the Big Woods,* in which Laura is six, are still reading about her when they are adolescents and Laura becomes a teacher (*Little Town on the Prairie*) and then marries Almonzo Wilder (*Those Happy Golden Years*) and finally settles with him on their South Dakota homestead (*The First Four Years*).

There are so many incidents in the Little House series that center around food, cooking, and eating that the books inspired Barbara Walker to compile the *Little House Cookbook.* Based on actual foods mentioned throughout the series, the recipes in Walker's book show how a little ingenuity is all that it sometimes takes to create wholesome meals and snacks, even if only the most basic ingredients and provisions are available. Food is certainly a labor of love in this caring and cared-for family.

The survival story is another type of historical fiction that lures children into the past and offers them adventure and suspense in the process. Survival stories usually tell of children who are thrust into a poignant human drama that forces them to contend with severe physical and emotional hardships. Often, the struggle to survive takes place outside the security of a familiar home environment and without the support of nurturing adults. In many survival stories, the authors focus on the grimmer chapters of history in order to expose the inhuman conditions that surface when some people lose sight of their responsibility to others by allowing political beliefs, self-interest, or greed to overshadow their concern for the rights, dignity, and worth of the individuals in a society. Given the authors' emphasis on political and social issues, these stories appeal to readers in the intermediate and upper grades who are becoming more aware of the world beyond their immediate environment and more conscious of universal moral concepts such as justice, human rights, and freedom.

In *The Slave Dancer,* Paula Fox explores a gruesome time in American history. In this Newbery Award novel, the author depicts the ordeal of a young adolescent who is kidnapped by the crew of a slave ship in 1840 and forced to play his fife for the slaves so they will exercise and therefore be in good physical shape when it comes time to sell them at the slave market. On his long and treacherous journey to Africa where the crew picks up its human cargo, Jesse has his first encounter with the kind of greed that causes men to regard human beings as nothing more than a profitable commodity. Jesse is forbidden to help these men, women, and children, and he is ridiculed when he expresses any concern for their plight as the slaves become more and more demoralized by the unrelenting degradation to which the ruthless crew subjects them.

Jesse can do nothing but watch the slaves become sick and diseased because of their paltry diet, which consists of meager rations of water and rice, and their confinement in the squalid, rat-infested hold of the ship. Stripped of their dignity, they are also denied the right to maintain their health and therefore the right to life itself. That injustice, Fox seems to say, is the real tragedy of the phenomenon of human slavery of any kind and in any era. Here, nutrition—or rather the lack of it—becomes an unforgettable human, moral, and political issue. It is also an issue of freedom, if one interprets freedom the way Elie Wiesel, winner of the 1986 Nobel Peace Prize and a survivor of the Buchenwald concentration camps, does: "Does there exist a nobler inspiration than the desire to be free? It is by his freedom that a man knows himself, by his sovereignty over his own life that a man measures himself. To violate that freedom, to flout that sovereignty, is to deny man the right to live his life, to take responsibility for himself with dignity."[31] Such a powerful concept becomes real and concrete for children in a book like *The Slave Dancer*.

Chester Aaron also depicts a grim chapter in American history in *Lackawanna*. It is the time of the Great Depression. A small group of abandoned, homeless children, who call themselves Lackawanna after the freight trains they are always hopping, have decided to live together in a deserted cellar room in New York City. Together they build a simple but comfortable life until nine-year-old Herbie is kidnapped by a hobo. Their search for Herbie leads the children into the heart of the country where, at every turn of their revealing journey, they come face-to-face with the terrible facts of America's economic collapse. Naturally, with so little substantial food available, the children are forced to beg for their meals, and when they reminisce about more secure times, their thoughts frequently center around food.

The Island on Bird Street by Uri Orlev also explores a dark period of history. Left on his own in a ruined house in the nearly abandoned Warsaw ghetto where Jews were confined during World War II, eleven-year-old Alex wonders if he can survive the conditions that constantly threaten his life, now that his mother has disappeared and his father, armed with a gun, has left, promising Alex that he will soon return. There is, first of all, the threat of being discovered by the Nazi soldiers who frequently search the ghetto for the few remaining Jews who will be transported to a death camp. But, even more pressing, there is the threat of starvation. Every morsel of food becomes a treasure for this unusually resourceful boy whose determination to stay alive helps to alleviate the panic and loneliness that fill his days until he is reunited with his father. Orlev, who survived the Holocaust as a young boy, has crafted a powerful story about cruelty as well as hope out of his own experiences during one of the most terrifying periods of history. By showing how the Holocaust all but shatters the life of one family, Orlev presents a poignant indictment of the madness that can take hold when a society comes under the control of people driven by prejudice and a total disregard for the sanctity of life. In the process, the author reminds his readers why they should never take the fulfillment of their basic human needs for granted.

Checklist for Evaluating Historical Fiction

1. Does the story hold your interest?
2. Do the characters think, act, feel, and look like people from the period of history the author is depicting?
3. Are the customs, values, and beliefs true to the period of history in which the story is set?
4. Are the details concerning such things as living conditions, transportation, and medical practices accurate and authentic in both the text and illustrations? Do they help you to visualize a culture?
5. Is there a theme? Is it thought provoking? Does it reveal as much about the human condition today as it does about conditions in the past?
6. Will the story and illustrations increase children's awareness and knowledge of the past as well as the present?

Summary

The best writers and illustrators of historical stories shape the past into a vivid, ongoing drama that involves all types of people. They make history accessible, relevant, and real for children by focusing on the experiences of young people who grew up in other times and places, but who had to face situations, make decisions, and work through feelings and conflicts that young people face in any age. Through historical stories that genuinely capture the complexities of personal, social, and family life, children can become aware of the ways ordinary and famous people in every era of history tried to live their lives and satisfy their basic human needs, sometimes under the pressures of hardship, oppression, and demeaning social injustice. Since the best writers and illustrators of historical fiction strive to present an accurate and authentic picture of the past from a human perspective, children who read these stories can learn about specific values, beliefs, and issues—many of them health-related—that characterized particular periods of history. They can begin to understand that history is not a dull subject made up only of facts about famous incidents and well-known "dead people," as one fourth grader put it, but a lively chronicle of how the human race has developed over time.

To explore life and living through exciting stories that tell of former times, people, and places is a pleasurable way to consider past mistakes that need to be avoided now and in the future and past successes that deserve the careful attention of anyone who believes that all of us have a responsibility to keep striving to build a better, more humane world for all peoples. Good historical stories can help to make children more sensitive to the world around them.

POETRY: HEALTH ISSUES IN SOUND AND MOTION

Well-written poems make us think about human experiences, ones we have had firsthand as well as those we may never have thought about until the poet sparked our imagination. Using just the right words and images, and just the right kind of tempo, pace, and rhythm, a sensitive poet can cast such a spell on us that, for the time being, our attention is captured and we get caught up totally in the poet's feelings about typical or extraordinary human situations and relationships. As Laurence Perrine puts it in *Sound and Sense,* "Poetry takes all life as its province. Its primary concern is not with beauty, not with philosophical truth, not with persuasion . . . but with all kinds of experience—beautiful or ugly, strange or common, noble or ignoble, actual or imaginary. . . . Poetry comes to us bringing life, and therefore pleasure."[32]

Poetry for young people captures a similar range of experiences, and the enjoyment and understanding it evokes can be just as rewarding. No matter how young or old we are, Alethea Helbig maintains, we read poetry in order to "feel more keenly, to see more sharply, and to know the world around us better because we have shared in some degree what the poet saw and felt."[33]

For poet Eve Merriam, a good poem can stimulate a thoroughly pleasurable kind of sharing and participation:

> **How to Eat a Poem**
> Don't be polite.
> Bite in.
> Pick it up with your fingers and lick the
>   juice that may run down your chin.
> It is ready and ripe now, whenever you are.
>
> You do not need a knife or fork or spoon
> or plate or napkin or table cloth.
>
> For there is no core
> or stem
> or rind
> or pit
> or seed
> or skin
> to throw away.*

Considering the negative experiences many students have with poetry, it may seem inconceivable that anyone could associate poetry reading with the type of enjoyment Eve Merriam envisions in "How to Eat a Poem." Raised on a steady diet of inappropriate poems and poor classroom

---

*From *JAMBOREE Rhymes for All Times* by Eve Merriam. Copyright © 1962, 1964, 1966, 1973, 1984 by Eve Merriam. All Rights Reserved. Reprinted by permission of Marian Reiner for the author.

experiences, many people begin early on to dislike, disregard, or even fear poetry in much the same way that they have a lifelong disdain for foods they were force-fed in childhood. Particularly with regard to poetry, many teachers seem to forget that interest, enjoyment, and the promise of a personal connection with literature are basic motivations for reading. It is hard for us to get excited about reading when the choices set before us offer little, if any, personal involvement.

The testimonies of hundreds of adult readers have provided some clues to the reasons why many readers develop an early aversion to poetry. For several years, we have asked the students and teachers with whom we work to write about and evaluate their experiences with literature from their earliest to their most recent memories of reading or being read to within and outside of school.[34] Consistently, many of these adults have indicated that they like poetry the least of all types of literature. Out of approximately one thousand students who have shared their histories with us, less than 5 percent reported that they now read or have a desire to read poetry for their own pleasure. It is not surprising that about 65 percent of the teachers in this population have indicated that they rarely share poetry with their students because, in addition to feeling unprepared to teach it, they don't know enough about it and have even less knowledge of poems which might turn their students on to this type of literature.

The majority of these students and teachers traced their disinterest in poetry to poor school experiences, with many indicating that they always felt uncomfortable with poetry because the poems they were asked to read were too difficult to understand. Another consistent complaint was about their lack of exposure to poetry. While only a few of these people could describe memorable experiences with poetry beyond the primary grades in elementary school, those who were exposed to poetry in later grades consistently criticized the inappropriateness of the subject matter of the poems they were assigned. The majority also described classroom practices that turned them off to poetry. For example, two classroom methods which many students criticized were teachers' line-by-line explanations of a poet's techniques and lectures about the meaning of the poems. They indicated that they felt cheated because they were given so few opportunities to talk about their personal responses to the poems.

Not all of these students had negative things to say about their school experiences with poetry. While few could recall specific poems that made a lasting personal impression, several described teachers who not only stimulated them to read poetry on their own, but also encouraged them to try their hand at writing poetry in order "to figure things out," as one future teacher put it. Positive experiences with poetry included open-ended discussions that welcomed different interpretations, exposure to poems that reflected readers' interests, putting together a collection of poems which students themselves chose, writing poetry, and having a choice concerning the types of poems read and discussed at school.

Ways to Make Poetry Enjoyable

The anecdotes detailed in these case studies can help point the way to some of the things teachers can do, as well as what they should not do, to encourage an interest in poetry. Perhaps the most important factor is the need to frequently and consistently introduce students to many different types of poems which stimulate involvement. As with any type of literature teachers bring into the classroom, poetry should speak to students about experiences that interest them, ones they can relate to and genuinely think about, given their immediate concerns and needs. However simple this interest principle may seem, it is one that is often overlooked, although the effort to surround children with poems they like is well worth a teacher's or parent's time and energy, since poems which appeal to children will keep them reading and asking for more of the same. Promoting an interest in literature should, after all, always be one of the primary goals of a reading program on every grade level.

It doesn't take much effort to discover scores of interesting poems for today's children. The fact that many of the poems which children enjoy are brief and therefore take only a few minutes to read aloud and discuss will be an added attraction to teachers who are understandably concerned with fitting poetry into a curriculum that often seems to be bursting at the seams with content. A health lesson or discussion about feelings, for example, could begin or end with responses to "I'm in a Rotten Mood!" one of the many brief poems in Prelutsky's very popular collection, *The New Kid on the Block,* which includes a variety of humorous verses about the ups and downs of childhood. The strong feelings of a child who's having a bad day also surface in "I Woke Up This Morning," another short poem, found in Kuskin's *The Rose on My Cake.* Kuskin reinforces her narrator's anger and frustration by increasing the size of the words as the intensity of this child's feelings grows. It is a poem that will require some practice to give it the type of oral reading that captures the full effect of the narrator's emotionally charged reactions to the constant demands of adults throughout the course of a terribly upsetting day.

Many other health-related topics can be approached through short poems which both interest young people and stimulate them to think about specific real-life experiences. To open a discussion on the hazards of smoking cigarettes, children in the intermediate or upper grades could listen to or read "Basic for Better Living" from *Finding a Poem,* a collection by Eve Merriam. Merriam, recipient of an Excellence in Poetry Award from the National Council of Teachers of English, uses tongue-in-cheek humor to point out the deleterious effects that substances like tar and nicotine have on the body. Humor is also at the heart of McGinley's "Reflections Dental," found in *Reflections on a Gift of Watermelon Pickle. . .,* an anthology by Dunning, Leuders, and Smith that has proved highly successful with older readers. In "Reflections Dental," a good poem to introduce when personal hygiene is the focus of attention, the poet ponders how perfect the teeth of TV personalities always look. In this same anthology, Langston Hughes considers depression and suicide in "Too Blue," a very melancholy journey that leads into the mind of a person afflicted with "those sad old weary blues."

While finding and sharing appealing poems is a good place to start developing student interest in poetry, it is just as important to sustain this interest with worthwhile and meaningful classroom experiences. As the testimonies of many students and teachers have suggested, the primary goal of these experiences with poetry should be to nurture and welcome the personal responses students have to poems that matter to them. In *Pass the Poetry, Please!*, a book filled with practical and exciting ways to bring children and poetry together, Hopkins advises teachers to avoid the "DAM approach" to poetry, which involves "dissecting, analyzing, and *meaninglessly* memorizing poetry to death."[35] Instead, in order to get children into the poetry habit, they need to frequently hear good poems read expressively in addition to reading aloud lots of poems themselves.

One quick and easy way to do this is to have an occasional short poetry break throughout the course of the school day. The poetry break is a simple but rewarding activity that exposes children to many different poems. The teacher or student reads to the whole group a poem about a topic that is either directly or indirectly related to the content of a particular classroom lesson. Following the reading, the listeners offer responses which can range from personal feelings and associations to remarks about favorite words, images, or other aspects of the poet's style or technique. When the subject of a health lesson is family life and living, for instance, children in a lower grade might hear and respond to "Mama Is a Sunrise" by Evelyn Tooley Hunt, "My Sister Jane" by Ted Hughes, or the traditional Eskimo verse, "Do not weep little one," all of which are found in the "Friends and Family" section of *The Scott, Foresman Anthology of Children's Literature,* edited by Sutherland and Livingston. Poems for older readers from this source include "Mother to Son" by Langston Hughes, which uses black dialect to tell of endurance and survival in the midst of life's hardships; "My Uncle Dan" by Ted Hughes, which characterizes an eccentric inventor; and "Taught Me Purple," a celebration of motherhood.

Things to Avoid When Sharing Poetry

- Poems that are difficult for children to understand.
- Poems unrelated to children's developmental needs, concerns, and life experiences.

- Adult-controlled selection of poetry.
- Infrequent exposure to poetry.
- Overanalysis of the techniques and devices used by the poet.
- Forced awareness of a single "correct" interpretation of a poem.
- Forced memorization of poetry.
- Forced, undirected writing of poetry.

During a poetry break, as well as with other types of poetry activities, it is important to accept the different responses and interpretations children have to a poem without judging their appropriateness or accuracy. This is a time for students to feel free to talk to the teachers and to each other about the feelings and thoughts a particular poem evokes in them. This is not to say that the teacher should not offer some suggestions or elicit further understanding through thoughtful questions, and thus serve as a model by revealing his or her own responses and questions, or by pointing out a few important features of the poem, but the principle here is that the teacher should act as a reader among other readers. In addition to the short time it takes to conduct a poetry break, another important advantage of this activity is that the students—hopefully along with the teacher—soon realize that they don't have to like each and every poem they hear or read. And, as with most skills, the more they have opportunities to listen to and read poetry, the better they get at being critical readers and thinkers by giving specific reasons for liking or disliking particular poems.

Things to Do When Sharing Poetry

- Select, often with student input, a wide variety of appealing poems.
- Incorporate health-related poems in all areas of the health program.
- Use recordings of poets reading their poems (for selections, see *A Multimedia Approach to Children's Literature,* edited by Mary Alice Hunt, published by the American Library Association).
- Encourage students to read aloud, record, and listen to poems they like.

- With clear directions for how to go about the process, encourage students to write their own poems. *A Celebration of Bees: Helping Children Write Poetry* by Barbara Esbensen (Winston Press, 1975), and *Pass the Poetry, Please!* by Lee Bennett Hopkins (Harper and Row, 1987) are two helpful sources of inventive poetry-writing activities that have proved successful with children of all ages.
- Feature a poet whose poems children like (see "Poetry Explained," a filmstrip by and about poet Karla Kuskin, distributed by Weston Woods, and "First Choice: Poets and Poetry," a set of filmstrips about the life and poetry of five children's poets, distributed by Pied Piper Productions).
- Demonstrate, with students' involvement, the process of reading and making sense of a poem.

The types of activities for motivating genuine involvement in poetry are as limitless as the teacher's imagination. Large-group choral reading, listening to either commercially prepared or student-prepared recordings of favorite poems, keeping a word bank of exceptional phrases and expressions found in particularly interesting poems, preparing an illustrated class anthology of original poems that are modeled on ones read and discussed, setting a poem to music as well as finding an appropriate musical background for specific poems, and dramatizing or pantomiming a story poem such as "Supermarket" by Felice Holman or "Sarah Cynthia Sylvia Stout Who Would Not Take the Garbage Out" by Shel Silverstein (both in *The Scott, Foresman Anthology*) are just a few approaches that can make poetry come alive.

Once children have had ample opportunity to listen to, read, and share many poems, they will be that much more receptive to discussions that focus on the characteristics and elements of poetry. In fact, as Amy McClure's research on classroom experiences with poetry has shown, when teachers introduce the ingredients of poetry through poems that interest children, students not only refer to these ingredients when responding to poetry, but they also tend to use some of them when writing their own poems.[36]

It is essential, therefore, that teachers know how poetry works in order to feel confident about drawing children's attention to the range of devices that poets use to communicate their thoughts and feelings to readers. It is also important to remember, though, that such information is best conveyed in the context of poems that capture children's attention and imagination. The goal is not to burden children with a list of terms that explain such things as figures of speech or types of poetry, such as the ballad, haiku, or free verse; the goal is to increase enjoyment and appreciation by first having them experience the poem and then showing them some of the devices and forms poets use to express themselves, to communicate their thoughts and feelings, and to keep a reader or listener interested.

Exploring the Characteristics of Poetry

If there is one word that best describes the way poets communicate their thoughts and feelings, that word is conciseness. Good poets, that is, are known for their ability to get to the heart of the matter without wasting words. "A single word in poetry," Rebecca Lukens maintains, "says far more than a single word in prose; the connotations and images hint at, imply, and suggest other meanings."[37] In *Sound and Sense,* Laurence Perrine describes the poet's economical use of language in a similar way: "The difference between poetry and other literature is one only of degree. Poetry is the most condensed and concentrated form of literature, saying most in the fewest number of words."[38] Since most children aren't accustomed to dealing with language that is so compact, that therefore implies so much more than the mere dictionary meaning of the poem's individual words, it usually takes them a while to get used to reading and listening between the lines. This is the reason it is so important to have them experience poems regularly, and to expose them to poems, or even light verses, related to their interests and experiences. When we share poems with children that are accessible and relevant to them, the chances are they will both enjoy the reading or listening experience and be better able to make sense of it.

A simple rule to follow is to begin with poems that spark children's interests and invite them to participate. For example, the rhythmic verses in Clyde Watson's *Father Fox's Pen-*

nyrhymes, accompanied by Wendy Watson's spirited illustrations that depict a large, content family and community of foxes at work and play, are a good introduction for younger children to the ways a poet suggests and implies a situation or experience with just a few carefully placed words and images. This brief verse from *Father Fox's Pennyrhymes* has an entire story to tell children about what it is like not to be hungry at mealtime:

> Oh, my goodness, oh my dear,
> Sassafras & ginger beer,
> Chocolate cake & apple punch:
> I'm too full to eat my lunch.*

Here, an adult can capitalize on the poem's conciseness and compression by inviting children to suggest reasons for the narrator's dilemma. Given the few details the poet has provided them, children could also practice some critical-thinking skills by making inferences about the age of the narrator, the setting of the poem, and the reactions of the narrator's parents and siblings to his or her predicament. This approach can also be used after reading "Keepsake," a poem for older children in Eloise Greenfield's *Honey, I Love,* which presents the basic ingredients of an endearing relationship between a child and an old person in just nine lines. With the help of a sensitive adult, children can fill in the gaps:

> Before Mrs. Williams died
> She told Mr. Williams
> When he gets home
> To get a nickel out of her
> Navy blue pocketbook
> And give it to her
> Sweet little gingerbread girl
> That's me
> I ain't never going to spend it.

"Aunt Roberta," from this same collection, could enhance a lesson or project that focuses on family life:

---

*"Oh My Goodness, Oh My Dear" from *FATHER FOX'S PENNYRHYMES*. Text copyright © 1971 by Clyde Watson. Illustrations copyright © 1971 by Wendy Watson. Reprinted by permission.

What do people think about
When they sit and dream
All wrapped up in quiet
    and old sweaters
And don't even hear me 'til I
Slam the door?

Rhythm, which gives poetry a musical quality, is another characteristic of poetry which can open the way to some exciting experiences with this type of literature. The rhythm of a poem is its distinctive beat, cadence, or movement. It must be carefully and thoughtfully developed by the poet to enhance the poet's subject matter and to reinforce the mood and feelings the poet is attempting to evoke. For example, the rhythm of "The Sidewalk Racer or On the Skateboard," from Morrison's *The Sidewalk Racer,* rushes along to capture the gracefulness and the exuberant energy and pace of the skilled skateboard enthusiast the poem depicts:

> Skimming
> an asphalt sea
> I swerve, I curve, I
> sway; I speed to whirring
> sound an inch above the
> ground; I'm the sailor
> and the sail, I'm the
> driver and the wheel
> I'm the one and only
> single engine
> human auto
> mobile.
> [p. 12]*

Similarly, the rhythm Greenfield has created for "Rope Rhyme," from *Honey, I Love,* is one of the key ingredients that makes this poem such an authentic and delightful picture of a child at play:

---

*Lillian Morrison, "The Sidewalk Racer or On the Skateboard" from *The Sidewalk Racer and Other Poems of Sports and Motion.* Copyright © 1977 by Lillian Morrison. Reprinted by permission of the author.

Get set, ready now, jump right in
Bounce and kick and giggle and spin
Listen to the rope when it hits the ground
Listen to that clappedy-slappedy sound
Jump right up when it tells you to
Come back down, whatever you do
Count to a hundred, count by ten
Start to count all over again
That's what jumping is all about
Get set, ready now,
                    jump
                         right
                           out!*

Both of these poems could help to enliven discussions that center on physical fitness and safety precautions while at play.

Even when the rhythmic pattern of a poem is not as obvious—or dramatic—as it is in Morrison's or Greenfield's poem, it can still be one of the essential elements which the poet uses to shape the subject of the poem and to contribute to the reader's engagement with it. In *Eats*, a collection of poems about food by Arnold Adoff, for example, the poet's celebration of the pleasure of eating chocolate is enhanced in the following excerpt from a longer poem by a soft and slow rhythm which complements the wonderful satisfaction a chocolate lover feels when savoring each delicious bite.

Chocolate
Chocolate
          i
love
     you so
          i
want
     to
marry
     you
     and

---

live
>forever
>>in the
>>flavor
>of your
>brown*

Rhyme also must be appropriate to the poet's attitude toward the subject of the poem and the response the poet expects from the reader. Rhyme functions primarily to shape the reader's perception of the topic, to underscore mood, and to help create a movement and pace which best support the poem's emerging tone and theme. When it is used—and it doesn't always have to be, as children are often surprised to learn—rhyme should have a clear, functional purpose. Used well, it can give a poem an inviting, contagious musical quality which attracts children and draws them into the experience. Like the element of rhythm, rhyme often stimulates children to participate spontaneously in an oral reading of a poem—even before a teacher or parent encourages them to do so.

Younger children in particular quickly memorize a poem that has a strong, distinct rhythm and rhyme, because they soon become familiar with the predictable language patterns these poems contain. During an oral reading of such poems, children frequently repeat whole lines or words, and they often guess at words which best fit the poem's rhyme scheme. This kind of active involvement should be encouraged at all age and grade levels, not only because it can increase children's enjoyment of poetry, but because it can also help them make sense of the poems they listen to as well as the ones they read on their own. When they participate in these ways, they are learning how to find the clues and signals in the text which enhance interpretation. For these same reasons, it is important for teachers and parents to read poems aloud expressively, even if this requires some practice beforehand.

Expressive oral reading serves as a powerful model for children, since an effective oral presentation of a poem shows

---

*"Chocolate" from *EATS* by Arnold Adoff. © 1979 by Arnold Adoff. Reprinted by permission of the author and Lothrop, Lee & Shepard (A Division of William Morrow & Co.).

them how one reader—in this case, an adult—discovered the specific features in a poem that led to an oral interpretation of it. Consistent experiences like these help children to become effective oral readers themselves.

Figurative language is another device poets use to express their thoughts and feelings. "Broadly defined," says Laurence Perrine, "a figure of speech is any way of saying something other than the ordinary way. . . of saying one thing and meaning another."[39] In this sense, most children and adults are familiar with figurative ways of using language. For example, it is not uncommon for someone to say "I was green with envy," or "It rained cats and dogs," or "there were a million kids on the bus," or "Sometimes my mind is like a sieve." As Perrine points out, the main difference between everyday figurative language and the kind poets create is one of degree; whereas ours is largely ordinary, the talented poet's is striking and unique—and reasonable. For example, as Dorothy Aldis demonstrates in "When I Was Lost," one of the 572 poems in Prelutsky's *The Random House Book of Poetry for Children,* a metaphor can transform a familiar feeling into a vivid and memorable image:

> Underneath my belt
> My stomach was a stone.
> Sinking was the way I felt.
> And hollow.
> And Alone.
> [p. 120]*

Sometimes a poet will extend a metaphor throughout the entire poem in order to create and sustain a mood, give a distinct kind of force and power to the topic, and make readers consider the subject of the poem from a fresh perspective. This is what Langston Hughes does in "Mother to Son," a poem from *The Selected Poems of Langston Hughes,* which compares the perseverance and courage needed to

---

*"When I Was Lost" by Dorothy Aldis reprinted by permission of G. P. Putnam's Sons from *ALL TOGETHER* by Dorothy Aldis, copyright 1925–28, 1934, 1939, 1952, copyright renewed 1953–56, 1962, 1967 by Dorothy Aldis.

survive life's problems and disappointments with the strength
and determination it takes to climb a difficult stairway:

> Well son, I'll tell you:
> Life for me ain't been no crystal stair.
> It's had tacks in it,
> And splinters,
> And boards torn up,
> And places with no carpet on the floor—
> Bare.
> But all the time
> I'se been a-climbin' on,
> And reachin' landin's,
> And turnin' corners,
> And sometimes goin' in the dark
> Where there ain't been no light.
> So, boy, don't you turn back.
> Don't you set down on the steps
> 'Cause you finds it kinder hard.
> Don't you fall now—
> For I'se still goin', honey,
> I'se still climbin',
> And life for me ain't been no crystal stair. [p. 187]*

Like a metaphor, a simile sets up a comparison between two
things. With simile, however, the comparison is less subtle
because it is expressed outright rather than implied as it is in a
metaphor. In "Back to School," from *Out in the Dark and
Daylight,* Aileen Fisher begins with a simile that compresses an
entire range of feelings about the coming of autumn into a
single, vivid image:

> When summer smells like apples
> and shadows feel cool
> and falling leaves make dapples
> of color on the pool
> and wind is in the maples
> and sweaters are the rule
> and hazy days spell lazy ways

---

*Copyright 1926 by Alfred A. Knopf, Inc. and renewed 1954 by Langston Hughes.
Reprinted from *THE SELECTED POEMS OF LANGSTON HUGHES,* by permission of the publisher.

it's hard to go to school.

But I go!
[p. 70]*

Effective similes stretch the imagination because they invite us to think about the ways dissimilar things are similar, due to the characteristics these things have in common. At the same time, similes can make abstract thoughts and feelings concrete. In "Some People," found in Ferris's *Favorite Poems Old and New,* for example, Rachel Field asks her readers to consider how people affect us either negatively or positively. The former, she says, can make "Your thoughts begin to shrivel up/Like leaves all brown and dried!" while the latter can cause you to have "thoughts as thick as fireflies/All shiny in your mind!" These are the kinds of images which children in particular can easily grasp because the references are so familiar to them. They are also believable and accurate images. Dry, dead leaves that have lost their color do in fact remind us of the negative emotions we associate with people who are always ready to do and say the kinds of things that cause us to feel bad, while a stream of fireflies, and the picture of pleasant summer nights which they bring to mind, evoke the good feelings we associate with people who encourage and support us.

Although it isn't necessary to have children analyze every figure of speech in the poems they listen to or read on their own, it is important for adults who share poetry with children to know about these techniques so they can expose children to a wide variety of interesting poems that contain a wide range of figurative language. Through such consistent exposure to poems that interest them, children can become accustomed to the ways in which poets, in contrast to other types of writers, depict human experiences. Occasionally, the adult may draw children's attention to figurative uses of language and other poetic devices, but this should be done only if it helps children become more aware and more knowledgeable of how such techniques encourage them to feel and think and imagine while reading and listening to poetry.

---

*"Back to School" from *OUT IN THE DARK AND DAYLIGHT* by Aileen Fisher. Illustrated by Gail Owens. Text copyright © 1980 by Aileen Fisher. Illustrations copyright © 1980 by Gail Owens. All selections reprinted by permission of Harper & Row, Publishers, Inc.

With children, analyzing a poem should never take precedence over their actual experience with it and their personal responses to it, just as children's knowledge of the rules and techniques related to a sport or game can never be as satisfying or enlightening as their involvement in it. Often, their active participation should suffice, since this type of unconscious delight is often the thing that keeps them playing—and reading. At other times, we can encourage them to tell us what they noticed or liked and disliked about a particular poem, but even then it may be more productive to have them express their responses through drama, art, or some other tactile, visual activity which utilizes their energies and nurtures their creativity. At other times, however, it should be enough to have children listen to poetry or to read it silently on their own without any postreading activity. As Eleanor Farjeon implies in the following poem, rather than always searching for how or why a poem affects us, we should enjoy the insights the poem provides us and the new ways of seeing which poetry can stimulate:

> **Poetry**
> What is poetry? Who knows?
> Not a rose, but the scent of the rose;
> Not the sky, but the light in the sky;
> Not the fly, but the gleam of the fly;
> Not the sea, but the sound of the sea;
> Not myself, but what makes me
> See, hear, and feel something that prose
> Cannot: and what it is, who knows?*

The shape a poem takes on the page is another characteristic that can help readers to make sense of a poem. In the best poems, visual characteristics such as shape, layout, and even the size of the words are not gimmicks; rather, they are clues to meaning. One critic refers to these typographic elements as "silent punctuation marks" which serve as signals to interpretation.[40] This type of visual play is evident in "I Woke Up This Morning" by Karla Kuskin. Here, the increasing size of the words is an appropriate reflection of a child's mounting anger:

---

*"Poetry" from *ELEANOR FARJEON'S POEMS FOR CHILDREN* by Eleanor Farjeon (Lippincott). Originally appeared in *SING FOR YOUR SUPPER,* copyright © 1938 by Eleanor Farjeon, renewed 1966 by Gervase Farjeon. All selections reprinted by permission of Harper & Row, Publishers, Inc.

I Woke Up This Morning

I woke up this morning
At quarter past seven.
I kicked up the covers
And stuck out my toe.
And ever since then
(That's a quarter past seven)
They haven't said anything
Other than "no."
They haven't said anything
Other than "Please, dear,
Don't do what you're doing,"
Or "Lower your voice."
Whatever I've done
And however I've chosen,
I've done the wrong thing
And I've made the wrong choice.
I didn't wash well
And I didn't say thank you.
I didn't shake hands
And I didn't say please.
I didn't say sorry
When passing the candy
I banged the box into
Miss Witelson's knees.
I didn't say sorry.
I didn't stand straighter.
I didn't speak louder
When asked what I'd said.

Well, I said
That tomorrow
At quarter past seven
They can
Come in and get me.

I'm Staying In Bed.*

---

*"I Woke Up This Morning" from *DOGS & DRAGONS, TREES & DREAMS* by Karla Kuskin. Originally published in *THE ROSE ON MY CAKE* by Karla Kuskin. Copyright © 1964 by Karla Kuskin. All selections reprinted by permission of Harper & Row, Publishers, Inc.

Sometimes poets actually show what they mean by forming the lines of the poem into a visual illustration of the subject of the poem that contributes to our understanding of it. This type of poetry, often referred to as "concrete" or "shape" poetry, is especially enjoyable for children to read, because it involves them visually in a type of puzzle that is fun to decipher. For example, the visual layout of "Supermarket"—found in *At the Top of My Voice and Other Poems,* a collection by Felice Holman—reflects the stacks of jars and cans among which a child is lost (see page 148).

In *Street Poems* and *Seeing Things,* collections of inventive shape poems by Robert Froman, the topics cover, among other things, the objects found in a garbage heap, pollution, and human emotions.

Checklist for Evaluating Poetry

1. Does the topic of the poem capture your interest? Will it capture the child's? Does the poem depict a genuine experience?
2. Does the poet respect the child's intelligence? Does he or she speak to, rather than down to, the child?
3. Do the rhythm, sounds, and other elements and techniques enhance the theme of the poem or detract from it? Are these elements appropriate to the thoughts and feelings explored by the poet?
4. Are the images created by the poet original and vivid? Will they cause children to see, hear, and feel with new insight and understanding?
5. Does the poem invite children to use their imaginations? Does it evoke strong responses?
6. Will the poem stand up to repeated readings? Does it read well aloud?

Children's Poetry Interests

Adults who dislike poetry because they have had consistently bad experiences with it usually find it hard to believe that children don't necessarily share their negative feelings. In

Supermarket

I'm
lost
among a
maze of cans,
behind a pyramid
of jams, quite near
asparagus and rice,
close to the Oriental spice,
and just before the sardines.
I hear my mother calling, "Joe,
Where are you, Joe? Where did you
Go?" And I reply in voice concealed among
the candied orange peel, and packs of Chocolate Dreams.

"I
hear
you, Mother
dear, I'm here–
quite near the ginger ale
and beer, and lost among a

                    maze
                of cans
           behind a
      pyramid of jams,
    quite near asparagus
  and rice, close to the
Oriental spice, and just before sardines."
                         But
                      still
                my mother
            calls me, "Joe!
          Where are you, Joe?
         Where did you go?"

"Somewhere
around asparagus
that's in a sort of
      broken glass,
           beside a kind of m-
                ess-
                  y jell
      that's near a tower of cans that f
                       e
                   l
                  l
and squashed the Chocolate Dreams." *

fact, children seem to be born with an instinct for playing with and imitating the rhythms, rhymes, and sounds that abound in poetry and verse. It is the rare infant or toddler, for instance, who doesn't respond to the playful chants, infectious rhymes, and fast-paced dramas that fill nursery rhymes. As many parents know, even before the youngest of children are capable of understanding what these verses mean, they will perk up and listen when daily activities are accompanied by the musical cadences of nursery rhymes. One recent collection with enough variety to satisfy any mood at any time of the day or year is *The Random House Book of Mother Goose,* a treasury of more than three hundred familiar and less familiar verses selected and illustrated with large, dramatic full-color pictures by Arnold Lobel. Bath time, for example, can become an adventure for a child when a parent sings or recites this humorous verse that tells of a voyage aboard a ship which contains some enticing treats and an interesting crew:

> **I Saw a Ship A-Sailing**
> I saw a ship a-sailing,
> A-sailing on the sea,
> And, oh, but it was laden
> With pretty things for thee.
>
> There were cookies in the cabin
> And applies in the hold;
> The sails were made of silk,
> and the masts were all of gold.
>
> The four-and-twenty sailors
> That stood between the decks
> Were four-and-twenty white mice
> With chains about their necks.
>
> The captain was a duck
> With a packet on his back,
> And when the ship began to move
> The captain said Quack! Quack!
> [p. 85]*

---

*"I Saw a Ship A-Sailing" reprinted by permission of Random House, Inc.

In this entertaining collection, there are also rhymes to accompany mealtimes, such as "Pat a cake, pat a cake, baker's man," "Betty Botter bought some butter," and "Polly, put the kettle on," as well as rhymes that can involve the child and the adult in acting out typical or unusual incidents such as "One, two, buckle my shoe," "It's raining, it's pouring/The old man is snoring," "Here we go round the mulberry bush," and "Blow, wind, blow! and go, mill, go!," which depicts the process of making bread out of freshly ground corn. Some of the Mother Goose verses, including "I do not like thee, Doctor Fell," "Little Miss Muffet," and "Punch and Judy/Fought for a pie," reveal and reinforce basic human emotions, while others, like "Jack and Jill went up the hill," "Solomon Grundy," and "Who killed Cock Robin?" familiarize children with human predicaments and struggles which, in some cases, lead to death.

Although nursery rhymes may entertain children, they also provide other rewards. As miniature narratives, these verses introduce children to the elements of story, since most of them depict different types of characters involved in a variety of situations and conflicts which cover a wide range of moods including humor, fear, suspense, and mystery. The language play and predictable rhythms and rhymes which fill these brief verses can also enhance children's language development and their appreciation for language. When children are invited to participate in these verses through clapping, movement, and other types of physical activity, they provide sensory-motor stimulation. Even more important are the security, reassurance, and other good feelings children can experience when a significant adult takes the time to share these rhymes with them, thus demonstrating, through the process of reading aloud and interacting with the child, that the child deserves this kind of focused attention. Finally, the more children are accustomed to hearing and responding to nursery rhymes and other types of verses from an early age, the more they will be prepared to move on to more demanding poetry as they grow older.

The pleasure and insights young children gain from poetry do not have to end the minute they enter school. The key to sustaining their interest in poetry is to find poems which match their concerns, feelings, needs, and experiences. Although this is best done by getting to know the children with whom one works each day, several studies of children's poetry preferences offer both teachers and parents some initial direction concerning types of poetry, as well as the content of poems which children themselves have said they like.

One team of researchers conducted a national survey of the poetry interests of boys and girls enrolled in first, second, and third grade.[41] The majority of the children indicated a preference for comical and nonsense poetry, and they liked poems about topics related to their own experiences and interests. Poems about animals as well as strange and fantastic events were at the top of their list. Regarding the forms of poetry, these primary grade children preferred narrative or story poems, limericks, and poems with strong musical elements like rhythm and rhyme.

Other studies have investigated the poetry preferences of students in the intermediate and upper grades.[42] Like students in the lower grades, these children demonstrated preferences for poems that depict familiar experiences and feelings, ones to which they can relate and with which they can identify. They, too, preferred humorous verse, but unlike younger students they favored contemporary, rather than traditional, poems, and they were more interested in realistic, rather than fantastic, poetry. Story poems, limericks, and poems that make use of obvious rhythm, rhyme, and sound were also the favorites of older students. For both groups— and for both males and females—the least-liked forms of poetry were free verse, lyric, and haiku.

Although these researchers emphasized how important it is for teachers to know about and respect children's preferences for poetry, they also have emphasized the narrow range of choices to which the children they surveyed were restricted. It may be that children's limited preferences reflect their lack of exposure to various kinds of poetry. In her national study, for example, Ann Terry found that more than 75 percent of teachers in the intermediate grades read poetry to their students only once a month. This hardly constitutes the kind of extensive exposure which will allow children to sample a wide variety of poems that cover a wide variety of topics, styles, and forms.

As Amy McClure found in her year-long study of a poetry program in a combined fifth and sixth grade classroom, when children regularly read, write, and share poetry in combination with a great deal of teacher encouragement, support, and the right kind of structure, they become better readers and writers, and they also develop a taste for, and appreciation of, many different kinds of poems and poets as well as the poetic techniques and elements these poets use. After being introduced to all sorts of poetic styles and forms during the school year, these fifth and sixth graders demonstrated an awareness of, and a preference for, a far wider range of poets and poems than students in previous studies. In addition to popular contemporary poets such as David McCord, Arnold Adoff, Eve Merriam, and Karla Kuskin, the children McClure queried listed Robert Frost, Carl Sandburg, Langston Hughes, Emily Dickinson,. and Robert Louis Stevenson among their favorites, many of whom have written both sophisticated free verse and deeply emotional poems that can be categorized as lyric poetry.[43] What McClure's study proves is that a poem's topic, not necessarily its form, is the main factor in determining children's interest in poetry. When a poem's subject matter genuinely interests them, children will more often than not accept the challenge of working through some fairly difficult poetry. This says a lot about the expectations teachers set for their students.

Something to Do

Make a list of several topics which you regularly cover in your classroom health program. In a public, school, or college library, find poems on these topics in either the *Subject Index to Poetry for Children and Young People,* compiled by Dorothy B. Frizzell Smith and Eva L. Andrews (Chicago: American Library Association, 1977), or the *Index to Poetry for Children and Young People, 1976–1981,* compiled by John Brewton, G. Meredith, and Lorraine Blackburn (New York: H. W. Wilson Co., 1983). Plan several poetry breaks around these poems, to cover a period of several months. Following each poetry break, briefly describe some student reactions as well as your observations about your own involvement. After a few months, review your notes to summarize any changes and development which took place from the first to the final poetry break.

Approaching Nutrition Through Poetry

The poems which teachers and parents can use to enliven factual information about nutrition as well as to help children consider attitudes and values about their diet cover a wide range of topics, types, and styles. There are, for example, selections with contagious rhythm and rhyme about overeating or the bad effects of eating unhealthy foods, humorous verse about the simple pleasures of eating good homemade foods, and inventive free-verse poems that celebrate the preparation and sharing of the kinds of foods we associate with holidays and other special occasions. As with poetry on any topic, poetry that focuses on food, eating habits, and nutrition can be found in three sources. The first is a collection of poems by one poet, such as Arnold Adoff's *Eats*. The second source, known as an anthology, contains selections by different people, such as *Poem Stew*, which was compiled by William Cole. The third source, usually appropriate for younger children, but by no means restricted to this audience, is a picturebook version of a single poem. Two examples of the illustrated single poem which children enjoy are *Jamberry* by Bruce Degen and *Mother Mother I Feel Sick Send for the Doctor Quick Quick Quick*, a fast-paced, comical narrative about the hazards of overeating by Charlip and Supree.

In the annotated lists that follow, we have described some popular, well-written collections, anthologies, and single-poem picturebooks which contain poems about a variety of nutrition-related topics and issues. Complete bibliographic citations for the selections will be found at the end of this chapter. The designations given for the grade levels of the children who might find the poems appealing in a particular book are only approximate recommendations. Many of the poems can be used either below or above the recommended grade levels.

Collections by One Poet

Eats. Arnold Adoff. Illustrated by Susan Russo. Grades three and up.

This collection contains more than forty free-verse poems which capture the smells, tastes, and other vivid sensations that make a family's favorite foods so enticing. The recipient of the 1988 Excellence in Poetry Award from the National Council of Teachers of English, Adoff combines fascinating images, sound play, and an inventive placement of words and sounds on the page to illustrate the joy and satisfaction of sharing good food among the members of an immediate and extended family. As an invitation to children to collect family recipes and shape them into free verse, the poet has included, in the form of poetry, several favorite recipes from his own family: "Sunday Morning Toast," "Grandma Ida's Cookie Dough for Apple Pie Crust," and "Peanut Butter Batter Bread." One of the poems can stimulate discussions about junk food:

> After Covering
> the continent
> of north america
> in
> sugar and bombing all
> our
> cities
> into surrender
> with their yellow cakes
> the giant landed on the white house lawn
> Twinkie
> and
> cream
> filled
> creatures
> demanded all our
> broccoli as their price
> for
> peace*

Is Anybody Hungry? Dorothy Aldis. Illustrated by Artur Marokvia. Grades K through five.

---

*"After Covering the Continent" from *EATS* by Arnold Adoff © 1979 by Arnold Adoff. Reprinted by permission of the author and Lothrop, Lee & Shepard (A Division of William Morrow & Co.).

In twenty-seven poems with surprising rhymes and rhythms, the poet looks closely at the eating habits and customs of animals and humans. The emphasis throughout is on eating as an essential fact of life. After hearing or reading "Cookout Night," students could share and then write about their own cookout experiences during a group or individualized writing activity.

Egg Thoughts and Other Frances Songs. Russell Hoban. Illustrated by Lillian Hoban. Preschool through grade two.
Based on the experiences of irrepressible Frances, the well-known, childlike badger in the Hobans' series about the trials and joys of living in a family, these brief poems depict the ways Frances tries to make sense of others, herself, and her place in the world. Several of the poems deal with food, particularly Frances's eating habits. Include "Sunny-Side Up" in a unit on food groups, or a discussion on children's most and least favorite foods.

How to Make Elephant Bread. Kathy Mandry and Joe Toto. Preschool through grade two.
The recipes for fifteen nutritious snacks are described in free verse. Large, multicolor illustrations help to whet the appetite. Young writers could model their own healthful snack verses on the poets' and collect them into an illustrated class book.

Munch. Alexandra Wallner. Illustrated by the author. Grades K through three.
Wallner lays out a delightful feast of more than thirty short, rhythmic verses that largely depict the consequences of overeating and food obsessions. Whimsical pen-and-ink pictures extend the content of the verses by showing a group of overweight animal characters in all sorts of zany predicaments caused by their overzealous appetites.

Pumpernickle Tickle and Mean Green Cheese. Nancy Patz. Illustrated by the author. Preschool through grade three.
To add some excitement to a trip to the store, Benjamin and Elephant play with words, rhymes, and puns that center around various foods.

Anthologies

How to Eat a Poem and Other Morsels. Selected by Rose H. Agree. Illustrated by Peggy Wilson. All ages.

More than seventy poems and light verses in a variety of poetic forms, tones, and moods focus on table manners, holiday foods, natural foods, snacks, overeating, and many other subjects. The selections are grouped by similar theme or topic such as "From Soup to Nuts," "Snacks," "Tutti-Frutti," and "Mind Your Manners." Many of the selections, including "Mr. East's Feast" and "The Baker's Boy," both by Mary Effie Lee Newsome, and Carson McCullers' "Slumber Party," can be interpreted collaboratively through reader's theater and large-group choral reading. "If All the World Was Paper," a traditional verse of unknown origin, is a case in point:

> If all the world was paper,
>   And all the sea was ink,
> If all the trees were bread and cheese,
>   What would we have to drink?
> *It's enough to make a man like me*
> *Scratch his head and think.* [p. 27]*

Poem Stew. Selected by William Cole. Illustrated by Karen Ann Weinhaus. Grades K through five.

Humor helps to reveal attitudes and feelings about food and eating found in the entertaining verses collected by Cole. These include language play based on the names of common foods ("Who Ever Sausage a Thing?" [author unknown], "A Man for All Seasonings" by Richard Wilbur), food aversions ("O Sliver of Liver" by Myra Cohn Livingston, "On Eating Porridge Made of Peas" by Louis Philips, "Artichokes" by Pyke Johnson, Jr.), eating habits ("Eat-It-All Elaine" by Kaye Starbird, "I Ate a Ton of Sugar" by Alice Gilbert, "The Friendly Cinnamon Bun" by Russell Hoban), the struggle to lose weight ("Father Loses Weight" by X. J. Kennedy), and behavior at the table ("Table Manners" by Gelett Burgess, "The Hot Pizza Serenade" by Frank Jacobs, "Piggy" by William Cole).

Munching. Selected by Lee Bennett Hopkins. Illustrated by Nelle Davis. Grades K through five.

Hopkins, a prolific collector with more than thirty poetry anthologies in print, has compiled over twenty delectable poems by modern and contemporary poets who focus mostly on people's

---

*"If All the World Was Paper" reprinted by permission of Random House, Inc.

experiences with common and uncommon foods, including pizza ("The Pizza" by Ogden Nash), popsicles ("Popsicles" by Cynthia B. Francis), artichokes ("The Artichoke" by Maxine W. Kumin), turtle soup ("Turtle Soup" by Lewis Carroll), and many more. A fourth grade teacher we know had her students perform some of the poems in *Munching* to conclude a two-week unit on nutrition. One group of students had created life-size props out of heavy cardboard for their presentation of "Sad Sweet Story" by Norah Smaridge:

> Eat up your carrots and drink up your milk;
> You'll have pearly-white teeth and a skin smooth as silk.
> Eat too much candy, you'll end up instead
> With a nutcracker jaw and no teeth in your head. [p. 16]*

General Collections and Anthologies

Breakfast, Books, & Dreams. Selected by Michael Patrick Hearn. Illustrated by Barbara Garrison. Grades one through six.

The twenty thoughtful poems in this anthology describe various experiences that involve children throughout the course of one day, from dawn following a night of dreaming to bedtime with its promise of the stories contained in dreams. Along the way, there is a poem which invites readers to help a child select the best school lunch from a menu filled with appealing choices ("Lunch" by Katy Hall), another about snacking ("Snack" by Lois Lenski), and a third told by a child who transforms the food on his plate into the material for a series of adventures—much to his parents' disapproval ("Trouble at Dinner" by J. A. Lindon).

The Random House Book of Mother Goose. Selected and Illustrated by Arnold Lobel. Preschool through grade three.

In this collection of more than three hundred familiar and lesser-known Mother Goose rhymes, food and eating are so much a part of the zany world depicted that it is hard *not* to find many references to these essential components of life. Caldecott medalist Lobel is especially skilled at giving fresh visual interpretations to the amusing and sometimes traumatic dilemmas and conflicts about food that involve such well-known characters as the frustrated old

---

*"Sad Sweet Story" by Norah Smaridge. Used by permission of the author, who controls all rights.

woman who lived in a shoe, Jack Sprat "who could eat no fat," the clumsy milkman who is literally covered in milk because he still hasn't learned how to keep the milk in his pots, Betty Botter who discovers a perfect solution to better batter in better butter, and exasperated Old Mother Hubbard whose wily dog refuses to be satisfied with the usual types of dog food. For all the nonsense these little stories-in-verse contain, they frequently capture important sentiments about human nature, as in this one about Hannah Bantry's private eating habits:

> Hannah Bantry, in the pantry,
> Gnawing at a mutton bone;
> How she gnawed it,
> How she clawed it,
> When she found herself alone. [p. 131]*

The Random House Book of Poetry for Children. Selected by Jack Prelutsky. Illustrated by Arnold Lobel. All grades.

Over five hundred poems and light verses are grouped by topic in fourteen sections including "Nature is...," "The Ways of Living Things," "Children, Children Everywhere," and "Some People I Know." The subject index is a great help to anyone who wishes to find poems on specific health-related topics such as emotions, body parts, death, the environment, relationships, and coping with illness. In "I'm Hungry," the section with poems about food and eating, the poets focus on vegetables ("Celery" by Ogden Nash, "I Eat My Peas with Honey" [author unknown]), fruits ("A Taste of Purple" by Leland Jacobs, "This Is Just to Say" by William Carlos Williams), and other types of foods ("Oodles of Noodles" by Lucia and James L. Hymes, "Meg's Egg" by Mary Ann Hoberman), as well as attitudes toward food and eating ("I Raised a Great Hulabaloo" [author unknown], "Pie Problem" by Shel Silverstein, "My Little Sister" by William Wise).

Read-Aloud Rhymes for the Very Young. Selected by Jack Prelutsky. Illustrated by Marc Brown. Preschool through grade three.

Presented here in large-book format are more than two hundred brief poems on subjects that interest young children. The brightly colored, dramatic illustrations will stretch children's imaginations in addition to helping them understand the poets' content and themes. Young children will participate in the rhythm and sound play in

---

*"Hannah Bantry" reprinted by permission of Random House, Inc.

"Crunch and Lick" by Dorothy Aldis, "Yellow Butter" by Mary Ann Hoberman, and "Toaster Time" by Eve Merriam. "The Meal" by Karla Kuskin, which describes an absurdly voracious appetite, could lead the way to discussions of well-balanced diets, while "The Picnic" by Dorothy Aldis and "Picnic Day" by Rachel Field could be used in conjunction with a presentation on nutrients, food sources, and calories. Children could then make drawings or collages of healthy and unhealthy foods consumed at picnics with family members and friends before they either write or tell personal experience stories about these outings.

Where the Sidewalk Ends. Shel Silverstein. Illustrated by the author. Grades three and up.

A popular poet with children and adults alike, Silverstein has a knack for capturing human foibles, predicaments, and off-beat experiences in rhythmic narrative poems and zany line drawings. Among the food-related poems in this collection are ones that tell of obsessions with different kinds of food ("I Must Remember," "Hungry Mungry," "Peanut Butter Sandwich"), problems with bad manners ("With His Mouth Full of Food"), and bizarre adventures with food ("Pancake?," "Spaghetti," "Sky Seasoning"). In *A Light in the Attic,* his second collection, children meet a polar bear who happily resides in a family's refrigerator which is well stocked with meat, fish, noodles, rice, and other ordinary foods ("Bear in There"), while "Wild Strawberries," which begins "Are wild strawberries really wild?," is an invitation to play with food names.

The Scott, Foresman Anthology of Children's Literature. Zena Sutherland and Myra Cohn Livingston. All grades.

This comprehensive collection of a wide assortment of children's literature from the past and present contains an extensive selection of poems organized around subject categories that match the developmental interests of children. Beginning with topics and concepts related to self, family, and relationships with people outside the family, the poets explore school experiences, common and uncommon objects, nature, physical activity, and the realm of the imagination and spirit. The section on food and eating includes Mother Goose rhymes, verses from the oral tradition, and a number of contemporary poems which can provide a feast of ideas related to dietary habits, the relationship between physical and emotional well-being, food choices, food groups, and food customs.

Father Fox's Pennyrhymes. Clyde Watson. Illustrated by Wendy Watson. Preschool through grade two.

Reflecting the style and tone of Mother Goose verses, Watson's brief rhymes depict everyday life within a tightly knit, fun-loving family and extended community of foxes. The detailed illustrations rendered in cartoon style heighten the comedy, add an active storyline with a wealth of visual comments about human relationships, and provide the kinds of interpretive details which keep young readers and listeners riveted to the page in search of the characters and actions the rhymes depict. In such a caring and loving family, food preparation and sharing are depicted as a particularly memorable demonstration of affection and concern.

The Illustrated Single Poem

Fresh Cider and Pie. Franz Brandenberg. Illustrated by Aliki. Preschool through grade three.
When spider grants a fly one last wish before he eats him, the crafty fly requests cider and apple pie, a treat which spider keeps making and eating until he is too full to eat his prey! Incorporated into this rhyming story are details about baking pies and using a cider press.

Mother Mother I Feel Sick Send for the Doctor Quick Quick Quick. Remy Charlip and Burton Supree. Illustrated by Remy Charlip. Preschool through grade four.
When the doctor arrives to help a young boy who has eaten too much, he finds in the boy's stomach a green apple, a ball, an entire birthday cake, a plateful of spaghetti, a flounder, cookies, and an odd assortment of other surprising objects. Silhouette drawings add to the humor of this exaggerated tale of woe and recovery.

Jamberry. Bruce Degen. Illustrated by the author. Preschool through grade three.
A musical verse tells of the wonderful day Bear has when he discovers all kinds of delectable berries.

Whiff, Sniff, Nibble and Chew: The Gingerbread Boy Retold. Charlotte Pomerantz. Illustrated by Monica Incisa. Preschool through grade three.
In this verse retelling of a traditional story, Gingerbread Boy is so determined not to be eaten that once he returns from his perilous trek around the farm, he jumps out of the farmer's stomach and runs away with the little old lady who made him in the first place.

Chicken Soup with Rice. Maurice Sendak. Illustrated by the author. Preschool through grade three.

While celebrating the joys of sipping chicken soup with rice, Sendak's cast of enthusiastic children move through the months of the year. The repetitive verse is featured in Sendak's musical film, *I'm Really Rosie* (Weston Woods), with music composed and sung by Carole King.

Summary

Like other imaginative writers, poets depict genuine human experiences, from typical incidents, thoughts, and feelings that are part and parcel of everyday life and living to ones that are difficult to accept and manage, including those that are intensely disturbing. By utilizing poetic techniques such as simile, metaphor, and hyperbole to create the compressed, concise language style which is one of poetry's most noticeable—and demanding—characteristics, the best poets shape their impressions and ideas into vivid images which capture our interest and stimulate us to see, think, and feel in new ways. Poets who write for children are no exception. They must be just as skilled in their art and craft as poets who write for adults, and, in addition to this, they should be sensitive to the things that matter to children and aware of the special ways children involve themselves in life's experiences as they try to make sense of the world around themselves and others. Poetry that focuses on health-related topics, issues, and problems can offer children the same rewards that can be gained from their involvement in any type of good poetry: better language, reading, and coping skills; the enjoyment that comes from hearing, reading, and responding to poems that genuinely interest them; and the satisfaction they experience when the poet captures their attention by amusing them or by giving them something personally meaningful to think about. If children are to associate poetry with pleasure and understanding, they need to hear and read and participate in a large variety of poems and light verse that truly appeal to them.

INFORMATIONAL BOOKS: HUMANIZING THE FACTS AND FIGURES OF HEALTH

Children can be remarkably curious about natural and manmade phenomena. Jim Trelease, author of *The Read-Aloud Handbook,* has called them "asking machines."[44] Trelease has described research findings which maintain that young children typically ask about thirty questions an hour! Of course, this statistic will not surprise teachers and parents, who often feel they should have been born with a mind like an encyclopedia in order to keep up with the questions children are apt to ask about everything from skydiving to sex, or from death to drugs. It is no easy task to satisfy children's natural inquisitiveness and to keep them looking for answers. To do these things, it takes a great deal of patience and a lot of knowledge, and it also helps if we know where to look for the many kinds of information children seek when we can't supply them with all the answers ourselves. We should also be able to direct them to a variety of reliable sources, so that they will know how to find information on their own without always needing our assistance. What our goal should be is to have children become independent, lifelong learners, for, as the TV commercial puts it, "A mind is a terrible thing to waste."

How simple it would be if all we had to do was to hand the child a list of facts. While it is essential to give children accurate, up-to-date information whenever they approach us with questions or problems, anyone who has worked with children knows that merely to respond to them with the facts of the matter is a far cry from the challenge teachers and parents face when attempting to make this information clear and understandable. In the first place, it is important to approach the issue or topic at hand from the child's point of view, with all that implies about the child's limited, but nonetheless significant, experience and background. It isn't, however, a matter of talking down to the child, for this is a sure way to lose any child's interest, nor is it merely a question of how to take complicated concepts and reduce them to their most basic and elementary form. This approach too often causes more confusion than understanding—not to mention what it implies about a lack of trust in, and respect for, children's capabilities and the awareness and insights they bring to the task. Instead, the amount and kind of information we share with children, as well as the words we choose and the examples we use to make concepts and ideas concrete and accessible for them, should be based on what we know about specific characteristics of their intellectual and personal development.

Another important ingredient in the process of helping children learn new things or reinforce information they already have acquired is the adult's genuine enthusiasm about learning. Not only is this kind of enthusiasm contagious; it can also serve as a memorable model which proves that learning can be exciting and enjoyable. To hold the child's interest, it also helps if the parent or teacher can make information available to children through a good story that teaches while it entertains. Far from distorting the truths or facts about a given subject, a story can contain information which is just as accurate and current as the information that fills textbooks and other types of factual resources. What a good story can do for facts and concepts and principles—and ways of discovering them—is to make them that much more interesting, relevant, and significant by showing children how these things are connected to, and stem from, human experience.

Writers who set out to share information with children face the same kinds of challenges. Like the authors of textbooks, they must be scrupulous in their effort to offer young readers the latest, most accurate information on a topic, but as writers of literature they need to utilize the various tools and techniques which imaginative writers of any type of literature use to entice readers into the world that exists between the covers of a book. On the one hand, then, these writers attempt to encourage children to make discoveries about topics, issues, and concepts, to acquire new knowledge or skills, to consider alternative ways of looking at issues based on concrete evidence, or to form opinions and attitudes about subjects that interest them. At the same time, exceptionally skilled writers of informational books, like truly gifted and inspiring teachers, are knowledgeable, enthusiastic guides or facilitators who have such control of their material that they are able to present it to children in inventive ways and therefore excite children about learning and prove to them that learning can be a fascinating, enjoyable, and challenging process. To qualify as a writer of effective informational literature—the "literature of fact," as John McPhee, an author of many acclaimed informational books, refers to this type of literature—a children's author faces quite a few challenging obligations and responsibilities.[45]

What Makes a Good Informational Book Good

In order to tell a good informational book for children from a less-effective one, teachers and parents need to consider such things as how the author organizes and develops the subject, the kind and amount of information the author includes, and the quality of the information to be shared with children. Like any illustrated children's book, the graphics in an informational book should also contribute to the child's understanding of the ideas the author presents. Knowing how these characteristics work in a number of well-written and effectively illustrated informational books which attempt to explain various aspects of human sexuality to children will help educators and parents to be aware of what to look for when they select health-related informational books for children.

In the first place, an informational book should offer children much more than a deluge of facts. In a good informational book, wisely chosen facts are organized to lead children to an understanding of theories, concepts, and principles related to a topic. In *Being Born,* for example, Sheila Kitzinger uses information gathered from prenatal psychology, ultrasound, and electronic recording of the fetal heart to explain the processes of gestation and birth from the fetus's perspective. With the help of Lennart Nilsson's stunning close-up photographs of the growth and development of a fetus, Kitzinger transforms documented facts about the characteristics of prenatal life into a startling story of what a fetus experiences deep inside the mother's body in order to convince children that, even before its actual birth, the baby can use some of its senses. If a good informational book is distinguished by how well an author and illustrator work together to sustain the interest of both the child and the adult, and teach them something valuable as well, then *Being Born* is a hallmark of excellence. The author's and illustrator's meticulous research emerges on every page of this carefully designed book, but they integrate the facts into a fascinating and memorable narrative that fosters a renewed respect for life.

Like all good literature, an informational book should also have a distinct style. An effective style not only makes the working out of concepts, opinions, and arguments easy to follow, clear, and understandable, it also keeps children involved whether they are reading the words or looking at the illustrations. The reason that so many textbooks quickly bore and frustrate readers of any age is because they are stripped of the color, vitality, and conviction of a writer's personal voice. Written or illustrated in an unnatural, monotonous style, textbooks frequently move along, piling one fact on top of the other, as though the author's main purpose was to prepare us for an objective test on the material. Simply put, the writer's use of language, including such elements as vocabulary choice, sentence complexity, length, and variety, and the illustrator's use of color, space, shape, line, and other visual ingredients determine the style of an informational picturebook. In *Wind Rose,* Crescent Dragonwagon explores the beauty of the love that leads to conception and birth through lyrical prose and vivid images. These are the means by which a father and mother explain the facts of life to their child while they also make her aware of how welcome she is in their life and what it means to be a family. The soft texture of Ronald Himler's subtle, though colorful, illustrations increases the warm emotional tone of an informative and sensitive portrait of the origins of life and the pleasures of family unity.

By contrast, Eric Johnson discusses sexuality in a direct, businesslike manner which resembles the forthright style of an Ann Landers column. Written for teenagers, *Love and Sex in Plain Language* is neither coldly clinical nor sentimental. Instead, Johnson presents documented facts, varying opinions, and well-known controversies about the physical and emotional aspects of sexuality and sexual behavior in honest, nonevasive terms, the point being that adolescents can make responsible choices only if they have a comprehensive understanding of what the issue of sex involves. In this straightforward, concerned, and nonjudgmental way, Johnson approaches male and female physiology, sexual intercourse, conception, gestation, birth, homosexuality, masturbation, contraception, sexually transmitted diseases, and other related issues.

Tone, which is closely related to style, is another important element to consider when evaluating the effectiveness of an informational book. Basically, tone reveals the author's point of view toward the topic as well as the reader, and in an informational book—as in any type of literature, for that matter—tone is an element which takes shape, and then shapes our attitudes and feelings, through the writer's manipulation of language, and, in the case of a picturebook, the illustrator's manipulation of the material included in the pictures and other graphic elements.

Just as an honest and truthful attitude on the part of both the writer and illustrator shows respect for children, a condescending tone underestimates their abilities, insights, and sensitivities, because underlying it is an assumption that ideas and concepts need to be watered down for children, or that they should be protected from "touchy," complicated, or controversial subjects. By showing just how complicated an issue the birth of a sibling can be for a child, Kathryn Lasky avoids these problems in *A Baby for Max.* Using her five-year-old son Max as the narrator of his own thoughts and feelings, Lasky gives her readers an authentic view of the ways her pregnancy and the baby's birth affected Max. Throughout, the tone is one of kind respect for Max's emotions, reactions, and concerns. Black-and-white photographs by the author's husband document the parents' tender regard for their son's feelings as he learns how to cope with his moods and to accept the changes which the birth will cause in his life. By following a family through the steps of a process which reveals each family member's manner of dealing with a complex situation, the book can serve as a model for children and adults of an honest, direct, and rational approach to solving human problems and working through the inevitable changes people of all ages must face.

The format and organization of an informational book are equally important, and should be closely examined. This is particularly true of books that provide a detailed discussion of a topic for children in the middle and upper grades. By using visual and typographical aids which clarify the sequence of the presentation and indicate the location of specific information, the author and illustrator help readers follow the discussion and make sense of it. *Sexual Abuse: Let's Talk About It,* by Margaret O. Hyde, is a good example of a thoughtfully arranged informational book for older children that contains a variety of useful and explicit aids for helping them process and comprehend the book's content. A table of contents, for example, provides a clear forecast of the organization, scope, and sequence of the material. There, readers learn that the author will develop the topic logically by moving from a general overview to a focus on specifics. Following an initial explanation of what sexual abuse is, as well as what it isn't, Hyde provides several case studies of sexually abused young people who mustered the courage to seek professional help. She then discusses in more detail productive ways to cope with sexual abuse and sensible ways to prevent it. Since Hyde does not attempt to cover all aspects of the subject—a good approach in informational books for the sake of establishing a sharper focus and preventing factual overlap—she ends with a description of materials for further study, including books, films, and audio cassettes. To further augment the book's usefulness, she includes information about the kinds of organizations that assist sexually—or otherwise—abused individuals, and a comprehensive index which facilitates the location of specific information in the text.

When writers of long informational books break up the chapters with meaningful headings and subheadings, they make it easier for children to follow the development of the discussion. For example, in each of the chapters in *Understanding AIDS,* a book geared to readers in grades two through five, author Ethan Lerner uses this technique to pave a clear path to the different topics and issues the book encompasses. Frequent chapter headings such as "How are infections spread?," "What is the connection between homosexuality and AIDS?," and "Is there a cure for AIDS?" serve as signposts to content, and help readers keep their bearings as they receive and assimilate new material. An interesting visual feature of this book derives from the way Lerner handles technical terms. The terms he highlights in the text in bold print are defined again in a concluding glossary. In addition to facilitating comprehension, techniques like these can come in handy for young writers when they prepare reports, provided the teacher spends some of the time examining the things professional authors do to present their material in clear and logical ways.

Illustrations and other types of graphics can also enhance comprehension by making details concrete and specific. Accuracy and currency are just as important in an informational book's graphics as they are in the written text. One of the reasons for the success of Kitzinger and Nilsson's *Being Born* is the care with which these collaborators document textual information with clear photographs, to which they have affixed simple captions in smaller print, to provide more technical facts than the text supplies. For instance, on the page where they explain the first stages of the formation of the fetus's body, the caption reads, "After 30 days you were 5 mm (1/5 inch) long." The inclusion of this kind of information clearly indicates that the author and photographer have done their research. It is a good way for authors or illustrators of an informational book to establish their knowledge of the subject.

Illustrations and other graphics should be placed close to the textual information they are meant to support. In *Teen Pregnancy* by Sonia Bowe-Gutman, for example, an explanation of the purpose, use, and reliability of various contraceptive aids is further enhanced by clear line drawings which, situated in breaks in the narrative, immediately demonstrate the correct use of the devices the text introduces. Explicit, thoughtfully designed, and carefully placed graphics like these help to prevent confusion.

This is particularly true of the way Miller and Pelham use

graphics in *The Facts of Life.* A visual feast of information, the book lays out the process of human reproduction and gestation with the use of intricate three-dimensional pop-up models and a reliable, smoothly written text that often utilizes metaphors (sperm compared with a "huge fleet," for example) to make the information particularly understandable to young children. The pop-up (scale is both explained and implied) show the workings of the reproductive organs, the growth of the fetus, the birthing process, and much more, and tabs can be manipulated to demonstrate the movement of chromosomes, the fertilized egg, and other pertinent features of the reproductive system. Furthermore, both the pop-ups and the movable tabs are numbered to correspond with a number in the more complex and technical information found in smaller print. As a result of this remarkable arrangement of visual aids, the book transforms an informative explanation of the reproductive process into an intriguing adventure for children of all ages as well as the adults who experience the book with them.

The best informational books are not only models for how to communicate and display information, they also demonstrate how people gather facts and other types of information in order to reach conclusions, make inferences, prove or disprove hunches, form opinions, and, in general, acquire knowledge. Sometimes, authors actually reveal the unfolding of the scientific process of investigation. Millicent Selsam does this in *All About Eggs,* an informational picturebook for young children. In order to prove that every creature and every human being comes from an egg, and to show where human birth fits in the world of living things, Selsam first observes and explains the origins of life for various animals before she introduces the phenomenon of birth for human babies.

In *It's a Baby,* another book for young children, George Ancona, who is both the author and the photographer, introduces some basic principles of the scientific method by showing how careful observation and an attention to detail are essential for capturing the growth and development of an infant during the first twelve months of life. In other instances, writers document the findings of researchers to show how conclusions are reached and problems are solved. For example, Alvin and Virginia Silverstein reserve a large part of *AIDS: Deadly Threat* for a discussion of the procedures, methods, and discoveries researchers used to put together the pieces of the AIDS puzzle before they were able to isolate the cause of the disease.

Authors of informational books who expect children to become aware of the scientific method of investigation will also distinguish between fact, opinion, and theory—between, that is, what is known, what is unknown, and what needs to be known about a subject. In *How You Were Born,* a book for young children with provocative descriptive illustrations by Hella Hammid, Joanna Cole lets her readers know that she is conjecturing about the things an unborn baby senses when she writes, "You probably heard your parents' voices talking and the sound of your mother's heart beating." Referring to a photograph which shows a four-and-one-half-month-old fetus sucking a thumb, she states, "Perhaps you sucked your thumb sometimes, like the unborn baby in the picture." Even for the youngest of readers, signals like these can clarify the differences between informed hunches and proven truths.

These distinctions should be made even more explicit for older readers. For instance, in his discussion of homosexuality in *Love and Sex in Plain Language,* Eric Johnson is careful to point out that, concerning the origin of the sexual preferences of homosexuals, "There is as yet no single theory on which all scientists agree." Words like "usually," "probably," "ordinarily," and "it is impossible to say" also show that a writer is acknowledging incomplete or inconclusive evidence or information. This kind of healthy skepticism not only helps to increase our belief in the accuracy of the information the author is providing us, it also raises our trust in the author. Naturally, we want to find other informational books by a writer who tells us the truth.

Of course, truthfulness and accuracy are two of the most important characteristics of a worthwhile informational book, for without these essential ingredients even the most beautifully designed and captivatingly written book is not worthy of a child's attention. When we know the subject well, the accuracy of the information is easy to detect. When we don't, we have to rely on elements in the text which help to verify the reliability of the information and the writer's qualifications. Fortunately, the habit among contemporary writers and publishers is to include such features as an introduction which, among other things, describes the author's particular approach to the topic in contrast to the approaches used by others, a list of consulted sources, and a list of recommended materials, should the child or adult want to pursue the subject further. All of these help to establish the author's authority.

Also, a quick check of the information included on the book jacket or at the end of the book will verify the author's background, experience, and expertise related to the subject. It helps to know, for example, that Sonia Bowe-Gutman, author of *Teen Pregnancy,* has written on this topic for the *Christian Science Monitor* and other award-winning newspapers, or that Oralee Wachter, author of *No More Secrets for Me,* a book about sexual abuse, and *Close to Home,* a treatment of child abduction, has received the National Mental Health Association's Award for Special Problems, and that the World Congress for Mental Health selected her film of *No Secrets for Me* as one of fifteen best films worldwide. That an author has concentrated on one subject area in which he or she has achieved an outstanding reputation as a writer who knows how to communicate with children is another good sign. Alvin and Virginia Silverstein, for example, had collaborated on many well-regarded books about the biological sciences prior to the publication of *AIDS: Deadly Threat.* The same is true of Margaret Hyde whose *AIDS: What Does It Mean to You?* was preceded by a number of notable publications, including *Mind Drugs, Cry Softly! The Story of Child Abuse,* and *Know About Smoking.*

There are other ways for authors of informational books to indicate that they have included accurate, up-to-date information. A list of the people the author consulted for advice and input is one. In *Feeling Safe, Feeling Strong,* which contains fictional accounts of acts of child abuse and information on handling such situations, Terkel and Rench acknowledge several authorities who have an insider's view of child

molestation and ways to deal with it. Joanna Cole, too, points
out that the suggestions of the Codirector of the Gesell
Institute for Human Development were incorporated into
The New Baby at Your House. Increasingly, authors also
include a foreword or preface by a leader in the field to show
that their books are endorsed by an expert. For example,
Donald Armstrong, M.D., Chief of the Infectious Disease
Service at the Memorial Sloan-Kettering Cancer Center,
wrote a foreword to support Elaine Landau's *Sexually Transmitted Diseases,* and, in his foreword, Vincent J. Fontana,
M.D., Medical Director of New York City's Foundling
Hospital and Chairman of the Mayor's Task Force on Child
Abuse, endorsed the approach to child sexual abuse prevention which Aho and Petras utilize in *Learning About Sexual
Abuse.* These may be small gestures, but they help to
guarantee the value of the information and the effectiveness
of an author's manner of handling a subject, particularly when
the child and adult have little personal experience and
knowledge on which to rely.

Checklist for Evaluating Informational Books

I. The Treatment of the Material

1. Do clear concepts emerge from the author's presentation of
   the material?
2. Is the author enthusiastic about the topic? Does the author
   use a fresh, inviting writing style that makes the reading
   experience interesting?
3. Do the author's style and tone demonstrate a respect for the
   child's intelligence, awareness, and experiences? Will the
   information, and the concepts it supports, be understood by
   the children for whom the book is intended?
4. Does the organization of the material enhance comprehension? When appropriate, are significant organizational aids
   included?
5. Do illustrations and other graphic elements support textual
   information? Do they enhance comprehension?

6. Does the author involve readers by providing them opportunities to solve problems, weigh decisions, and consider alternative points of view? Is independent thinking encouraged?

II. Approaches to the Information

1. If appropriate, does the author demonstrate methods of scientific investigation?
2. Does the author distinguish between fact, theory, and opinion?
3. Does the author make an effort to show how the information is relevant to everyday life and how it affects the quality of life? Does the author discuss the effects of the subject, and the issues raised by it, on individuals and institutions?

III. Quality and Quantity of Information

1. Are the author's qualifications made known? Are there indications that the information is accurate and current?
2. Does the author establish a clear focus for the presentation? Is the author's point of view easily detected?
3. Does the reader gain an understanding of significant information about the topic?
4. If appropriate, does the author include significant controversies about the topic?
5. Does the book contain an adequate representation of gender, race, and age in both the writing and illustrations? Are stereotypes and gross generalizations avoided?

IV. Additional Considerations

1. Will the book encourage interaction among children and between children and adults?
2. Does the book stimulate the reader to want to pursue the topic further? Are additional resources suggested?

The Range of Informational Books for Children

In the past fifteen years or so, informational books for children have undergone a number of noticeable changes. In addition to marked improvements in the quality of the writing and the illustrations in books for younger children, informational books currently encompass a much wider range of topics in a much more varied range of attractive formats than in previous years. Never before have so many knowledgeable individuals from so many different fields found their way into the children's book world, where they have discovered a fertile field in which to explore their ideas and an enthusiastic audience with which to share them.

Many of these writers have excellent reputations for producing quality books on subjects and issues that pertain to the well-being of children. By knowing who writes the best of these informational books, parents, teachers, and librarians can be confident that they are choosing books which reflect the high standards we have discussed in this chapter. The extensive Bibliography in Chapter 6 will assist them in their search. In addition to naming some notable authors who have focused on health topics, the Bibliography contains examples of some of the health areas these authors have addressed, the approximate grade levels to which their books are geared, and examples of the books they have written.

Although there are many other contemporary nonfiction writers whose books deal with health issues, the ones we have pointed out have produced an impressive variety of quality books that have a great deal to say to children as well as adults about the measures all people must take to ensure a healthful lifestyle. A quick and easy way to find out about other health issues which these notable authors have addressed is to check the descriptions of their books in several book selection aids which are available in the reference area of most school and public libraries. For example, *Best Books for Children*, edited by Gillespie and Gilbert, and *The Elementary School Library Collection*, edited by Winkel, contain brief descriptions of recommended books—classics as well as contemporary examples—which are listed under major subject headings. Since selection guides such as these are frequently revised, it is important to ask for the latest edition.

Parents, teachers, and librarians can also learn about current health-related informational books by checking into the various awards and honors which are given to outstanding authors and illustrators of nonfiction. The Eva L. Gordon Award for

Children's Science Literature, for example, is given annually by the American Nature Study Society to an author or illustrator whose books are scientifically sound, stimulate children to understand the interrelationships among concepts and ideas, and encourage them to become independent, critical thinkers who are capable of using the scientific method to make their own discoveries about scientific principles. Similarly, the Children's Science Book Award was established by the New York Academy of Sciences to single out quality children's books in various sciences. Other awards that frequently feature health-related informational books are the Please Touch Book Award, given to an author or illustrator of a picturebook that effectively explains a concept, and the Washington Post/Children's Book Guild Nonfiction Award, which honors an author or illustrator who has made a lasting contribution to the area of informational children's books.

Something to Do

Using one of the book selection guides, find several informational books on the same health topic for children at a particular age or grade level. To determine which is the best book among the ones you have chosen, evaluate the books by using the criteria listed on the Checklist for Evaluating Informational Books (see page 172).

Nutrition in Informational Books

As the old saying puts it, "You are what you eat." Although this oversimplifies a complex issue, there is still a great deal of wisdom in the warning this statement implies. Obviously, we are much more than the foods we consume, but a good, thoughtful diet can certainly help us to function in healthy and productive ways. Of course, childhood is the best time to become aware of the importance of proper nutrition, for that is when lasting habits are formed and valuable attitudes toward nutrition are established. In order to develop wholesome habits and attitudes, children need to receive consistent messages about nutrition, both at home and at school.

As always, actions speak louder than words when it comes to making children aware of what it takes to lead a healthy life, but words—in this case, the words discovered in interesting, accurate informational books that speak to children about nutrition in terms they can relate to and understand—can also contribute to the things they need to know in order to make intelligent, informed decisions and choices about their diet. Today's children can have access to an ever-increasing variety of fresh, inventive, and up-to-date informational books that make learning about such things as balanced diets, food sources, the chemistry of different kinds of foods, eating disorders, and weight control an enjoyable and informative experience. The more adults know about various types of good informational books on nutrition, the more confident they will be in recommending specific books to specific children at the right time.

Categories of Informational Books on Nutrition

The types of informational books described here fall into five categories: survey books, how-to books, self-help books, informational picturebooks, and social history books.

The purpose of a survey book is to present a general introduction to basic facts and concepts about a topic. Survey books are a good place to begin a search for information when a reader has little or no background on the topic. The best of these books make complex topics understandable and interesting without sacrificing accuracy. In the area of nutrition, for example, *Vitamins—What They Are, What They Do,* by Judith Seixas, introduces younger readers to the ways vitamins work in the body. The author has included an easy-to-follow vitamin chart, a true-and-false test about vitamins, consumer tips, and information about vitamin safety. In *The Good Food Book* by the Bergers, children in the intermediate grades can learn basic information about such topics as digestion, the effects of overeating, wise food buying, food production and marketing, and world hunger. In addition to a comprehensive index which makes the search for specific topics easy, *The Good Food Book* also contains informative illustrations that have been placed in close proximity to the textual material they are intended to explain. This is also an example of a survey book that can serve as a springboard for more in-depth study, since the authors provide a list of books for further reading.

Good for Me! by Marilyn Burns is intended for older children searching for information about some of these same topics. Subtitled, "All About Food in 32 Bites," *Good for Me!* emphasizes the ways a variety of lifestyle factors affect a person's health. The author discusses the roles consistent exercise, calorie intake, and snacks play in a person's effort to maintain a healthful lifestyle. Characteristic of informational books in the Brown Paper School Book series, *Good for Me!* conveys information with a breezy, comical writing style and busy cartoon illustrations. *Foodworks,* a publication of the Ontario Science Centre, also uses a comical tone to entice children (from grades three to eight) into a consideration of the seriousness of what and how they eat. Clearly and entertainingly written, the book is like a survival manual that includes a discussion of what food does inside the body, and contains science experiments that focus on food, quick and easy nutritious recipes which children can safely prepare, and information about eating habits in other cultures.

How-to books, as their name implies, are intended to stimulate active learning and participation through doing or making things related to a particular topic. The emphasis in these books is on learning-by-doing, and the underlying attitude toward children is that accomplishment and achievement are essential for attaining self-esteem. The child-centered cookbook is the most obvious example of a how-to book that centers on nutrition. In addition to healthful recipes, cookbooks for children should contain safety precautions and advice and clear, logical directions that won't frustrate the child.

An outstanding series that meets these and other criteria is the Little Chef series, all by author and illustrator Liz Martin, for children in the primary grades. Using illustrations with bold lines and primary colors as well as a minimal text, each book in the series clearly describes every step of the cooking process for one type of food (pizza, muffins, and pretzels, for example). The books are spiral bound for easy handling, and durable laminated pages make them so easy to clean that the child need not feel guilty for the kind of messiness that typically and naturally is part of preparing different kinds of foods. An equally thoughtful series of cookbooks for children in the intermediate and upper grades is the Ethnic Menu series published by Lerner Publications. In this case, food customs and traditions of a variety of countries serve as the background for simple, though frequently exotic, recipes. Each book in this continuing series, which now includes foods of Korea, China, Mexico, and several African and Caribbean nations, features full-color photographs, occasional line drawings, a metric conversion chart, safety hints, and an index. *Cooking the Italian Way* by Bisignano is a characteristic example of the care that went into the publication of this series.

A number of cookbooks for children have been inspired by popular classics from the world of children's books. Arnold Dobrin, for example, based the recipes in *Peter Rabbit's Natural Foods Cookbook* on references to food found in Beatrix Potter's books for young children. From start to finish, the recipes reflect the spirit of simple goodness which characterizes Potter's unforgettable animal community. Similarly, *The Little House Cookbook* by Walker and *The Louisa May Alcott Cookbook* by Anderson offer children in the intermediate grades a number of period recipes and thus place food and nutrition within a specific cultural context. These are good cookbooks to introduce to children after they have listened to, or read independently, the literature that led to the recipes.

Closely related to the how-to book is the self-help book, sometimes called the survival book. In self-help books, young readers find advice for living based on sound scientific principles. Largely popular with preteen and teenage readers, the best self-help books encourage readers to understand the facts of an issue or topic before they make decisions about which course of action to follow. *Bodyworks* by Bershad and Bernick is a case in point. As a "Guide to Food and Physical

Fitness," the book discusses, among other things, the ways different foods affect the body and the characteristics of a well-balanced diet. Sara Gilbert focuses on similar concerns in *Fat Free: Common Sense Guide for Young Weight Worriers,* which approaches the topic first by describing the science of body fat, and then by discussing specific guidelines for determining whether or not a person is in fact overly fat. The author uses humor to lessen anxiety, a conversational, yet intimate writing style to make the reading experience that much more personal, and includes a calorie-carbohydrate chart for monitoring consumption, a subject index, and a listing of books for those who want to pursue the topic further.

Recent companions to *Fat Free* are *Too Fat? Too Thin? Do You Have a Choice?* by Arnold and *How To Be a Reasonably Thin Teenage Girl* by Lukes, both of which provide a down-to-earth approach to weight loss based on realistic personal goals, hints about developing wise eating habits and planning low-calorie meals, and the need to set reasonable short-term and long-term goals. Arnold also discusses some of the latest studies and theories on weight control which consider heredity as well as personal habits in determining an individual's weight. A much more serious tone characterizes *Eating Disorders* by Ellen Erlanger, which explains the emotional and psychological motivations for anorexia nervosa and bulimia nervosa through compassionate attention to warning signs, symptoms, dangers, and, finally, organizations that can offer help.

The recent proliferation of informational picturebooks is one of the most noticeable trends in nonfiction books for children. In books of this type, the illustrations should clarify and interpret the ideas and concepts the child finds in the text. In the past, the majority of informational picturebooks used drawings and paintings to help explain the information, but more and more of them now use photographs to make the information concrete. While many informational picturebooks with photographs are appropriate for younger readers in the primary grades, just as many are geared to the interests and development of older readers, who also appreciate the kind of help vivid, carefully placed photographs can give them when they are trying to understand the facts and issues related to particular subjects.

Whether they contain drawings or photographs, good informational picturebooks about nutrition offer children important facts and concepts in an attractive visual format. These books have the advantage of making nutritional information easy to understand, because the visuals not only help to make facts and concepts concrete, but they frequently also relate them to everyday human experience. Quite a few of these books focus on one type of healthful food. In *The Popcorn Book,* for example, Tomie dePaola presents to younger readers a potpourri of facts and legends surrounding this popular food. As one young boy reads from a textbook on popcorn, another prepares a bowlful of the real thing which they later share. *Popcorn* by Millicent Selsam, a book for slightly older readers which takes a more scientific approach to the topic, traces the history of popcorn and describes the life cycle of the plant while explaining, with the help of Wexler's clear color photographs, the difference between popcorn and other variations of corn. Using a similar format, this award-winning team has focused on fruits in *The Apple and Other Fruits.*

A more detailed look at the apple can be found in *Apples, How They Grow* by Bruce McMillan. Using richly textured black-and-white photographs and a compelling writing style, McMillan shows the life cycle of the apple while explaining the many uses of this versatile fruit. Younger children can follow the apple's progress from bud to fruit by looking at the wordless sequence of photographs on the pages to the right, while older children with a more advanced reading vocabulary can focus on the detailed, scientific information contained in the captioned photographs and text that appear on the left.

Informational picturebooks about different kinds of vegetables also range from the simple to the complex. For example, in *Growing Vegetable Soup,* written and illustrated by Lois Ehlert, readers observe a father and son as they plant seeds and then cultivate, harvest, and prepare a variety of vegetables for a delicious soup. Bright primary colors and large, bold print make the experience, and the good feelings that go with it, that much more accessible to primary grade readers who, by following the steps in the process, are also introduced to the elements of a simple story structure with a predictable pattern. Cultivating vegetables is also the main topic of *A Book of Vegetables* by Harriet Sobol, which features fourteen vegetables, and *Corn Is Maize* by Aliki, which, among other things, describes the facts and legends that grew out of the American Indians' dependence on this staple.

Often, authors of informational picturebooks will integrate facts and concepts into an interesting story. In *The Growth of the Potato,* for example, Millicent Selsam reveals a wealth of fascinating facts about the complicated process of cultivating a potato crop in a story that tells of a young person's visit to a potato farm and market, where she learns about the care and attention potato plants need to grow properly. In *The Shopping Basket,* Burningham introduces younger children to simple math concepts as well as some common foods through a humorous fantasy story about a child's eventful trip to a neighborhood market. On his way to and from the market, the child imagines that he meets, and outwits, a variety of animals that want him to share his goods. In *Pumpkin Pumpkin,* Titherington tells of a young boy who watches a pumpkin grow full-cycle from seed to mature vegetable to seed. The author used soft colored-pencil drawings to give a dreamy feel to Jamie's experiences in nature and to capture his genuine, childlike interest in the natural phenomena that unfold around him while he tends to his garden with rapt attention.

Another category of children's informational books is made up of books that depict the history of a specialized topic. Appropriate for readers in the intermediate and upper grades who have reached the concrete operations stage in their development and therefore have a firm grasp of the concept of time, these books provide information by placing a topic or issue within a historical and social context.

In the area of nutrition, the social history informational book gives children the opportunity to explore changing customs, beliefs, and attitudes about nutrition and different types of foods. For instance, they can trace America's culinary history in Perl's *Slumps, Grunts, and Snickerdoodles: What Colonial America Ate and Why,* Hunter's *Stew and Hangtown*

Fry: What Pioneer America Ate and Why, and *Junk Food, Fast Food, Health Food: What America Eats and Why.* In addition to providing authentic regional recipes from these three periods, Perl offers a wealth of information about geography, the domestic life of the time, the social climate, local mores and manners, and the ways people used and adapted to available ingredients. Each of the books contain maps, notes about measurements, recipe charts, a thorough index, and an annotated list of books for further research and reading.

Some social history books are more specific in scope. *Scoop After Scoop* by Krensky, for example, focuses on the history of ice cream from ancient to modern times, while *Milk,* by Giblin, traces the centuries-long effort to make milk a pure and safe product. With the use of prints, photographs, interesting anecdotes, and well-documented facts, Giblin describes the composition of milk, the people who have cultivated it, the various ways it has been marketed, and standards of purity. In *From Hand to Mouth: Or, How We Invented Knives, Forks, Spoons, & Chopsticks, & the Table Manners to Go with Them,* Giblin reveals the history of eating utensils and table manners of various cultures with the same vivacious style, attention to detail, and respect for the intelligence of his readers which characterize the best informational books for children.

Summary

Due to the increased quality and quantity of informational books, today's children have access to a wonderful array of attractive and accurate books that invite them to become excited about the process of learning. The best informational books draw the child into a world where people their own age investigate, from a child's perspective, the facts, beliefs, and attitudes that are related to a specific subject.

When children are learning about personal and community health issues, good informational books can help to answer their questions, clarify concepts and personal values, reinforce the accurate information they are receiving from informed parents and teachers, and demonstrate how health concepts truly influence the way people choose to live. When health-related information is placed within a human context, particularly through the art of an effective story, the facts become less remote from everyday experience and much more immediate.

Imaginative informational books also offer children a well-deserved break from the language and format of textbooks. Unlike many of the texts they must read, informational books offer variety. Since there are many different informational trade books on the same subject, children can choose the most appealing from among them. Knowing that other books on a topic are available, children can reject one book if it doesn't interest them in favor of another, and, when it seems appropriate, they can be asked to compare and contrast different authors' and illustrators' treatments of the same or similar topic. Such variety also makes it possible for students of health at different grade levels to find and enjoy all sorts of books that genuinely match their interests, tastes, and abilities. Finding a book that truly speaks to them personally about health issues and matters of wellness, they will feel they have something important to contribute to the discussions that take place whenever their own health or the health of others is being discussed.

Also, factually sound and effectively designed informational books can be models to children as they are learning ways to use language to express their ideas. The best informational books lay out a process of discovery and demonstrate how facts, theories, and opinions differ. They show children how information can be explained in a lively, interesting way without detracting from the responsibility to be accurate and honest. As Jo Carr reminds us, an outstanding book of nonfiction can lead a child ". . . by way of facts and beyond facts—to awakened understanding."[46]

BIOGRAPHY: HEALTH ISSUES IN THE LIVES OF REAL PEOPLE

As the story of an individual's life, a biography is a direct route into the workings of human behavior. As a type of literature that chronicles the experiences of many different kinds of people, biography reveals the circumstances that shape people's lives—including the values and beliefs people espouse, the problems they face, the moral dilemmas they confront, the relationships they form, and the choices they make. A well-written biography provides readers with an inside view of a person's private and public world. What attracts both children and adults to biography is the opportunity this type of literature offers readers to witness the unfolding of a human drama, not only for the pleasure of it, but also for the insights into human nature that can be gained from observing people living their lives.

Biography has a number of implications for fostering healthful behaviors and attitudes among children. First, by depicting the lives of others, biography can make children aware of the forces that influence the course of a person's life and the things people do to enhance or hinder their own well-being and the well-being of others. Second, because biography reveals the ways all sorts of people deal with life's problems and challenges, it demonstrates effective and ineffective ways to cope with stressful situations. Third, since biography often describes the ways people lose or gain control of the course of their lives, it reveals to children behaviors and attitudes that either promote or prevent personal health. Fourth, biography can help to make children conscious of the factors that contribute to a person's self-concept and self-esteem. Finally, as a window to the variety of characteristics that make people both different from and like each other, biography can alert children to the needs people have in common as well as the things that make people unique. Biography, then, can help to nurture children's sense of the human family at the same time as it widens their tolerance for different kinds of people.

The Range of Biographies for Children

Increasingly, children's biographies have become much more diverse than they were. Contemporary biographers for children are less restrictive than they were in former years, concerning not only the kinds of people children are interested in reading about but also the aspects of a person's life which can be revealed to children and the sophistication with which the material can be handled. There are, for example, many more biographies of women, members of cultural groups of all types, and popular contemporary figures, such as sports and political figures, as well as rock music stars and TV and film personalities. For instance, *Homeward the Arrow's Flight,* a biography for older children by Marion Brown, tells the inspiring story of Susan La Flesche, the first American Indian woman to become a doctor, while the biographies in the *Women of Our Time* series, published by Viking Kestrel, introduce the seven-to-eleven age group to a number of well-known twentieth-century figures, including Martina Navratilova, Dolly Parton, Betty Friedan, and Winnie Mandela.

There also is a wider selection of picturebook biographies for younger children. In *The Story of Johnny Appleseed,* for example, Aliki presents the intriguing exploits of the legendary conservationist, and in *A Weed Is a Flower,* the same author/illustrator tells of George Washington Carver's personal journey from slavery to his role as a preeminent research scientist. For slightly older readers, there is the award-winning series by Jean Fritz which depicts the foibles and achievements of famous historical figures such as Benjamin Franklin, Paul Revere, and Christopher Columbus. With their breezy style, droll humor, and focus on both the strengths and weaknesses of flesh-and-blood human beings, Fritz's picturebook biographies make good read-alouds which show children that even famous people have idiosyncrasies and need to contend with personal and social problems.

Some picturebook biographies, designed for early independent readers, use a limited vocabulary and a simple writing style to focus on both ordinary and dramatic incidents in a person's life. A good example is *The One Bad Thing About Father,* by F. N. Monjo, with lively illustrations by Rocco Negri, which provides glimpses of Teddy Roosevelt's active professional and family life as seen through the eyes of his son Quentin, a youngster who wishes that his loving father wasn't quite so preoccupied with the presidency of the United States.

Characteristics of Biography

Many of the ingredients of a good informational book are also found in well-written biographies. The most important of these is meticulous accuracy. "A good biographer," Sutherland and Arbuthnot point out, "resembles a good detective, following clues, interviewing people, hearing what the subject has to say, and then—and only then—reaching a tentative conclusion that is presented to readers, who serve as the jury."[47] That is, the biographer should make every effort to paint as accurate a portrait of the subject as research will allow. To have control of as many aspects of the person's life as possible, the biographer needs to research all of the known pieces of the individual's life as well as the characteristics of the time and place in which the individual lived. This applies to the illustrator as well. In *Christopher Columbus* by Cesarani, for example, Piero Ventura's watercolors of the setting, the style of clothing, and other important visual details clearly place the story in the late fifteenth century and thus enhance both the facts and spirit of the written text.

As a way to assure their readers that they have done their homework, it is standard procedure for biographers to point out some of the sources they consulted as they delved into the person's life. Others demonstrate their research by distinguishing fact from opinion and fictionalized from actual incidents and dialogue. In his Newbery Award picture biography of Lincoln, Russell Freedman concludes with a variety of information which offers further facts about Lincoln's life and verifies the biographer's expertise. In addition to listing a selection of books by and about Lincoln, Freedman provides documented quotations from Lincoln's speeches and correspondence, a detailed tour of Lincoln memorials, monuments, and museums, and a description of the scholars, curators, and other people who guided his research. In a less elaborate way, Jean Fritz uses brief endnotes to verify, expand, and explain certain facts and ideas. For example, at the conclusion of *Where Do You Think You're Going, Christopher Columbus?*, Fritz explains that native Americans had discovered the New World thousands of years before Columbus arrived. Such thoroughness and care not only demonstrates a respect for the intelligence and curiosity of children, but also provides insight into what a writer must do to create a full and accurate portrait of the subject.

An accurate portrait is a truthful one. Biographers should take care to offer a balanced picture of the individuals they depict, presenting examples of successes as well as failures, attributes as well as shortcomings and vices, and the pleasant as well as the harsh realities of a person's life. The best biographies depict the whole person, not only those characteristics which we want children to emulate. For example, the Lincoln who emerges in *Me and Willie and Pa,* a picturebook biography by Monjo, is indeed a caring family man and an astute politician, but he also is a real individual who makes jokes, loses his temper, tells stories, gets frustrated and annoyed, and sometimes cries. Similarly, in *Martina Navratilova* by Knudson, the tennis superstar from Czechoslovakia is characterized as determined and disciplined, but also as a person with unpredictable emotions, who sulks when her game is not up to par and is inclined to panic when she muffs a play.

Good biographies also draw the reader in with an inviting writing style that complements the writer's purpose and the spirit and tone of the person's life. The restrained and dignified style of Coerr's writing and Himler's illustrations in *Sadako and the Thousand Paper Cranes* are well-suited to the seriousness and sadness of this emotional biography of a Japanese girl who dies of leukemia as a result of radiation sickness from the bombing of Hiroshima. *Growing Older* by Ancona, on the other hand, abounds with vivid, humorous details that add vitality to the remembrances and anecdotes of a group of spunky elderly Americans.

Authentic dialogue also helps to create a memorable writing style which sustains interest. Biographers must often invent dialogue, but the best of them do this by rooting this speech in a thorough understanding of the language of the time as well as the temperaments and relationships of the individuals they are depicting. For example, never does the reader doubt the authenticity of the invented dialogue which fills *Grand Papa and Ellen Aroon, Being an Account of Some of the Happy Times Spent Together by Thomas Jefferson and His*

Favorite Granddaughter because the author, F. N. Monjo, has his subjects speak in a manner that seems a natural outgrowth of what is known about their personalities.

Finally, in the hands of a perceptive biographer, the characteristics of one person's life lead the way to a fundamental theme or concept about human nature. Frequently, the title signifies the theme that has emerged from a careful study of an individual's life. In *The Disease Fighters,* for example, Aaseng focuses on the value of determination and risk-taking by exploring the efforts of several Nobel Prize winners who battled against tuberculosis, diabetes, diphtheria, and other diseases. At the heart of *Dreams into Deeds: Nine Women Who Dared* by Peavy and Smith, there is an endorsement of the urge to follow one's inspiration and intuition. The book celebrates the talents, drive, and self-esteem of several outstanding women including Rachel Carson, Margaret Mead, and Babe Didrickson Zaharias, who chose early on to lead the lives they envisioned for themselves. Similarly, the title of *Sure Hands, Strong Heart: The Life of Daniel Hale Williams* by Patterson points up the lesson Williams learned from his father about the need to develop both his physical skills and his mind. In a very prejudiced period of American history, Williams was one of the youngest blacks to become a physician and was the first U.S. surgeon to perform open-heart surgery. By unifying the story of a person's life around a central idea or theme that best characterizes the subject's personality, the biographer moves beyond specific facts and incidents and implies that each life has a pattern and shape that give it meaning.

Checklist for Evaluating Biography

1. Does the biographer provide enough details to give a full picture of the subject's life? Are memorable incidents and interesting anecdotes included?
2. Is there a clear sense of the characteristics of the historical period in which the subject lived, including social, political, and economic background?
3. Is the writing style fresh and inviting? Are colorful details and pertinent information integrated naturally into the narrative?

Is the dialogue authentic and believable even when it is invented?
4. Does the biographer interpret the subject's life story and provide a fundamental statement about human nature based on evidence?
5. Does the biography evoke strong thoughts and feelings that can deepen a child's understanding of human nature?
6. Is there specific evidence that the author and illustrator have thoroughly researched the subject's life? Is fact distinguished from opinion?
7. Does the biographer present a balanced view of the subject's life? Are strengths as well as flaws described? Does the biographer include both ordinary and momentous incidents?

Biography and Health Issues

Many biographies and autobiographies deal directly with issues and concerns that should be standard fare in a comprehensive health program. Consider, for example, the area of mental and emotional health which might encompass such behaviors as dealing with stress, developing problem-solving skills for resolving conflicts and personal problems, respecting the rights of others, and achieving a positive self-concept. Biography can serve as a catalyst for discussions of these topics. In the brief biographies included in *Winners Never Quit: Athletes Who Beat the Odds* by Aaseng, upper-grade children meet several sports figures who overcame mild or severe physical, psychological, and social obstacles in order to excel, while the obstacle for Mary Lou Retton, in Sullivan's account of her career, was low self-esteem. This successful gymnast needed to overcome a negative perception of herself as stocky and short before she could achieve the status of a world-class competitor.

Provocative autobiographies also can prompt children to think about the emotional and psychological aspects of health. For example, *Childtimes: A Three-Generation Memoir* by Eloise Greenfield and Lessie Jones Little, contains the childhood memories of three black women—a grandmother, mother, and daughter—who tell of the joys of growing up in a close, secure extended family while having to endure the agony of blatant bigotry. As David Kherdian shows in *Deep River Run,* the warmth of family ties and the reassurance offered by his loving relatives also helped him to survive the turmoil and alienation he experienced as a first-generation child growing up in America. For Cynthia Rylant, who grew up in the 1960s, it was the absence of her estranged mother and father that became the central issue of her childhood—one that caused her pain and filled her with longing. In *But I'll Be Back Again,* Rylant not only describes her early and enduring sorrows, such as her father's bout with alcoholism and her mother's decision to leave her with her grandparents while she studied nursing, but she also shares her feelings about boyfriends and girlfriends, her first kiss, her infatuation with the Beatles, her career as a writer, her failed marriages, and many other things that give life its true substance.

A number of biographies tell about people who have coped with disease. Several, including Aaseng's *The Inventors,* McCoy's *The Cancer Lady: Maud Slye and Her Heredity Studies,* Ranahan's *Contributions of Women: Medicine,* and Shiels's *Winners: Women and the Nobel Prize,* focus on the achievements and efforts of professionals in medicine and other sciences involved in disease prevention. Others capture the experiences of those afflicted with disease. In *Child of the Silent Night,* for example, Hunter traces Laura Bridgman's history from her bout with scarlet fever, which left her blind and deaf, to her successful attempt to read and communicate with others as a result of the rehabilitation she received at Boston's Perkins Institute. *Babe Didrikson: The World's Greatest Woman Athlete* by Schoor focuses on the phenomenal accomplishments of a multitalented sports figure who was just as well known for her courageous fight against cancer as she was for her athletic skills, and in *Alan Alda: An Unauthorized Biography,* Bonderoff lays out this actor's route from his crippling childhood illness to his accomplishments in film and television.

Environmental health is another issue that biography can make children aware of. For children in the intermediate grades, there is Swift's *From the Eagle's Wing: A Biography of John Muir,* which tells of Muir's respect for nature and his need to live in open spaces because of the peace they provided him. Critical-reading skills can be nurtured by having the same readers compare Swift's interpretation of Muir's sentiments about the natural environment with Dines's more recent interpretation in *John Muir,* a book that underplays Muir's life as a conservationist and highlights his career as an inventor. Older readers could be involved in a similar activity by contrasting the style and tone of Aliki's picturebook biography of Johnny Appleseed and Hunt's more detailed and less romantic account in *Better Known as Johnny Appleseed,* which is based on legend and actual reminiscences of this conscientious pioneer and missionary who is well known for his love of nature. Older readers will also learn about the effort and knowledge needed to protect our natural resources when they read about the contributions of the professional conservationists depicted in *To the Rescue: Seven Heroes of Conservation* by Vandivert.

Something to Do

Read a biography or autobiography which is not described in this chapter. Referring to the Health Education Curricular Progression Chart found in Chapter Two, select specific topics and concerns which the book you have read raises directly or indirectly about health.

Summary

To read biography from a health perspective is to learn about real-life circumstances, attitudes, and behaviors that either enhance well-being or contribute to a generally unhealthy state or illness. By providing children with concrete examples of significant conditions, actions, and decisions that actually affect people's health, biography places health-related issues and concerns of various degrees of severity in a very real human context. The more children are exposed to specific evidence of how the positive and negative conditions in a person's life truly have an impact on health and sickness, the more they will know about the psychological, social, and biological aspects of health and illness, and the better they will be at figuring out how to cope with these conditions and possibly to control them. From hearing and reading true stories of the ways people succeed or fail to manage their lives, children will at least have a greater opportunity to learn how to manage their own lives successfully.

PLAYS: HEALTH ISSUES ON STAGE

One of the most exciting current trends in children's literature is the increase in the number of high-quality plays. In contrast to the plays and dramatic skits found in school textbooks, or the ones children themselves write and perform, the plays which contribute to this trend are written largely by professional playwrights who hope to have their work produced by skilled artists who, in turn, make their living at performing plays for audiences of children and adolescents.

Because of this increased interest in professional children's theatre as a legitimate form of theatre, there are many more good plays to choose from than were available in the past—whether one is looking for thoughtful, provocative plays for children to experience in the theatre or ones they can read and perhaps dramatize at school or at home. Many of these plays contain young characters who are involved in the kinds of situations with which children can identify and from which they can learn something valuable about themselves and others. For anyone concerned with children's health, the important thing about contemporary children's plays is that more and more of them are addressing many of the prevailing conditions which either enhance well-being or prevent people from attaining a healthy lifestyle. Plays, then, constitute yet another type of literature which can make children conscious of human conditions and personal choices which either enhance wellness or contribute to illness.

Finding Good Plays

Although there are a variety of good children's plays on specific health topics and issues, finding these plays can be a difficult and frustrating business. Unlike all of the other types of children's literature, plays simply have not become a major concern of mainstream publishers that specialize in children's books. Only occasionally do any of these publishers publish a play. In addition, although new plays appear annually, the best of the lot rarely make it into anyone's list of highly recommended or outstanding books of a given year. A hidden type of literature, plays also are seldom reviewed in professional journals where critics highlight readable, well-written children's books.

Since it is the rare child who is not drawn to any type of literature which offers an opportunity to dramatize interesting situations, particularly ones that are filled with conflicts and problems, this lack of interest in plays on the part of mainstream publishers and critics of children's books usually comes as a surprise to anyone who is responsible for the care and development of children. As many child-development specialists have shown, children simply like to pretend and to act out roles. It is one of the things they do continually in their play as a way to make sense of life's situations and gain some kind of control over them. And it is one of the ways language and literature, plays included, can come alive for them.

Given children's natural affinity for drama, why then are not more of the mainstream publishers providing children with many more plays that speak to their needs, concerns, and interests? One of the main reasons seems to stem from the fact that, unlike the other types of children's literature which we share with children, plays are not merely meant to be read; rather, they are meant to be performed. Perhaps, then, mainstream publishers feel that since the full impact of a play can only be made in a theatre, plays may have little interest for readers and will, therefore, not sell. Yet, even theatre professionals begin the production process by reading a play privately and, later, by reading it aloud with the other people who are involved in a performance of the play. It is in the imagination of a director, actor, designer, and many other people that a play performance first takes shape. And this is based on the discoveries these people make about character, story, conflict, theme, and other elements as they read, study, and discuss the play as literature in its written form. With proper guidance, children, too, can make similar discoveries as they read a play script and put their imagination to work.

On the other hand, publishers and critics may also believe that plays are too difficult for children to read because of the distinctive characteristics of a play script. True, the format of a play script does demand a different reading strategy and different reading skills than do other types of literature, but this also can be said of poetry or, for that matter, any type of literature. In each case, one of the goals of a conscientious teacher or parent is to help children become familiar with the unique demands various types of literature make on them as readers. Plays are no different.

Finally, people often feel that they need special training in the dramatic arts in order to adequately introduce plays to children. However, the fact that these same adults may not have had any training as poets, novelists, or biographers doesn't prevent them from providing children opportunities to experience these types of literature. As with any subject they are not adequately prepared to teach or discuss, the best teachers do some preparatory work to fill in the gaps and learn along with children. Discussing and dramatizing plays need not be the exception, because plays can help children acquire important reading and life skills throughout the course of their development.

With so few plays available from mainstream publishers of children's books, teachers, parents, and librarians must look elsewhere to find good plays on health-related topics. A good place to begin is with the *Index to Children's Plays in Collections.* The most recent edition of this guide, by Trefny and Palmer, lists more than four hundred one-act plays and skits which were published between 1975 and 1984. Although the authors made no attempt to select plays on the basis of literary merit, the listing does provide a good introduction to a wide variety of plays which have been indexed according to playwright, title, and subject area.

Plays Magazine is an ongoing resource for actual scripts. Published monthly from October to May, *Plays Magazine* usually contains easy-to-read short plays, skits, monologues, and dramatized classics. Although the magazine steers clear of controversial and serious topics, some of the material deals with health-related topics and issues. Those who subscribe to the magazine can perform the plays without paying a royalty fee. The publisher of this magazine, Plays, Inc., also has published a number of thoughtful collections of royalty-free plays, such as *Plays from Folktales of Africa and Asia* by Winther and *Folk Tale Plays from Round the World* by Nolan, both of which contain several entertaining selections that can complement health concepts and information.

Perhaps the quickest way to find out about the best contemporary and classical plays for children is to examine the recent catalogs of publishers who supply scripts to children's theatre professionals. These publishers are noted in the list of plays at the end of this chapter. Typical of publisher's catalogs, the ones that advertise plays offer a brief description of the play and the characters involved in it. Any type of performance of theatre scripts, whether within or outside a legitimate theatre, is subject to a modest royalty fee.

The problem with plays published by a company that specializes in theatre scripts is one of format and appearance. Because theatre scripts are published for play producers and performers rather than young play readers, they do not have—and should not be expected to have—the visual appeal of typical, mainstream children's books. They rarely contain illustrations of any sort, and when they do, the illustrations usually consist of one or two photographs of what the play looked like in performance. For readers of any age, a more serious problem is the way such scripts are printed. Unlike the clear, bold print and good paper that mainstream publishers must use if they expect to sell their books, most theatre scripts are printed in small type sizes on inexpensive paper. This can make them somewhat difficult to read and handle, particularly for beginning readers who are just getting used to the way a play script works. Until more major children's book publishers give attention to plays, however, theatre scripts will have to remain one of the main sources of plays for children.

In recent years, a few major publishers of children's books have made a small number of plays available to children in the type of attractive format that makes a play easy to read. Several of these are anthologies and collections that contain good examples of various types of plays that have proven successful onstage. The ones listed are particularly worthwhile resources which include several highly readable plays with health-related themes.

Children's Plays from Beatrix Potter. Rona Laurie.
Potter narrates five of the six short plays about family concerns, feelings, and communication which contain plots, dialogue, and stage directions taken from Potter's stories. The large print, illustrations, and different typeface for dialogue and stage directions make the plays appropriate for beginning readers and actors.

Dramatic Literature for Children: A Century in Review. Edited by Roger L. Bedard.
Bedard traces the development of children's theatre in America with commentaries geared to adult critics and students and thirteen examples of representative, influential plays, all of which have proven appealing to young audiences. Among the plays children of various ages might read on their own or with others are Frances Hodgson Burnett's dramatization of *The Little Princess,* which shows a young girl coping successfully with personal misfortune; *The Birthday of the Infanta,* a study of death as well as a haunting story of a princess who, hurried into adulthood by the rules of royalty, has become a cynical, hardened individual; Aurand Harris's *Androcles and the Lion,* an energetic, comical drama that explores friendship and responsibility; and Joanna Kraus's *The Ice Wolf,* a provocative look at the effects of rejection and a society's unwillingness to accept a young person who doesn't fit its expectations.

How to Eat Fried Worms. Thomas Rockwell.
In addition to the title play, an adaptation of Rockwell's zany novel about the pranks of a group of mischievous boyhood friends, this collection contains three humorous plays that can lead intermediate graders into discussions about relationships.

Picture Book Theatre. Beatrice de Regniers.

Two short plays about relationships in an illustrated text have been thoughtfully designed for young readers and performers. In *The Magic Spell,* a young girl breaks the hex that has turned her brother into a cat.

Plays Children Love. Edited by Coleman A. Jennings and Aurand Harris. Illustrated by Susan Swann.

This anthology contains more than twenty recent and older plays by some of the best children's playwrights. The editors divided the selections into ones recommended for adult performers and those appropriate for children to perform, though children will certainly find plays to read in each of these sections. Among the selections which should interest parents, teachers, and librarians who are looking for plays on health topics and concerns are these: Judith Martin's *Ma and the Kids,* a play in several episodes for younger children to read or perform, which depicts with biting humor the strained relationship between an indulgent mother and her demanding children, and, for older children, Suzan Zeder's *Step on a Crack,* which follows the tribulations of an imaginative ten-year-old who, while trying to adjust to a new stepmother, learns a great deal about herself.

In *Plays Children Love Volume II,* Jennings and Harris provide a similar collection of both amusing and serious drama. *Dandelion,* by Judith Martin, is a prize-winning fantasy review of songs and scenes for all ages about evolution, the life cycle, and culture, while *Who Laughs Last?* by Nellie McCaslin is an entertaining dramatization of a Polish folktale for intermediate graders that focuses on two old people who devise a clever plan in order to survive after they have been forced to retire, and, in the process, win the respect of the king and queen they once served.

Theatre for Youth: Twelve Plays with Mature Themes. Edited by Coleman A. Jennings and Gretta Berghammer.

The full-length plays contained within this anthology cover a wide range of serious topics, including problems of aging, death and dying, friendship, courage, conformity, sexuality, maturation, and struggles with moral decisions.

Two Plays about Foolish People. Patricia Miles Martin.

Resolving conflicts is one of the topics in both *An Invitation to*

Supper and *Little Hoo and the Foolish Ones*. For children in the intermediate grades.

Walk Together. Nancy Henderson.
Human rights and individuality are explored in five one-act plays suitable for older children to read as well as perform. In one, a contemporary close-knit Mexican family attempts to survive with dignity, and in another a group of children who have been programmed by a computer struggle to maintain their personal integrity.

Wish in One Hand, Spit in the Other, A Collection of Plays by Suzan Zeder. Edited by Susan Pearson-Davis.
A contemporary award-winning playwright, Zeder is known for her professional integrity as well as her honest, and demanding depictions of the problems and concerns of young people. The six plays in this collection include *Wiley and the Hairy Man*, which explores how a young boy eventually overcomes his fears; *Doors and Other Doors*, which examine the effects of divorce on a child and his parents; and *Mother Hicks*, which lays out the course of a young orphan girl's emerging self-awareness and also addresses the value of an honest, supportive relationship.

Several mainstream publishers have also published a small number of single-play books. The themes explored in a few of these plays can alert children to values, attitudes, and behaviors that enhance physical well-being and emotional health. For example, *Hattie, Tom, and the Chicken Witch*, an I-Can-Read play book written and illustrated by Dick Gackenbach, features Hattie Rabbit, who rightfully wins the respect of her friends when she accidentally lands a major part in an Easter play from which she was initially excluded. She does a superlative job as the play's narrator. The play itself, which reveals how a group of hens devises a master plan to outsmart a greedy pig who extorts all their eggs, is an amusing study of effective ways to handle stress and solve a problem. By beginning with a prose story that leads naturally into a play that in turn uses a storyteller and features the same characters found in the story, Gackenbach makes it easier for beginning readers to become familiar with the characteristics of a play script. The script also distinguishes the stage directions and speakers' names from the lines they speak by using different colors for the print.

Another recent play script in picturebook format for beginning readers is *Starring Francine and Dave,* written and illustrated by Ruth Young. Here, a little boy and girl take to the stage to dramatize three brief episodes about the cooperation needed to prepare and share food. In "Peanut Butter and Jelly" and "Lemonade" they experiment with the necessary ingredients before coming up with the right thing, and in "Chocolate Cake" they negotiate the size of the piece in order to be sure that each one receives a fair share. Vivid illustrations that demonstrate emotions, gestures, and interpretations of specific lines and a glossary that explains how to produce a play provide children with some good suggestions for how to create their own performances.

Several single-play books can also provide upper-grade children with some fresh insights into important health topics. When considering such issues as a person's responsibility to others or the ways in which one person's behavior can help or harm others, older children might read or act out selected scenes from *When the Rattlesnake Sounds,* Alice Childress's one-act play about an incident in Harriet Tubman's life. Set in a hotel laundry room where Tubman works with two of her friends, the play contains emotionally charged scenes that focus on the effects of prejudice, the pressures and benefits of freedom, and one's responsibility to self and others. Similar themes are woven into *Escape to Freedom,* Ossie Davis's biographical play which traces the struggles of Frederick Douglass to defy the injustices which demeaned the black people of his time. In *Street* by Joan Aiken, the central issue is society's responsibility to the environment. Once a quiet town, Street is now a bedlam of deafening traffic and lethal pollution, because one group valued profit and progress more than they valued the health of the town's inhabitants and the natural environment. Aiken uses suspense and exaggerated realism to demonstrate the consequences of making poor choices.

Society's predicament is just as extreme in *The Door in the Wall,* a play based on De Angeli's Newbery Medal novel of the same name. In the play, which is set in thirteenth century

England, young handicapped Robin learns how to survive the confusions and conflicts which a massive plague has thrust on his homeland. A good way to ease students into the characteristics of a play script is to have them compare the play with the novel.

Characteristics of Plays

Compared with other types of literature in which a narrator provides the essential story elements, a play script requires readers or performers to supply many pertinent story details as they transform written language into appropriate sounds, gestures, and visual images. The script of a play consists mostly of dialogue, a sequence of events, and a limited description of a setting. Therefore, in order to make a play come alive, whether in a corner of a classroom or in an actual or imagined theatre, play readers and performers of any age must use their imagination while paying close attention to textual details. They must decide how to visualize the setting and time period of the play, how to develop the action through appropriate pacing, and how to supply characters with a distinctive personality and equally distinctive gestures and movements based on an understanding of the characters' emotions, thoughts, and relationships.

In all the other types of literature discussed in this chapter, a narrator told the story. In a play, the actors *show* the story—largely through action and dialogue. Play readers do the same kind of things on the stage that exist in their imagination. To demonstrate this key difference between narrative and dramatic literature and to note some of the other characteristics of a script, compare a scene from a narrative story with the same scene from the play version of the story. Here, for example, is a section from the beginning of *A Bear Called Paddington* by Michael Bond, a story which, among other things, captures the joys of living in a loving family. Following the narrative version is the same section as scripted by Michael Bond and Alfred Bradley in *Paddington on Stage*.

Mrs. Brown clutched at her husband. "Why, Henry," she exclaimed, "I believe you were right after all. It *is* a bear!"

She peered at it closely. It seemed a very unusual kind of bear. It was brown in colour, a rather dirty brown, and it was wearing a most odd-looking hat, with a wide brim, just as Mr. Brown had said. From beneath the brim two large, brown eyes stared back at her.

Seeing that something was expected of it the bear stood up and politely raised its hat, revealing two black ears. "Good afternoon," it said, in a small, clear voice.

"Er . . . good afternoon," replied Mr. Brown, doubtfully. There was a moment of silence.

The bear looked at them inquiringly. "Can I help you?"

Mr. Brown looked rather embarrassed. "Well . . . no. Er . . . as a matter of fact, we were wondering if we could help you."

Mrs. Brown bent down. "You're a very small bear," she said.

The bear puffed out its chest. "I'm a very rare sort of bear," he replied, importantly. "There aren't many of us left where I come from."

"And where is that?" asked Mrs. Brown.

The bear looked around carefully before replying. "Darkest Peru. I'm not really supposed to be here at all. I'm a stowaway!"

"A stowaway?" Mr. Brown lowered his voice and looked anxiously over his shoulder. He almost expected to see a policeman standing behind him with a notebook and pencil, taking everything down.

"Yes," said the bear. "I emigrated, you know." A sad expression came into its eyes. "I used to live with my Aunt Lucy in Peru, but she had to go into a home for retired bears."

"You don't mean to say you've come all the way from South America by yourself?" exclaimed Mrs. Brown.

The bear nodded. "Aunt Lucy always said she wanted me to emigrate when I was old enough. That's why she taught me to speak English."

"But whatever did you do for food?" asked Mr. Brown. "You must be starving."

Bending down, the bear unlocked the suitcase with a

small key, which it also had around its neck, and brought out an almost empty glass jar. "I ate marmalade," he said, rather proudly. "Bears like marmalade. And I lived in a lifeboat." [pp. 8–10]*

Mrs. Brown   (*humouring him*) Very well. (*She peers behind the parcels*) Why Henry, I believe you were right after all! It is a bear!

(*Paddington stands up suddenly. He is wearing a bush hat with a wide brim and has a large luggage label around his neck.*)

Paddington   Good afternoon (*He raises his hat*).

Mr. Brown   Er . . . good afternoon.

Paddington   Can I help you?

Mr. Brown   Well . . . no. Er, not really. As a matter of fact, we were wondering if we could help you.

Mrs. Brown   (*Taking a closer look*) You're a very unusual bear.

Paddington   I'm a very rare sort of bear. There aren't many of us left where I come from.

Mr. Brown   And where is that?

Paddington   Darkest Peru. I'm really not supposed to be here at all. I'm a stowaway.

Mrs. Brown   A stowaway?

Paddington   Yes, I emigrated you know. I used to live with my Aunt Lucy in Peru, but she

---

*Excerpt from *A Bear Called Paddington* by Michael Bond. Copyright © 1958 Michael Bond. Reprinted by permission of Houghton Mifflin Company.

	had to go into a Home for Retired Bears.
Mrs. Brown	You don't mean to say you've come all the way from South America by yourself?
Paddington	Yes. Aunt Lucy always said she wanted me to emigrate when I was old enough. That's why she taught me to speak English.
Mr. Brown	But whatever did you do for food? You must be starving.
Paddington	(*Opening his suitcase and taking out an almost empty jar*) I ate marmalade. Bears like marmalade. And I hid in a lifeboat. [pp. 17–18]*

In a sense, the task of a play reader or performer is like a narrator's task, for each of them reveals, controls, and orchestrates the events of a story. In the narrative version of the story, the setting as well as many of the characters' thoughts and feelings are supplied by an all-knowing narrator. In the script, however, the playwright, as a type of narrator, offers only a few suggestions in brief stage directions about the environment of the play and what a character is thinking or feeling. Instead, it is the dialogue which serves as the main source of information about plot development and character reaction and interaction. To be effective, the dialogue in a play must be more economical and organized than the leisurely or random conversation we are used to. A good playwright creates dialogue that contains sufficient clues and suggestions for how to transform written language into the sights and sounds of a story that always happens in the present. The dialogue should contain believable and authentic language, and it also must be deliberately designed to

---

*Excerpt from *Paddington on Stage* by Michael Bond and Alfred Bradley. Copyright © 1974 Michael Bond and Alfred Bradley. Reprinted by permission of Houghton Mifflin Company.

demonstrate a pattern of events that acquires meaning and reveals a character's motives and attitudes. What a narrator can reveal about these elements in elaborate descriptions, a playwright must show through what the characters say and how they act. Onstage, they will physicalize their thoughts, feelings, and attitudes based on the clues they find largely in the dialogue.

Both on the page and the stage, a play should also contain a clear conflict or problem which motivates the characters to act and requires a solution. When the characters have something important at stake, when they are consistent, interesting, and involved in the action of the plot, they capture and keep the interest of the reader or audience member. We get caught up immediately in the problem Paddington Bear presents, especially because the playwright makes him such a lovable character. Will he be caught by the police he fears and be sent back to Peru? Can he survive without his aunt's care? Where and how will he live? Will the Browns be able or willing to adopt him? A good play alerts us to a genuine problem or dilemma within its opening minutes, and we read or watch and listen with concern and interest until this problem is solved.

Entertainment, of course, should be one of the rewards of reading or seeing a play. But a good play also raises important issues. A good play sharpens our awareness by having us explore a significant theme. In an effective play, all the play's elements support this theme. Children's plays are no exception. As theatre for young people has matured, more and more playwrights have realized that children not only like plays that provide escape and a good dose of lively entertainment. They are also interested in plays that provoke them to think about serious problems and issues. For example, in *The Boy Who Talked to Whales,* Webster Smalley invites children to consider conflicting human values. In the play, a boy proves he can communicate with whales and contrives to save them from extinction at the hands of a group of greedy whale hunters. In *Special Class,* Brian Kral uses a blend of comedy and drama to explore the dreams and disappointments of the handicapped child in our society.

The Bridgework Theater of Goshen, Indiana, has also shown that children of all ages respond sensitively to plays that portray serious themes. Several of Bridgework Theater's plays, created by Don Yost in collaboration with the theatre's actors, provide children with strategies for preventing sexual abuse. *Little Bear* introduces young children to information and skills that can make them less vulnerable to sexual abuse, and *Out of the Trap,* a drama for older children, emphasizes how a better understanding of personal rights and boundaries can help children prevent abusive incidents. Since both plays are available in script form and as videotaped productions, children read and discuss the plays before they see them performed. The plays are accompanied by a comprehensive curriculum guide that is sensitive to the way children should be introduced to topics of this nature.

Checklist for Evaluating Plays

1. Does the play contain a story that appeals to the interests of the children for whom the play is intended? Is the story revealed mainly through appropriate action and incident rather than through wordy explanations? Does it show rather than tell the story?
2. Does the playwright provide a clear description of place and time?
3. Do the stage directions and dialogue provide readers and performers with sufficient suggestions for making the play come alive? Is the dialogue believable? Does it stretch the imagination?
4. Are the characters interesting? Does the reader or performer get to know their thoughts and feelings? Are they involved in resolving a significant conflict or solving a meaningful problem? Are they revealed by what they do and how they interact?
5. Does the play's action develop according to a thoughtfully arranged pattern of events which shapes the reader's, performer's, or audience's understanding of the situation?
6. Does the play raise important issues for children to think about? Does it explore a significant theme that enlightens children about their concerns, needs, and interests?

Plays and Health Issues

By comparison with other types of children's literature, there are relatively few plays on health-related topics. But their number is rapidly increasing, and so is their quality. As more and more playwrights break free from the restrictions of the past to experiment with content, style, and theme, more plays are appearing that address the kinds of personal and social issues that concern children and frequently influence the course of their everyday lives. Many of these plays illustrate a process of maturing that leads a young person to a better sense of identity. For Karen in *East of the Sun, West of the Moon,* adapted by Brian Kral from the Norwegian folktale of the same name, this process is laid out as a perilous journey through a dark Scandinavian wilderness populated by magical trolls, mysterious hags, and talking gargoyles. To save a young man from the curse that makes him a bear by day and a man by night, Karen battles these supernatural forces and emerges from the struggle a more self-realized individual. Comparing the play with the tale on which it is based, children in the intermediate grades can explore the significance of the heroine's decision to help another human being and the personal rewards she gained by doing so.

A journey that leads to self-identity is also at the heart of *The Princess Who Was Hidden from the World,* a dramatization of a West African folktale by Winther, and *The Voyage of the Dragonfly,* an original fantasy play by Max Bush. The first play illustrates the problems which an overly protective parent can cause a child. In this case, the child is a naive, completely dependent, and vulnerable princess who has been secluded from the world by her father. En route to her arranged marriage, her servant forces her to exchange roles with her so that she—the servant—can marry the prince. When the princess finally asserts herself and refuses to be pushed around, she changes her fate and gains true autonomy. The remark her father makes at the end of the play has a timeless and familiar ring to it: "Now I realize that I should have taught my daughter more about the world!" In *The Voyage of the Dragonfly,* young Queen Meaghan goes on a quest to retrieve a mystical flame whose power is the only thing that can save her land from being destroyed. The conflicts that result are both internal and external, and the voyage becomes a passage of self-discovery as each character finds a new personal vision.

A large number of plays explore the roles and interactions of individuals within families. Some of these plays portray incidents and problems that typically surface in an average family. For example, in *Five Little Peppers,* based on a classic for younger children and adapted to the stage by Rosemary Musil, a family of poor, mischievous children joins forces with a family of even more mischievous wealthy children for some good-hearted fun. Underlying their antics are themes of parental support, personal ambition, and the obligation wealthy people have to help others. *Family Talk,* a fast-paced drama for older children by Megan Terry, examines some effective ways to establish good interpersonal communication among family members.

Children's playwrights are also conscious of the problems many families must confront. This is evident by the number of plays in which the dramatic issue is a tense, though usually solvable, family crisis. With the eloquence and inventive theatrical style that have characterized each of her other plays, Joanna Kraus, in *Kimchi Kid,* paints an honest picture of the troubles a contemporary American couple encounter when they adopt a Korean child. Through honest talk and, even more importantly, out of mutual respect for each other's feelings and concerns, Hak Soo and his parents begin to understand what it takes to form a genuine family. In *Medea's Children* by Lysander and Osten, a divorce is the problem that radically changes a brother and sister's life. Set in both ancient Corinth and a contemporary home, the play contrasts parallel situations which show how two sets of siblings try to make sense of the troubles that have caused their respective parents' relationships to disintegrate. *Wilma's Revenge* by Ross depicts an unsettling family situation addressed by many children's plays—sibling rivalry. Here, the rivalry motivates a young girl to search for elaborate, foolproof plans and strategies that will teach her older brother, a relentless bully who taunts her, a lesson or two. Although the play's comedy relieves some of the tension, it never detracts from the playwright's concern for the stress Wilma must endure or the message the play drives home about the way one person's behavior can affect another.

Formerly a taboo subject in any type of children's literature, death is now a central issue in a number of children's plays that are sensitive to children's needs and feelings. *The Arkansaw Bear,* by Aurand Harris, makes a reassuring statement about death. Saddened and confused by her grandfather's imminent death, Tish, not unlike many young children, uses fantasy to cope with a difficult problem. In her fantasy world she meets Dancing Bear who is running away from death. Through the insights she gains from hearing Dancing Bear's story, Tish learns about the ongoing cycle of life and death, which helps her to clarify her feelings and accept an inevitable fact of life. Harris blends realism and fantasy, pathos and humor, and music, pantomime, dance, and magic to dramatize a universal truth in terms that children of all ages can understand and images to which they can relate. Fantasy is also a vehicle for coping with death in *You Don't See Me* by Kathryn Schultz Miller. In this play, Stephanie finds her way through her brother's death by creating a fantasy in which he appears as a mime. Until she is ready to accept his loss, acknowledge her grief, and realize that she will be able to go on living without him, she needs his help to prepare for the science fair. The Readers Theatre Script Service has developed a poignant play about death in *Johnny Pye and the Footkiller,* an adaptation of a story by Stephen Vincent Benet. Appropriate for older children, this Readers Theatre script follows Johnny Pye from boyhood to old age as he tries to escape death.

The touchy subject of suicide is handled delicately in two plays for older readers. In *Apologies* by Brian Kral, the family and friends of a teenager who has taken her own life sort through the events leading up to her tragic decision in an effort to understand it. Given the fact that suicide is the third leading cause of death among today's adolescents, this compelling and honest drama deserves the attention of anyone concerned with the welfare of young people. *Suicide,* developed by Living Stage Theatre of Washington, D.C., is just as uncompromising in its depiction of the topic. Here, the surviving member of a teen suicide pact struggles through his complicated feelings, as the ghost of his girlfriend urges him to take his own life. With proper guidance, these plays allow young people to take a hard look at the influence of peer pressure and alternative ways to cope with life's tensions and problems. Both plays have proven highly successful with young audiences.

Something to Do

First read a children's play that has been adapted from a narrative story. Then read the story. What are the differences and similarities between the two? How does the play version involve you in the story, compared with the narrative version? How might these similarities and differences influence the way you involve children in plays? For adaptations on health-related topics, see *The Three Little Kittens* by June Barr (family cooperation), *The Velveteen Rabbit* by James Still (responsibility to others; self-acceptance), *Charlotte's Web* by Joseph Robinette (friendship; death), *Androcles and the Lion* by Aurand Harris (friendship; responsibility to others), *Wiley and the Hairy Man* by Suzan Zeder (fears; self-concept), and *Ozma of Oz* by Suzan Zeder (aging; relationship between young and old person).

Summary

Whether children are reading a play on their own, hearing it read aloud, or seeing it unfold in a theatre, good plays provide them with an opportunity to observe characters involved in a variety of real-life situations. From stage directions to dialogue, the language of a play is meant to be seen, heard, and shared. When children discuss and improvise play scenes or prepare more polished oral readings, they are actively discovering how language, within specific social contexts, can express a range of ideas, emotions, and moods. Through play reading, they not only learn about, but also demonstrate, the power words have to make meaning out of our experiences. The criteria used to find quality fiction apply to plays as well. An interesting story, a well-paced plot, recognizable and believable characters, plausible language, and a distinct style are essential characteristics that engage children's interests and provide them with a pleasurable reading experience.

Increasingly, children's plays are addressing a wide range of health-related concerns and issues. In addition to plays that depict everyday experiences regarding family life, friendship, responsibility to self and others, and the process of growing up and achieving a positive self-image, there are also plays that deal with more difficult issues, such as rejection, divorce, death and dying, suicide, and substance abuse. Children's plays, like other types of meaningful literature, are a fine source of valuable themes and topics that can make children aware of conditions, circumstances, and personal decisions that can support their well-being or work against it.

BOOK SELECTION

Numerous studies have shown that when children are provided uninterrupted periods of time for both private and shared reading, together with access to a wide variety of reading materials that genuinely interest them, not only are they motivated to read and read well, but they also develop a lasting attraction to books.[48] And, as the Commission on Reading pointed out in *Becoming a Nation of Readers,* a recent state-of-the-art report on reading instruction in the United States, the amount of time children read and the availability of materials they enjoy are factors that also enhance the development of such reading skills as comprehension, fluency, and a positive attitude toward reading.[49] "Increasing the proportion of children who read widely and with evident satisfaction," the Commission maintained, "ought to be as much a goal of reading instruction as increasing the number who are competent readers."[50] How might parents and educators reach this goal? Among other things, advised the Commission, they should surround children with developmentally appropriate books that fit their interests and needs and satisfy their natural curiosity.

Opportunities like these may be more the exception than the rule for many American children. In an era such as ours, the resounding cry for higher standards and educational excellence is all too frequently translated into a school reading program that requires slavish adherence to daily practice in isolated language skills, so that students can pass standardized tests and teachers can satisfy the demands of accountability. According to recent estimates, American children are spending up to 70 percent of the time reserved for reading instruction immersed in skillsheets, workbook exercises, and other types of commercially published classroom materials that focus largely on literal level subskills.[51] Practices like these greatly limit children's exposure to good literature. When schools allocate thousands of dollars for the purchase of costly commercial reading programs, there often remain enough funds to buy a very limited number of children's books. In 1985, for example, the ratio in school budgets which was spent on basal programs and trade books was 100 to 1, or $350,000,000 for commercial materials to $3,000,000 for library trade books.[52] What is so surprising— if not bewildering—about these priorities is how such choices ignore the substantial body of research which suggests that having children do workbook exercises or other types of activities that involve them in language outside the context of experiences with meaningful, relevant books does not make them better readers.[53] As with any other language skill, children become proficient readers by being read to and by reading many different kinds of materials.

Sadly, the preoccupation with a drills-and-skills approach to reading instruction does not leave much time for the amount of reading children need to do in order to become competent readers who not only know how to read, but also choose to read. In a recent survey of life in a variety of American schools, Goodlad found that students in grades K through six spent approximately 6 percent of the school day actually reading, while in junior high the figure dropped to less than 3 percent.[54] That is about seven to ten minutes a day for reading! The amount of time children reserve for reading out of school may not be much greater. When one team of researchers investigated the leisure time activities of fifth graders, it was discovered that the majority of these young people used only 1 percent of their free time for reading from books, while one hundred minutes of their day were consumed by television viewing.[55]

Another recent survey, conducted by the National Assessment of Educational Progress, revealed a significant decline in inferential comprehension skills among secondary school students and a marked decrease in the degree to which young people value and enjoy reading by the time they reach high school.[56] Is it surprising, then, that, according to fairly current estimates, sixty million Americans are functionally illiterate, and that the United States ranks as low as forty-ninth in literacy levels among 158 United Nations countries?[57] Surely, it is reasonable to wonder about the value of reading programs that spend so much money, time, and energy on reading instruction and yet produce questionable results.

If the amount of reading that children do is in fact the best predictor of which children read well and develop a positive attitude toward reading, there can be no question that children need ample time to experience a large number of worthwhile books from every type of literature. Rather than seeing literature merely as a pleasant diversion from more serious learning tasks, or as a supplement to a reading program, or, worse yet, as the type of material that children should have access to only during special periods reserved for language arts instruction, teachers—as well as parents— would do well to make literature the focus around which all subjects revolve. When children read for pleasure, and when they develop specific tastes and specific strategies for choosing books, a wonderful foundation exists for increasing learning and understanding. This foundation can be used to develop basic skills as well as skills that go far beyond the basics.

Approaches to Book Selection

For anyone who works with children, the first step toward making this foundation a sturdy one is to become familiar with a wide variety of children's books in each of the categories we discussed in the first part of this chapter. With a large variety of the best children's books in mind—and readily available in home, school, and public library collections—parents and teachers will be better prepared to choose quality books to share with children, to try out new and interesting titles, and to lead children to many different kinds of books so that they, too, can begin to become familiar with the wonderful and varied treasures that await them in good books. Children can't be expected to be hooked by books, to develop their tastes for different types of literature, and to acquire new reading skills if they aren't aware of, and don't have access to, a vast number of books from which to choose the ones that really excite them. The more parents and teachers know about the best titles, authors, and illustrators from among the forty thousand or so children's books now in print, the more children will know about them, too.

It is important for parents, teachers, and librarians to feel that the literature they select with and for children represents the best of the lot. When adults believe strongly in the value of the books they select for read-aloud sessions, or for any of the extension activities that are meant to evoke responses from children while they are in the process of making sense of literature, it is more likely that adults will be interested in the books they have chosen and that their sincere excitement about literature and reading will be apparent to children. The adult's enthusiasm for reading can cause children to realize that reading is worth the effort because one's involvement with literature can be personally rewarding and satisfying. Perhaps more than anything else parents and teachers can say about the value of reading, it is their genuine excitement about literature that does the most to motivate children to develop the reading habit. Anyone who was turned on to reading at a young age by a librarian, teacher, or parent with a love of literature knows how inspiring such an individual is, and what an enduring model—one that often remains a vital link to a reader's life-long attraction to books.

Although book selection begins with an awareness of many quality books, it is a disservice to children to have book selection end there. When children are exposed solely to the types of literature the adults in their lives approve of or critics sanction, they could be turned off to books. In limiting young people's choices to literature that reflects only adult tastes, preferences, and interests, there is the danger that children's own interests will not be respected and satisfied. Since a major goal of book selection is to make children aware of a wide range of literature that can capture and hold their attention and therefore motivate them to keep reading, the urge to insure that children read critically acclaimed contemporary literature and enduring classics needs to be balanced with a sincere and constant effort to provide them with books that satisfy their interests, appeal to their tastes, and reflect characteristics of children at various stages in their development.

Working from a developmental perspective, the adult selects books with and for children by taking into account what human-development specialists have revealed about various aspects of children's physical, emotional, social, moral, and intellectual development, among others. For example, in Chapter Four, where we describe the kinds of books that can complement the health-related topics and issues which are contained in the Growing Healthy Curriculum, we use selected developmental characteristics of children to help guide book selection. There, we suggest that children will more likely be interested in books that directly or indirectly reflect their needs and concerns in developmentally appropriate ways.

When it comes to choosing books that children will enjoy for their appealing content and relevant themes, no method of selecting literature is as reliable as the one in which children are invited to sample a number of books and to decide which ones they like or dislike. Numerous researchers have used this method, not only to investigate specific aspects of children's reading interests, but also to explore such things as the literary elements and aesthetic features of the types of literature that children of various ages feel motivated to read, what and who influences their book choices, the quality and quantity of the books they read, the role of instruction in their reading lives, and the nature of their responses to various types of literature.

Anyone who selects literature with and for children can use

the results of these studies to become more aware of the kinds of literature that truly matter to children of all ages and therefore be better prepared to recommend books to children which other children their own age have endorsed. While most of these studies have shown children's interests and tastes to be remarkably diverse, they also have consistently revealed a number of factors that influence children's book choices across age groups and contribute to their changing tastes and interests. The most useful of these for individuals who select literature for and with children include the following:[58]

1. Children's tastes and interests in literature become more diverse when they have access to a wide range of books and literary types.
2. Both their peers and the adults in their lives influence children's book choices.
3. Although children's interests and responses change according to age, younger children read and comprehend challenging literature.
4. Interest is gender-related, and the most noticeable differences between the books males and females choose to read begin when children are in the intermediate grades.
5. Although bright children read more and better books than less bright children, there are few differences in the reading interests of these two groups.
6. The physical and graphic characteristics of books (illustrations, length, cover, type of print, and so on) influence book choices.
7. Children prefer literature which reflects their developmental characteristics and concerns.
8. Children like literature that explicitly teaches a lesson.
9. Children choose and enjoy books in which the characters have empathy for one another.
10. Children are interested in various types of plot structures. The stories they like have cause-and-effect arrangements as well as linear and episodic structures.

Concerning the topics that appeal to children, and the types or categories of books that interest them, research has shown children's tastes and preferences to be so eclectic that it is impossible to come up with definitive lists of books which are certain to appeal to all children all the time. For example, when Sebesta compared the books which children from around the country selected for the 1978 Children's Choices list with the books they did not select, he discovered that children will read about almost any topic as long as it is presented in a concrete fashion.[59]

The heterogeneous nature of children's literary interests is further underscored by the discrepancies and conflicting findings in studies of their book choices. Some of these discrepancies are highlighted in Sebesta's recent analysis of children's favorite books of poetry.[60] For instance, contrary to studies which reported that children ranked poetry among their least favorite types of literature of all the types made available to them, Sebesta's study of a number of Children's Choices lists revealed that children of all ages do in fact find poetry of various tones, moods, types, forms, and content to be appealing. Further, the characteristics of many of the poems children favored contradicted what other studies have revealed about their preferences for such characteristics. For example, in contrast to many of these studies, Sebesta's analysis showed that among the poems children favor, there are traditional poems, serious poetry, free verse, and poems with extended figures of speech, such as personification and metaphor. In other words, children's tastes and interests are much more diverse than previous studies had indicated, and, as Sebesta proves, this range of interests surfaces when children have access to a wide range of literature from which they are invited to freely choose the most appealing.

While discoveries such as Sebesta's provide important insights into the diversity of children's interests and tastes in literature, they also call attention to the value and usefulness of a method of book selection—like the one used in the Children's Choices project—that makes a number of books available to children and gives them the freedom to decide which books currently matter to them and which books they do not find relevant or enjoyable. As a child-centered method of book selection, a program like Children's Choices not only serves parents, teachers, and librarians in their search for different types of high-interest literature of varying levels of complexity likely to appeal to children at specific grade levels; such a program also suggests a sensible approach to book selection that those who choose literature with and for children will want to use—and use continually—if they intend to motivate children to read and to keep them reading. In addition to making a large number of books of all types available to children, an important feature of the Children's Choices approach is the opportunity it gives children to be the ultimate critics of what they read. The children, students in kindergarten through eighth grade in schools in various regions of the country, read any number of books and evaluate them on ballots, with the younger students who can't yet write dictating their responses. From the outset, the children know that their opinions of the books matter because their evaluations will be used to recommend books to other children.

Another important feature of the approach is that, except for suggested, nonrestrictive age level designations, no effort is made to group the books according to their difficulty or appropriateness. As a result, it is not uncommon for certain books to be shared among children of varying ages and, one assumes, abilities. In fact, one of the standard sections of the annual Children's Choices list reports on books enjoyed by "all ages." In light of the many restrictions that are often placed on children's book selections, there is much to praise and emulate in a reading program that motivates children to read and read widely by simply inviting them to read, listen to, respond to, and discuss many different kinds of books. Imagine the excitement for literature and reading that would be generated throughout this country if, as part of every book selection process, each child, regardless of ability, socioeconomic status, or any other factor, were given a similar opportunity to become immersed in interesting books! Shouldn't this be every child's right?

Children's Book Choices on Health Issues

Our examination of the books children approved for the Children's Choices lists of 1984 to 1988 revealed a significant increase in the number of books that contain health-related content. During these five years, the percentage of health-related books rose from 18 percent to 39 percent, which is an indication that children are searching for information and answers about health matters. What this suggests is that children of the 1980s have a real and growing concern for understanding themselves and their relationship to others and to the world around them. Although children did choose some books that provide a lighthearted look at childhood, many favored books that illuminate problems and concerns plaguing their young society. A number of these books, particularly those in the informational books category, are intended to dispel myths surrounding drug, alcohol, and physical abuse as well as sexuality and sex-role stereotyping. As Sebesta discovered about children's reading interests in general, a common thread running through these health-related books is a sense of warmth, caring, and honesty. Another feature of the books is that no subject area seems taboo for a specific age or grade level. This affirms Sebesta's finding that children of any age will read on any topic if the author presents the topic in a specific and concrete way. This suggests that adults may be overly concerned with matching books with the age or ability of a particular group of children.

The chart on pages 219–25 indicates broad, health-related content areas and matches them with books chosen by children who participated in the Children's Choices programs from 1984 to 1988. Although we have grouped the books according to age and grade level, it is important to remember that children often exhibit a much wider range of interests and abilities than specific age or grade levels indicate. If books are made accessible to children by health educators, parents, and librarians who have presented and discussed the books with children in an inviting literacy environment, a fruitful relationship between child and book can be fostered.

Children become proficient and sensitive readers by hearing good literature and by reading all sorts of meaningful books from the entire spectrum of literary types and categories. When children are continually surrounded by many examples of quality books that reflect their needs and concerns and spark their interest, it is the rare child who is not enticed by at least some of the experiences and situations writers and illustrators depict between the covers of their

(continued on page 226)

Grade/Suggested Reading Level	Health-Related Content Areas	Literature Suggestions from Children's Choices, 1984–1988*
K–2 beginning independent	developing/dealing with emotions	*Ernie's Little Lie.* Dan Elliot. Illus. John Mathieu. Random, 1983 (lying, anxiety). *Snap! Snap!* Colin and Jacqui Hawkins. Illus. Colin Hawkins. Putnam, 1984 (bedtime fears). *Waiting for Mom.* Linda Wagner Tyler. Illus. Susan Davis. Viking, 1987 (bravery). *Where Is Nicky's Valentine?* Harriet Ziefert. Illus. Richard Brown. Puffin, 1987 (being forgotten).
	self image	*Bear's Picture.* Daniel Pinkwater. Dutton, 1984 (individuality). *Grandpa Bear.* Bonnie Pryor. Illus. Bruce Degen. Morrow, 1985 (sense of size). *Barber Bear.* Bernard Wiseman. Little, Brown, 1987 (getting cleaned up). *Bird's New Shoes.* Chris Riddell. Holt, 1987 (what's right for self). *Bossyboots.* David Cox. Crown, 1987 (seeing aggression in self). *Here Are My Hands.* Bill Martin, Jr. and John Archambault. Illus. Ted Rand. Holt, 1987 (rhyming to teach body parts). *Norma Jean, Jumping Bean.* Joanna Cole. Illus. Lynn Munsinger. Random, 1987 (self image). *So Hungry!* Harriet Ziefert. Illus. Carol Nicklaus. Random, 1987 (preparing and eating food).

---

*Unless otherwise indicated, the author is also the illustrator.

Grade/Suggested Reading Level	Health-Related Content Areas	Literature Suggestions from Children's Choices, 1984–1988
	childhood experiences	*Get Well, Clown Arounds!* Joanna Cole. Illus. Jerry Smath. Parents, 1983 (illness, wellness).
		Random House Book of Poetry for Children. Sel. by Jack Prelutsky. Illus. Arnold Lobel. Random, 1983 (poetry on childhood themes).
		Patrick and Ted. Geoffrey Hayes. Four Winds/Macmillan, 1984 (friendship, separation).
		Secrets of a Small World. Richard J. Margolis. Illus. Donald Carrick. Macmillan, 1984 (poetry on childhood themes).
		Best Friends. Sel. by Lee Bennett Hopkins. Illus. James Watts. Harper, 1986 (poetry on childhood themes).
		Freckles and Willy: A Valentine's Day Story. Margery Cuyler. Illus. Marsha Winborn. Holt, 1986 (friendship).
		Grover and the New Kid. Jennifer Smith. Illus. Tom Cooke. Random, 1987 (friendship).
		I Want to Be Somebody New. Robert Lopshire. Random, 1986 (being yourself).
		Why Are You So Mean To Me? Deborah Hautzig. Illus. Tom Cooke. Random, 1986 (revenge).
		Harry Takes a Bath. Harriet Ziefert. Illus. Mavis Smith. Viking, 1987 (cleanliness).
		Pookins Gets Her Way. Helen Lester. Illus. Lynn Munsinger. Houghton, 1987 (selfishness).
		Too Many Lollipops. Robert Quackenbush. Golden, 1987 (diet).

realistic family situations	*Hat.* David Lloyd. Illus. Gill Tomblin. Random, 1984 (family situations). *The Crack-of-Dawn Walkers.* Amy Hest. Illus. Amy Schwartz. Macmillan, 1984 (jealousy). *Joey Runs Away.* Jack Kent. Prentice, 1985 (running away from home). *Goodbye House.* Frank Asch. Prentice, 1986 (moving away). *Where Are You Going, Little Mouse?* Robert Kraus. Illus. Jose Aruego and Ariane Dewey. Greenwillow, 1986 (running away from home). *The Farmer in the Soup.* Freya Littledale. Illus. Molly Delaney. Scholastic, 1987 (role reversal). *Daddy Makes the Best Spaghetti.* Anna Grossnickle Hines. Illus. by author. Clarion, 1987 (working parents).
3–4 younger readers	family; relationships	*Maude and Sally.* Nicki Weiss. Greenwillow, 1983 (friendship). *Tee-Tee.* Stephen Cosgrove. Illus. Robin James. Price/Stern/Sloan, 1983 (belonging/independence). *The Pain and the Great One.* Judy Blume. Illus. Irene Trivas. Bradbury, 1984 (sibling rivalry). *What to Say to Clara.* Barney Saltzberg. Atheneum, 1984 (shyness). *The Patchwork Quilt.* Valerie Flournoy. Illus. Jerry Pinkney. Dial, 1985 (family, elderly). *The Perfect Family.* Nancy Carlson. Illus. by author. Carolrhoda, 1985 (large families). *A Weekend with Wendell.* Kevin Henkes. Greenwillow, 1986 (assertiveness). *A Place for Ben.* Jeanne Titherington. Greenwillow, 1987 (sharing).

Grade/Suggested Reading Level	Health-Related Content Areas	Literature Suggestions from Children's Choices, 1984–1988
	fears; strange and fantastic	*What's Under My Bed?* James Stevenson. Greenwillow, 1983 (independence, belonging).
		Anna Banana and Me. Lenore Blegvad. Illus. Erik Blegvad. McElderry, 1985 (fear, fearlessness).
		The Ghost-Eye Tree. Bill Martin, Jr. and John Archambault. Illus. Ted Rand. Holt, 1985 (facing fears).
		Spider's First Day at School. Robert Kraus. Illus. by author. Scholastic, 1987 (facing fears).
	developing social empathy	*Amy: The Story of a Deaf Child.* Lou Ann Walker. Illus. w/photographs by Michael Abramson. Lodestar, 1985 (deafness).
		Willy the Wimp. Anthony Browne. Knopf, 1985 (self esteem).
	humorous stories	*A Stitch in Time for the Brothers Rhyme.* Julie Brinckloe. Raintree, 1985 (humor, role reversal, rhyme).
		Class Clown. Johanna Hurwitz. Illus. Sheila Hamanaka. Morrow, 1987 (fitting in).
	animal stories	*It's Not Easy Being a Bunny.* Marilyn Sadler. Illus. Roger Bollen. Random, 1983 (identity).
		Peabody. Rosemary Wells. Dial, 1983 (adjusting to a new baby).
		Pamela Camel. Bill Peet. Houghton, 1984 (unattractiveness).
		The Foundling Fox. Irina Korschunow. Trans. James Skofield. Illus. Reinhard Michl. Harper, 1984 (sharing and commitment).
		Andy Bear: A Polar Bear Cub Grows Up at the Zoo. Ginny Johnston and Judy Cutchins. Illus. with photographs by Constance Noble. Morrow, 1985 (bonding).

| 5–6 | middle/older readers | | self image | |

Making the Team. Nancy Carlson. Carolrhoda, 1985 (physical size and ability).

Oscar Mouse Finds a House. Moira Miller. Illus. Maria Majewska. Dial, 1985 (finding a home).

So Many Raccoons. Jan Wahl. Illus. Beth Lee Weiner. Caedmon, 1985 (running away, family).

The Story of Poppyseed. Barbi Sargent. Grosset, 1985 (loneliness).

P.J. the Spoiled Bunny. Marilyn Sadler. Illus. Roger Bollen. Random, 1986 (selfishness).

The Puppy Who Wanted a Boy. Jane Thayer. Illus. Lisa McCue. Morrow, 1986 (role reversal).

Bon Appetit, Mr. Rabbit! Claude Boujon. McElderry, 1987 (diet).

Goodbye, Max. Holly Keller. Greenwillow, 1987 (death of a pet).

Beanpole. Barbara Park. Knopf, 1983 (self image).

Behind the Attic Wall. Sylvia Cassedy. Crowell, 1983 (self image).

How Do You Lose Ninth Grade Blues? Barthe DeClements. Viking Kestrel, 1983 (insecurity, belonging).

If This Is Love, I'll Take Spaghetti. Ellen Conford. Four Winds, 1983 (teen problems).

Anastasia, Ask Your Analyst. Lois Lowry. Houghton, 1984 (teen problems).

Friends Are Like That. Patricia Hermes. Scholastic/Apple, 1984 (friendship; peer acceptance).

Beauty and the Beast. Retelling by Warwick Hutton. Illus. by reteller. McElderry, 1985 (recognizing inner beauty).

A, My Name Is Ami. Norma Fox Mazer. Scholastic, 1986 (self awareness and belonging).

Dancer in the Mirror. Winifred Morris. Atheneum, 1987 (self image).

Mufaro's Beautiful Daughters: An African Tale. John Steptoe. Illus. by author. Lothrop, 1987 (vanity and true beauty).

Grade/Suggested Reading Level	Health-Related Content Areas	Literature Suggestions from Children's Choices, 1984–1988
	independence; nonconformity	*Bummer Summer.* Ann Martin. Holiday, 1983 (independence). *The Leftover Kid.* Carol Snyder. Putnam, 1986 (independence). *A Horse to Love.* Nancy Springer. Harper, 1987 (independence, trust). *Johnny May Grows Up.* Robbie Branscum. Illus. Bob Marstall. Harper, 1987 (growth, responsibility).
	factual advice re painful issues	*Ramona Forever.* Beverly Cleary. Illus. Alan Tiegreen. Morrow, 1984 (coping with death). *A Sheltering Tree.* Mary Ann Whitley. Walker, 1985 (physical abuse). *Abby, My Love.* Hadley Irwin. McElderry, 1985 (incest). *Locked in Time.* Lois Duncan. Little, 1985 (dealing with fear, anxiety). *Sweetly Sings the Donkey.* Vera Cleaver. Lippincott, 1985 (family disintegration). *What Is the Sign for Friend?* Judith E. Greenberg. Illus. with photos by Gayle Rothschild. Watts, 1985 (deafness). *Kevin Corbett Eats Flies.* Patricia Hermes. Illus. Carol Newsom. HBJ, 1986 (belonging; dealing with loss). *Robyn's Book.* Robyn Miller. Scholastic, 1986 (disability, dealing with death). *Adventures in Babysitting.* Elizabeth Faucher. Scholastic, 1987 (depression). *Double Trouble.* Barthe DeClements and Christopher Greimes. Viking, 1987 (family disintegration). *The Girl With the Crazy Brother.* Betty Hyland. Watts, 1987 (mental illness). *The Lawrence Taylor Story.* Howard Liss. Illus. with photos. Enslow, 1987 (drug abuse).

Maybe by Then I'll Understand. Jane McFann. Avon, 1987 (alcoholism).

Rabble Starkey. Lois Lowry. Houghton, 1987 (mental illness).

The Secret Garden. Frances Hodgson Burnett. Adapted by James Howe. Illus. Thomas B. Allen. Random, 1987 (disability).

social awareness

Always Faithful. Patricia Baeher. NAL/Signet Vista, 1983 (values).

Megan's Beat. Lou Willett Stanek. Dial, 1983 (values).

Molly's Pilgrim. Barbara Cohen. Illus. Michael J. Deraney. Lothrop, 1983 (other cultures).

Take Back the Moment. Janice Stevens. NAL/Signet Vista, 1983 (juvenile crime).

Different, Not Dumb. Margot Marek. Illus. with photos by Barbara Kirk. Watts, 1985 (learning disability).

Life Is Not Fair. Stephen Manes. Illus. Warren Miller. Dutton, 1985 (injustice).

Rasco and the Rats of NIMH. Jane Leslie Conly. Illus. Leonard Lubin. Harper, 1986 (ecology).

Germy Blew It. Rebecca C. Jones. Dutton, 1987 (nonconformity).

People Like Us. Barbara Cohen. Bantam, 1987 (religious differences).

nonstereotyping; sex roles

A Blue-Eyed Daisy. Cynthia Rylant. Bradbury, 1985 (feminine identity).

The Agony of Alice. Phyllis Reynolds Naylor. Atheneum, 1985 (role models).

The Great Mom Swap. Betsy Haynes. Bantam, 1986 (sex roles).

Almost Fifteen. Marilyn Sachs. Dutton, 1987 (sexual identity).

There's a Boy in the Girl's Bathroom. Louis Sachar. Knopf, 1987 (sexual identity).

books. For children as for adults, the best literature, in all its forms, styles, and categories, provides an ongoing record of, and a means to explore, humanity's concerns, problems, struggles, and joys. Good literature entertains, but it also sheds light on the business of being human.

In school at least, many children do not have access to the rich and varied worlds in literature's many domains. As one children's literature critic put it recently, and as research affirms:

> The worlds of poetry and story are, unfortunately, too often lost along the way. In our adult eagerness to have children understand "the way the world really works," we sometimes forget that literature is itself an authentic and essential way of knowing through feeling, which is just as critical to today's life as scientific knowledge.[61]

This urge to treat science as the main source of information about life's processes can be particularly limiting for children when they are asked to focus their attention on matters of health and illness, for science may divorce these matters from a human context, which is the element that helps to make concepts and life's experiences concrete for children. Like all the other arts, literature allows us to view well-being and sickness as human conditions that involve and affect the whole person. For children as for adults, literature relates information, attitudes, and decisions about health to daily life.

Unless children have access to many different kinds of books, literature's rewards will be unavailable to them. The adults with whom children live and work can make literature accessible to them by knowing and recommending many good books, by providing ample opportunities for them to express and explore their thoughts and feelings about the books they like and dislike, and by creating a wholesome, supportive environment for reading, learning, and relating where children will feel safe and respected, where their opinions, concerns, and interests are genuinely welcomed and valued, and where they can freely choose or reject books. In *The Hurried Child,* David Elkind gives some reasons for the need to provide such opportunities for all children:

But education—true education—is coincident with life
and is not limited to special skills or concepts and
particularly not to test scores. True education does not
come packaged or sequenced. Much of it is spontaneous, an outgrowth of openness and curiosity. It is this
attitude toward learning, this openness to questioning
and curiosity that parents need to impart to their
children.[62]

NOTES

1. Betsy Hearne, *Choosing Books for Children* (New York: Laurel, 1981),
   p. 7.
2. Paul Hazard, *Books, Children and Men* (Boston: Horn Book, 1944),
   p. 49.
3. For several authors who make such claims, see Dorothy Butler, *Cushla
   and Her Books* (Boston: Horn Book, 1980); David Elkind, *The Hurried
   Child* (Reading, MA: Addison-Wesley, 1981); and Denny Taylor and
   Dorothy S. Strickland, *Family Storybook Reading* (Portsmouth, NH:
   Heinemann, 1986).
4. Jim Trelease, *The Read-Aloud Handbook,* rev. ed. (New York: Philomel, 1985), p. 27.
5. Jim Trelease, "Introduction," in *Once Upon a Time . . .* (New York:
   Putnam, 1986), p. 11.
6. Zena Sutherland and May Hill Arbuthnot, *Children and Books,* 7th ed.
   (Glenview, IL: Scott, Foresman, 1986), p. 42.
7. Lillian Smith, *The Unreluctant Years* (New York: Viking, 1967), p. 37.
8. Hearne, *Choosing Books for Children,* pp. 92–93.
9. Bruno Bettelheim, *The Uses of Enchantment* (New York: Knopf,
   1976).
10. David Anspaugh, Gene Ezell, and Karen Nash Goodman, *Teaching
    Today's Health,* 2d ed. (Columbus, OH: Merrill, 1987), pp. 259–75.
11. Cited in Jane Yolen, *Touch Magic* (New York: Philomel, 1981), p. 49.
12. Sheila A. Egoff, *Thursday's Child: Trends and Patterns in Contemporary
    Children's Literature* (Chicago: American Library Association, 1981),
    p. 80.
13. Jane Yolen, *Writing Books for Children,* rev. ed. (Boston: The Writer,
    1983), p. 54.
14. Anthony L. Manna and Sue Misheff, "What Teachers Say About Their
    Own Reading Development," *Journal of Reading* 31 (October 1987):
    160–68.
15. Rebecca Lukens, *A Critical Handbook of Children's Literature,* 3d ed.
    (Glenview, IL: Scott, Foresman, 1986), p. 113.
16. Yolen, *Writing Books for Children,* p. 72.
17. Nicholas Tucker, *The Child and the Book: A Psychological and Literary*

Exploration (Cambridge: Cambridge University Press, 1981), pp. 62–66; 100–104.

18. Bettelheim, *Uses of Enchantment*, p. 46.
19. Ibid., p. 47.
20. Yolen, *Writing Books for Children*, pp. 92–93.
21. Sutherland and Arbuthnot, *Children and Books*, p. 332.
22. Lukens, *A Critical Handbook of Children's Literature*, p. 111.
23. Sutherland and Arbuthnot, *Children and Books*, p. 333.
24. For an overview of this holistic approach to health, see *The Holistic Health Movement* by Kristine Beyerman Alster (University of Alabama Press, 1989). Holistic medical practice has been described in *Minding the Body, Mending the Mind* by Joan Borysenko, M.D. (Addison-Wesley, 1986) and *Love, Medicine, and Miracles* by Bernie Siegel, M.D. (Harper and Row, 1986). For a journal which regularly discusses personal holistic health management, see *Medical Self-Care Magazine*, P.O. Box 1000, Point Reyes, CA 94956.
25. Wallace E. Lambert and Otto Klineberg, *Children's Views of Foreign People: A Cross-National Study* (New York: Appleton-Century-Crofts, 1967).
26. J. DeWolf and E. Jack, "Weight Control in Adolescent Girls," *Journal of School Health* 54 (October 1984): 347–49.
27. Charlotte S. Huck, Susan Hepler, and Janet Hickman, *Children's Literature in the Elementary School*, 4th ed. (New York: Holt, Rinehart and Winston, 1987), p. 465.
28. Geoffrey Trease, "The Historical Novelist at Work," in *Writers, Critics, and Children*, eds. Geoff Fox, et al. (New York: Agathon Press, 1976), p. 40.
29. Geoffrey Trease, *Writers, Critics, and Children*, p. 44.
30. Arthur Schlesinger, "The Cycles of American History," speech given at the Midland Center for the Arts, Midland, MI, 12 July 1987.
31. Elie Wiesel, "What Really Makes Us Free," *Parade Magazine*, Dec. 27, 1987, p. 6.
32. Laurence Perrine, *Sound and Sense*, 2d ed (New York: Harcourt, Brace and World, 1963), p. 9.
33. Alethea Helbig, "Maybe the Gallows, But Not a Tin Ear," *The ALAN Review* 14 (Spring 1987): 4–7.
34. Manna and Misheff, "What Teachers Say About Their Own Reading Development," pp. 160–68.
35. Lee Bennett Hopkins, *Pass the Poetry Please!* rev. ed. (New York: Harper and Row, 1987), p. 11.
36. Amy Anderson McClure, "Children's Responses to Poetry in a Supportive Literary Context," (Ph.D. dissertation, The Ohio State University, 1985).
37. Rebecca Lukens, *A Critical Handbook of Children's Literature*, p. 195.
38. Laurence Perrine, *Sound and Sense*, p. 10.
39. Ibid., p. 54.
40. Donna Norton, *Through the Eyes of a Child* (Columbus, OH: Merrill, 1983), p. 328.

41. Carol Fisher and Margaret Natarella, "Young Children's Preferences in Poetry: A National Survey of First, Second, and Third Graders," *Research in the Teaching of English* 16 (Dec. 1982): 339–54.

42. Ann Terry, *Children's Poetry Preferences: A National Survey of the Upper Elementary Grades,* 2d ed. (Urbana, IL: National Council of Teachers of English, 1984). See also Amy Anderson McClure, "Children's Responses," and Chow Loy Tom, "Paul Revere Rides Ahead: Poems Teachers Read to Pupils in the Middle Grades," *The Library Quarterly* 43 (Jan. 1973): 27–38.

43. Amy Anderson McClure, "Children's Responses to Poetry in a Supportive Literary Context," p. 331.

44. Jim Trelease, "Introduction," in *Read-Aloud Rhymes for the Very Young,* Jack Prelutsky, sel. Illustrated by Marc Brown (New York: Knopf, 1986), p. 1.

45. Cited in Jo Carr, "The Literature of Fact," *The Horn Book Magazine* 62 (Oct. 1981): 514.

46. Jo Carr, "The Literature of Fact," p. 515.

47. Sutherland and Arbuthnot, *Children and Books,* p. 440.

48. These claims are discussed in the following: Richard C. Anderson, et al., *Becoming a Nation of Readers:The Report of the Commission on Reading* (Champaign, IL: Center for the Study of Reading, 1985); Nancie Atwell, *In the Middle* (Portsmouth, NH: Heinemann Educational Books, 1987); Daniel Fader, *Hooked on Books* (New York: Berkley, 1966); Anthony L. Manna and Sue Misheff, "What Teachers Say About Their Own Reading Development," *Journal of Reading* 31 (Oct. 1987): 160–68; Gordon Wells, *The Meaning Makers* (Portsmouth, NH: Heinemann Educational Books, 1986); and Regie Routman, *Transitions. From Literature to Literacy* (Portsmouth, NH: Heinemann Educational Books, 1988).

49. Anderson, et al., *Becoming a Nation of Readers,* pp. 76–78.

50. Ibid., p. 15.

51. C. Fisher, et al., *Teaching and Learning in Elementary Schools: A Summary of the Beginning Teacher Evaluation Study* (San Francisco: Far West Regional Laboratory for Educational Research and Development, 1978), p. 124.

52. Patrick Shannon, *Broken Promises. Reading Instruction in Twentieth-Century America* (Granby, MA: Bergin and Garvey, 1989), p. 38.

53. Anderson, et al., *Becoming a Nation of Readers,* pp. 75–76.

54. John Goodlad, *A Place Called School* (New York: McGraw-Hill, 1984), p. 125.

55. L. G. Fielding, et al., "A New Focus on Free Reading: The Role of Trade Books in Reading Instruction," in *Contexts of Literacy,* ed. T. E. Reynolds and R. Reynolds (New York: Longman, 1990).

56. Cited in Nancie Atwell, *In the Middle,* p. 153.

57. Jonathan Kozol, *Illiterate America* (Garden City, NY: Anchor Press/Doubleday, 1985), p. 4.

58. Concerning items one and two, see Amy Anderson McClure, "Children's Responses to Poetry in a Supportive Literary Context" (Ph.D.

dissertation, The Ohio State University, 1985) and Barbara Kiefer, "The Responses of Primary Children to Picture Books" (Ph.D. dissertation, The Ohio State University, 1982). For examples of young children's interactions with complex literature, see Gayle Goodman, "James' Grandfathers," *Language Arts* 64 (Jan. 1987): 40–53; Nina Mikkelsen, "The Power of Story," *Language Arts* 64 (Jan. 1987): 61–72; and Dorothy Butler, *Cushla and Her Books* (Boston: The Horn Book, 1980). Good sources concerning the role of gender and ability are Alan Purves and Richard Beach, *Literature and the Reader: Research in Response to Literature, Reading Interests, and the Teaching of Literature* (Urbana, IL: National Council of Teachers of English, 1972); David Russell, *Children Learn to Read* (Boston: Ginn, 1961); and, from a different perspective, Elizabeth Segel, "Choices 'For Girls'/'For Boys': Keeping the Options Open," *School Library Journal* 28 (Mar. 1982): 105–107. Information regarding item six can be found in Barbara Kiefer, "The Responses of Primary Children to Picture Books." A developmental perspective is discussed in Andre Favat, *Child and Tale: The Origins of Interest* (Urbana, IL: National Council of Teachers of English, 1977) and Nicholas Tucker, *The Child and the Book: A Psychological and Literary Exploration* (Cambridge: Cambridge University Press, 1981). Items eight, nine, and ten are discussed in Sam Leaton Sebesta, "What Do Young People Think About the Literature They Read?" *Reading Newsletter* 8 (1979).

59. Sam Leaton Sebesta, "What Do Young People Think About the Literature They Read?" p. 32.
60. Sam Leaton Sebesta, "Choosing Poetry," in *Children's Choices,* eds. Nancy Roser and Margaret Firth (Newark, DE: International Reading Association, 1983).
61. Kay E. Vandergrift, *Child and Story: The Literary Connection* (New York: Neal-Schuman, 1980), p. 7.
62. David Elkind, *The Hurried Child* (Reading, MA: Addison-Wesley, 1981), p. 67.

CHILDREN'S BOOKS CITED IN CHAPTER 3*

Introduction

Donovan, John. *I'll Get There, It Better Be Worth the Trip.* Harper & Row, 1969.
•Krementz, Jill. *How It Feels When a Parent Dies.* Knopf, 1981.
•———. *How It Feels When Parents Divorce.* Knopf, 1984.

---

*Unless otherwise indicated, in all books cited, the author is also the illustrator. A bullet (•) denotes those books that depict multicultural experiences.

Lindgren, Astrid. *Pippi Longstocking.* Translated by Florence Lamborn. Illus. Louis S. Glanzman. Viking, 1950.
•Maruki, Toshi. *Hiroshima No Pika.* Lothrop, 1980.
Sendak, Maurice. *Outside Over There.* Harper & Row, 1981.
Seuss, Dr. *The Butter Battle Book.* Random House, 1984.
Shulevitz, Uri. *Dawn.* Farrar, Straus, 1971.
Silverstein, Alvin, and Silverstein, Virginia B. *Heartbeats: Your Body, Your Heart.* Harper & Row, 1983.
Smith, Doris Buchanan. *Return to Bitter Creek.* Viking Kestrel, 1986.

Folktales

"The Ash Lad Who Had an Eating Match With the Troll." In *Favorite Folktales From Around the World.* Edited by Jane Yolen. Pantheon, 1986.
Beauty and the Beast. Deborah Apy, reteller. Illus. Michael Hague. Henry Holt, 1983.
"Being Greedy Chokes Anansi." In *Favorite Folktales From Around the World.* Edited by Jane Yolen. Pantheon, 1986.
The Bun: A Tale from Russia. Marcia Brown. Harcourt, 1972.
"The Corn in the Rock." In *The Monkey's Haircut and Other Stories Told by the Maya.* Edited by John Bierhorst. Illus. Robert Andrew Parker. Morrow, 1986.
The Crane Wife. Sumiko Yagawa. Illus. Suekicki Akaba. Morrow, 1981.
dePaola, Tomie. *Strega Nona.* Prentice-Hall, 1975.
"The Enormous Genie." In *Three Apples Fell from Heaven, Armenian Tales Retold.* Virginia Tashjian. Illus. Nonny Hogrogian. Little, Brown, 1971.
The Funny Little Woman. Arlene Mosel. Illus. Blair Lent. Dutton, 1972.
The Gingerbread Boy. Paul Galdone. Seabury, 1975.
Hansel and Gretel. Rika Lesser, reteller. Illus. Paul O. Zelinsky. Dodd, Mead, 1984.
Hans in Luck. Grimm Brothers. Illus. Felix Hoffman. Atheneum, 1975.
"How the Peasant Helped His Horse." In *Three Rolls and One Doughnut: Fables from Russia.* Mirra Ginsburg. Illus. Anita Lobel. Dial, 1970.
Jack and the Wonder Beans. James Still. Illus. Margot Tomes. Putnam, 1977.
"The King of Ireland's Son." In *Favorite Folktales From Around the World.* Edited by Jane Yolen. Pantheon, 1986.
"The Lad Who Went to the North Wind." In *East of the Sun and West of the Moon, and Other Tales.* Peter Christian Asbjornsen and Jorgen E. Moe. Illus. Tom Vroman. Macmillan, 1963.
Little Red Riding Hood. Paul Galdone. McGraw-Hill, 1974.
The Magic Cooking Pot. Faith Towle. Houghton Mifflin, 1975.
"The Magic Pear Tree." In *Favorite Folktales From Around the World.* Edited by Jane Yolen. Pantheon, 1986.
The Magic Porridge Pot. Paul Galdone. Clarion, 1976.
"The Marvelous Pear Seed." In *Tales the People Tell in China.* Robert Wyndham. Illus. Jay Yang. Messner, 1971.

"The Pancake." In *The Scott, Foresman Anthology of Children's Literature.*
    Zena Sutherland and Myra Cohn Livingston. Scott, Foresman, 1984.
Rapunzel. Barbara Rogasky. Illus. Trina Schart Hyman. Holiday House,
    1982.
Rumpelstiltskin. Donna Diamond, reteller. Holiday House, 1983.
Sawyer, Ruth. *Journey Cake, Ho!* Illus. Robert McCloskey. Viking, 1953.
Snow White and the Seven Dwarfs. Translated by Randall Jarrell. Illus.
    Nancy Ekholm Burkert. Farrar, Straus and Giroux, 1972.
"The Talking Fish." In *Once There Was and Was Not, Armenian Tales Retold.*
    Virginia Tashjian, reteller. Illus. Nonny Hogrogian. Little, Brown, 1966.
The Three Little Pigs. Paul Galdone. Seabury, 1970.
The Three Wishes. Paul Galdone. McGraw-Hill, 1961.
The Three Wishes. Margot Zemach. Farrar, Straus and Giroux, 1986.
Tom Tit Tot. Joseph Jacobs. Illus. Evaline Ness. Scribner's, 1965.
"The Wee Bannock." In *English Fairy Tales.* Flora Annie Steel. Illus.
    Arthur Rackham. Macmillan, 1962.
The Wolf and the Seven Little Kids. Grimm Brothers. Translated by Anne
    Rogers. Illus. Otto S. Svend. Larousse, 1977.

Fantasy and Science Fiction

Andersen, Hans Christian. *The Ugly Duckling.* Trans. R. P. Keigwin. Illus.
    Adrienne Adams. Scribner's, 1965.
Bond, Michael. *A Bear Called Paddington.* Illus. Peggy Fortnum. Houghton
    Mifflin, 1960.
Bond, Nancy. *The Voyage Begun.* Atheneum, 1981.
Burton, Virginia Lee. *The Little House.* Houghton Mifflin, 1942.
Engdahl, Sylvia Louise. *The Far Side of Evil.* Illus. Richard Cuffari.
    Atheneum, 1971.
Erickson, Russell E. *Warton and the Castaways.* Illus. Lawrence DiFiori.
    Lothrop, 1982.
Grahame, Kenneth. *The Wind in the Willows.* Illus. E. H. Shepard.
    Scribner's, 1940.
Hoban, Russell. *A Baby Sister for Frances.* Illus. Lillian Hoban. Harper &
    Row, 1964.
————. *A Bargain for Frances.* Illus. Lillian Hoban. Harper & Row, 1970.
————. *Bedtime for Frances.* Illus. Garth Williams. Harper & Row, 1960.
————. *A Birthday for Frances.* Illus. Lillian Hoban. Harper & Row, 1968.
————. *Bread and Jam for Frances.* Illus. Lillian Hoban. Harper & Row,
    1964.
Hoover, H. M. *This Time of Darkness.* Viking, 1980.
Lobel, Arnold. *Frog and Toad Together.* Harper & Row, 1972.
McCully, Emily Arnold. *First Snow.* Harper & Row, 1985.
————. *Picnic.* Harper & Row, 1985.
Marshall, James. *Yummers!* Houghton Mifflin, 1973.
————. *Yummers Too.* Houghton Mifflin, 1986.

Merrill, Jean. *The Pushcart War*. Illus. Ronni Solbert. W. R. Scott, 1964.
O'Brien, Robert C. *Mrs. Frisby and the Rats of NIMH*. Illus. Zena
   Bernstein. Atheneum, 1971.
————. *Z for Zachariah*. Atheneum, 1975.
Pinkwater, Daniel M. *Attila the Pun*. Four Winds, 1981.
————. *Fat Men From Space*. Dodd, Mead, 1977.
————. *The Magic Moscow*. Four Winds, 1980.
————. *Slaves of Spiegel*. Four Winds, 1982.
Potter, Beatrix. *The Tale of Peter Rabbit*. Warne, 1902.
Rodgers, Mary. *Freaky Friday*. Harper & Row, 1972.
————. *Summer Switch*. Harper & Row, 1982.
Selden, George. *The Cricket in Times Square*. Illus. Garth Williams. Farrar,
   Straus and Giroux, 1960.
Sendak, Maurice. *Where the Wild Things Are*. Harper & Row, 1963.
Seuss, Dr. *The Five Hundred Hats of Bartholomew Cubbins*. Vanguard, 1938.
White, E. B. *Charlotte's Web*. Illus. Garth Williams. Harper & Row, 1952.
Williams, Margery. *The Velveteen Rabbit*. Illus. William Nicholson. Dou-
   bleday, 1922. Illus. Alan Atkinson. Knopf, 1983. Illus. Michael Hague.
   Holt, 1983. Illus. Ilse Plume. Godine, 1983.
Wrightson, Patricia. *The Dark Bright Water*. Atheneum, 1979.
————. *The Ice Is Coming*. Atheneum, 1977.
————. *Journey Behind the Wind*. Atheneum, 1981.

Realistic Fiction

Alexander, Martha. *Nobody Asked Me If I Wanted a Baby Sister*. Dial, 1971.
————. *When the New Baby Comes, I'm Moving Out*. Dial, 1979.
Alexander, Sue. *Nadia the Willful*. Illus. Lloyd Bloom. Pantheon, 1983.
•Andrews, Jan. *Very Last First Time*. Illus. Ian Wallace. Atheneum, 1986.
Byars, Betsy. *After the Goat Man*. Illus. Ronald Himler. Viking, 1974.
Cleary, Beverly. *Ramona and Her Mother*. Illus. Alan Tiegreen. Morrow,
   1979.
DeClements, Barthe. *How Do You Lose Those Ninth Grade Blues?* Viking,
   1983.
————. *Nothing's Fair in Fifth Grade*. Viking, 1981.
•dePaola, Tomie. *Watch Out for the Chicken Feet in Your Soup*. Prentice-
   Hall, 1974.
•Friedman, Ina R. *How My Parents Learned to Eat*. Illus. Allen Say.
   Houghton Mifflin, 1984.
Froelich, Margaret Walden. *Reasons To Stay*. Houghton Mifflin, 1984.
•Greenfield, Eloise. *She Come Bringing Me That Little Baby Girl*. Illus. John
   Steptoe. Harper & Row, 1974.
Hall, Lynn. *The Solitary*. Scribner's, 1986.
•Hamilton, Virginia. *A Little Love*. Philomel, 1984.
Kerr, M. E. *Dinky Hocker Shoots Smack*. Harper & Row, 1972.
Lipsyte, Robert. *One Fat Summer*. Harper & Row, 1977.

Lowry, Lois. *Anastasia Krupnik.* Houghton Mifflin, 1979.
————. *A Summer to Die.* Illus. Jenni Oliver. Houghton Mifflin, 1977.
Radley, Gail. *CF in His Corner.* Four Winds, 1984.
Roy, Ron. *Breakfast With My Father.* Illus. Troy Howell. Houghton Mifflin, 1980.
Rylant, Cynthia. *The Relatives Came.* Illus. Stephen Gammell. Bradbury, 1985.
Viorst, Judith. *Alexander and the Terrible, Horrible, No Good, Very Bad Day.* Illus. Ray Cruz. Atheneum, 1972.
Vogel, Ilse-Margaret. *My Twin Sister Erika.* Harper & Row, 1976.
Wersba, Barbara. *Fat, A Love Story.* Harper & Row, 1987.
————. *Love Is the Crooked Thing.* Harper & Row, 1988.
Williams, Vera B. *The Great Giant Watermelon Birthday.* Greenwillow, 1980.
Zolotow, Charlotte. *Timothy Too!* Illus. Ruth Robbins. Houghton Mifflin, 1986.

Historical Fiction

Aaron, Chester. *Lackawanna.* Lippincott, 1986.
Aliki. *A Medieval Feast.* Crowell, 1983.
Collier, James Lincoln, and Collier, Christopher. *My Brother Sam Is Dead.* Four Winds, 1974.
Conrad, Pam. *Prairie Songs.* Harper & Row, 1985.
Forbes, Esther. *Johnny Tremain.* Illus. Lynd Ward. Houghton Mifflin, 1946.
•Fox, Paula. *The Slave Dancer.* Illus. Eros Keith. Bradbury, 1973.
Hall, Donald. *The Ox-Cart Man.* Illus. Barbara Cooney. Viking, 1979.
•Harvey, Brett. *Immigrant Girl.* Illus. Deborah Kogan Ray. Holiday House, 1987.
————. *My Prairie Year.* Illus. Deborah Kogan Ray. Holiday House, 1986.
Lasker, Joe. *Merry Ever After.* Viking, 1976.
•Orlev, Uri. *The Island on Bird Street.* Translated by Hillel Halkin. Houghton Mifflin, 1984.
Trease, Geoffrey. *Mist Over Athelney.* Illus. R. S. Sherriffs and J. L. Stockle. London: Macmillan, 1958; as *Escape to King Alfred.* Vanguard Press, 1958.
Wilder, Laura Ingalls. *By the Shores of Silver Lake.* Illus. Garth Williams. Harper & Row, 1953.
————. *The First Four Years.* Illus. Garth Williams. Harper & Row, 1971.
————. *Little House in the Big Woods.* Illus. Garth Williams. Harper & Row, 1953.
————. *Little House on the Prairie.* Illus. Garth Williams. Harper & Row, 1953.
————. *Little Town on the Prairie.* Illus. Garth Williams. Harper & Row, 1953.

————. *On the Banks of Plum Creek*. Illus. Garth Williams. Harper & Row, 1953.

————. *Those Happy Golden Years*. Illus. Garth Williams. Harper & Row, 1953.

Poetry

Adoff, Arnold. *Eats*. Illus. Susan Russo. Lothrop, 1979.

Agree, Rose H. *How To Eat a Poem and Other Morsels*. Illus. Peggy Wilson. Pantheon, 1967.

Aldis, Dorothy. *Is Anybody Hungry?* Illus. Artur Marokvia. Putnam, 1964.

Brandenberg, Franz. *Fresh Cider and Pie*. Illus. Aliki. Macmillan, 1973.

Charlip, Remy, and Supree, Burton. *Mother Mother I Feel Sick Send for the Doctor Quick Quick Quick*. Illus. Remy Charlip. Parents, 1966.

Cole, William, compiler. *Poem Stew*. Illus. Karen Ann Weinhaus. Harper & Row, 1983.

Degen, Bruce. *Jamberry*. Harper & Row, 1983.

Dunning, Stephen; Leuders, Edward; and Smith, Hugh. *Reflections on a Gift of Watermelon Pickle and Other Modern Verses*. Scott, Foresman, 1966.

Ferris, Helen, ed. *Favorite Poems Old and New*. Illus. Leonard Weisgard. Doubleday, 1957.

Fisher, Aileen. *Out in the Dark and Daylight*. Illus. Gail Owens. Harper & Row, 1980.

Froman, Robert. *Seeing Things*. Crowell, 1974.

Froman, Robert. *Street Poems*. Dutton, 1971.

•Greenfield, Eloise. *Honey, I Love*. Illus. Leo and Diane Dillon. Harper & Row, 1978.

Hearn, Michael Patrick, compiler. *Breakfast, Books, and Dreams*. Illus. Barbara Garrison. Warne, 1981.

Hoban, Russell. *Egg Thoughts and Other Frances Songs*. Illus. Lillian Hoban. Harper & Row, 1972.

Holman, Felice. *At the Top of My Voice and Other Poems*. Scribner's, 1970.

Hopkins, Lee Bennett, compiler. *Munching*. Illus. Nelle Davis. Little, Brown, 1985.

•Hughes, Langston. *Selected Poems of Langston Hughes*. Knopf, 1954.

Kuskin, Karla. *The Rose on My Cake*. Harper & Row, 1964.

Livingston, Myra Cohn. *The Way Things Are and Other Poems*. Illus. Jenni Oliver. Atheneum, 1974.

Lobel, Arnold. *The Random House Book of Mother Goose*. Random House, 1986.

Mandry, Kathy, and Toto, Joe. *How to Make Elephant Bread*. Pantheon, 1971.

Merriam, Eve. *Finding a Poem*. Illus. Seymour Chwast. Atheneum, 1970.

————. *It Doesn't Always Have to Rhyme*. Illus. Malcolm Spooner. Atheneum, 1964.

•Morrison, Lillian. *The Sidewalk Racer and Other Poems of Sports and Motion*. Lothrop, 1977.

Patz, Nancy. *Pumpernickel Tickle and Mean Green Cheese*. Watts, 1978.
Pomerantz, Charlotte. *Whiff, Sniff, Nibble and Chew: The Gingerbread Boy Retold*. Illus. Monica Incisa. Greenwillow, 1984.
Prelutsky, Jack. *The New Kid on the Block*. Illus. James Stevenson. Greenwillow, 1984.
————, editor. *The Random House Book of Poetry for Children*. Illus. Arnold Lobel. Random House, 1983.
————, compiler. *Read-Aloud Rhymes for the Very Young*. Illus. Marc Brown. Knopf, 1986.
Sendak, Maurice. *Chicken Soup With Rice*. Harper & Row, 1962.
Silverstein, Shel. *A Light in the Attic*. Harper & Row, 1981.
————. *Where the Sidewalk Ends*. Harper & Row, 1974.
Smith, William Jay. *Laughing Time*. Illus. Fernando Krahn. Delacorte, 1980.
•Sutherland, Zena, and Livingston, Myra Cohn. *The Scott, Foresman Anthology of Children's Literature*. Scott, Foresman, 1984.
•Turner, Ann. *Street Talk*. Illus. Catherine Stock. Houghton Mifflin, 1986.
Wallner, Alexander. *Munch*. Crown, 1976.
Watson, Clyde. *Father Fox's Pennyrhymes*. Illus. Wendy Watson. Crowell, 1971.

Informational Books

Aho, Jennifer S., and Petras, John W. *Learning About Sexual Abuse*. Enslow, 1985.
•Aliki. *Corn Is Maize*. Harper & Row, 1976.
•Ancona, George. *It's a Baby*. Dutton, 1979.
Anderson, Gretchen. *The Louisa May Alcott Cookbook*. Illus. Karen Milone. Little, Brown, 1985.
Arnold, Caroline. *Too Fat? Too Thin? Do You Have a Choice?* Morrow, 1984.
Bershad, Carol, and Bernick, Deborah. *Bodyworks*. Illus. Heidi Selig. Random House, 1981.
Berger, Melvin, and Berger, Gilda. *The Good Food Book*. Illus. Byron Barton. Crowell, 1978.
Berger, Melvin. *Why I Cough, Sneeze, Shiver, Hiccup, and Yawn*. Illus. Holly Keller. Harper & Row, 1983.
Bisignano, Alfonse. *Cooking the Italian Way*. Photographs by Robert and Diane Wolfe. Illus. Jeanette Swofford. Lerner, 1982.
Bowe-Gutman, Sonia. *Teen Pregnancy*. Lerner, 1987.
Burningham, John. *The Shopping Basket*. Crowell, 1980.
Burns, Marilyn. *Good for Me!* Illus. Sandy Clifford. Little, Brown, 1978.
Cole, Joanna. *How You Were Born*. Illustrated with photographs by Hella Hammid. Morrow, 1984.
————. *The New Baby at Your House*. Illustrated with photographs by Hella Hammid. Morrow, 1985.

dePaola, Tomie. *The Popcorn Book*. Holiday House, n.d.; Scholastic, 1978.

Dobrin, Arnold. *Peter Rabbit's Natural Foods Cookbook*. Illus. Beatrix Potter. Warne, 1977.

Dragonwagon, Crescent. *Wind Rose*. Illus. Ronald Himler. Harper & Row, 1976.

Ehlert, Lois. *Growing Vegetable Soup*. Harcourt, 1987.

Erlanger, Ellen. *Eating Disorders*. Lerner, 1988.

George, Jean Craighead. *One Day in the Alpine Tundra*. Illus. Walter Gaffney-Kessell. Harper & Row, 1984.

Giblin, James Cross. *From Hand to Mouth: Or, How We Invented Knives, Forks, Spoons, & Chopsticks, & the Table Manners to Go With Them*. Crowell, 1987.

————. *Milk*. Crowell, 1986.

Gilbert, Sara. *Fat Free: Common Sense Guide for Young Weight Worriers*. Macmillan, 1975.

Haskins, James. *Who Are the Handicapped?* Doubleday, 1978.

Hyde, Margaret O., and Forsyth, Elizabeth H. *AIDS: What Does It Mean to You?*, rev. ed. M. D. Walker, 1987.

————. *Cry Softly! The Story of Child Abuse*. Westminster, 1980.

————. *Know About Smoking*. Illus. Dennis Kendrick. McGraw-Hill, 1983.

————. *Mind Drugs*, 5th ed. Dodd, Mead, 1986.

————. *Sexual Abuse: Let's Talk About It*, rev. ed. Westminster, 1987.

Johnson, Eric W. *Love and Sex in Plain Language*, 4th ed. Harper & Row, 1985.

Kitzinger, Sheila. *Being Born*. Illus. Lennart Nilsson. Grosset & Dunlap, 1986.

•Krementz, Jill. *How It Feels When Parents Divorce*. Knopf, 1984.

Krensky, Stephen. *Scoop After Scoop*. Illus. Richard Rosenblum. Atheneum, 1986.

Landau, Elaine. *Sexually Transmitted Diseases*. Enslow, 1986.

Langone, John. *Dead End: A Book About Suicide*. Little, Brown, 1986.

Lasky, Kathryn. *A Baby for Max*. Illustrated with photographs by Christopher G. Knight. Scribner's, 1984.

Lauber, Patricia. *Too Much Garbage*. Garrard, 1974.

Lerner, Ethan A. *Understanding AIDS*. Illus. Mark Wilken. Lerner, 1987. (Also available in Spanish language edition.)

LeShan, Eda. *When a Parent Is Very Sick*. Atlantic, 1986.

Lukes, Bonnie. *How to Be a Reasonably Thin Teenage Girl*. Illus. Carol Nicklaus. Atheneum, 1986.

McMillan, Bruce. *Apples, How They Grow*. Houghton Mifflin, 1979.

Martin, Liz. *Little Chef Series*. Viking Kestrel, 1986.

Meltzer, Milton. *The American Revolutionaries*. Crowell, 1987.

Miller, Jonathan, and Pelham, David. *The Facts of Life*. Illus. Harry Willock. Viking, 1984.

Nourse, Alan E. *Menstruation: Just Plain Talk*. Watts, 1980.

Ontario Science Centre. *Foodworks*. Addison-Wesley, 1987.

Perl, Lila. *Junk Food, Fast Food, Health Food: What America Eats and Why*. Clarion, 1980.

————. *Hunter's Stew and Hangtown Fry: What Pioneer America Ate and Why.* Illus. Richard Cuffari. Seabury, 1977.

————. *Slumps, Grunts, and Snickerdoodles: What Colonial America Ate and Why.* Illus. Richard Cuffari. Clarion, 1975.

Pringle, Laurence. *Death Is Natural.* Four Winds, 1979.

Rockwell, Anne, and Rockwell, Harlow. *Happy Birthday to Me.* Macmillan, 1981.

Seixas, Judith S. *Vitamins—What They Are, What They Do.* Illus. Tom Huffman. Greenwillow, 1986.

Selsam, Millicent. *All About Eggs.* Illus. Stephanie Fleischer. Addison-Wesley, 1980.

————. *The Apple and Other Fruits.* Illustrated with photographs by Jerome Wexler. Morrow, 1973.

————. *The Growth of the Potato.* Illus. Ben Shecter. Harper & Row, 1972.

————. *Popcorn.* Illustrated with photographs by Jerome Wexler. Morrow, 1976.

Showers, Paul. *You Can't Make a Move Without Your Muscles.* Harper & Row, 1982.

Silverstein, Alvin, and Silverstein, Virginia B. *AIDS: Deadly Threat.* Enslow, 1986.

————. *The Skeletal System: Framework for Life.* Illus. Lee J. Ames. Prentice-Hall, 1972.

•Siska, Heather Smith. *People of the Ice.* Illus. Ian Bateson. Douglas and McIntyre, 1980.

Sobol, Harriet. *A Book of Vegetables.* Dodd, Mead, 1984.

Terkel, Susan Neiburg, and Rench, Janice E. *Feeling Safe, Feeling Strong.* Lerner, 1984.

Titherington, Jeanne. *Pumpkin Pumpkin.* Greenwillow, 1986.

Wachter, Oralee. *Close to Home.* Scholastic, 1986.

————. *No More Secrets for Me.* Illus. Jane Aaron. Little, Brown, 1983.

Walker, Barbara M. *Little House Cookbook.* Illus. Garth Williams. Harper & Row, 1979.

Biography

Aaseng, Nathan. *The Disease Fighters.* Lerner, 1987.

————. *The Inventors.* Lerner, 1988.

•————. *Winners Never Quit: Athletes Who Beat the Odds.* Lerner, 1980.

•Aliki. *A Weed Is a Flower, The Life of George Washington Carver.* Prentice-Hall, 1965.

————. *The Story of Johnny Appleseed.* Prentice-Hall, 1963.

Ancona, George. *Growing Older.* Dutton, 1978.

Bonderoff, Jason. *Alan Alda: An Unauthorized Biography.* New American Library, 1982.

•Brown, Marion Marsh. *Homeward the Arrow's Flight.* Abingdon, 1980.

Cesarani, Gian Paolo. *Christopher Columbus*. Illus. Piero Ventura. Random House, 1979.

•Coerr, Eleanor. *Sadako and the Thousand Paper Cranes*. Illus. Ronald Himler. Putnam, 1977.

Dines, Glen. *John Muir*. Putnam, 1974.

•Freedman, Russell. *Lincoln: A Photobiography*. Clarion, 1987.

Fritz, Jean. *And Then What Happened, Paul Revere?* Illus. Margot Tomes. Coward, McCann, 1973.

―――. *Where Do You Think You're Going, Christopher Columbus?* Illus. Margot Tomes. Putnam, 1980.

―――. *What's the Big Idea, Ben Franklin?* Illus. Margot Tomes. Coward, McCann, 1976.

•Greenfield, Eloise, and Little, Lessie Jones. *Childtimes: A Three-Generation Memoir*. Harper & Row, 1979.

Hunt, Mabel Leigh. *Better Known as Johnny Appleseed*. Illus. James Daugherty. Lippincott, 1950.

Hunter, Edith. *Child of the Silent Night*. Houghton Mifflin, 1963.

•Kherdian, David. *Deep River Run*. Illus. Nonny Hogrogian. Carolrhoda, 1984.

Knudson, R. R. *Martina Navratilova*. Illus. George Angelini. Viking Kestrel, 1986.

McCoy, J. J. *The Cancer Lady: Maud Slye and Her Heredity Studies*. Thomas Nelson, 1977.

Monjo, F.N. *Grand Papa and Ellen Aroon, Being an Account of Some of the Happy Times Spent Together by Thomas Jefferson and His Favorite Granddaughter*. Illus. Richard Cuffari. Holt, 1974.

―――. *Me and Willie and Pa*. Illus. Douglas Gorsline. Simon & Schuster, 1973.

―――. *The One Bad Thing About Father*. Illus. Rocco Negri. Harper & Row, 1970.

•Patterson, Lillie. *Sure Hands, Strong Heart: The Life of Daniel Hale Williams*. Abingdon, 1981.

Peavy, Linda, and Smith, Ursula. *Dreams into Deeds: Nine Women Who Dared*. Scribner's, 1985.

Ranahan, Demerris C. *Contributions of Women: Medicine*. Dillon, 1981.

Rylant, Cynthia. *But I'll Be Back Again*. Orchard, 1989.

Schoor, Gene. *Babe Didrikson: The World's Greatest Woman Athlete*. Doubleday, 1978.

Shiels, Barbara. *Winners: Women and the Nobel Prize*. Dillon, 1985.

Swift, Hildegarde Hoyt. *From the Eagle's Wing: A Biography of Jon Muir*. Morrow, 1962.

Vandivert, Rita. *To the Rescue: Seven Heroes of Conservation*. Warne, 1982.

Plays

Aiken, Joan. *Street*. Illus. Arvis Stewart. Viking, 1978.

Barr, June. *The Three Little Kittens*. In *Plays Children Love, Vol. II*. Edited by Coleman A. Jennings and Aurand Harris. St. Martin's, 1988.

Bedard, Roger L., ed. *Dramatic Literature for Children: A Century in Review.* Anchorage, 1984.

Benet, Stephen Vincent. *Johnny Pye and the Footkiller.* Readers Theatre Script Service, 1984.

Bond, Michael, and Bradley, Alfred. *Paddington on Stage.* Houghton Mifflin, 1977.

Bush, Max. *The Voyage of the Dragonfly.* Anchorage, 1989.

•Childress, Alice. *When the Rattlesnake Sounds.* Coward, McCann, 1975.

•Davis, Ossie. *Escape to Freedom.* Viking, 1976.

De Angeli, Marguerite. *The Door in the Wall.* Doubleday, 1969.

de Regniers, Beatrice. *Picture Book Theatre.* Clarion, 1982.

Gackenbach, Dick. *Hattie, Tom, and the Chicken Witch.* Harper & Row, 1980.

Harris, Aurand. *Androcles and the Lion.* Anchorage Press, 1964.

———. *The Arkansaw Bear.* Anchorage, 1980.

•Henderson, Nancy. *Walk Together.* Messner, 1972.

Jennings, Coleman A., and Harris, Aurand, eds. *Plays Children Love.* Illus. Susan Swann. Doubleday, 1981.

———. *Plays Children Love, Volume II.* St. Martin's, 1988.

•Jennings, Coleman A. and Berghammer, Gretta, eds. *Theatre for Youth: Twelve Plays with Mature Themes.* University of Texas, 1986.

Kral, Brian. *Apologies.* Anchorage, 1988.

———. *East of the Sun and West of the Moon.* Anchorage, 1987.

———. *Special Class.* Anchorage, 1981.

Kraus, Joanna Halpert. *The Ice Wolf.* New Plays, 1982.

•———. *Kimchi Kid.* New Plays, 1985.

Laurie, Rona. *Children's Plays from Beatrix Potter.* Warne, 1980.

Living Stage Theatre Company, 6th and Maine Avenue, S.W., Washington, DC 20024. *Suicide.*

Lysander, Per, and Osten, Suzanne. *Medea's Children.* Translated by Anne-Charlotte Harvey. New Plays, 1985.

Martin, Patricia Miles. *Two Plays about Foolish People.* Putnam, 1972.

Miller, Kathryn Schultz. *You Don't See Me.* Coach House, 1984.

Musil, Rosemary G. *Five Little Peppers.* Anchorage, 1940.

•Nolan, Paul T. *Folk Tale Plays from Round the World.* Plays, Inc., 1982.

Pearson-Davis, Susan, ed. *Wish in One Hand, Spit in the Other. A Collection of Plays by Suzan Zeder.* Anchorage, 1988.

Robinette, Joseph. *Charlotte's Web.* Dramatic Publishing, 1983.

Rockwell, Thomas. *How to Eat Fried Worms.* Delacorte, 1980.

Ross, Monica Long. *Wilma's Revenge.* Anchorage, 1989.

Smalley, Webster. *The Boy Who Talked to Whales.* Anchorage, 1980.

Still, James. *The Velveteen Rabbit.* Available from Emmy Gifford Children's Theatre, 3504 Center Street, Omaha, NE 68105.

Terry, Megan. *Family Talk.* Available from Omaha Magic Theatre, 1417 Farnam Street, Omaha, NE 68102.

•Winther, Barbara. *Plays from Folktales of Africa and Asia.* Plays, Inc., 1976.

Yost, Don. *Little Bear.* Bridgework Theater, 113½ East Lincoln Avenue, Goshen, IN 46526.

————. *Out of the Trap.* Bridgework Theater, 113½ East Lincoln Avenue, Goshen, IN 46526.
Young, Ruth. *Starring Francine and Dave.* Orchard, 1988.
Zeder, Suzan. *Ozma of Oz.* Anchorage, 1981.
————. *Wiley and the Hairy Man.* Anchorage, 1978.

4. Integrating Literature with the School Health Program

> Childhood has its own way of seeing, thinking, and feeling, and nothing is more foolish than to try to substitute ours for theirs.—*Jean-Jacques Rousseau*, **Emile**[1]

Literature's domain is human experience, and literature's intent is to awaken people of all ages to new or different ways of seeing themselves, the world, and others. Every encounter with meaningful literature is an invitation to explore significant human issues and examine the conditions, beliefs, and values which any type of well-written literature brings to light. Children, too, will have access to literature's rewards when the books they are encouraged to read reflect their interests and concerns, and contain accurate and honest perceptions of the human condition. Far from providing only an entertaining break from serious school tasks and the important business of life, literature has the potential to enhance learning, to motivate children to make valuable discoveries about life and living, and to encourage them to apply to their own lives the insights and understanding they gain from reading.

At a crucial time in a child's life, when habits, values, attitudes, and beliefs are being formed, a story, poem, informational book, or any other type of literature can reveal to the child a wide range of powerful truths about human experience. Some of these are:

• Personal and social dilemmas, problems, and conflicts are persistent aspects of the life process.

- Personal and social change, derived from reason as well as intuition, is possible.
- Although there are few easy or final solutions to the problems and dilemmas life poses, a person can discover effective ways to cope, heal, persevere, and exercise at least some control over his or her life.
- Alternatives and options are a law of life, as is the need to develop meaningful relationships and to survive.
- Intense feelings and thoughts are normal.
- The desire for trusting relationships is a basic human need.
- No experience is the same for everyone, and multiple interpretations and perspectives concerning human experience are natural.
- The urge to achieve a clear sense of personal identity is a life-long process.

Whenever children are encouraged to step back from a selection of literature they have read or heard in order to reflect on it, they can consider the issues which have surfaced, the recognitions and realizations the literature has evoked, and the insights they may have gained about the ways the writer or illustrator has captured and affirmed the pleasure or pain or mystery of some aspect of the situations through which people of all ages live out their lives. This capacity to reveal life's circumstances and to provide vital information about the physical, social, and emotional aspects of human growth and change aligns literature with the issues and concerns that ought to be at the heart of every health education program. Whether students are exploring the influence their peers can have on their behavior, effective ways to cope with stress, loss, and conflict, the nature of human relationships, community health problems, the causes and prevention of sexually transmitted diseases, or the consequences and characteristics of a healthful diet, literature endows health-related principles and concepts with human concern, human motivation, and human behavior. This, in turn, demonstrates how health issues truly influence a person's potential and performance.

In schools which consider the physical, psychological, emotional, and social well-being of students to be a primary concern and responsibility, children are not only provided

occasional opportunities to acquire health-related information and skills, but they also are given consistent, concrete,
and age-appropriate messages about health issues, ones they
need to be alerted to as well as ones that immediately concern
them. In schools like these, health education consists of much
more than a sequence of brief, isolated lessons that concen-
trate largely on publicized health crises or basic facts about
body systems and nutrition. Rather, the skills, attitudes, and
behaviors that contribute to health filter into each and every
aspect of school life, and the well-being of students—as well
as that of teachers and staff—becomes everyone's concern
each school day. Recent reports on various conditions which
currently affect the health of American children indicate the
kinds of real-life issues a comprehensive school health program might address:[2]

1. Approximately sixty percent of American children have used
   alcohol by eighth grade.
2. More than seventy percent of American teachers report that
   poor health and undernourishment cause significant problems
   for their students.
3. Mental disturbances and emotional disorders afflict approximately 7.5 million American youths; twelve percent of them
   are under the age of 18.
4. One out of seven adolescents has attempted suicide, the chief
   cause being depression.
5. The U.S. has the highest teenage birthrate in the Western
   world.
6. Two-and-a-half million teenagers in the U.S. contract sexually
   transmitted diseases annually.
7. More than half of all U.S. teenagers have had intercourse by
   the age of seventeen and less than half of these adolescents
   regularly use contraception.

In responding to the problems which many students face, the
Carnegie Corporation's Task Force on the Education of
Young Adolescents urges the schools to take a leadership role
in nurturing students' well-being. "If you're hungry, have an
abscessed tooth, or struggle with an emotional disorder," the
Task Force maintains, "your prospects of success in school lie
somewhere between remote and nonexistent."[3]

To have an impact on children, a school health program must offer direct instruction in health, but it also must move beyond the topics that are covered in health lessons and encompass other appropriate content areas if the goal of the program is to make students conscious of the decisions, conditions, and options that influence health. It is not only the need to impart cognitive information to children which must drive the health education program forward; subject matter competency without human understanding and a personal recognition of the importance of living healthfully will give children only half the picture. As children themselves pointed out in a recent study of the ways they handle stress,[4] cognitive activities do not head their list of coping behaviors. Rather, these children indicated that they first sought the support of friends and parents, or avoided or expressed their feelings before employing what the researchers called cognitive strategies, such as rationally figuring out what to do about the stressful situation and the feelings it called forth. Many of the children also indicated that the strategies they use are not very effective. It would seem then that, in addition to involving children in textbook lessons on ways to handle life's difficulties, they need to explore and evaluate various coping strategies as they unfold in specific human contexts. In this way, they can weigh options and repercussions, and examine the significance of behaviors, values, and attitudes.

Of the many content areas in a school curriculum which are likely to promote such awareness, literature holds particular promise. When teachers enrich health issues and concepts with various types of literature, they provide a "human-sense" context for the health-related experiences that directly concern or at least interest children. Given opportunities to consider the life issues, moral concerns, and themes that writers fathom, children can explore situations that either enhance or hinder healthful living. By framing these topics for inspection and reflection, literature has the capacity to help children make informed decisions about the many situations they or others may encounter or are actually confronting.

This chapter introduces a wide variety of literature that can alert children to many of the conditions that influence their health. In conjunction with brief profiles of children's characteristics at each stage in their development, the topics which constitute the Growing Healthy Curriculum served as a guide for selecting various types of literature that can reveal and give human shape to the different factors which affect physical, emotional, and social well-being.

BOOK SELECTION AND CHILDREN'S DEVELOPMENT

The task—and challenge—of selecting appropriate literature for children begins with a firm understanding of the characteristics children bring to the reading process at each stage in their development. A child will more likely be drawn into literature in a personal way and make sense of the experience when the situations and themes that the writer depicts are somehow related to the child's capabilities and interests and address his or her concerns and needs. The more we know about the characteristics of the children with whom we work, the better equipped we will be to provide them with content and classroom experiences that help to nurture their intellectual, emotional, and social development.

In the table that follows (pages 247–55) the developmental patterns of childhood identified by the American School Health Association provides a basic guideline for ensuring that the selections of literature which correspond with the topics in the Growing Healthy curriculum are developmentally appropriate.[5] According to the American School Health Association, child development encompasses physical, emotional, social, and intellectual characteristics. In turn, each of these characteristics suggests a number of developmental needs that can lead the way to realistic instructional goals and other reasonable expectations for students. These childhood needs also contain implications for book selection.

The table presents the growth and development patterns which the American School Health Association has endorsed. The examples of children's books included in each category can help to enhance many of the needs which the various developmental characteristics imply. Further information about these books, including a brief description of their content, can be found in the next section of this chapter, *Correlating Literature and Health Issues*. It should be kept in mind that no developmental chart can ever capture individual differences in mental abilities, learning rates and styles, and other unique characteristics that one always finds among groups of children. The following chart provides only general principles and trends rather than strict, inflexible norms or standards that all children should be expected to fit or demonstrate on schedule. There simply is no substitute for observing particular groups of children and interacting with them in order to gain a sense of who they are and what concerns them. As Maxine Green has pointed out, "Anyone who has reared a child or taught a child knows full well that generalizations about stages and structures cannot capture the many nuances of child development, and the possibilities very often outreach predictions."[6]

*Growth and Development Characteristics**

Grades K–3   Ages 5–8

PHYSICAL CHARACTERISTICS	NEEDS
Growth relatively slow.	To develop large muscle control through motor skills.
Increase in large muscle coordination, beginning of development of small muscle control.	To have play space and materials. To use instructional tools & equipment geared to stage of
Bones growing.	development.
Nose grows larger.	
Permanent teeth appearing or replacing primary teeth; lower part of face more prominent.	To establish basic health habits: toileting, eating, covering nose and mouth with cough, etc.
Hungry at short intervals; may overeat and become fat.	To have snack time and opportunity to develop social graces.
Enjoys active play—climbing, jumping, running.	To have plenty of sleep and rest, and exercise interspersed with rest.

---

*From *A Pocketguide to Health and Health Problems in School Physical Activities*, pp. 4–9. Edited by Barbara Petroff. Kent, OH: American School Health Association, 1981. Used by permission of the American School Health Association.

Susceptible to fatigue and limits
self.
Visual acuity reaches normal.
Susceptible to respiratory & communicable diseases.

To have health examinations and
follow-up.
To have visual and auditory
checks.
To have dental attention.

Running with Rachel/Asch; *The Berenstain Bears Visit the Dentist*/Berenstain; *Keeping Clean*/Cobb; *When I See My Doctor*/Kuklin; *Gregory, the Terrible Eater*/Sharmat; *Alexander's Midnight Snack*/Stock; *Exercise: What It Is, What It Does*/Trier.

EMOTIONAL
CHARACTERISTICS

NEEDS

Self-centered, desires immediate
attention to his/her problem—
wants to be first.
Sensitive about being left out.
Sensitive about ridicule, criticism
or loss of prestige.
Easily aroused emotionally.
Can take responsibility but needs
adult supervision.
Parent image strong; also
identifies with teacher.
Expresses likes and dislikes
readily.
Questioning attitude about sex
differences.

To receive encouragement,
recognition, ample praise,
patience, adult support.
To express inner feelings,
anxieties and fears.
To feel secure, loved, wanted,
accepted (at home & at school).
To be free from pressure to
achieve beyond capabilities.
To have a consistent, cooperative-
ly planned program of classroom control. Must have
guidance.
To develop self-confidence.
To have some immediate
desirable satisfactions.
To know limitations within which
she can operate effectively.
To develop realistic expectations
of self.

Dinosaurs Divorce/Brown; *Aaron's Shirt*/Gould; *Evan's Corner*/Hill; *They Really Like Me!*/Hines; *Mama One, Mama Two*/MacLachlan; *I Want To Be Big*/McPhail; *Foolish Rabbit's Big Mistake*/Martin; *Ira Sleeps Over*/Waber.

SOCIAL CHARACTERISTICS	NEEDS

Lack of interest in personal grooming.

Engages in imitative play.

Friendly, frank, sometimes aggressive, "bossy," assertive.

Generally tolerant of race, economic status, etc.

Gradually more socially oriented and adjusted.

Boys and girls play together as sex equals, but aware of sex differences.

To have satisfactory peer relationships; receive group approval.

To learn the importance of sharing, planning, working and playing together—both boys and girls.

To have help in developing socially acceptable behavior.

To learn to assume some responsibility; to have opportunities to initiate activities, to lead.

To work independently and in groups.

To accept sex role.

To develop an appreciation of social values, such as honesty, sportsmanship, etc.

Always and Forever Friends/Adler; *Phoebe's Revolt*/Babbitt; *A Mouse Called Junction*/Cunningham; *Hansel and Gretel*/Grimm; *Frog and Toad Are Friends*/Lobel; *Come On, Patsy*/Snyder; *So What If I'm a Sore Loser*/Williams; *William's Doll*/Zolotow.

INTELLECTUAL CHARACTERISTICS	NEEDS

Varied intellectual growth and ability of children.

Interested in things that move, bright colors, dramatizations, rhythmics, making collections.

Interested in the present, not the future.

Learns best through active participation in concrete, meaningful situations.

Can abide by safety rules.

Wants to know "why."

Attention span short.

To experience frequent success and learn to accept failure when it occurs.

To have concrete learning experiences and direct participation.

To be in a rich, stable, challenging environment.

To have time to adjust to new experiences and new situations.

To learn to follow through to completion.

To develop a love for learning.

To learn without developing feelings of hostility.

To communicate effectively.

Two Under Par/Henkes; *Happy Birthday, Sam*/Hutchins; *Poems for Fathers*/Livingston; *The Inch Boy*/Morimoto; *Henry and Mudge*/Rylant; *Ira Says Goodbye*/Waber; *It Could Always Be Worse*/Zemach; *Someone New*/Zolotow.

Growth and Development Characteristics

Grades 4–6   Ages 8–11

PHYSICAL CHARACTERISTICS

Growth slow and steady.
Girls begin to forge ahead of boys in height and weight.
Extremities begin to lengthen toward end of this period.
Muscle coordination improving.
Continued small muscle development.
Bones growing, vulnerable to injury.
Permanent dentition continues.
Malocclusion may be a problem.
Appetite good, increasing interest in food.
Boundless energy.
Tires easily.
Visual acuity normal.
Menarche possible toward end of this period.

NEEDS

To develop and improve coordination of both large and small muscles.
To have plenty of activities and games which will develop body control, strength, endurance, and skills-stunts (throwing, catching, running, bicycles, skates).
To have careful supervision of games appropriate to strength and developmental needs; protective equipment.
To have competitive activity with children of comparable size.
To have sleep, rest, well-balanced meals.
To have health examinations and follow-up.
To have visual and auditory checks.
To have dental attention.

I Am the Running Girl/Adoff; *Human Body*/Bruun; *Tennis Is For Me*/Dickmeyer; *The Hospital Book*/Howe; *Zanballer*/Knudson; *Sleep and Dreams*/Silverstein; *Body Sense, Body Nonsense*/Simon; *Body Maintenance*/Ward.

EMOTIONAL CHARACTERISTICS	NEEDS
Seeks approval of peer group.	To begin seriously to gain a
Desire to succeed.	realistic image of self and
Enthusiastic, noisy, imaginative,	appreciate uniqueness of
desire to explore.	personality.
Negativistic (early part of period).	To be recognized for individual
Begins to accept responsibility for	worth; to feel self-assurance
clothing and behavior.	and self-esteem.
Increasingly anxious about family	To receive encouragement and
& possible tragedy.	affection; to be understood and
Increasing self-consciousness.	appreciated.
Sex hostility.	To exercise self-control.
Becomes "modest" but not too	To talk about problems and
interested in details of sex.	receive reasonable explana-
	tions. To have questions
	answered.

Is Anybody There?/Bunting; *Good-bye, Chicken Little*/Byars; *Dear Mr. Henshaw*/Cleary; *The Dream Keeper and Other Poems*/Hughes; *In Charge*/Kyte; *It Ain't All for Nothin'*/Myers; *Waiting to Waltz*/Rylant; *The Kids' Book of Questions*/Stock.

SOCIAL CHARACTERISTICS	NEEDS
Learns to cooperate better in	To be recognized and accepted by
group planning and group play	peer groups; receive social
and abides by group decisions.	approval.
Interested in competitive activ-	To have relationships with adults
ities and prestige.	which give feelings of security
Competition keen.	and acceptance.
Begins to show qualities of	To assume responsibilities, have
leadership.	increased opportunities for
Developing interest in	independent actions and
appearance.	decisions.
Strong sense of fair play.	To develop appreciation for
Belongs to a gang or secret club;	others and their rights.
loyal to group.	To learn to get along with others
Close friendships with members	and accept those different from
of own sex.	self.
Separate play for boys and girls.	

The Secret Garden/Burnett; *Where in the World Is the Perfect Family?*/Hest; *Altogether, One at a Time*/Konigsburg; *Lucky Charms & Birthday Wishes*/McDonnell; *Return to Bitter Creek*/Smith; *Mufaro's Beautiful Daughters*/Steptoe.

INTELLECTUAL CHARACTERISTICS

Likes to talk and express ideas.
High potential of learning—in science, adventure, the world.
Eager to acquire skills.
Wide range of interests; curious, wants to experiment.
Goals are immediate.
Demands consistency.
Generally reliable about following instructions.
Attention span short.

NEEDS

To experiment, explore, solve problems, challenges, use initiative, select, plan, evaluate.
To receive individual help in skill areas without harmful or undue pressure.
To have opportunities for creative self-expression.
To have a rich environment of materials and the opportunity to explore it.
To participate in concrete, real-life situations.
To be able to accept one's self with strengths and weaknesses.

The Inventors/Aaseng; *M.C. Higgins, the Great*/Hamilton; *A Ring of Endless Light*/L'Engle; *Hatchet*/Paulsen; *Straight Talk about Drugs and Alcohol*/Ryan; *But I'll Be Back Again*/Rylant; *Robinson and Friday*/Schneider; *Delmore's Brainstorm*/Shorto.

Growth and Development Characteristics

Grades 7–9   Ages 11–14

PHYSICAL CHARACTERISTICS

Accelerated, uneven growth.
Individual differences most prominent; girls continue rapid growth, are taller and heavier than boys in early period.

NEEDS

To have adequate nourishment for growth spurt and daily energy.
To understand developmental change of adolescence.
To recognize wide physical differences as normal.

Muscular growth toward adult size begins toward end of period.
Variable coordination.
Bones growing, vulnerable to injury.
Onset of puberty generally at the beginning of this age range for girls and at the end for boys.
Dental caries common.
Permanent dentition—28 teeth.
Malocclusion may be present.
Appetite ravenous but may be capricious.
Enjoys vigorous play.
Tires easily, particularly girls.
Visual problems increase.
Variations in development of secondary sexual characteristics. Menarche.
Skin problems, voice changes, etc.
Reproductive organs growing.

To have good protective equipment in games.
To have physical activity interspersed with rest.
To have health examinations and follow-up.
To have visual and auditory checks.
To have dental attention.

Growing Strong/Fodor; *Better Physical Fitness for Girls*/Jacobs; *A Different Season*/Klass; *American Sports Poems*/Knudson; *The You Can Do It! Kids Diet*/Matthews; *Overeating*/Sanchez; *Angel Dust Blues*/Strasser.

EMOTIONAL CHARACTERISTICS

NEEDS

Emotional instability; sudden and deep swings in mood.
Strong feelings of like and dislike, negative and positive attitudes.
Sensitive, self-critical but cannot take criticism.
Overanxious about health; thinks s/he has a gruesome disease.
Over-concerned about physical and emotional changes.
Striving for independence from adults.
Hero worship.
Searching for sensational emotional experiences.

To express volatile emotions, grief, anger, disappointment, likes, dislikes.
To assume responsibility for own conduct.
To achieve more independence.
To feel secure, wanted, loved, trusted, adequate, capable.
To have privacy respected.
To exercise self-discipline.
To experience success, receive individual recognition.
To identify with a friendly adult (teacher, parent, older friend).
To be alone occasionally.

Self-conscious.
Shows growing restraint in
  expressing feelings.
Unique sense of humor.

To feel the support, firm guidance
  and assurance of an adult.
To differentiate between reality
  and fiction, fact and fiction.

The Crazy Horse Electric Game/Crutcher; *And I Heard A Bird
Sing*/Guy; *Why Me? Coping With Family Illness*/Kosof; *The
Language of Goldfish*/Oneal; *You'll Survive*/Powledge; *In a
Room Somewhere*/Zeder.

SOCIAL CHARACTERISTICS

NEEDS

Interested in competitive sports
  as participant and spectator.
Developing good sportsmanship.
Socially insecure.
Very peer-conscious.
Desires freedom with security.
Argues against authority but
  wants it.
Sensitive to appearance (clothes,
  skin).
Imitative fads in clothing, speech,
  etc.
Wishes to conform to clearly
  defined pattern of good school
  citizenship.
Assumes responsibility for
  personal and group conduct.
Beginning to discriminate right
  from wrong.
Aware of opposite sex, chivalry,
  rivalry, teasing.
Separating into groups by sex:
  boys into large groups, girls into
  small groups, then gradually
  mixed groups.

To see one's self as a socially
  accepted, important person.
To relate to members of the same
  and opposite sex.
To receive recognition from and
  acceptance by peers.
To work and play with different
  age groups.
To recognize the importance of
  leadership as well as being a
  follower.
To have congenial social settings.

Straight Talk about Love and Sex for Teenagers/Burgess-Kahn;
Tinker Autumn/Denson; *Love and Sex in Plain Language*/
Johnson; *Ishi: Last of His Tribe*/Kroeber; *Izzy, Willy-Nilly*/
Voigt; *Life Without Friends*/White.

INTELLECTUAL CHARACTERISTICS	NEEDS
Eager to learn, curious, alert exploring.	To determine individual motives, goals, standards and ideals.
Reads widely.	To satisfy curiosity, desire to
Wider range of abilities and interests.	know; to experiment.
Wants to succeed.	To express one's self verbally, manually and through activities
Wants precise assignments and meaningful experiences.	such as dance, music, clubs, debate, etc.
Skeptical, demands facts.	To appreciate the value of work
Unrealistic in passing judgment.	and products of work.
Overconfident in own information.	To know the satisfaction of achieving to the extent of one's
Increasing span of attention and concentration.	ability.

Johnny May Grows Up/Branscum; *A Year in the Life of Rosie Bernard*/Brenner; *Born Different*/Drimmer; *The Leaving*/Hall; *Smart Choices*/Kolodny; *Throwing Shadows*/Konigsburg; *To the Rescue: Seven Heroes of Conservation*/Vandivert.

CORRELATING LITERATURE AND HEALTH ISSUES

As discussed in Chapter Two, the Growing Healthy Curriculum introduces children in grades kindergarten through seven to basic skills and behaviors that can promote a healthy lifestyle. Based on principles and concepts drawn from biological, behavioral, sociological, and health sciences, the curriculum attempts to involve children in a hands-on, multimedia program which nurtures critical-thinking abilities and problem-solving skills, the objective being to provide children with tools that will maximize their potential for leading healthy and productive lives. Developed by the National Center for Health Education with the endorsement of the U.S. Centers for Disease Control and the American Lung Association, the Growing Healthy Curriculum focuses on selected aspects of personal and social health in ten major content areas from which the specific topics and concepts in each grade level derive:

A. Growth and development
B. Mental and emotional health
C. Personal health
D. Family life
E. Nutrition
F. Disease prevention and control
G. Safety and first aid
H. Consumer health
I. Drug use and abuse
J. Community health

The topics that constitute each of these categories are laid out across the grades in a cumulative and sequential manner. Many of the topics introduced at one grade level are later explored from a different perspective within the context of a different subject area category. For example, in the personal health category one teaching objective in grade five is to make students aware of the ways peers and family members might influence their health behaviors and habits. A similar topic is also explored in the family life category in kindergarten ("things that parents do to promote health in the family"), grade one ("ways each family member can help the family work together as a unit"), grade two ("why family members should be considerate of each other" and "ways friends help each other"), and grade three ("the responsibilities and privileges of each family member" and "different kinds of friendship").

Similarly, after students are introduced to the function and structure of teeth and gums in kindergarten, and the eye and ear in second grade (each within the area of growth and development), they are given opportunities to apply this basic information to the situations presented in their study of personal health habits at grade two ("ways to protect the eyes, ears, gums, and teeth") and, also at grade two, to their exploration of the causes and prevention of different types of diseases ("diseases and disorders of the eyes, ears, gums, and mouth" and the "functions of mechanical aids for vision, hearing and dental health"). Carefully planned sequences of this sort make it possible to reinforce the skills and attitudes students have learned in previous grades. This will help to ensure their achievement, their confidence as learners, and the kind of personal satisfaction that mastery over content entails.

The variety of children's literature accommodates this type of curricular sequencing. Because there are many different books on the same or similar health topics for students of all ages and abilities, teachers can usually find books with similar content for each grade level in order to further reinforce the information and insights students acquire in previous and subsequent grades. In addition, it is possible to select different children's books on the same topic that not only approach the material from varying perspectives, but also match children's varying abilities and interests.

Another noteworthy characteristic of the Growing Healthy Curriculum is its flexibility. The lifestyle goals and curriculum level objectives consist of broad, general subject categories which can accommodate a wide array of topics that either evolve out of students' immediate concerns, interests, and needs, or develop spontaneously from classroom discussions of the fundamental issues on which the curriculum focuses. For example, a discussion of disease prevention and control in the third grade could serve as the catalyst for an exploration of the actions individuals can take to help solve or prevent community health problems. Here, the teacher could motivate discussion by introducing the students to *Sadako and the Thousand Paper Cranes,* a picturebook biography by Eleanor Coerr, with illustrations by Ronald Himler, which tells of a young Japanese girl who dies of leukemia as a result of the bombing of Hiroshima. In the upper grades, where the issue is sexually transmitted diseases, students might explore some of society's attitudes and impressions about people who contract a communicable disease. In this case, they could be encouraged to consider various characters' reactions to Alex, a teenager afflicted with ARC (AIDS-related complex) in *Good-Bye Tomorrow,* by Gloria Miklowitz.

The following charts provide examples of literature that

relate in both direct and indirect ways to the concepts and issues found in the ten areas of the Growing Healthy Curriculum. Accompanying the learning objectives for each grade level is an annotated list of appropriate children's books about the topics in a particular section of the curriculum. More comprehensive lists of books that relate to these topics can be found in Chapter Six. Throughout, books about a particular cultural group have been identified with the bullet symbol (•).

The booklists in Chapter Six also draw attention to several topics that the Growing Healthy Curriculum does not specifically include, but which nonetheless concern children. These extensions to the Curriculum focus on four areas: the experiences of people with handicaps and disabilities, death and dying, suicide, and abusive situations. Given the alarming rate of both attempted and successful suicides among young people, it would seem that the issues surrounding suicide need to be discussed at appropriate times in the elementary school classroom. Although the National Center for Health Statistics does not as yet report suicide figures for children under ten, the *Encyclopedia of Suicides* maintains that increasing numbers of children between the ages of two and ten are in fact attempting suicide.[7] Also, it is estimated that one out of seven adolescents has attempted suicide, and that approximately seventy percent of these teenagers, as well as fifty percent of those who died, were either drunk or high on drugs.[8] National statistics concerning abusive situations such as physical neglect and sexual and emotional abuse are no less alarming. According to the National Committee for Prevention of Child Abuse, approximately one million American children are the victims of some type of abuse annually. More than 2,000 of these children die.[9]

When selecting books for particular health-related issues it is important to remember that just as a work of literature can suggest several themes, it also can deal with several topics, thereby making it possible to integrate a particular selection of literature into several curricular areas. This is particularly feasible when there are only a few books about a specific subject. For example, relatively few children's authors have addressed issues specifically related to consumer health, one of the Growing Healthy topics (section H in the curricular chart). However, when students are considering consumer issues such as sources in reliable health information as well as legitimate health products and services, they could focus on the treatment given these topics in the numerous examples of literature about personal health (section C), nutrition (section E), disease prevention and control (section F), safety and first aid (section G), and drug use and abuse (section I). Even a brief examination of the booklists in this chapter will reveal the large number of books with topics that are suitable for discussion beyond the topical category to which they have been assigned.

GROWING HEALTHY:HEALTH EDUCATION CURRICULAR PROGRESSION CHART

A. *Growth and Development*

A.I. Grades K–3

Lifestyle Goals

The individual:

- Appreciates the contribution of each of the body systems to the survival and health of the total system;
- Views growth and development as a lifelong process fostered by responsible behavior.

Curriculum Level Objectives

The student:

1. Describes the growth and development of healthy teeth and gums.

2. Explains the structure and function of teeth.

1. Names major body parts.

2. Describes the kinds of information provided by each of the senses.

Source: From Growing Healthy Health Education Curricular Progression Chart, 1985. Used by permission of the National Center for Health Education.

    1. Describes the structure and
    function of the eye and ear.

    1. Lists characteristics common to all
    living things.

    2. Describes the balanced rela-
    tionships among body
    systems.

    3. Illustrates ways the skeletal and
    muscular systems work together.

Aliki. *My Five Senses*. Rev. ed. Crowell, 1989. K–3. Captures the excitement and wonder of a child's discovery of ordinary things by focusing on
such sensations as licking an ice cream cone, petting a dog, and hearing
a fire engine. Full-color illustrations. A Let's-Read-and-Find-Out Science
Book.

Balestrino, Philip. *The Skeleton Inside You*. Illus. Don Bolognese. Crowell,
1971. K–4. Harper & Row paperback, 1987. The shape, structure, and
function of bones explained simply with the accompaniment of vivid
pictures. A Let's-Read-and-Find-Out Science Book.

Cole, Joanna. *The Magic School Bus Inside the Human Body*. Illus. Bruce
Degen. Scholastic, 1989. 1–4. When Arnold eats the shrunken Magic
School Bus during a class outing in the science museum, his classmates
enjoy a trip into the stomach, heart, bloodstream, lungs, brain, nasal
cavity, and other body parts. Accompanying scientific facts help to
explain how the body turns food into energy.

LeSieg, Theo. *The Tooth Book*. Illus. Roy McKie. Random House, 1981.
Pres–2. A Bright & Early Book. Children's Choice. Entertaining rhymes
explain the reasons for teeth and ways to care for them.

Oxenbury, Helen. *I Touch*. Random House, 1986. Pres.–K. With the use
of simple, full-color drawings, the author/illustrator depicts a cheerful
toddler exploring ordinary objects and concepts. The series of sturdy
board books includes *I Can, I See,* and *I Hear.*

————. *729 Curious Creatures*. Harper & Row, 1980. Children's Choice.
K–3. Since the pages of this heads-bodies-and-legs-book are cut into
thirds, children can make interesting combinations of the pictures and
words.

•Rothman, Joel. *This Can Lick a Lollipop: Body Riddles for Kids/Esto Goza
Chupando un Carmelo: Las Partes del Cuerpo en Adivinanzas Infantiles.*
Spanish text by Argentina Palacios. Photographs by Patricia Ruben.
Doubleday, 1979. K–3. Rhyming riddles, with answers provided in the
photographs, that identify parts of the body.

Showers, Paul. *How Many Teeth?* Illus. Paul Galdone. Harper & Row,
1962. Grades K–3. Harper & Row paperback, 1987. The function and
types of teeth, from infancy to adulthood, explained in a story format
with the help of informative and amusing illustrations.

•Showers, Paul. *Look At Your Eyes*. Illus. Paul Galdone. Crowell, 1962. Pres–3. Harper & Row paperback, 1987. The daily activities of a child demonstrate how the parts of the eye work and why eyes are different colors.

Showers, Paul. *You Can't Make a Move Without Your Muscles*. Illus. Harriet Barton. Crowell, 1982. 1–3. The role of the body's muscles explained in simple terms and experiments.

A.II. Grades 4–6

Curriculum Level Objectives

1. Describes the functions of body cells in the production of energy.

2. Explains how growth and development occurs at the level of the cell.

3. Describes the structure and function of the digestive system.

1. Explains the physiological needs of a cell.

2. Describes interdependence among body systems.

3. Describes the structure and function of the respiratory system.

1. Differentiates among kinds and functions of body cells.

2. Explains how body systems are interrelated in their functioning.

3. Identifies the role of blood in meeting cell needs for nourishment and excretion.

4. Describes the structure and function of the circulatory system.

Adams, Anthony. *The Living Cell.* Readers Theatre Script Service, n.d. 5-up. A dramatization of recent scientific knowledge about the cell.

Baldwin, Dorothy, and Lister, Claire. *Your Body Fuel.* Watts, 1984. 4–7. Describes the digestive system, the uses of enzymes, and the organs involved in processing food.

Cole, Joanna. *The Human Body: How We Evolved.* Illus. Walter Gaffney-Kessell. Morrow, 1987. K–4. A noted science writer describes how our eyes, teeth, hands, feet, brain, and bones have changed over the past five million years.

Evans, Ifor. *Biology.* Watts, 1984. 5–8. With the aid of color illustrations, the author presents a lively overview of the biological sciences that includes an explanation of the cells of plants and animals, the dynamics of living communities, DNA, evolution, microorganisms, and taxonomy. A glossary of key terms and ideas is included.

Kramer, Stephen. *Getting Oxygen.* Illus. Felicia Bond. Crowell, 1986. 3–6. An explanation of how and why plants and animals, from one-celled organisms to complex mammals, breathe. Complemented by black and white illustrations, diagrams, and a list of books for further reading on this and related topics.

Miller, Jonathan. *The Human Body.* Designed by David Pelham. Illus. Harry Willock. Viking, 1983. 6-up. A clearly written technical text and three-dimensional pop-up pictures explain body parts and their functions.

Silverstein, Alvin, and Silverstein, Virginia B. *Heartbeats: Your Body, Your Heart.* Illus. Stella Ormai. Lippincott, 1983. 4–6. An exploration of the circulatory system, defects of the heart, and current research on ways to overcome heart disease, with a focus on disease prevention and control and the importance of diet and exercise. Diagrams, pencil drawings, and an index.

———. *The Excretory System: How Animals Get Rid of Waste.* Illus. Lee J. Ames. Prentice-Hall, 1972. 4–6. How skin, lungs, and the digestive system work in animals and humans.

Simon, Seymour. *About the Foods You Eat.* Illus. Dennis Kenrick. McGraw-Hill, 1979. 4–8. An overview of digestion and nutrition. Includes easy-to-follow experiments.

———. *About Your Lungs.* McGraw-Hill, 1978. 2–5. An introduction to the nature of the human lung and the respiratory system.

A.III. Grade 7

Curriculum Level Objectives

1. Compares the functions of the cell to the functions of the total organism.

2. Explains the function of the nervous system in controlling

and coordinating body
systems.

3. Explains the function of
   hormones in regulating body
   systems.

4. Describes the basic structure
   and function of the nervous
   system.

Bruun, Ruth Dowling, and Bruun, Bertel. *The Brain—What It Is, What It Does*. Illus. Peter Bruun. Greenwillow, 1989. 2-up. Two doctors explain how the brain makes the body work, how we think and learn, and how the brain deals with feelings and sleep. A brief chapter on animal brains, a glossary of terms, and explanatory diagrams help enhance this introduction to the importance of the brain.

————. *The Human Body: Your Body and How It Works*. Illus. Patricia J. Wynne. Random House, 1982. 5-up. An Outstanding Science Trade Book. An introduction to the eight areas of the human body and its major systems—skeletal, respiratory, circulatory, urinary, endocrine, and reproductive. Clearly labeled and color-coded illustrations complement and extend the explanation.

Kalina, Sigmund. *Your Nerves and Their Messages*. Illus. Arabelle Wheatley. Lothrop, Lee & Shepard, 1973. 3-up. The complicated patterns and networks of nerve cells are explained with the help of informative diagrams and illustrations.

Kettelkamp, Larry. *Your Marvelous Mind*. Westminster, 1980. 4–7. A brief summary of research on the brain, its power, types of memory, and selected techniques of memorization.

Miles, Betty. *The Trouble with Thirteen*. Knopf, 1979. 4–6. Children's Choice. Two teenage friends reveal their ambivalent feelings about the physical and emotional changes they are undergoing.

Noble, Iris. *Contemporary Women Scientists of America*. Messner, 1979. 6-up. A discussion of the lives and careers of nine leaders in science fields such as nuclear physics, astronomy, and genetics, with a focus on problems of discrimination and the importance of intelligence and determination.

Nourse, Alan E. *Hormones*. Watts, 1979. 6-up. Discusses the function and production of hormones and substances the body manufactures to keep its vital functions operating.

Seuling, Barbara. *You Can't Sneeze With Your Eyes Open & Other Freaky Facts About the Human Body*. Lodestar, 1986. 6-up. Illustrated with the author's tongue-in-cheek line drawings, this collection reveals many startling, but true, facts about the human body.

Silverstein, Alvin, and Silverstein, Virginia B. *Sleep and Dreams*. Harper & Row, 1974. 5–8. A familiar human state is made fascinating through an explanation of the science of sleeping and dreaming.

Williams, Barbara. *So What If I'm a Sore Loser?* Harcourt, 1981. K–3. An explanation of how to control one's anger in order to look for alternatives to conflict resolution.

B. Mental/Emotional Health

B.I. Grades K–3

Lifestyle Goals

The individual:

- Exhibits a positive self concept;
- Expresses emotions comfortably and appropriately;
- Weighs potential benefits against possible consequences before choosing one action over another;
- Communicates and cooperates effectively with others;
- Develops and maintains interpersonal relationships.

Curriculum Level Objectives

The student:

1. Names ways in which people are the same as and different from other people.

2. Describes the relationship between feelings and senses.

3. Defines the meaning of friendship.

1. Explains ways people are unique.

2. Describes positive qualities of self and others.

3. Differentiates between acceptable and unacceptable behavior.

1. Differentiates between pleasant and unpleasant emotions.

2. Compares responsible with irresponsible expressions of emotions.

3. Illustrates ways emotions are revealed through physical reactions.

1. Describes how one person's behavior can help or harm others.

2. Illustrates similarities and differences among people.

3. Describes personal health responsibilities.

de Regniers, Beatrice Schenk. *The Way I Feel . . . Sometimes.* Illus. Susan Meddaugh. Clarion, 1988. 1–4. Witty poems that capture the changing and changeable emotions of children, from feelings about the days of the week and a pet goldfish to friendship.

Elting, Mary. *The Macmillan Book of the Human Body.* Illus. Kirk Moldoff. Aladdin, 1987. 3–7. A lively investigation, with dramatic full-color art, of the major body systems including how they function, the various organs within each of them, scientific discoveries, and amazing facts. A glossary and index are included.

•Gray, Nigel. *A Country Far Away.* Illus. Philipe Dupasquier. Orchard Books, 1989. Pres–3. Side-by-side pictures depict the similarities and differences between the lives and cultures of two boys, one in a Western country, the other in a rural African village.

Hopkins, Lee Bennett, Selector. *Best Friends.* Illus. James Watts. Harper & Row, 1986. K–3. Poems about the joys and tribulations of friendship.

Langton, Jane. *The Hedgehog Boy.* Illus. Ilse Plume. Harper & Row, 1985. K–5. A Latvian folktale of a lonely boy with the skin of a hedgehog who is rebuffed by society, but perseveres and wins the love of a caring princess. Love is the catalyst for his transformation.

Lobel, Arnold. *Frog and Toad Are Friends.* Harper & Row, 1970. Two devoted friends share their problems.

Simon, Norma. *Why Am I Different?* Illus. Dora Leder. Whitman, 1976. K–2. A focus on some of the differences among people in growth, abilities, culture, family situations, and beliefs. The author emphasizes the need for a realistic self-image and individuality.

•Sneve, Virginia Driving Hawk, Selector. *Dancing Tepees: Poems of American Indian Youth.* Illus. Stephen Gammell. Holiday House, 1989. 1–4. Poems from the oral tradition of various tribes of North American Indians that capture themes of youth from birth through adolescence.

•Spier, Peter. *People.* Doubleday, 1980. All grades. A large, wordless book that introduces many different kinds of people from around the world.

Steig, William. *Spinky Sulks.* Farrar, Straus & Giroux, 1988. Pres.-3. A young boy copes with feelings of rejection, but his loving, patient family helps him cope.

Zolotow, Charlotte. *The Quiet Mother and the Noisy Little Boy.* Illus. Marc Simont. Harper & Row, 1989. Pres.–3. A noisy little boy discovers the pleasure of a quiet moment with his mother after his very noisy cousin pays a visit to their home.

B.II. Grades 4–6

Curriculum Level Objectives

1. Illustrates the importance of physical and psychological need satisfaction.

2. Explains the relationship between physical well-being and mental/emotional health.

1. Describes positive personality traits.

2. Explains the influence of peer pressure on behavior.

1. Analyzes the influence of peer pressure on health choices.

2. Identifies positive and negative effects of stress.

3. Describes constructive ways to help reduce stress.

4. Explains the significance of the problem-solving process in making health-related choices.

•Bergman, Tamar. *The Boy from Over There*. Translated by Hillel Halkin. Houghton Mifflin, 1988. 3–6. A fictional account of the experiences of several Israeli children during the years immediately following World War II, and the difficult patterns of human growth which parallel the turbulent division of British Palestine and the birth of the modern state of Israel.

•Cameron, Ann. *More Stories Julian Tells*. Illus. Ann Strugnell. Knopf, 1986. 3–6. Short stories in which a black child tells of his experiences with family members and his best friend, Gloria.

Gilbert, Sara. *Get Help: Solving the Problems of Your Life*. Morrow, 1989. 6-up. Thirteen categories of problems, from abuse to eating disorders, and specific, step-by-step advice for coping with them. Provides information on agencies which can help as well as how to communicate with agency personnel.

Hinton, S.E. *Rumble Fish*. Delacorte, 1975. 6-up. A novel that features a young adolescent's first-person account of a harsh life among street gangs.

Holl, Kristi D. *Perfect or Not, Here I Come*. Atheneum, 1988. 3–7. Tara learns some important lessons about teamwork, leadership, fairness, and the standards she sets for herself to impress her busy, perfectionist parents.

LeShan, Eda. *When Grownups Drive You Crazy*. Macmillan, 1988. 3–7. A close look at the conflicts and misunderstandings that occur between children and adults from the child's point of view. Offers advice on ways to deal with anger, confusion, embarrassment, fear, and other feelings. The sequel to *When Your Kids Drive You Crazy*. (Macmillan, 1985).

Roberts, Willo Davis. *Megan's Island*. Atheneum, 1988. 3–7. Suspense and

self-discovery blend in the story of an eleven-year-old's search for the
secret of her identity.

Stine, Jovial Bob, and Stine, Jane. *The Sick of Being Sick Book.* Illus. Carol
Nicklaus. Dutton, 1980. 3–6. Children's Choice. Tips on how to cope
with sickness.

•Turner, Glennette Tilley. *Take a Walk in Their Shoes.* Illus. Elton C. Fox.
Cobblehill, 1989. 4-up. Brief biographies of fourteen blacks who
achieve success despite the odds against them. Includes skits about them
to act out.

•UNICEF Declaration of the Rights of Children. *A Child's Chorus.* Illus.
various artists. Dutton, 1989. 4-up. A bill of rights that celebrates the
essential and universal needs of children the world over. Artists from
around the world provide visual interpretations of these needs.

B.III. Grade 7

Curriculum Level Objectives

1. Analyzes the interrelationship
   among physical, mental/
   emotional and social well-
   being.

2. Describes the function of
   emotions in producing and
   relieving tension.

3. Describes the importance of
   setting realistic personal goals.

•Berry, James. *A Thief in the Village (and Other Stories).* Orchard Books,
1988. 7-up. Short stories about the experiences of present-day boys and
girls in a seaside village close to Kingston, Jamaica. Themes center on
coming of age, conflicts derived from opposing values, the humiliation of
a boy who is physically different, and other topics.

Bush, Max. *The Voyage of the Dragonfly.* Anchorage, 1989. 4-up. Set in
medieval times, this fantasy play depicts the perilous journey of a strong
young queen to retrieve a mystical flame that can save her kingdom from
destruction. The voyage leads to self-discovery as each character finds a
new vision.

•Childress, Alice. *Rainbow Jordan.* Howard, McCann, 1981. 6-up. The love
and compassion a fourteen-year-old learns to accept from others help
her to cope with her mother's neglect.

Curtis, Robert H. *Mind and Mood.* Scribner's, 1989. 6-up. This self-help
guide provides interpretations of scientific research in the physiology
and psychology of human emotions, a discussion of physical ailments

that may be psychosomatic, and advice on controlling emotions, ways to get help when needed, and achieving emotional maturity.

Danzinger, Paula. *Can You Sue Your Parents for Malpractice?* Delacorte, 1979. 7-up. Children's Choice. At fourteen, Lauren, nearly overwhelmed by a plague of personal problems, starts finding some solutions when she takes a course in law for young people and meets Zack, an eighth grader.

•Hamilton, Virginia. *Anthony Burns: The Defeat and Triumph of a Fugitive Slave.* Knopf, 1988. 7-up. Put on trial under the Fugitive Slave Act, a young black man reveals the brutality of slavery as well as the political, racial, and social tensions of the times.

•Hotze, Sollace. *A Circle Unbroken.* Clarion, 1988. 7-up. Rachel, captured as a child in 1838 by a band of renegade Indians, is recaptured at seventeen by her minister father. She attempts to convince him that she was not raised by a group of heathens, but by a loving, caring family that she misses.

Norman, Jane. *The Private Life of the American Teenager.* Rawson, Wade, 1981. 7-up. School, sex, siblings, friends, drugs, and other concerns are discussed by adolescents who participated in a nationwide survey.

Rylant, Cynthia. *A Kindness.* Watts, 1988. 7-up. Unwilling to share his single mother with the baby she is about to have, a fifteen-year-old learns the difference between support and interference and the need to let go.

Shaw, Diana. *Make the Most of a Good Thing: You!* Little, Brown, 1985. 6–8. An Outstanding Science Trade Book. Advice for teenage girls about peer pressure, uncertainty, identity, and other matters. Charts and diagrams help to focus the reader's attention.

C. Personal Health

C.I. Grades K–3

Lifestyle Goals

The individual:

• Adheres to a lifestyle that promotes personal well-being;

• Pursues leisure time activities that promote physical fitness and relieve mental and emotional tension;

• Follows health care practices that prevent illness and maintain health.

Curriculum Level Objectives

The student

1. Defines the meaning of personal health practices.

2. Describes ways that health care practices promote physical, mental, and social health.

1. Identifies personal health practices that can protect the health of self and others.

2. Explains the importance of regular visits to health advisors.

1. Explains benefits of personal health care practices.

2. Lists reasons for regular visits to the dentist.

3. Describes ways to protect the eyes, ears, gums, and teeth.

1. Explains individual needs for exercise, relaxation, and sleep.

2. Describes physical, mental, and social implications of cleanliness.

3. Defines the meaning of personal fitness.

4. Identifies characteristics of good posture.

Cobb, Vicki. *Keeping Clean.* Illus. Marilyn Hafner. Harper & Row, 1989. K–3. Describes the origins of soap and water, toothpaste and toothbrush, and comb and brush, and how they help to keep us clean.

Drescher, Joan. *Your Doctor, My Doctor.* Walker, 1987. 1–3. The author/artist identifies various people in the medical professions, showing them as human beings with their own individualities.

Isenberg, Barbara and Jaffe, Marjorie. *Albert the Running Bear's Exercise Book.* Illus. Diane de Groat. Houghton Mifflin, 1984. K–3. A friend convinces Albert that he can become a much better runner by doing additional exercises. Outlines an exercise program with varying levels of difficulty.

Kessler, Leonard. *The Big Mile Race.* Greenwillow, 1983. K–3. Children's Choice. A group of friendly animals prepares for and wins a difficult race. Includes training guidance, proper nutrition, and warm-ups.

Kuklin, Susan. *When I See My Dentist . . .* Bradbury, 1988. Pres.–1. A photo essay that follows Erica to the dentist where her teeth are cleaned, treated with fluoride, and X-rayed. Clear descriptions and photographs of the instruments and the process.

Neff, Fred. *Running Is for Me.* Lerner, 1980. 2–5. With photographs and a clear, simple text, the author describes young Stephanie's jogging experiences with her mother, the need to stay in condition, and the value of warm-up exercises.

Reit, Seymour. *Jenny's in the Hospital.* Illus. Nina Barbaresi. Golden, 1984. K–3. When Jenny has an accident while playing, she is taken to the emergency room of a nearby hospital where the doctors discover that she

has broken her arm. Her overnight hospital stay provides a detailed
description of examination rooms, medical instruments, hospital rooms,
and hospital routines and procedures.

Silverstein, Alvin, and Silverstein, Virginia B. *The Mystery of Sleep*. Illus.
Nelle Davis. Little, Brown, 1987. 2–5. Explores dreams, nightmares,
snoring, insomnia, sleep habits, and many other sleep-related facts.

C.II. Grades 4–6

Curriculum Level Objectives

1. Illustrates correct dental health practices.

2. Analyzes the relationship between fitness and diet.

1. Explains how personal health behavior is influenced by that of peers and family members.

2. Describes physical advantages of good posture and regular exercise.

1. Describes physical, social and emotional benefits of regular exercise and fitness.

2. Compares immediate and long-range effects of personal health care choices.

Bershad, Carol, and Bernick, Deborah. *Bodyworks: The Kids' Guide to Food
and Physical Fitness*. Illus. Heidi Johanna Selig. Random House, 1981.
5–8. How good nutrition and exercising help to keep the body fit.

Braden, Vic, and Phillips, Louis. *Sportsathon: Puzzles, Jokes, Facts & Games*.
Illus. Andrea Eberbach. Penguin, 1986. 4-up. Baseball, basketball,
football, tennis, and other sports provide the subjects for puzzles, jokes,
and other challenges.

Flandermeyer, Kenneth L. *Clear Skin: A Step-By-Step Program to Stop
Pimples, Blackheads, Acne*. Illus. Monique M. Davis. Little, Brown, 1979.
5-up. The causes and treatment of minor skin problems.

Knudson, R.R. and Swenson, May, eds. *American Sports Poems*. Orchard
Books, 1988. 5-up. More than 180 poems cover feelings, sights, and
sounds associated with all kinds of popular sports. In addition to a
title/author index, the collection includes a subject index.

Kozuszek, Jane Everly. *Hygiene.* Watts, 1978. 3–5. Why it's important to keep clean and ways to do it.

Lewis, Nancy and Lewis, Richard. *Keeping in Shape.* Watts, 1976. 4–6. Advice and facts about ways to get in shape and stay fit.

•McLoughlin, John C. *Holy Secrets.* Lothrop, Lee & Shepard, 1988. 5-up. Subtitled "A History of Medicine from Shaman to Surgeon," this historical survey of the healing arts traces the age-old effort of human beings to cure injury and disease. Illustrated with dramatic black and white drawings.

•Patterson, Lillie. *Sure Hands, Strong Heart: The Life of Daniel Hale Williams.* Illus. David Scott Brown. Abingdon, 1981. 5-up. Williams was one of the first black physicians to perform open heart surgery. His career and times are described.

Schneider, Tom. *Everybody's a Winner: A Kid's Guide to New Sports and Fitness.* Illus. Richard Wilson and the author. Little, Brown, 1976. 4–6. The term "new" refers to lifetime rather than competitive team sports. Running, weight training, swimming, physical games, and other activities are described.

Settel, Joanne and Baggett, Nancy. *Why Does My Nose Run?* Illus. Linda Tunney. Atheneum, 1985. 2–6. Answers to common questions about the human condition.

C. III. Grade 7

Curriculum Level Objectives

1. Identifies areas in which personal patterns of health care may need improvement or change.

2. Synthesizes a plan combining regular physical activity with personal health habits that promote and maintain total health.

Browne, David. *Crack and Cocaine.* Illus. Ron Howard Associates. Gloucester, 1987. 7-up. A discussion of the nature of these drugs, the risks in using them, and efforts to prevent production and distribution.

Cavallaro, Ann. *Blimp.* Lodestar, 1983. 7-up. In this novel a high school student finally plans to do something about her weight problem.

Davis, Julie. *Sweet Dreams Body Book.* Bantam, 1983. 6-up. A guide to diet, nutrition, and exercise for teenage females. Features a list of low-calorie snacks, a diet and exercise plan for tight schedules, instructions and illustrations for fitness and spot reducing, and one hundred diet tips, recipes, and suggestions for maintaining proper weight.

Eagan, Andrea Boroff. *Why Am I So Miserable If These Are the Best Years of My Life?* Avon, 1988. 7-up. A *School Library Journal* Best Book of the Year. Common sense advice about the concerns of young women, from hygiene, menstruation, birth control, pregnancy, relationships with opposite sex, and legal rights for women.

Harder, Eleanor, and Harder, Ray. *The Trouble with Derek.* Pioneer Drama Service, 1980. 7-up. Using two Luann comic strip characters, this play focuses on Luann and Delta's attempts to convince Bernice that Derek, the new student, is carrying drugs in his gym bag.

Kolodny, Nancy J., Kolodny, Robert C., and Bratter, Thomas E. *Smart Choices.* Little, Brown, 1986. 7-up. A sourcebook of information about aspects of adolescent family, school, and social life including coping with divorce, pregnancy, and the suicide of a friend, and making friends or using drugs. The emphasis is on decision-making and considering options.

Levine, Saul, and Wilcox, Kathleen. *Dear Doctor.* Lothrop, Lee & Shepard, 1987. 7-up. Based on letters written to the authors, two doctors, for their "Youth Clinic" column in the *Toronto Star,* the book offers responses to many adolescent concerns including homosexuality, drugs, depression, and eating disorders. Indexed and headlined for easy reference.

Lyttle, Richard B. *The New Physical Fitness: Something for Everyone.* Watts, 1981. 6–8. Why exercising is important, along with suggestions for how to get started.

Madaras, Lynda. *Lynda Madaras' Growing Up Guide for Girls.* Newmarket, 1986. 6-up. Tips on responsible self-care as well as quizzes, exercises, and space to record thoughts and feelings. Also see the author's *What's Happening to My Body* series for males and females.

Simon, Nissa. *Don't Worry, You're Normal.* Crowell, 1982. 6-up. Teens themselves selected the topics in this self-health guide, which provides information based on medical research about the physical and psychological characteristics of adolescence.

D. Family Life and Health

D.I. Grades K–3

Lifestyle Goals	Curriculum Level Objectives
The individual:	The student:
• Respects the rights and privileges of every family member;	1. Describes things that parents do to promote the health of the family.

- Adjusts appropriately to changing physical, mental and social roles, responsibilities and privileges as they occur throughout the life cycle;

- Deals comfortably and appropriately with the demands of his or her own gender;

- Communicates effectively as a member of a family or society;

- Supports the belief that the health of all children is an individual, family, and community responsibility.

1. Explains the function of a family.

2. Describes various kinds of families.

3. Explains ways each family member can help the family work together as a unit.

1. Explains why family members should be considerate of each other.

2. Explains ways family membership changes.

3. Describes ways friends help each other.

1. Explains the responsibilities and privileges of each family member.

2. Identifies unique social and physical characteristics of girls and boys.

3. Describes different kinds of friendships.

Ackerman, Karen. *Song and Dance Man.* Illus. Stephen Gammell. Knopf, 1988. K–4. 1989 Caldecott Medal. When the children pay a visit to their Grandpa, he takes them to the attic, shows them the costume he wore in vaudeville, and performs one of his routines for them. Colored pencil drawings enliven the experience.

Brown, Laurence Krasny, and Brown, Marc. *Dinosaurs Divorce.* Little, Brown, 1986. Pres.-3. "A Guide for Changing Families" that helps young children deal with the situations and difficulties a divorce is likely to bring. The advice focuses on coping with feelings, living in two homes, sharing the ordeal with friends, and living with stepparents.

Bunting, Eve. *The Big Red Barn.* Illus. Howard Knotts. Harcourt, 1979. 1–4. When his mother dies, and when his father later brings home a new wife, a young boy uses the family barn as refuge. After the barn burns, the boy's grandfather helps him realize that barns and families can be rebuilt.

•Flournoy, Valerie. *The Patchwork Quilt.* Illus. Jerry Pinkney. Dial, 1985. 1–4. The quilt that grandma is making as a labor of love parallels the events in a warm and loving family.

•Pomerantz, Charlotte. *The Chalk Doll.* Illus. Frank Lessac. Lippincott, 1989. Pres.-3. While Mother tucks Rose in for her nap on the day Rose has a cold, she tells her daughter about growing up in Jamaica. The cozy dialogue between Rose and her mother is illustrated with affectionate, brightly colored paintings by a West Indian artist.

•Simon, Norma. *All Kinds of Families.* iiius. Joe Lasker. Whitman, 1976. K–2. A picturebook essay on the diversity of family life in a multicultural world. Family love is emphasized in both the writing and illustrations.

•Sobol, Harriet Langsam. *We Don't Look Like Our Mom and Dad.* Photographs by Patricia Agree. Coward, McCann, 1984. 2–5. This photo essay depicts the family life of two Korean-born children who are adopted. Honest discussions about their culture, the circumstances of their adoption, and their biological parents.

•Strete, Craig Kee. *When Grandfather Journeys into Winter.* Illus. Hal Frenck. Greenwillow, 1979. K–3. The meaning of life and death is woven into a powerful story of a relationship between a Native American grandfather and his grandson.

Titherington, Jeanne. *A Place for Ben.* Greenwillow, 1987. Pres.-3. Soft pictures and minimal text tell of Ben's relationship with his baby brother.

Waxman, Stephanie. *What Is a Girl? What Is a Boy?* Crowell, 1989. Pres-2. A candid explanation of the physical differences between boys and girls.

D.II. Grades 4–6

Curriculum Level Objectives

1. Describes the growth spurt that occurs during adolescence.

1. Explains the function of the reproductive system.

2. Describes the progression of the individual through the cycle of life.

1. Describes changes in physical, social, and mental/emotional characteristics that occur during adolescence.

Coats, Laura Jane. *Mr. Jordan in the Park.* Macmillan, 1989. K–4. Time, change, and the pleasure of sharing memories are at the heart of Mr. Jordan's stories about his experiences in a park from infancy to old age. Watercolor illustrations evoke the moods and feelings of the past and present.

•Drucker, Malka. *Celebrating Life: Jewish Rites of Passage.* Holiday House,

1984. 4–6. An exploration of the ways in which birth, puberty, marriage, and death connect the generations. Includes photographs, a glossary, an appendix, and an index.

Kleeberg, Irene Cumming. *Latchkey Kid.* Illus. Anne Canevari Green. Watts, 1985. 5-up. Advice on ways latchkey children can manage their lives when they're alone. Safety tips and activities are suggested.

Madaras, Lynda. *The What's Happening to My Body? Book for Boys.* Newmarket, 1987. 5–8. In a straightforward manner, the author describes different views of the physical and emotional changes that occur during puberty. Advice on how to deal with these changes is interspersed throughout the text.

———. *The What's Happening to My Body? Book for Girls.* Newmarket, 1987. 5–8. A guide to pubertal changes for females.

Mayle, Peter. *"What's Happening to Me?"* Illus. Arthur Robins. Lyle Stuart, 1975. The process and predicaments of puberty explained through cartoon-style illustrations and humorous incidents.

Miller, Jonathan, and Pelham, David. *The Facts of Life.* Illus. Harry Willock. Viking Kestrel, 1984. 4-up. Detailed three-dimensional pop-up illustrations parallel scientific explanations of human reproduction and birth.

Nilsson, Lennart. *How Was I Born? A Photographic Story of Reproduction and Birth for Children.* Delacorte, 1975. 3–7. Candid, detailed explanations and large, explicit photographs trace the process from conception to birth.

Rosenberg, Ellen. *Growing Up Feeling Good.* Puffin, 1989. 4-up. A guide to helping preteens and teenagers cope with the changes, pressures, confusions, and decisions that are part of growing up. Topics include friendship, family life, drugs, AIDS, suicide, and physical changes.

Shreve, Norma. *Family Secrets: Five Very Important Stories.* Illus. Richard Cuffari. Knopf, 1979. 3–7. The death of a pet, the suicide of a neighbor, an aging grandparent, a relative's divorce, and cheating in math class are the situations a boy and his family face.

D.III. Grade 7

Curriculum Level Objectives

1. Describes the reproductive processes.

2. Explains why some adolescents begin the growth spurt earlier than others.

3. Analyzes the effect of the mother's health on prenatal development and birth of her child.

4. Identifies ways to cope with family conflicts common during adolescence.

5. Identifies social and cultural forces in the development of responsible health behavior.

•Bell, Ruth, and others. *Changing Bodies, Changing Lives.* Random House, 1988. An American Library Association Best of the Best Books 1966–1988. 7-up. A comprehensive examination of the sexual and emotional changes of adolescence, which draws on the thoughts and feelings of actual teenagers. Topics explored include adolescent pregnancy and its alternatives, AIDS and other sexually transmitted diseases, gay sexuality, and sexual identity.

Boston Hospital Children's Hospital Staff. *What Teenagers Want to Know About Sex—Questions and Answers.* Little, Brown, 1988. 6-up. Using a question and answer format, the authors discuss sex and sexuality, including sexually transmitted diseases.

Brown, Fern G. *Teen Guide to Childbirth.* Watts, 1988. 6-up. Three case studies explain medical procedures and some of the options of delivery, including hospital birth, a birthing center, and home delivery. Key terms are explained in a glossary, and an index facilitates the search of specific information.

Davis, Ken. *How to Live with Your Parents Without Losing Your Mind.* Zondervan, 1988. 7-up. A pastor and counselor uses biblical and personal stories to provide advice to adolescents on how to communicate effectively with parents and siblings.

•de Jenkins, Lyll Becerra. *The Honorable Prison.* Dutton, 1988. 7-up. When their journalist father is put under house-arrest a Latin American family attempts to deal with the pressures of living in complete isolation.

Greenberg, Harvey R. *Emotional Illness in Your Family.* Macmillan, 1989. 6-up. Written by a medical doctor, the entries in this reference book describe many of the illnesses an adolescent might encounter, including Alzheimer's disease, bi-polar disorder, depression, and drug abuse.

Janeczko, Paul B., compiler. *Strings: A Gathering of Family Poems.* Bradbury, 1984. 6-up. More than one hundred poems by numerous American poets that explore relationships in nuclear and extended families.

Johnson, Eric W. *Love & Sex in Plain Language.* Illus. Russ Hoover. Rev. ed. Harper & Row, 1985. 7-up. A frank discussion of the physical, emotional, and moral aspects of sex and relationships. The glossary references places in the text where topics and issues are discussed, and a test is included to assess the reader's mastery of the material.

McCoy, Kathy. *Teenage Body Book Guide to Sexuality.* Pocket Books, 1983. 7-up. Emphasizing values, beliefs, and feelings, the author of *The Teenage Body Book* discusses such issues as contraception, sexually transmitted diseases, and personal choice.

Zindel, Paul. *The Effects of Gamma Rays on Man-in-the-Moon Marigolds.* Harper & Row, 1971. 7-up. A poignant play about the troubled relationship between an alcoholic mother and her two adolescent daughters.

E. Nutrition

E.I. Grades K–3

Lifestyle Goals

The individual:

- Eats a daily diet that provides adequate nutrients for the maintenance of health;

- Selects food representative of a wide range of food stuffs;

- Balances calorie intake with energy needs;

- Avoids dependence upon food fads as the sole criterion for diet choices or meal planning.

Curriculum Level Objectives

The student:

1. Names foods that contribute to strong bones and teeth.

2. Lists many kinds of foods.

1. Lists sources of commonly eaten foods.

2. Explains the role of breakfast in providing energy for work and play.

3. Identifies appropriate foods for healthful snacks.

1. Describes individual and ethnic variations in food choices.

2. Describes sources of different kinds of foods.

3. Explains how certain foods can be harmful to oral health.

1. Classifies foods according to their principal nutrients.

2. Illustrates food combinations that provide a balanced daily diet.

3. Explains why certain foods have limited nutritional value.

Dragonwagon, Crescent. *This Is the Bread I Baked for Ned.* Illus. Isadore Seltzer. Macmillan, 1989. K–3. A playful, cumulative, and rhythmic verse-story about various types of good food and the good feelings that come from sharing them.

Hayes, Sarah. *Eat Up, Gemma.* Illus. Jan Ormerod. Lothrop, Lee & Shepard, 1988. Pres.-1. Reluctant Gemma is coaxed into eating through her older brother's clever plan.

Hiser, Constance. *No Bean Sprouts, Please!* Illus. Carolyn Ewing. Holiday House, 1989. 2–5. A mystery unfolds when James and his friends discover that James's magic lunch box, which turns healthy foods into junk food, has disappeared.

•Lattimore, Deborah. *Why There Is No Arguing in Heaven.* Harper & Row, 1989. 1–5. The first Creator God of the Mayas challenges Lizard House and Moon Goddess to create a being to worship him, but the Maize God is the only one to succeed—and thus corn comes into being. The author's full-color illustrations capture the textures and moods of a Mayan myth.

•Nathan, Joan. *The Children's Jewish Holiday Kitchen.* Schocken, 1986. K–6. A cookbook that introduces special foods and customs associated with Jewish holidays.

•Ontario Science Centre. *Foodworks.* Addison-Wesley, 1987. 3-up. A discussion of the role and function of food and eating customs and habits in various parts of the world. Food-related science activities and recipes are included.

Readers Theatre Script Service. *Jingle Jangle Jingle.* N.d. K–3. A script that encourages recognition of vocabulary related to numbers, days, and foods.

Sharmat, Mitchell. *Gregory, the Terrible Eater.* Macmillan, 1980. K–3. According to his parents, Gregory, a goat, should be eating old shoes, tires, and other trash, but he prefers fruit and vegetables.

Smaridge, Norah. *What's On Your Plate?* Illus. C. Imbior Kudrna. Abingdon, 1982. 1–3. Children's Choice. Story poems that encourage healthful eating habits and personal hygiene.

•Turner, Dorothy. *Milk.* Illus. John Yates. Carolrhoda, 1989. 1–4. The history of milk, the process that brings it to our tables, and a description of how milk is prepared in various parts of the world. Also provided are nutritional information and some recipes. The same format can be found in three other books by the author: *Eggs, Potatoes,* and *Bread.*

E.II. Grades 4–6

Curriculum Level Objectives

1. Names energy sources common to all living things.

2. Describes the functions of the major nutrients.

3. Identifies factors that influence personal food choices.

4. Analyzes the nutritional worth of food choices for meals and snacks.

1. Explains why a variety of foods is needed every day.

2. Explains how diet choices based upon food fads may provide inadequate nourishment.

1. Explains why nutrition requirements vary from person to person.

2. Illustrates the function of nutrients in building strong bodies.

3. Interprets physical and mental consequences of a poorly balanced diet.

Adoff, Arnold. *Chocolate Dreams.* Illus. Turi MacCombie. Lothrop, Lee & Shepard, 1989. 3-up. Poems that celebrate chocolate in its many forms. Illustrated in chocolate tones.

Branscum, Robbie. *Johnny May Grows Up.* Illus. Bob Marshall. Harper & Row, 1987. 4–8. Thirteen-year-old Johnny attempts to deal with a catalog of personal problems, not the least of which is her tendency to gain weight when she eats the foods she likes.

Clark, Elizabeth. *Meat.* Illus. John Yates. Carolrhoda, 1989. 3–6. In addition to the history of meat, the book provides information about the processes involved in preparing meat for the market, nutritional facts, and easy healthful recipes. Other books in the Foods We Eat series are *Vegetables* and *Citrus Fruits* by Susan Wake, and *Fish* by Elizabeth Clark.

Cohen, Lila B. *The King Who Loved Lollipops.* Dramatic Publishing, 1973. 3-up. When the king can find no one to make the chocolate-covered, coconut-coated, peanut butter lollipops he adores, a peasant woman tells him her daughter knows how even though she doesn't. When the daughter becomes his queen, she must rely on a wily gnome who will provide the treat only if she gives him her first child. A play based on "Rumpelstiltskin."

Fodor, R.V. *What to Eat and Why.* Morrow, 1979. 4–6. Photographs and diagrams help to provide basic information about good nutrition.

Gaskin, John. *Eating.* Illus. Elaine Mills. Watts, 1985. 3–6. The fundamentals of proper nutrition as well as how the body digests and uses food.

Proddow, Penelope. *Demeter and Persephone.* Illus. Barbara Cooney. Doubleday, 1972. 2–6. A retelling of the Greek myth that explains the origins of the seasons and of crops.

Seixas, Judith S. *Junk Food—What It Is, What It Does.* Illus. Tom Huffman. Greenwillow, 1984. 3–5. A lively introduction to the forms and effects of a variety of unhealthy foods.

•Shorto, Russell, and Cwiklik, Robert. *Carrots and Kings.* Illus. Matt Faulkner. Kipling, 1990. 5-up. A series of interconnected stories that focus on food customs to explain the history and culture of various ancient and modern societies, including China, Italy, France, the Philippines, and America. Recipes are interspersed.

E.III. Grade 7

Curriculum Level Objectives

1. Evaluates individual diets according to nutritional requirements of adolescents.

2. Explains the relationship between calorie intake and level of activity to body weight.

3. Analyzes implications of dependence on food fads and fallacies in selecting a diet.

4. Describes ways to lose weight safely.

Benjamin, Carol Lee. *Nobody's Baby Now.* Macmillan, 1984. 6–9. Through a supportive relationship with her grandmother, Olivia, overweight, depressed, and feeling unloved, develops a new sense of self.

•Fine, John Christopher. *The Hunger Road.* Atheneum, 1988. 7-up. A look at hunger and homelessness in a variety of cultures. Illustrated with candid photographs.

•Giblin, James Cross. *From Hand to Mouth: Or, How We Invented Knives, Forks, Spoons, & Chopsticks, & the Table Manners to Go With Them.* Crowell, 1987. 4–7. A history of utensils and table etiquette with a focus on the cultures in which they developed and the reactions of those cultures to new, often bizarre, customs. Copious photographs, a bibliography of books to read on these topics, and an index round out an intriguing study.

Janeczko, Paul B., compiler. *This Delicious Day.* Orchard Books, 1987. 6-up. More than sixty poems that feature different kinds of meals and foods.

Lukes, Bonnie L. *How to Be a Reasonably Thin Teenage Girl.* Illus. Carol Nicklaus. Atheneum, 1986. 7-up. The author, a weight loser herself, offers sensible, down-to-earth advice about setting realistic personal goals concerning a diet, developing short-term and long-term strategies, and dealing with well-meaning friends and family members.

Perl, Lila. *Junk Food, Fast Food, Health Food: What America Eats and Why.* Houghton Mifflin, 1980. 6-up. An examination of the effects of twentieth-century technology on the food industry and eating habits. Provides information about marketing techniques, consumerism, ingredients, and additives. Recipes are included in addition to a list of books for further exploration of the subject.

Sanchez, Gail Jones, and Gerbino, Mary. *Overeating: Let's Talk About It.* Illus. Lucy Misiewicz. Dillon, 1986. 5–8. What causes young people to overeat? What are the consequences? What is a realistic plan for changing one's eating habits?

Tchudi, Stephen. *The Burg-O-Rama Man.* Delacorte, 1984. 6–9. A story of how the TV promotional campaign of a fast food chain affects a high school community.

F. Disease Prevention and Control

F.I. Grades K–3

Lifestyle Goals	Curriculum Level Objectives
The individual:	The student:
• Adheres to a lifestyle that promotes well-being and minimizes exposure to known risk factors;	1. Describes germs. 2. Names ways to avoid germs.
• Maintains immunizations of self and family at recommended levels of effectiveness;	1. Explains the difference between illness and wellness. 2. Names ways to break the communicable disease cycle.
• Seeks preventive measures such as examinations at specified intervals.	1. Differentiates between communicable diseases and chronic-degenerative diseases. 2. Describes preventive measures for injuries to bone and muscle tissue.

1. Names diseases and disorders
   of the eyes, ears, gums, and
   mouth.

2. Explains the functions of
   mechanical aids for vision,
   hearing, and dental health.

3. Explains ways sound health
   habits help prevent disease.

Amadeo, Diana M. *There's a Little Bit of Me in James.* Illus. Judith Friedman. Whitman, 1989. 1–4. Although Brian worries about Jamey, his younger brother who has leukemia, he wishes his parents could spend less time at the hospital and more time with him.

Baldwin, Anne. *A Little Time.* Viking, 1978. 3–6. A ten-year-old begins to understand her feelings and those of her family toward her younger brother, who has Down's syndrome.

Corey, Dorothy. *A Shot for Baby Bear.* Illus. Doug Cushman. Whitman, 1988. Pres.-1. Baby Bear's fears cannot be assuaged when he learns that he has to get a shot.

Gaes, Jason. *My Book for Kids with Cancer: A Child's Autobiography of Hope.* Melius & Paterson, 1987. 3-up. American Cancer Society Courage Award. Young Jason describes his painful treatment and remarkable recovery. The text contains Jason's hand-printed words as well as his cartoon-style drawings.

Hausherr, Rosmarie. *Children and the AIDS Virus.* Clarion, 1989. 1–5. The true stories of a five-year-old boy who contracted the human immuno-deficiency virus (HIV) that causes aids from a blood transfusion, and a ten-year-old girl who was born to a mother with AIDS, are at the center of the author's description of the immune system and the HIV. Also addressed is the issue of contact with non-infected children and the search for a cure. Thirty black-and-white photographs give the text added candor.

Kibbey, Marsha. *My Grammy.* Illus. Karen Ritz. Carolrhoda, 1988. 1–4. While explaining Alzheimer's disease, this story shows that Amy can still love Grammy despite the changes the disease has caused in her grandmother.

Payne, Sherry Neuwirth. *A Contest.* Illus. Jeff Kyle. Carolrhoda, 1982. K–3. A child with cerebral palsy describes his experiences and feelings.

Rabe, Berniece. *Where's Chimpy?* Photographs by Diane Schmidt. Whitman, 1988. Pres.-2. With the help of her father, a child with Down's syndrome finds the toy monkey she has lost on a busy day. Now it's her turn to help her father find his missing glasses. Basic concepts are woven into the storyline.

Sabin, Francene. *Microbes and Bacteria.* Illus. Alexis Batista. Troll, 1985. 3–5. An introduction to the world of microbes and bacteria, including scientific discoveries about these tiny creatures, their importance to our daily life, viral diseases, possible cures, and questions scientists are still trying to answer.

Showers, Paul. *No Measles, No Mumps for Me.* Illus. Harriet Barton. Crowell, 1980. 1–3. A story reveals the nature of germs and viruses and the need for vaccinations.

F.II. Grades 4–6

Curriculum Level Objectives

1. Identifies problems and diseases that may interfere with the functioning of the digestive system.

2. Explains the importance of good dental practices in the prevention of problems of the mouth, teeth, and gums.

3. Explains ways digestive upsets and diseases may be avoided.

1. Describes ways to prevent diseases of and injuries to the respiratory system.

2. Explains how lifestyle choices help reduce the risk of cancer.

1. Describes disorders and diseases that may harm the circulatory system.

2. Analyzes the relationship of certain risk factors to the occurrence of heart disease.

3. Explains how lifestyle choices help reduce the risk of heart disease.

Aaseng, Nathan. *The Disease Fighters.* Lerner, 1987. 5-up. An Outstanding Science Trade Book for Children. Aaseng details many life-saving medical discoveries including insulin, the cause of malaria, and the cures for diphtheria and tuberculosis made by researchers who were awarded the Nobel Prize in medicine.

Bates, Betty. *Tough Beans.* Illus. Leslie Morrill. Holiday House, 1988. 3–7.

With the help of his best friend Cassie, fourth grader Nat Berger learns how to cope with the effects of diabetes.

Brown, Fern G. *Hereditary Disease*. Watts, 1987. 4–9. What hereditary diseases are and efforts to combat them.

Fine, Judylaine. *Afraid to Ask: A Book for Families to Share about Cancer*. Lothrop, Lee & Shepard, 1986. 5-up. Based on actual case studies, this book describes research in the causes of various types of cancer, ways to prevent and treat them, and survival rates.

Ostrow, William, and Ostrow, Vivian. *All About Asthma*. Illus. Blanche Sims. Whitman, 1989. 2–6. With humor, the author describes his struggles with asthma: the initial attack, causes, ways to avoid and cope with an attack, and learning about the myths that surround the condition.

Patent, Dorothy. *Germs!* Holiday House, 1983. 5-up. The nature of germs as well as how they attack and affect the body, what the body does to combat them, and research in disease control and prevention. Enhanced with photographs.

Roy, Ron. *Move Over, Wheelchairs Coming Through*. Clarion, 1985. 4–6. Profiles of seven handicapped young people that reveal their courage, determination, and the help they receive from family members and friends.

Seixas, Judith S. *Living with a Parent Who Drinks Too Much*. Greenwillow, 1979. 5-up. Advice concerning ways to deal with the behavior of an alcoholic parent and the family problems that are likely to ensue.

Warren, C. *Understanding and Preventing AIDS*. Children's Press, 1988. 5-up. A survey of the history and symptoms of the disease, and a discussion of how it spreads, how it may be prevented, and how it may be cured.

Wiles, Julian. *The Boy Who Stole the Stars*. Dramatic Publishing, 1981. 4-up. While attempting to come to grips with the effects of Alzheimer's disease on his grandfather, Nicholas learns about love and friendship in a play that explores some difficult concerns.

F.III. Grade 7

Curriculum Level Objectives

1. Describes measures for the prevention and control of chronic and neurological disorders.

2. Explains the function of immunization in preventing disease.

3. Describes ways to prevent or control sexually transmitted diseases.

Bach, Alice. *Waiting for Johnny Miracle*. Harper & Row, 1980. 7-up. Set in a hospital, this novel explores the relationships among several people, including an adolescent, who are victims of cancer.

Gravelle, Karen, and John, Bertram A. *Teenagers Face to Face with Cancer*. Messner, 1986. 6-up. Teenagers discuss their struggles with the disease as well as their relationships with family members and friends and their thoughts about death. Includes information about the disease, a glossary keyed to terms introduced in the text, and a bibliography of books on cancer and efforts to cure it.

Hughes, Barbara. *Drug-Related Diseases*. Watts, 1987. 4–9. A discussion of several drug-related diseases, the risks involved, and ways to prevent them.

Hughes, Monica. *Hunter in the Dark*. Atheneum, 1983. 5–8. While Mike hunts alone for a white-tail buck, his thoughts turn to his bout with leukemia and his relationships.

Lambert, Mark. *Medicine in the Future*. Bookwright, 1986. 6-up. Conjectures on probable and possible medical advancements related to transplants, prolongation of life, and the use of modern technologies within the medical fields.

Madaras, Lynda. *Lynda Madaras Talks to Teens about AIDS*. Newmarket, 1988. 7-up. The author stresses the need to make wise choices based on available information. It could save lives.

Miklowitz, Gloria D. *Good-Bye Tomorrow*. Delacorte, 1987. 7-up. As a result of a blood transfusion, Alex contracts AIDS-related complex (ARC). This novel focuses on the reaction of his friends, girlfriend, and family, and the controversy about him that shakes the entire community once his condition is revealed in a local newspaper.

Nilsson, Lennart, and Lindberg, Jan. *The Body Victorious*. 6-up. Using high-magnification photographs and informative captions within a lucid text, the authors illustrate the workings of the immune system.

Strasser, Todd. *Friends Till the End*. Delacorte, 1981. 7-up. As his friend struggles with leukemia, an adolescent discovers some truths about life.

G. Safety and First Aid

G.I. Grades K–3

Lifestyle Goals	Curriculum Level Objectives
The individual:	The student:
• Takes steps to correct hazardous conditions when possible;	1. Identifies safety hazards at home, at school, and in between.

- Follows rules and procedures recommended for safe living;
- Avoids unnecessary risk-taking behavior;
- Applies correct emergency treatment when appropriate.

2. Names places and people who can provide help if needed.

1. Explains the importance of having playground safety rules.

2. Describes how the senses help protect us from accidents and injury.

3. Explains how to obtain help in an emergency.

1. Explains how to prevent accidental eye, mouth, and ear injuries.

2. Differentiates between hazards and accidents.

3. Describes basic first-aid treatment of eye, mouth, and ear injuries.

1. Explains the need for obeying safety rules at home, school, work, and play.

2. Describes personal responsibility for reducing hazards and avoiding accidents.

3. Explains accepted procedures of safe bicycle travel.

Arnold, Caroline. *Who Keeps Us Safe?* Illus. by the author, with photographs by Carole Bertol. Watts, 1982. Pres.-3. How police, firefighters, and other emergency personnel aid their communities.

Brown, Marc, and Krensky, Stephen. *Dinosaurs, Beware! A Safety Guide.* Little, Brown, 1982. Pres.-3. American Library Association Notable Children's Book of 1982; *Booklist* Children's Editors' Choice of 1982. Approximately sixty safety tips are demonstrated by dinosaurs in situations at home, during meals, camping, in the car, and in other familiar places.

Charlip, Remy, and Supree, Burton. *Mother Mother I Feel Sick Send for the Doctor Quick Quick Quick.* Illus. Remy Charlip. Parents Press, 1966. K–3. In a rhythmic verse story a child who has consumed an odd assortment of objects is helped by a doctor.

Chlad, Dorothy. *When I Ride in a Car.* Children's Press, 1983. Pres.-2. Ways to stay safe while riding in a car.

Cole, Joanna. *Cuts, Breaks, Bruises, and Burns.* Illus. True Kelley. Crowell,

1985. 2–5. With the aid of humorous pictures, the author explains how specialized cells in the body help to heal simple wounds and injuries. Provides first aid suggestions for minor injuries.

Gore, Harriet Margolis. *What to Do When There's No One But You.* Illus. David Lindroth. Prentice-Hall, 1974. 2–4. A series of stories that depicts common first aid problems and illustrated procedures for caring for injuries.

Leaf, Munro. *Safety Can Be Fun.* Lippincott, 1961. Harper & Row paperback, 1988. Pres.-2. The Nit-Wits in this book willingly get involved in a variety of dangerous situations, only to prove how much smarter it is to play it safe.

Martin, Charles E. *Island Rescue.* Greenwillow, 1985. 1–3. When a child is injured on a school picnic everyone lends a hand.

Older, Jules. *Don't Panic! A Book about Handling Emergencies.* Illus. J. Ellen Dolce. Western, 1986. Safety advice including ways to get help.

Rinkoff, Barbara. *No Pushing, No Dunking: Safety in the Water.* Illus. Roy Doty. Lothrop, Lee & Shepard, 1974. K–3. Two children learn the importance of safety rules for swimming and boating.

G.II. Grades 4–6

Curriculum Level Objectives

1. Describes ways to handle and store foods in a sanitary manner.

2. Explains reasons for appropriate fire safety measures.

1. Demonstrates the ability to provide rescue breathing.

2. Describes procedures for saving a choking victim.

3. Explains the importance of playing safely in and around water.

1. Describes the importance of following appropriate first-aid measures for bleeding and shock.

Baker, Eugene. *Bicycles.* Illus. Tom Dunnington. Creative Education, 1980. 3–5. Presents safety suggestions for riding a bicycle.

Banks, Ann. *Alone at Home: A Kid's Guide to Being in Charge.* Illus. Cathy Bobak. Puffin, 1989. 3–7. A workbook, in a large format, with safety tips for children to complete and keep handy when they're alone at home.

Bauer, Marion Dane. *On My Honor.* Clarion, 1986. 6-up. 1987 Newbery Honor Book. On a dare, Tony and Joel attempt to swim across a dangerous river. When Tony drowns, Joel faces his remorse and the need to tell both sets of parents why the accident occurred.

Chaback, Elaine, and Fortunato, Pat. *The Official Kids' Survival Kit: How to Do Things on Your Own.* Illus. Bill Ogden. Little, Brown, 1981. 4-up. Alphabetically arranged with numerous cross references, this guide offers safety tips for such situations as traveling, being alone at home, dealing with sexual advances and people who make you feel uncomfortable, being followed, and taking measures to ensure a secure home environment. Also presented is advice on accident prevention, nutrition, settling arguments, and coping when both parents work.

Chlad, Dorothy. *Matches, Lighters, and Firecrackers Are Not Toys.* Illus. Lydia Halverson. Childrens Press, 1982. 3–5. How these things can be hazardous.

Freeman, Lory. *A Kid's Guide to First Aid.* Parenting Press, 1983. K–5. Life-saving skills in story format for children to use when there are no adults around.

Hubbard, Kate, and Berlin, Evelyn. *Help Yourself to Safety.* Franklin Press, 1985. 1–6. A guide to avoiding sexual assault and preventing abduction.

Vandenberg, Mary Lou. *Help: Emergencies That Could Happen to You and How to Handle Them.* Illus. R.L. Markhem. Lerner, 1975. 1–4. Ways to deal with emergencies such as a fire, lightning, and animal and insect bites as well as swimming and skating accidents.

Ward, Brian R. *First Aid.* Watts, 1987. 5-up. Some skills for handling emergencies at home, school, or in the community. Includes a glossary of important terms.

Wolf, Bernard. *Firehouse.* Morrow, 1983. 5-up. A description of the people and machines that fight fires. Photographs help to make the information concrete.

G.III. Grade 7

Curriculum Level Objectives

1. Lists, in order, the first-aid steps to be taken when accidents occur.

2. Explains the relationship between unnecessary risk taking and accidents.

Haskins, James. *Street Gangs, Yesterday and Today*. Hastings House, 1974. 7-up. Newspaper accounts, interviews, and sociological studies explain gang life from colonial times to contemporary times.

Holman, Felice. *The Wild Children*. Viking, Kestrel, 1985. 6–9. After Russian troops arrest his parents and sister following the Bolshevik Revolution of 1917, Alex is forced to join a band of other homeless children whose safety and survival are always at risk.

Kyte, Kathy S. *Play It Safe: The Kids Guide to Personal Safety and Crime Prevention*. Illus. Richard Brown. Knopf, 1983. 5-up. Practical skills to use at home and school.

Moeri, Louise. *Downwind*. Dutton, 1984. 6-up. A possible radiation leak from a nearby nuclear power plant causes a community to panic.

Paulsen, Gary. *Hatchet*. Bradbury, 1987. 6-up. Newbery Award Honor Book. By learning how to keep his wits about him, a boy survives alone in the Canadian wilderness for fifty-six days.

Petersen, P.J. *Going for the Big One*. Delacorte, 1986. 6-up. Abandoned by their stepmother, three teenagers trek across the Canadian wilderness in search of their father. Their journey becomes a struggle for survival.

Phipson, Joan. *Hit and Run*. Atheneum, 1985. 7-up. In anger, sixteen-year-old Roland steals a car that hits a baby carriage. While hiding in the Australian countryside, he comes to a powerful understanding of what he must do with his life.

Richmond, Sandra. *Wheels for Walking*. Atlantic Monthly, 1985. 7-up. Eighteen-year-old Sally attempts to regain the control of her life and body after a car accident leaves her paralyzed.

Rickman, Ivy. *Night of the Twisters*. Crowell, 1984. 6-up. Ways to cope with a natural disaster are woven into a fictionalized account of the tornadoes that nearly devastated Grand Island, Nebraska, in 1980.

Voigt, Cynthia. *Izzy, Willy-Nilly*. Atheneum, 1986. 7-up. On the way home from a party, fifteen-year-old Izzy is involved in a car wreck because her date is drunk. Her leg is amputated, and now she must rebuild her life.

H. *Consumer Health*

H.I. Grades K–3

Lifestyle Goals	Curriculum Level Objectives
The individual:	The student:
• Chooses health products and services on the basis of valid criteria;	1. Lists health products people commonly purchase.
	2. Names people whose job it is to help keep us well.

- Accepts only that health information provided by recognized health authorities;

- Utilizes services of qualified health advisors in the maintenance and promotion of his/her own health.

1. Explains ways TV advertising influences choices of foods and other products.

1. Describes the many kinds of health advisors.

1. Identifies advertising methods used to promote the sale of health-related products.

2. Analyzes reasons for choosing health products commonly used.

Field, Rachel. *General Store.* Illus. Giles Laroche. Little, Brown, 1988. Pres.-3. Using a cut-paper technique, Laroche interprets a classic narrative poem in which a young shopkeeper reveals the many goods and services provided in an old-fashioned general store.

Gertz, Susanna. *Teddy Bears Go Shopping.* Four Winds, 1982. K–3. Children's Choice. When they lose their shopping list, four bears, who can remember only the last item, end up buying three kinds of ice cream.

Heide, Florence Parry. *The Problem with Pulcifer.* Illus. Judy Glasser. Lippincott, 1982. 2–4. Instead of staying glued to the television set like everyone else, Pulcifer prefers to read. Even a book-aversion therapist cannot motivate Pulcifer to mend his ways! Cartoon-style drawings enhance the tongue-in-cheek humor.

•Kuklin, Susan. *When I See My Doctor. . . .* Bradbury, 1988. Pres–1. Four-year-old Thomas's first-person account of his trip to the doctor for a physical checkup. Complete with color photographs of the instruments, a phonetic spelling of key terms, and a conversational writing style.

Marino, Barbara Pavis. *Eric Needs Stitches.* Photographs by Richard Rudinski. Addison-Wesley, 1979. K–3. The step-by-step process, from bicycle accident to an emergency room where a doctor and nurse care for him, and then the pleasure of an ice cream cone. A matter-of-fact style.

Oxenbury, Helen. *The Checkup.* Dial, 1983. K–3. A young boy causes havoc in the doctor's office while having his annual checkup.

Reit, Seymour. *Some Busy Hospital!* Illus. Carolyn Bracken. Golden, 1985. 1–3. Procedures, instruments, care givers, staff, and departments are explained.

Seixas, Judith S. *Vitamins—What They Are, What They Do.* Illus. Tom Huffman. Greenwillow, 1986. 1–4. What vitamins are, how they were discovered, how they work, and whether or not they are safe. A vitamin chart and a true/false test for readers are included.

Wolf, Bernard. *Michael and the Dentist.* Four Winds, 1988. K–3. Photographs document Michael's first experience of having a cavity cleaned and filled. Vivid illustration of the office setting, dental equipment, and procedures involved.

H.II. Grades 4–6

Curriculum Level Objectives

1. Interprets the meaning of nutritional information provided on food labels.

2. Explains how information contained on a label can be used in selecting health products.

1. Analyzes methods used to sell health products and services.

2. Differentiates between health quackery and sound medical practice.

1. Explains why prescriptions for medications and other professional advice must be carefully followed.

2. Identifies sources of reliable health information and services.

3. Identifies sales appeals used in media promotion of health-related products.

Arnold, Caroline. *What Will We Buy?* Illus. Ginger Giles. Watts, 1983. 4-up. A survey of the goods and services available from a variety of stores. Discusses how shoppers pay for their purchases.

Byars, Betsy. *The TV Kid.* Illus. Richard Cuffari. Viking Kestrel, 1976. 4–6. The problems eleven-year-old Lennie, a friendless boy, faces as a result of his obsession with television viewing.

Crofford, Emily. *Frontier Surgeons: A Story About the Mayo Brothers.* Illus. Karen Ritz. Carolrhoda, 1989. 3–6. Traces the efforts of the Mayo brothers to establish the field of cooperative medicine, from the opening of their small hospital in 1888 to the development of the largest medical clinic in the world, which continues today as a mecca for surgeons eager to study new techniques.

Howe, James. *The Hospital Book.* Photographs by Mal Warshaw. Crown, 1981. 2–4. An introduction to procedures, equipment, terminology, staff, reasons for hospitalization, and the fears that people are likely to have about hospitalization.

Kelley, Alberta. *Lenses, Spectacles, Eyeglasses, and Contacts.* Elsevier, 1979.

5-up. A history of vision aids, from the Middle Ages to the present. Black-and-white photographs and drawings serve to document facts, anecdotes, and scientific advancements.

Kyte, Kathy S. *The Kids' Complete Guide to Money.* Illus. Richard Brown. Knopf, 1984. 4–6. In addition to raising awareness about consumerism, the author offers advice on ways to earn, save, and spend money effectively.

Nourse, Alan E. *The Tooth Book.* McKay, 1977. 5-up. An explanation of various dental problems, proper care, decay, and the structure and function of teeth.

Taylor, Paula. *The Kids' Whole Future Catalog.* Random House, 1982. 5-up. A look at some of the products and living conditions such as jet-powered backpacks and underground cities which future technologies may produce. Large-book format with numerous black-and-white illustrations. Includes a section on places to contact for information on the products described in the text.

Wolfe, Bob, and Wolf, Diane. *Emergency Room.* Carolrhoda, 1983. 3–5. Black-and-white action photographs document cases, the work of hospital staff, the function of equipment, and procedures.

H.III. Grade 7

Curriculum Level Objectives

1. Describes the role and function of official consumer protection agencies.

2. Identifies criteria for the selection of an appropriate health advisor.

3. Interprets data provided on prescription and over-the-counter drug labels.

Angell, Judie. *A Word From Our Sponsor or My Friend Alfred.* Bradbury, 1979. 5–7. A group of boys move into the world of big business and learn about the challenges of consumerism.

Berger, Melvin. *Consumer Protection Labs.* Harper & Row, 1975. 6-up. How various government and private testing labs work to protect the consumer.

Fisher, Leonard Everett. *The Hospitals.* Holiday House, 1980. 5-up. Dramatic scratchboard illustrations augment this history of hospitals and attitudes toward hospitalization in the U.S., from early pesthouses to the emergence of more sophisticated institutions in the nineteenth century.

Fleischman, Paul. *Path of the Pale Horse.* Harper & Row, 1983. 6-up.

During the yellow fever epidemic in Philadelphia in the late eighteenth century, a doctor's apprentice learns about the pressures and rewards of medical practice as well as the influence of medical superstitions and quackery.

Haskins, James. *The Consumer Movement.* Watts, 1975. 7-up. A detailed account of consumer rights, legislation, and other efforts to protect the consumer, with a discussion of the actions people can take to ensure solutions to problems and dangers.

•Levy, Elizabeth. *Lawyers for the People: A New Breed of Defenders and Their Work.* Knopf, 1974. 7-up. The efforts of Eleanor Holmes Norton to promote and protect consumers' rights are highlighted along with the work of eight other lawyers who focus on various aspects of public-interest issues, including the rights of juveniles, the poor, prison inmates, and women.

•Mails, Thomas E., with Dallas Chief Eagle. *Fool's Crow.* Discus Books, 1980. 7-up. Practices related to medicine and healing among the Teton Sioux are described by Fool's Crow, a ceremonial chief and medicine man.

Olsen, James T. *Ralph Nader, Voice of the People.* Childrens Press, 1974. 5-up. The life, philosophy, and work of a pioneer in the consumer-rights movement.

Schmitt, Lois. *Smart Spending.* Scribner's, 1989. 5–9. With the aid of case studies, the author focuses on such issues as advertising, mail-order schemes, the protection inherent in labels and warranties, and ways to seek compensation for unsatisfactory goods and services.

I. Drug Use and Abuse

I.I. Grades K–3

Lifestyle Goals	Curriculum Level Objectives
The individual:	The student:
• Adheres to medical recommendations in the use of drugs and medications;	1. Names hazardous substances that people use or abuse.
	2. Explains reasons for consulting adults before using an unknown substance.
• Refrains from the abuse of potentially harmful drugs;	
• Obeys laws and regulations regarding the use of controlled substances.	1. Describes correct uses of medicine.
	2. Explains how use of unknown substances can be hazardous.

3. Names methods of identifying potentially hazardous substances.

1. Defines the term *drug*.

2. Explains why people choose to avoid certain mood modifiers such as tobacco.

1. Explains the difference between use and abuse of drugs.

2. Predicts the effect of certain drugs on physical, mental, and social functioning.

Christopher, Matt. *Tackle Without a Team*. Illus. Margaret Sanfilippo. Little, Brown, 1988. 3–7. Can Scott trap the person who put the marijuana in his duffel bag? With the help of a tape recorder, he tracks down the culprit, clears his name, and is reinstated on the football team.

Cleary, Beverly. *Ramona and Her Father*. Illus. Alan Tiegreen. Morrow, 1975. 2–5. The trials and tribulations of seven-year-old Ramona include a father who has lost his job, a mother who, now employed, spends much time away from home, and a campaign to get her father to quit smoking.

Jance, Judith A. *Welcome Home*. Franklin Press, 1986. 1–5. The goal of this guide is to let children know that they are not the cause of a parent's alcoholism. The author encourages her readers to seek help. Part of The Children's Safety Series.

Kenny, Kevin, and Krull, Helen. *Sometimes My Mom Drinks Too Much*. Illus. Helen Cogancherry. Raintree, 1980. K–3. The emphasis is on alcoholism as a disease in a story about an eight-year-old's struggle to understand her alcoholic mother and the confused feelings her mother's illness evokes.

Seixas, Judith S. *Alcohol—What It Is, What It Does*. Illus. Tom Huffman. Greenwillow, 1977. 1–3. Provides basic information about alcoholism and alcoholics: liquids that contain alcohol, the reasons people choose to drink or abstain, the hazards, physical effects, myths and misconceptions, and sources of help for alcoholics and their families.

———. *Tobacco—What It Is, What It Does*. Illus. Tom Huffman. Greenwillow, 1981. 1–3. The effects of cigarette smoking on the body and the factors involved in starting and quitting.

Taylor, Paula. *Johnny Cash*. Illus. John Keely. Creative Education, 1975. 2–5. The famous country singer's bout with drug addiction and the difficult road to recovery once he kicks the habit.

Vigna, Judith. *I Wish Daddy Didn't Drink So Much*. Whitman, 1988. Pres.–3. A story that tells of young Lisa's reactions to her father's illness.

I. Drug Use and Abuse

I.II. Grades 4–6

Curriculum Level Objectives

1. Describes effects of drugs on organs of the body.

2. Identifies similarities and differences between drugs and foods.

3. Explains the relationship between drug use and nutritional status.

1. Analyzes the effects of drugs on the functioning of body systems.

2. Describes effects of the use of drugs that may be inhaled.

3. Explains the necessity of sound decisions concerning the use of any drug.

1. Describes hazards associated with the use of any drug.

2. Describes reasons why some people abuse drugs.

Berger, Gilda. *Smoking Not Allowed: The Debate.* Watts, 1987. 6-up. Following a brief history of smoking, this book examines the known and potential effects on health, increased regulations to prohibit smoking in public places, and the debate over individual rights.

Claypool, Jane. *Alcohol and You.* Rev. ed. Watts, 1988. 6-up. Statistics about teenage drinking, some of the consequences and prevention strategies, and advice on treatment are among the topics treated. Also included are an index and a bibliography of books and other resources on alcohol and related subjects.

Fox, Paula. *Moonlight Moon.* Bradbury, 1982. 5–8. While visiting her estranged father who often drinks too much, fifteen-year-old Catherine must face her feelings and the need to get on with her life.

Holland, Isabelle. *Now Is Not Too Late.* Lothrop, Lee & Shepard, 1980. 5–8. Eleven-year-old Cathy discovers that the artist for whom she is a model is really her mother, the woman who, as an alcoholic, abused and abandoned her when Cathy was an infant. Is it too late for a reconciliation?

Leiner, Katherine. *Something's Wrong in My House.* Photographs by Chuck Gardiner. Watts, 1988. 5-up. Eight young people describe life in families in which alcohol is a problem and their efforts to cope with the situation. Includes further reading for children of alcoholics and places to go for help.

Madison, Arnold. *Drugs and You.* Rev. ed. Messner, 1982. 4-up. A comprehensive survey of various kinds of drugs, from stimulants to depressants, including alcohol, LSD, glue, caffeine, and nicotine, with a focus on efforts to control drug trafficking and cure drug addiction.

•Myers, Walter Dean. *It Ain't All for Nothin'.* Viking, 1978. 6–8. Twelve-year-old Tippy resorts to drinking when he is forced to live with his contentious, ne'er-do-well father. When he finally reveals the bleak conditions of his life to Mr. Sylvester, he begins to sense the possibility of a hopeful future and the privilege of choice.

Seixas, Judith S. *Living with a Parent Who Takes Drugs.* Greenwillow, 1989. 5-up. How to understand and cope with a parent who takes drugs, how and where to seek help, children's rights and responsibilities, and laws related to drugs.

Ward, Brian R. *Drugs and Drug Abuse.* Watts, 1988. 4–7. Addictive drugs defined, along with a discussion of their attraction and dangers and the legal aspects of taking drugs.

Washton, Arnold W., and Boundy, Donna. *Cocaine and Crack.* Enslow, 1989. 6-up. A discussion of these two highly addictive drugs and their effects on the body and mind of the user.

I.III. Grade 7

Curriculum Level Objectives

1. Analyzes physical, mental, and social effects of drug abuse.

2. Identifies variables that modify the effect of a given drug dose.

3. Explains reasons for laws regulating drug use (including OTC, prescription, alcohol, tobacco, as well as illicit drugs).

4. Describes alternatives to the use of mood modifiers as a means to solving problems and initiating good feelings.

Berger, Gilda. *Crack: The New Drug Epidemic!* Watts, 1987. 6-up. What it is, what it does to the body and mind, and how an addict is treated.

Berger, Gilda. *Drug Abuse: The Impact on Society.* Watts, 1988. 6-up. The emphasis is on the effects of illegal drug use on families, society, and the use. Also discussed are issues related to personal health and drug use, including a chapter on AIDS, legal repercussions, and drug testing and trafficking.

Brooks, Bruce. *No Kidding.* Harper & Row, 1989. 7-up. Set in Washington, D.C., midway through the twenty-first century when sixty-nine percent of the adult population is alcoholic, this novel focuses on the scheme of a willful and cunning adolescent to control his mother, an alcoholic, and his brother. Control, he learns, is an illusion.

DeClements, Barthe. *No Place for Me.* Viking Kestrel, 1987. 6–8. Having been forced to move from one relative to another because of her mother's alcoholism, Copper finds the solace, affection, and hope she longs for as a result of her relationship with Aunt Maggie.

Edwards, Gabrielle. *Coping with Drug Abuse.* Illus. Nancy Lou Gahan. Rosen, 1983. 7-up. Types of drugs and their effects on the body.

•Guy, Rosa. *The Disappearance.* Delacorte, 1979. 7-up. A Harlem teenager is caught between his responsibility to his alcoholic mother, the violence and squalor of ghetto life, and his will to survive.

Hyde, Margaret O., ed. *Mind Drugs.* Fifth revised edition. Dodd, Mead, 1986. 7-up. The contributors, authorities who have worked with young people and drugs, address such issues as cocaine use and its effects, ways young people can help to get drunk drivers off the road, and new attitudes toward alcohol.

Martin, Thomas. *Private High.* Anchorage Press, 1986. 6-up. A tense contemporary drama focused on teenage alcohol and drug abuse.

Newman, Susan. *You Can Say No to a Drink or a Drug.* Putnam, 1987. 7-up. Straightforward talk about the dangers, documented with nine true case stories and photographs.

Snyder, Zilpha Keatley. *The Birds of Summer.* Atheneum, 1984. 7-up. When Summer suspects that her irresponsible mother is involved with growing marijuana, she becomes determined to make a better life for herself and her sister.

J. Community Health Management

J.I. Grades K–3

Lifestyle Goals	Curriculum Level Objectives
The individual:	The student:
• Obeys laws and regulations designed to protect the health of the community;	1. Defines *pollution*. 2. Names sources of air pollution.

- Contributes to community programs designed to promote community health;

- Accepts responsibility as a citizen in supporting the activities and programs of community health workers;

- Avoids any personal action that might contribute to the deterioration of the environment.

3. Explains how people can work together to solve problems.

1. Describes characteristics of a healthy community.

2. Names groups who help maintain and promote community health.

3. Describes ways the senses can be protected from air pollution.

1. Differentiates among kinds and sources of environmental pollution.

2. Describes ways to avoid hearing loss due to noise pollution.

1. Identifies ways health agencies help in protecting health and the environment.

2. Describes ways individuals can help keep a healthy school environment.

3. Identifies ways to help health agencies in the promotion of health.

Cooney, Barbara. *Miss Rumphius*. Viking Kestrel, 1982. K–3. To make the world a more beautiful place, Miss Rumphius plants lupines throughout the countryside.

Cutchins, Judy, and Johnson, Ginny. *The Crocodile and the Crane*. Morrow, 1986. 3–6. An introduction to the science of captive breeding and other methods of keeping rare birds from extinction.

Evernden, Margery. *The King of the Golden River*. Coach House, 1955. 3–6. Southwest Wind, Esq., punishes Hans and Schwartz for their greed by drying up their valley, but Gluck, their considerate brother, restores its fertility with the help of the King of the Golden River. Play version of a classic story.

Gates, Richard. *Conservation*. Childrens Press, 1982. 1–4. An introduction to what can be done to conserve energy and preserve nature.

Kellogg, Steven. *Johnny Appleseed*. Morrow, 1988. 3–5. Lively, impressionist illustrations help to capture the adventures of the American pioneer whose efforts to beautify nature are legendary.

Peet, Bill. *The Wump World*. Houghton Mifflin, 1970. K–3. When the

Pollutants arrive on the planet Wump, their technology nearly destroys the natural environment.

Seuss, Dr. *The Lorax*. Random House, 1971. K–3. The Lorax, a little brown creature, tries in vain to ward off pollution and ecological blight.

Turner, Ann. *Heron Street*. Illus. Lisa Desimini. Harper & Row, 1989. 1–4. A lyrical tale that tells both the sadder side of what progress has done to nature and the wonders it has created for people.

Vigna, Judith. *Nobody Wants a Nuclear War*. Whitman, 1986. 1–4. Candid information about the havoc a nuclear war might cause, along with hopeful reassurance to children who might fear such a war.

Wilcox, Charlotte. *Trash!* Photographs by Jerry Bushey. Carolrhoda, 1988. K–4. An exploration of what happens to the more than 100,000 garbage-truck loads of trash Americans throw away each day. Statistics, full-color photographs, and vivid writing present a picture of landfills, recycling methods, conservation, and methods of trash pickup.

J.II. Grades 4–6

Curriculum Level Objectives

1. Identifies causes of water pollution.

2. Describes community facilities and procedures that ensure safe water supplies and sanitary trash and sewage disposal.

1. Describes methods used to control environmental pollution.

2. Identifies individual and community responsibilities in the control of environmental problems.

1. Explains the role of community health agencies in protecting and promoting the health and safety of community members.

2. Describes ways in which improving the environment can enhance physical, mental, and social health.

Amon, Aline, ed. *The Earth Is Sore: Native Americans on Nature.* Atheneum, 1981. 4-up. Native American poetry that both celebrates nature and pleads for its preservation. Collages of prints made from natural materials grace the pages, and a description of the poems and their sources is included.

Anderson, Madelyn Klein. *Environmental Diseases.* Watts, 1987. 5-up. A discussion of the diseases which such factors as radiation and toxic waste may cause.

Finney, Shan. *Noise Pollution.* Illus. Anne Canevari Green. Watts, 1984. 6-up. Noise pollution in its many forms, how it affects us, and what can be done to combat it.

Hoover, H.M. *Children of Morrow.* Four Winds, 1973. 5-up. The state of Earth several hundred years after all life, except for two isolated populations, has been suffocated by pollutants in the atmosphere.

Lambert, Mark. *The Future for the Environment.* Bookwright, 1986. 6-up. How can we slow down or stop some of the changes that are affecting the world's natural environments?

Pringle, Laurence. *Living in a Risky World.* Morrow, 1989. 5–8. The author examines the ways the risks that are hazardous to human and environmental life are detected, identified, and assessed, the effect of the media in shaping public opinion, and the role of the federal government.

Vandivert, Rita. *To the Rescue: Seven Heroes of Conservation.* Warne, 1982. 6-up. The lives of seven men who have made important contributions to the preservation of endangered species.

Williams, Gene B. *Nuclear War, Nuclear Winter.* Watts, 1987. 5-up. Following a brief history of the arms race, the author considers the probable effects of a nuclear war and worldwide efforts for disarmament, particularly the Star Wars program.

J.III. Grade 7

Curriculum Level Objectives

1. Describes community efforts in preventing and controlling disease.

2. Describes the importance of individual participation in community health activities.

3. Identifies career opportunities in the health field.

Gay, Kathlyn. *Silent Killers: Radon and Other Hazards.* Watts, 1988. 7-up. In addition to radon, Gay describes asbestos, dioxin, formaldehyde, mercury, and other environmental hazards that affect people within and outside the home. She uses news reports, statistics, and government documents to defend her theories and opinions. A bibliography of articles concludes the discussion.

Helgerson, Joel. *Nuclear Accidents.* Watts, 1988. 7-up. The causes and consequences of several known accidents are described, Chernobyl included.

Kerrod, Robin. *The World of Tomorrow.* Watts, 1980. 4–8. As we move toward the twenty-first century, what types of social, political, and environmental issues should concern us?

Lambert, Mark. *Future Sources of Energy.* Bookwright, 1986. 7-up. Part of the Tomorrow's World series. As nonrenewable sources of energy are depleted, new ones must take their place in order for humankind to survive. The author considers research in the development of new energy sources as well as ways to conserve present sources.

Pringle, Laurence. *Lives at Stake.* Macmillan, 1980. 6-up. Part of the Science for Survival series. Pringle discusses documented and potential hazards that are detrimental to the human environment. In looking at the science and politics of environmental health, he describes the dangers in food, products, pollutants, drugs, and the types of hazards found in places of employment. He outlines a plan of action for citizens, industry, and government agencies.

———. *Nuclear Energy.* Macmillan, 1989. 7-up. The author of *Nuclear Power: From Physics to Politics* examines the history, development, and current status of nuclear technology, including safety concerns and the possible future of nuclear power throughout the world.

———. *Restoring Our Earth.* Enslow, 1987. 7-up. What private and public organizations and agencies are doing to replenish water, air, and land. Contains a glossary, a list of books on the subject of environmental problems and solutions to them, and an index.

———. *What Shall We Do With the Land? Choices for America.* Crowell, 1981. 7-up. Ways to conserve and preserve the natural environment.

Strieber, Whitley. *Wolf of Shadows.* Knopf, 1985. 7-up. Set in the not-so-distant future, this novel traces the journey of a wolf that instinctively leads his pack and two humans to a refuge after a nuclear war.

Tchudi, Stephen. *The Green Machine and the Frog Crusade.* Delacorte, 1987. 7-up. David Morgan's campaign to save a woodland marsh from being converted into a shopping mall. Provides a view of ecology, community concern, and the political process.

NOTES

1. Jean-Jacques Rousseau, *Emile* (New York: Dutton, 1957), p. 26.
2. Items 1, 2, 3, and 4 are reported in "The State of the Kids," *American Health* 8 (October 1989): 43–56. Items 5, 6, and 7 are discussed in George Howe Colt, "Teen Sexuality," *Life* 12 (July 1989): 24.

3. As reported in "The State of the Kids," p. 50.

4. As reported in "How Kids Cope," *American Health* 8 (October 1989): 90.

5. Barbara Petroff, editor, *A Pocketguide to Health and Health Problems in School Physical Activities* (Kent, OH: American School Health Association, 1981).

6. Maxine Green, "Landscapes and Meanings," *Language Arts* 63 (December 1986): 777.

7. Glen Evans and Norman L. Faberow, *The Encyclopedia of Suicides* (New York: Facts on File, 1988), p. 1.

8. Ibid., p. 5.

9. National Committee for Prevention of Child Abuse, *It Shouldn't Hurt to Be a Child* (Chicago: National Committee for Prevention of Child Abuse, 1986), p. 4.

5. Experiencing Literature with Children

> More than helping them to read better, more than exposing them to good writing, more than developing their imagination, when we read aloud to children we are helping them to find themselves and to discover some meaning in the scheme of things.—*Jim Trelease,* **The Read-Aloud Handbook**[1]

If recent surveys of reading instruction in American schools have painted an accurate picture of the techniques many teachers are using to involve students in literature, for the majority of American children, involvement in literature may amount to little more than a movement through a rigid program of skills-and-drills.[2] This picture includes images of small groups of students of similar ability sounding out words, taking turns reading aloud from a story in a prescribed, ability-level textbook, searching through a paragraph to find a word on a vocabulary list, the main idea, or an example of a supporting detail, or describing, predicting, or making a diagram of the sequence of events in a story. The picture also shows individual students at their desks practicing some of these same skills in exercises found in paperback workbooks and dittoed skill sheets. Finally—and only when time allows—the picture might reveal several students reading silently from books they have brought to school or ones they have borrowed from the school's media center.

That children also read for enjoyment as well as to gain some understanding of themselves, others, and "the scheme of things" are, as these recent surveys have found, rarely considered important priorities in school curricula. Consistently, the surveys trace this inordinate concern for literal-level skills and subskills, often to the complete exclusion of the skills readers of all ages use to gather meaning from what they read, to a prevalent philosophy about reading instruction that emphasizes a "teach/test/reteach/retest instructional cycle" and equates competency with the ability to decode the most basic features of written language, namely, syllables and words.[3] Such practices, however necessary they may be for equipping children with rudimentary skills, give students few opportunities to read self-selected books for sustained periods of time, opportunities which can help them refine their skills, expand their tastes, and develop an appreciation for many different types of literature.

For the majority of American teachers, reading instruction is a matter of overseeing the smooth operation of a skills-and-drills program that, for all intents and purposes, approaches reading as though it were a scientific operation. According to recent estimates, commercial programs are used in 90 percent of our classrooms, with students spending up to 70 percent of the time reserved for reading instruction on workbook exercises and fill-in-the-blank worksheet drills that reduce their experiences with literature to a monotonous ritual that mainly involves a search for "right" answers.[4] Although it has been shown that children have many valuable things to say about books that interest them, current practice in reading instruction leaves little time for interaction with literature and with other readers. Meaningful discussion known to enhance comprehension, confidence, and self-esteem, is perceived as a pleasant diversion from the more serious work at hand.[5]

COMMERCIALIZED READING INSTRUCTION

The Basal Reading Program

In addition to workbooks and worksheets, a school district receives an impressive number of materials when it purchases (at a staggering cost) a basal reading program. As the Commission on Reading has pointed out, "An entire basal reading program would make a stack of books and papers four feet high."[6] The bulk of the program for each elementary school grade consists of literature anthologies which are graded to suit children of different reading abilities. Whether the literature has been specially written to highlight the skills introduced in particular lessons, or purchased from professional authors, in order for basal publishers to sell their product they must make sure that the difficulty level of the selections, in terms of vocabulary, sentence structure, and concept, match the ability level of the children for whom the selections are intended. With few exceptions, this means that the selections are altered according to a readability formula which measures sentence length and the complexity of the words. Having analyzed the literature selections in a sixth-grade basal text published in 1987, one reading specialist found ". . . that 40% of the selections of literature had been altered in some way. . . ."[7] The more important discovery, however, had to do with the content of what was cut in the effort to make the literature uniform. "The publishers," the specialist discovered, ". . . often omit setting, characterization, and descriptive detail and leave a 'bare bones' plot while adding stylized illustrations."[8] This kind of tampering, as Patrick Shannon notes, clearly suggests that the ". . . anthologies may be produced more for opportunities to practice word recognition than to understand one's life better or to find pleasure in reading."[9]

At the heart of the basal program is a teacher's manual. This is intended to be a fail-safe guide to procedures for managing the program in a systematic, sequential fashion. Studies of the ways in which teachers use the manual have indicated that it is followed with very little deviation from the prescribed methods.[10] In terms of actual practice, then, reading lessons are fairly uniform in most classrooms. Students are grouped by ability and work within an anthology and other materials geared to their level of proficiency. In these groups they work on skills such as word analysis, summarizing, and recalling details, and each student reads orally as a check on mastery of words and oral fluency. Comprehension checks also are done through the questions the basal manual directs the teacher to ask. Preceding or following a group session, students are given time to work alone on workbooks or worksheet exercises intended both to assess their understanding and provide opportunities for practice in the skills covered in group sessions. It is customary for students at any grade level to complete up to one thousand workbook pages annually.[11] Finally, further assessments are made with objective tests. Although basal publishers encourage teachers to give students opportunities to read independently in order to have them apply their skills, the usual practice among teachers is to skip this part of the lesson, apparently because of time restrictions.[12]

For many American students reading instruction is a repetitive cycle that, for the most part, involves diagnosis and prescription. In general, the cycle includes:

- Reading tightly controlled and contrived texts.
- Summarizing incidents.
- Looking for correct answers to questions sanctioned by the basal program guidebook.
- Completing exercises that assess understanding of isolated skills.

The cycle allows children few opportunities to read "real" literature. In fact, it has been estimated that students read approximately forty-three consecutive words before they are interrupted with questions or corrections,[13] despite evidence which suggests that the amount of time students spend reading independently significantly influences reading achievement.[14] Even more important perhaps are the attitudes toward literature and the process of reading which the typical pattern of instruction may instill in children. For example, the workbook activities that take up most of the instructional time require, as the Commission on Reading has pointed out, a ". . . perfunctory level of reading. Children rarely need to draw conclusions or reason on a higher level. Few activities foster fluency, or constructive and strategic reading. Almost none require any extended writing."[15] Although there have been many attempts to implement more holistic approaches to reading instruction, the prescriptive, textbook-centered approach has become an American tradition, with the format and structure of the established cycle having been closely followed for more than twenty-five years.

Reactions to Commercial Reading Programs

In light of the increasing number of illiterate Americans and the increasing number of children who possess the basic skills but show little interest in reading, many literacy experts, along with concerned classroom teachers, have begun to question the value of practices that require such an investment of time and money but yield such negligible results. Their concern has focused on the inconsistencies between classroom methods and the findings revealed by classroom research, as well as long-term experiences with children about successful ways to empower students to become self-motivated and proficient readers and writers. Several of these inconsistencies in reading instruction have received special attention:[16]

- The amount of time students spend on workbook exercises has little effect on reading achievement.
- Although the amount of time children devote to independent reading significantly enhances literacy development, students in the primary grades are given only seven to eight minutes a day for independent reading, while an average of fifteen minutes is allocated for independent reading in the intermediate grades.
- Lack of sufficient funding to support independent reading in contrast to the amount of funds spent on commercial basal materials (a 100-to-1 ratio in school budgets in 1987).
- The use of "controlled" reading materials despite evidence which suggests that (a) "made-for-school" materials may hamper rather than enhance comprehension, and (b) children are capable of reading natural language texts—even before they enter school.
- Exposure to limited types of literature (predominately brief, abridged, and "controlled" stories), while research suggests that reading widely provides experiences with and the neces-

sary background knowledge for handling increasingly complex
reading materials.
- Limited opportunities for response to literature, despite research findings about even young children's abilities to express
  high-level types of responses (interpretive and evaluative, for
  example) and the effects of exposure to a variety of response
  modes (writing, drama, art, and music activities) on reading
  skills and enjoyment.
- Limited discussion about literature despite research which
  shows that the interactions promoted by discussions enhance
  comprehension.
- Ability grouping in the face of evidence for the positive effects
  of heterogeneous grouping on reading skills, interest in literature, and the inclination to reach beyond ability levels when
  interest in reading materials is intense.

In his study of representative basal anthologies, Patrick
Shannon found that, in addition to limiting students to stories
and poetry (more than two-thirds of the selections in basal
texts for grades one through six), most of the selections
present a stereotypical view of children, childhood, and
realities of everyday life. He comments about the characteristics of these stories:

> Girls are often sweet, demure, and bookish; boys are
> gregarious, active, and funny. Like Disney movies, the
> characters contribute unrealistically to events in the
> world, relegating the actual concerns of children to the
> unimportant. At once, the stories are found to be glib,
> sexist, and demeaning.[17]

Shannon also draws attention to some of the most glaring
problems in the types of one-sided interactions between
teachers and students that the typical basal manual sanctions.
For example, although it has been shown that children are
quite capable of asking questions about the literature they
hear and read, observations of sixty basal lessons revealed that
students did not ask one question. They were, however,
required to supply answers—one-word answers or para-
phrases that matched the answers in the teacher's manual—
for up to forty questions the teacher asked.[18] Shannon further

notes that ". . . students read orally for no other purpose than to receive feedback from their teacher . . . the entire activity is disconnected from students' lives and even other parts of the reading lesson."[19]

Left to the devices of the basal reading program and the ways in which its directions and principles are translated into classroom practice, children are likely to develop a false or incomplete notion of the reading process. If the basal approach is all they have to go by, as it so often is, they will soon sense that reading, at least for success in school, is an act of extracting fixed and absolute meanings from a text rather than infusing a text with private and shared meanings, and, in the process, making sense of it by drawing on what they know and feel and have experienced as they form their responses to incidents, characters, point of view, mood, facts and concepts, or any of the other elements writers lay before them.[20] The process of reading is much more constructive and interactive than commercial materials would have readers believe.

If commercial materials, at least in terms of how they are used in countless classrooms, are in fact detrimental to children's development as readers, why have they become the standard means of reading instruction? The reasons are complex because they are rooted in long-standing economic, political, and instructional principles and attitudes. For example, many teachers believe, or are trained to believe, that despite what research and common sense tell them and what classroom experiences have revealed, students need to learn a set number of skills before they can read or write. Commercial materials address this issue by arranging and classifying skills and competencies according to a clearly defined sequence that gives parents, teachers, and administrators the impression that learning is progressing, or not progressing, in a systematic and orderly fashion. Given the large number of students with varying abilities, needs, experiences with reading, and expectations which teachers face each day, a program that promises to regulate and systematize instruction and learning for *all* students can be seen as a real blessing, particularly when teachers must deal with the pressures of accountability. For teachers who work in self-contained classrooms, the challenge of having to teach all or most of the subjects, and to teach them well, makes it tempting to resort to programmed materials and textbooks which supposedly are developed by experts. Even though a basal program strips teachers of their professional privilege, it does offer them a sense of security and the kind of control that many parents, administrators, and teachers themselves equate with true professionalism.

When teachers first make the switch to more literature-based instruction, it can seem as though security and control have been traded for confusion and lack of definite direction as far as skills are concerned. For teachers who are accustomed to teaching with a manual, or who are unfamiliar with children's literature, even the most rudimentary picture book can appear to be a threat as well as a challenge, and the time and energy it will take to organize, implement, and sustain a literature-based program can seem like an overwhelming responsibility. To develop a truly worthwhile and effective literature program in any area of the curriculum, teachers first need to read or at least know about a wide variety of literature. They need to have a firm understanding of specific books in order to plan and implement strategies for whole-group instruction that generate interest and enthusiasm, develop students' reading and literacy skills, facilitate an awareness of the characteristics of different types of literature, and provide opportunities for personal engagement with literature and personal response through meaningful activities and projects.

In light of the value of having children choose their own books for independent reading and small-group reading activities, the reading teacher must also accept the responsibility for satisfying the tastes and interests of particular children. The payoff for these efforts will be enthusiastic, competent, and willing readers who turn to literature for pleasure and to learn something about themselves and the world, but, even to teachers who acknowledge the benefits of literature for their students and themselves, the challenge of placing literature at the center of the curriculum can force them to retreat to "basalized" instruction.

CURRENT ATTEMPTS AT REFORM

While it seems unlikely that the authority and control that commercial reading programs have in American schools will give way to sweeping changes in current instructional practice, there are signs of a renewed interest in more literature-based curricula. With the support of numerous technical studies as well as teachers' and parents' testimonies about the value of literature, increasing numbers of teachers throughout the country are becoming convinced that children will develop into eager, self-motivated, and proficient readers when they have ready access to various types of "real" literature that address their needs, concerns, and interests, and consistent opportunities to refine and extend their responses to literature with enrichment activities. Also, several publishers have developed literature-based reading programs that keep the literature intact and emphasize the notion of teaching language and reading skills in the context of high-interest literature selections. For example, "Bridges: Moving from the Basal into Literature," published by Scholastic, and the programs developed by Sundance Publishers endorse an interactive approach to literature which incorporates writing, listening, and speaking.

The insights gained from studies of children's actual interactions with literature have been particularly influential in providing a direction for literature-based instruction. In contrast to technical investigations that place children in made-for-research situations in order to study specific phenomena, the most revealing studies of literacy and reading development have been those in which the researcher observes children for an extended period of time as they interact in natural situations such as the home or classroom. The purpose of this naturalistic or ethnographic research is to provide educators, parents, and anyone else interested in children's development with realistic and relevant information about the ways children actually learn and use language when reading, writing, speaking, and listening. Because it is based on "real-world" insights into children, teachers in particular are often drawn to the discoveries that naturalistic research uncovers.

Three types of naturalistic investigations have added a number of significant insights to our understanding of children and the conditions which enhance their literacy development. The first type reports the findings of researchers, such as university professors, who come from outside the setting in which children are observed. For example, *Children's Responses to Poetry in a Supportive Literary Context,* a study by Amy McClure, chronicles the experiences of fifth and sixth graders who, with their teachers serving as facilitators, read, listened to, wrote, and shared various types of poetry.[21] McClure spent an entire school year as a participant/observer in their classroom. The second type of naturalistic study is done by parents. In *Prelude to Literacy,* for example, Maureen and Hugh Crago document their daughter's encounters with the picture books and stories she was exposed to between the ages of twelve months and five years, and in *Cushla and Her Books* Dorothy Butler tells the remarkable story of how her handicapped granddaughter's interactions with literature and with the supportive family who constantly read to her, helped her to develop mental and emotional capabilities that doctors feared she would never be able to acquire.[22] The third category consists of the testimonies of teachers who describe the situations in their own classrooms. *In the Middle* by Nancie Atwell and *Transitions* by Regie Routman provide honest, informative accounts of the benefits and problems two teachers experienced when they developed and implemented a literature-based reading and writing program after years of restricting their students to the strategies prescribed in commercial materials.[23] Atwell works with junior high school students, while Routman is a reading specialist in the primary grades. Both books describe current theory but also offer a realistic view of classroom management, organization, procedures, activities, relationships between students and teachers, and much more.

Consistently, naturalistic studies have identified a number of conditions which support and promote the development of literacy through and with literature. The researchers have focused on such issues as the attributes of readers, the roles of adults, the context for experiences with literature, the nature of response to literature, the acquisition of specific literacy skills, involvement in the literature/reading process, and the social characteristics of reading, listening to, and interpreting literature, and of relating to the situations and ideas which texts or illustrations reveal.

The Value of Time

If, as Regie Routman points out, true "literacy implies using reading, writing, thinking, and speaking daily in the real world, with options, appreciation, and meaningful purposes in various settings and with other people," then children should have consistent opportunities not only to hear many types of literature read aloud and to self-select books, but also to reflect on the literature they hear and read through writing, discussion, and other meaningful activities that encourage them to express, refine, and extend their thoughts and feelings.[24] In keeping with the way people interact with literature and language "in the real world," there should be periods of time in both classrooms and libraries for entire groups of children to gather together and, in light of the give-and-take spirit modeled by the teacher or librarian, to set out to make personal sense of a story, biography, play, or informational book through genuine conversation.

With their attention and commitment captured in this way, children can be encouraged to focus on specific characteristics of various types of literature and specific techniques which writers use to draw readers into the worlds they have shaped with language and their imagination. They can also develop and refine specific reading skills such as noticing and describing details, tracing sequences, learning and using new words, making predictions about the course of events, a conflict or problem, or the development of a character, and relating the experiences in literature to their own lives. When these things are done consistently within the context of genuine, rather than contrived, literature that interests and excites children, reading skills and strategies have a greater chance of being remembered, used, and refined over time.

This same spirit of inquiry should characterize small-group experiences with literature. It is more likely that students will be motivated to read, to find pleasure in the experience, and to willingly commit themselves to the task when these groups are formed to work on activities and extended projects that relate to specific types of literature, or a topic, theme, or issue, or an author or illustrator for whom the members of the group have expressed a particular interest. Routman and others have shown that grouping of this sort, in contrast to ability grouping, has a positive effect on students with language and reading problems.[25] Interest grouping allows students to recommend books to one other and to help each other interpret the literature they read together. This approach gives "problem" readers something to reach for. These are important discoveries with many implications for teachers and parents. In the traditional approach to reading instruction, children designated as low-ability readers are frequently removed from their classroom and, instead of being exposed to the kinds of books that could suit their interests and needs, turn them on to reading, perhaps for the first time, and make them aware of the skills they already know, are given a heavy dose of isolated skills through workbook exercises and other strategies.

Literacy development is also influenced by the amount of time children spend reading books of their own choosing. At times, these choices may be guided by a parent, teacher, or librarian who draws attention to an author or illustrator, a type of literature, or many types of literature centered around a topic or issue that children will find interesting and relevant to their own lives and experiences. Bulletin boards and other displays can help to make children aware of the literature that is available. At other times, individualized reading is free reading, with the child being given access to books in the classroom, school, or public library. By promoting individualized and free reading, adults foster the reading habit and make children conscious of how and why people choose or reject certain books.

If there is one element of instruction that deeply concerns today's educators, it is the element of time. There are good reasons for their anxiety. Classrooms are busy places, and there is much to do in the course of one brief school year. The concept of time-on-task-on-schedule is firmly established as the educational order of the day, as is the need to prove that students are in fact learning specific, measurable skills. As one teacher recently pointed out about the pressures she contends with each day, "I have no time to relate to kids; I have to get them ready for the Iowa [tests of basic skills]." It is not surprising, then, that a commercial basal program, with its clear-cut and linear scope and sequence, should be attractive—regardless of the problems it frequently causes children. If for no other reason than the fact that children do indeed perform adequately on standardized tests of reading and writing after they have been involved in a literature-based literacy program, teachers and administrators need to reconsider their priorities.[26] If current practice is responsible, at least to some degree, for even relatively small numbers of students who have turned off and tuned out as far as reading is concerned, or who, as a recent report from the National Assessment of Educational Progress indicates, are unable to effectively interpret what they read, then it seems appropriate—and vital—to consider some viable alternatives to what now goes on in far too many classrooms.[27]

An Environment for Reading and Sharing Literature

The setting where books are read, shared, and discussed significantly helps to foster children's desires to read and to enhance the pleasure they derive from books. All aspects of the environment, whether in the home, school, or library, send signals to children about reading and literature. The environment can indicate whether literature is treasured or not, and whether children's personal engagement with books is valued or unimportant. Every environment expresses obvious and subtle attitudes toward reading, literature, and children.

One of the most important features of an environment that nurtures literacy is the collection of books it contains. Although it may contain a limited number of books, the collection should first of all be diverse—in terms of accommodating the varying abilities and interests of the children it is intended to serve, the various ethnic, racial, and religious cultures it should expose children to, the types of literature it should introduce, and the uses and styles of language and art it can make children aware of. In addition to literature that challenges children and gives them something to reach toward, it is important that the collection contains what G. Robert Carlsen calls the "peanuts and popcorn" of a reading diet, such as the "easy" books in the Stepping Stone series published by Random House, or the Fourth Floor Twins series published by Viking Kestrel.

It often surprises parents and teachers to see how diverse children's tastes in literature can be, but, like adult readers, their tastes and interests can develop only when they know about the many kinds of books that are available for increasing their awareness about life and living, for information, for relaxation, or for a quick-and-easy reading experience. Often, adults work from the assumption that books that deal with complex moral, social, or personal issues and questions may be too demanding for children to grasp, and so they presume that children will not or cannot read them. As we have shown throughout this book, the problems and issues many children have to contend with are in fact complicated and challenging. Because literature can serve as a powerful means to help children clarify and cope with life's challenges and difficulties, they need books that take an honest look at these difficulties and reveal realistic and authentic ways of dealing with and perhaps resolving them.[28] Children certainly need to be introduced to books by Norman Bridwell, Jack Kent, Shel Silverstein, and Judy Blume, but they also are capable of responding to the situations and themes presented in the literature of Chris Van Allsburg, Paul Goble, Myra Cohn Livingston, Virginia Hamilton, Mildred D. Taylor, and H. M. Hoover—when we give them opportunities to do so and when we truly listen to what they have to say about the discoveries they are making. The books we choose for any type of literature collection ultimately indicate the nature of our respect for children.

Teachers can do several things to build a diverse collection and help children widen their tastes, the most basic and essential being a willingness to become familiar with a wide range of children's books. A good place to start is by using the literature selection aids which are listed in Appendix II. These will help to ease the effort to find books on particular topics and themes that match children's interests and needs, many of which are health related. Teachers should not overlook the value of publishers' catalogs for promoting an interest in books. Available free of charge during the fall and spring publishing seasons, these catalogs contain announcements of new books, a list of the awards and honors the company's authors and illustrators have received, a description of new works by the publisher's current authors and illustrators, a brief biographical sketch of these artists, and photographs of them. These can be used, for example, when developing bulletin boards or displays that feature authors or illustrators. Just as children like to collect information about their favorite sports and entertainment personalities, they like to find out about the writers and artists who interest them. For young children this kind of information can make them aware of the fact that books do not appear miraculously in finished form; instead, they are written and illustrated by people, and are part of a long production process that involves considerable amounts of planning and revision. That professional writers and artists work hard at what they do; that they sometimes change what they have written and drawn throughout the process; that their books reflect their personal experiences—these can be very inspiring facts for young writers and budding artists.

There are other things parents and teachers and librarians can do to create an environment where books are valued and tastes can develop. They can:

- Take risks with selections of literature that are unfamiliar to them and the children with whom they work.
- Provide a comfortable, quiet, and special place for individualized reading.
- For classroom reading experiences, develop a flexible environ-

ment that can accommodate collaboration on literature activities and projects and other interactions with books.

- Test a selection to see how children respond to it. If it is unappealing to the majority, look for one that is more appealing. Discuss the reasons readers have for rejecting a book for a "better" one.
- Introduce books that other children (perhaps former students or the children who participate in the Children's Choices project) have liked.
- Invite older students to present booktalks about selections that interested them when they were younger.
- Entice children into books with frequent booktalks of your own, revealing just enough of the details of the selection to capture their attention. Do this often with new books.
- Allow children to give their own booktalks. Encourage them to critique new books, using a form like the one used in the Children's Choices program, which can serve as an opening to a book conference or a longer piece of writing (see p. 319).
- Display books attractively, with the cover facing outward.
- Make books accessible by developing a lending library in the classroom.
- Have children suggest books for the classroom library.
- Include books that children write in the classroom collection.
- Help children become aware of different types of literature by involving them in organizing and classifying the books and other reading materials in the classroom collection.

Even if it contains only a limited number of paperback books, a classroom library can do much to promote reading. For example, Dona Bolton, a preschool teacher in Ohio, has discovered that children have more to say when books are readily available, particularly the books introduced in literature sessions that involve the entire group.[29] Her students often reach for familiar books spontaneously in order to reread them (even before they can read in the conventional sense of the word), to share them with their peers, and to use them to lend a kind of authority to points they want to make during the planned and incidental discussions about content and concepts that unfold throughout the course of the day. Once Dona Bolton organized her relatively small collection into a lending library, spontaneous conversations about the books increased as the children talked to one another about

Children's Choices 1985

Tuesday's Child
BOOK TITLE

5th
GRADE

Rootstown Elem
SCHOOL NAME

Rootstown
SCHOOL DISTRICT

I like the book   ✓

The book was O.K.   ___

I did not like the book   ___

Jason
STUDENT NAME

Mrs. Flick
TEACHER NAME

I liked the book because
COMMENTS ABOUT THE BOOK
it tells you how to talk
with your parents about
problems in the world.

the content of the books they had borrowed or intended to borrow. "A healthy kind of competition had developed around the lending library," she points out, "because the children argue over who should be allowed to take a book home. Naturally, the popular books receive the most attention. When this happens I make sure to recommend similar books or other books by the same author."

The lending library also promotes greater parent awareness of the reading program and the literature children like to hear and read. It broadcasts the message that "Books Are Read Here!" For example, it is not uncommon for Mrs. Bolton's students to talk with their parents about the books they plan to borrow, and, in the process, to review the topics in a given book or summarize a plot. In this way, they reveal their reading interests and their tastes in literature. The borrowed books, of course, are the ones children expect their parents to read to them at home. For children from disadvantaged homes or homes where few or no books are available, the classroom lending library is often the only source of good literature. Research has also shown that the quality of children's responses to literature is influenced by how accessible books are during whole-group discussions and small-group activities.[30] It pays, then, to make the effort to build a substantial classroom collection over time and to stock it with multiple copies for use during whole-group and small-group experiences with literature.

The ways in which books are shared and discussed is another important aspect of a reading environment. In contrast to the one-way, teacher-dominated approach to literature which many commercial reading programs set up, the majority of children's experiences with literature should foster genuine interaction. Depending on the tone established by the adult, the types of questions asked, and the comments made, children will soon recognize whether or not it is appropriate to reveal their thoughts and feelings about the literature they read or hear. When every experience with literature turns into a literal-level or word-level skills lesson, or an exchange directed only by a series of generic questions—regardless of the types of thinking these questions are intended to nurture—children are programmed to believe that their personal responses to the literature are not welcomed or valued, at least not in the classroom. The classroom, they learn by such practices, is no place to talk about or be excited about literature. It is, instead, a place where you take texts apart by "attacking" words, or developing story maps, or finding correct information. That literature might also have something to do with genuine human experience, or personal awareness and understanding, or the joy of discovering new information, is seldom considered an essential focus in a commercial reading program's agenda, and it is seldom recommended as one of the reasons that people read. The problem with many school reading programs is that they encourage teachers to teach reading without teaching the child, or, worse, to teach as though the reader does not exist.[31]

While children are involved in read-aloud sessions and after they have finished reading a poem, or folktale, or informational book, they need to spend at least some of the time engaged in open-ended conversation about what the experience has meant to them. To teachers who are accustomed to a programmed approach to reading instruction, conversation may at first seem a waste of time or too simplistic an activity to constitute a legitimate instructional strategy. For busy parents, conversation is often regarded as a luxury. But, as numerous studies have shown, the dialogue that revolves around literature greatly enhances children's comprehension, their awareness of what readers actually do to make sense of print, and their ability to make personal connections with literature both heard and read.[32]

There are good reasons for the positive influence that meaningful conversation has on children's reading abilities. In *Children Talk about Books,* an illuminating study of the responses of children of varying ages and abilities to books that interest them, Donald Fry found that talk about literature is connected to the reader's self-concept:

> Our perceptions of ourselves as readers illuminate by analogy our perceptions of ourselves as learners, people who live through experiences and interpret them . . . if we encourage children to talk about what happens as *they* read—and all the children in this study do that in their different ways—then they will grow into an aware-

ness of themselves reading, which is another way of
coming to understand how they learn, how they live,
how they are.[33]

The exchange of thoughts and opinions about literature which
dialogue promotes can also help to clarify children's sense of
the reading process. Guided, meaningful talk about literature
is a type of collective thinking. It is a way for both children
and adults to deal with the problems they may be having with
understanding words or concepts. It is a time to reason,
speculate, debate, revise, and figure things out; a time, that is,
to construct private and shared meanings based on clues and
elements discovered in both the text and illustrations. In
conversations about books with an adult and with siblings or
peers, children will often have their thoughts and opinions
affirmed and broadened. With proper direction, they can
acquire the habit of noting specific elements in the text that
support a response or question it. They can learn that not
every opinion can be validated by the elements a particular
story, poem, or biography contains, but, at the same time, that
each work of literature can evoke a number of different
responses and interpretations.

Although teachers, parents, and librarians perform a valuable service for children by being attentive to what children
are thinking and feeling in response to literature, and although they need to encourage children to express their
thoughts, feelings, and opinions about literature, they also
need to demonstrate that response to literature is not merely
a free-for-all or a pursuit where anything goes. When the
adult facilitates, structures, and orchestrates these exchanges,
and also participates in them as a reader among readers, he or
she can help children recognize the ways people read,
respond to, use, and interpret works of literature. Many
reading skills can be learned from the dialogue that evolves
out of and centers on books that capture children's attention,
and, as Marilyn Cochran-Smith's and Harriet Ennis's studies
have shown, this applies to both very young children and
adolescents.[34] Parents and teachers who are themselves
readers know that these exchanges about literature are
important for readers of all ages.

The Adult as Role Model

The adult who reads motivates children to read, just as the adult who writes inspires children to write. Children will be motivated to read when they are surrounded by good books that appeal to them, but an adult can help them along the way by being a reader for whom literature is a passion and not only a pastime. What also helps to motivate and encourage children to read is the parent's or teacher's genuine interest in literature that interests children. If parents and teachers are familiar with and enthusiastic about children's literature and the writers and illustrators who create it, children will sense that this literature is valuable and worthy of their attention. Adults can actually demonstrate this interest through booktalks, "gossip" about authors and illustrators, their willingness to talk about effective or powerful images, passages, and techniques in children's books, and especially by showing how children's literature affects them personally. By doing these things, they model what it is like to be hooked on books. This can be particularly motivating to reluctant readers as well as children who like to read but have learned that school is not the place to satisfy their interest.

Adults can also model how a reader makes sense of literature, and thus take some of the mystery out of the reading process. They can make children aware of what Donald Fry calls "readerly behaviour."[35] They do this, once again, through demonstration, through what they do, say, and think as they get caught up in the reading process. In their investigations of the roles adults play during storytime events, for example, Roser and Martinez found that parents and teachers can be instrumental in helping young children use the types of high-level cognitive abilities, such as inferring and evaluating, which curriculum guides typically reserve for older students.[36] Parents and teachers helped to guide children through texts and enrich their responses by assuming three roles:

- As a "co-responder" who stimulates interaction and response by revealing personal responses to the literature, noting details in texts and illustrations, modeling reader behaviors, and encouraging children to share their responses;

- As an "informer/monitor" who asks questions, makes comments, and supplies background information for helping children who are having difficulties and for encouraging children to pay close attention to details and perceive connections that relate to cause and effect and reasonable conclusions;
- As a "director" who, among other things, manages the session by introducing a selection of literature and structuring and overseeing discussion.

Roser and Martinez maintain that "it may be crucial that adults extend the roles they have typically assumed during instructional interaction with readers. For if young children can respond in broadly divergent ways to literature . . . certainly even more can be expected from older readers." A parent or teacher, they believe, must serve as a "partner who shares books and who thinks aloud in response to literature."[37] The beneficiaries will be children who acquire a new or different awareness of reading as a process that involves remaking the literature according to one's sense of things.

Whether literature is shared in the home, school, or library, the adult can demonstrate "readerly behaviors" by:

- *Reading aloud expressively; encouraging children to do the same.* Expressive reading is interpretive reading. Inflection, pitch, volume, tone, and other elements of oral reading demonstrate an understanding of the characteristics of literature such as styles of language and illustration, conflict, action, underlying tone, point of view, and characterization. Expressive reading on the part of an adult also reflects the nature and degree of involvement in literature and can influence children's oral reading of literature.
- *Having children read silently before they read orally.* During silent reading we begin to "listen to" the text, to make it come alive as our awareness of character, relationships, conflict, setting, and the like develops. Silent reading is therefore a rehearsal for oral reading.
- *Thinking aloud about the feelings, thoughts, and associations specific features of the text and illustrations are evoking.* This demonstrates for children how readers personally engage and interact with the images and ideas authors and illustrators provide. It encourages children to make personal connections with literature and to feel free to share them.

- *Revealing genuinely tentative understandings of, confusions over, or problems with the meaning and significance of incidents, language, relationships, character motivation and intention, the sequence of events, the causes for specific thoughts, feelings, and actions as well as their effects, and the beliefs and values the author invites the reader to consider.* When adults show how readers muse, wonder, and predict and then keep reading for affirmation or the need to revise initial responses, they demonstrate reading strategies and the ways in which writers capture and sustain a reader's interest. Further reading and thinking also help to answer some of the questions and solve some of the problems readers have as they work through a selection of literature and gain more information and develop further insights. Children need to experience these strategies in order to internalize them. They can then serve children whenever they read.

- *Being responsive to children's unsolicited and unexpected responses.* Children are more likely to become confident readers when they sense that their ideas, feelings, and opinions about literature are valued and respected. They will learn to trust themselves as readers if they are encouraged to take risks and if they feel that a reaction to literature which doesn't match the adult's expectations is not a mistake or a misreading. To support risk-taking, the teacher or parent must, first of all, be attentive to what the child is saying about the literature and genuinely respond to the thoughts and feelings the literature is causing the child to have. At times, the child's questions or musings can set the direction for a lesson, a read-aloud session, group discussion, an activity, or even a literature-related project. For example, when a group of fourth graders was discussing one of the chapters in *Racso and the Rats of NIMH,* Conly's sequel to *Mrs. Frisby and the Rats of NIMH,* several children commented on Racso's attraction to junk food. Rather than proceed with her agenda, the teacher pursued this response and led a discussion on the motivations behind Racso's attraction. This was later followed up with a unit on nutrition that included dramas about the eating habits of story characters. In another classroom, at the preschool level, the teacher read aloud *The Day Our TV Broke Down* by Wright, in order to make her students aware of the bad effects of inordinate television viewing. For one child in the group, however, a minor incident in the book, the fact that the main character was living with one parent and visited the other parent on weekends, prompted a concern about divorce. By attending to this response, the teacher discovered that it was actually the teacher's own divorce which had concerned and confused the child, causing her to wonder if her parents would also divorce. The teacher then planned a unit on different kinds of families.

• *Respecting a reader's privacy.* Sometimes literature evokes a deeply personal reaction which the reader may want to keep private. The need to simply enjoy the experience without verbalizing one's response may be at the heart of the matter, or it may be that the selection has elicited a painful memory or a troublesome concern that the child may not want to reveal. Adults should not expect every response to be overt and observable, and they should sense when it is appropriate to respect a reader's right to his or her privacy. This is particularly significant when selections of literature deal with highly personal or private health issues. In one eighth grade, the issue was death. The teacher, Melanie Dye, had developed a teaching unit in which she and her students explored death and dying by first reading a number of stories, poems, and nonfictional accounts, including *The Red Pony* by Steinbeck, *The Pigman* by Zindel, *You Shouldn't Have to Say Goodbye* by Hermes, *Death Be Not Proud* by Gunther, and "Dirge Without Music" by Edna St. Vincent Millay. In conjunction with the unit, the teacher used a brief questionnaire (participation was voluntary) to determine her students' feelings about death and about the subject of death in literature. "It should be noted," she wrote at the completion of the unit, "that one student had a very intense reaction to the questions:"

> This student, a boy, sat with tears streaming down his face before he even received the questionnaire at his desk. The boy's father had died two years ago and obviously the pain of that situation is still fresh in his memory. He did manage to circle responses to the first three questions, and, oddly enough, for number three, his reply read "I have not had to deal with death of someone close to me." Did his tears convey his true reply?

The teacher decided that it was best not to probe.

• *Comparing and contrasting various selections of literature.* The more we read, the more we realize that particular events, characters, themes, images, symbols, and story types and structures reappear in various selections of literature (many are noted in Chapter Three). Magical transformations that accompany a new awareness about human relationships appear in tales from around the world such as "Beauty and the Beast," "The Frog Prince," "Sleeping Beauty," and "The Theft of Fire." A sly trickster who tries to outwit others, but is himself outwitted, can be found in folktales from Africa (*The Dancing Granny* by Ashley Bryan; "Anansi's Hat-Shaking Dance"), Jamaica ("Anansi and the Old Hag"), and the American South (Brer Rabbit in *The Tales of Uncle Remus* and *More Tales of Uncle Remus* by Julius Lester), as well as in contemporary stories such as *Flossie and the Fox* by McKissack. Journeys that take characters out of their environment, transport them to an unfamiliar place where they are tested, contend with difficulties, and learn something about themselves and others, and then lead them back home again provide the structure in children's plays, picture books, novels, and poems. Magical objects; seasonal images of death and renewal; symbols of hope and despair; patterns of imprisonment, escape, and freedom; fortune gained, lost, and regained; survival despite the odds; underdogs, helpers with special powers, and unlikely heroes and heroines—these are some of the elements that appear and reappear in classics, comics, cartoons, films, paintings, and advertisements. By developing shared-book sessions, classroom units, library story hours, and literature-related activities and projects that focus on these elements and compare and contrast them in various types of literature, teachers and librarians can help to bring some order to a massive body of literature, foster an awareness of the characteristics of literature, and alert children to some of the same conditions that have concerned people in different cultures throughout the world. For three good sources that take a comparative approach to the study of literature, see *Fairy Tales, Fables, Legends, and Myths* by Bosma, *The Family of Stories* by Moss and Stott, and *The Child as Critic* by Sloan.

In relation to a unit on nutrition, Geri McGill, a fourth grade teacher, encouraged her students to compare three folktales that feature a magical cooking pot by having them collaborate on developing a chart which highlighted specific story elements.[38]

Comparison Chart Based on Story Structure

Book	*The Magic Pot* by Patricia Coombs	*Tripple-Trapple* by Manning-Sanders	*The Wonderful Pot* by ACE
Setting			
Where	in the country	in the country	in the country
When	once	once upon a time	once
Characters	funny little demon; poor man and wife; rich man	merry devil; poor man and wife; rich man	pot; stranger; poor man and wife; rich man
Problem	Rich man would not give man work or bread	Rich man would not help them	Rich man would not help them
Action 1	Found pot by side of road and takes it	Finds pot by side of road and takes it	Trades his cow to stranger for pot
Action 2	Pot goes hucka-pucka to rich man's house and returns full of stew	Pot tripple-trapples to rich man's house and returns full of porridge	Pot skips to rich man's house and returns full of pudding
Action 3	Pot goes hucka-pucka to rich man's house and returns with butter	Pot tripple-trapples to rich man's house and returns with butter	Pot skips to rich man's house and returns with wheat
Action 4	Pot goes hucka-pucka to rich man's house and returns with silver	Pot tripple-trapples to rich man's house and returns with silver spoons	Pot skips to rich man's house and returns with gold
Action 5	Pot goes hucka-pucka to rich man's house and returns with gold	Pot goes tripple-trapple to rich man's house and returns with gold	Pot skips to rich man's house where rich man jumps on it
Action 6	Pot goes back to rich man's house	Pot goes back to rich man's house	
Resolution	Rich man dumps mud and stones in pot. Pot lifts him high. Never seen again.	Rich man dumps mud in pot. Pot lifts him high. Takes him to hell.	Rich man cannot get off. Pot carries him to the North Pole.

A visual aid of this sort can promote thinking, for it encourages children to consider the connections, commonalities, and differences among different selections of literature. It also provides children with a concrete picture of the entire story by making them aware of where and how the pieces—particularly the events and characters—fit in the overall scheme of things. In some classrooms, students illustrate the sequence of a selection's events on a long sheet of newsprint. As the author introduces new actions or situations, the students add these to their illustration of what happens in the selection, to whom it happens, and how situations and conflicts are resolved. This type of activity is also helpful for reviewing a selection. In a second grade unit that explored children's fears, for example, an oral reading of the "Dragons and Giants" chapter in Lobel's *Frog and Toad Together* was followed up with the construction of a story map that reviewed the course of events and the characters' responses to them (see diagram below).

To model reading behaviors and strategies, the adult demonstrates how a reader works through a selection of literature in order to comprehend it. Demonstrations show children how a reader becomes involved in a constructive, meaning-making process by following clues, gathering evidence, drawing on life experiences as well as experiences with other literature, responding to images, descriptions, incidents, beliefs, and values, pursuing hunches, confusions, and questions, revising an earlier response, enjoying, feeling deeply, or sometimes abandoning a selection for a more

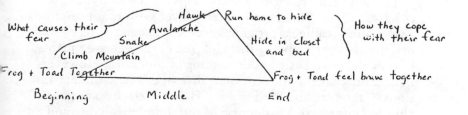

interesting, appropriate, or serviceable one. Demonstrations can also serve as invitations to children to join in so that the reading process is a collaborative venture. As many studies have shown, the nature and quality of these collaborations that involve children and an adult strongly influence children's notion of reading, the ways in which they approach literature, and their movement toward literacy. Several researchers have found that students of different ages also imitate the types of questions teachers ask and the ways in which they search through a test for details and evidence.[39]

That children follow the adult's lead and imitate the reading behaviors and strategies they are shown was brought home in Mrs. Bolton's preschool classroom. One of the group's favorite folktales was *The Three Billy Goats Gruff,* the version illustrated by Marcia Brown. The children frequently asked to hear this story during literature sessions that involved the entire group, and most of them would join in, both physically and orally, as their teacher read it aloud. During one of the free play periods when the children worked on projects and activities at various interest centers, a small group of children spontaneously improvised a series of dramas based on the tale. Taking turns, one child would serve as the narrator/director whose task was to "read" the tale expressively, oversee the correct development of events, give the actors directions, and supply them with the proper dialogue. The oral reading clearly imitated the teacher's actual handling of the book (even when the book was held upside down), the way she interacted with her audience, and her varying intonation, pitch, tone, and volume; and the actors' manner of confronting the troll also reflected the teacher's dramatic encounters with this fearsome creature during her many oral readings.

The skills children use in these transactions with literature reach far beyond the type of literal-level skills that prescriptive reading-readiness programs typically assign to preschoolers, the assumption being that children of this age are capable of only the most basic understanding of literature. However, in order to make literature come alive in effective dramatizations of the sort observed in Mrs. Bolton's classroom, young children must have a firm grasp of the complete picture and a

more than superficial understanding of how the events build
and the characters develop and relate to one another. In this
instance, the adult served a critical role in promoting literacy
through literature. In the questions she asked and answered
and the enthusiasm she showed, in the way she led her
students through the text by examining specific words and
phrases and specific characteristics of the illustrations, in her
manner of stating, inviting, and responding to opinions and
other reactions, and in her eagerness to take the time for
repeated readings and to reflect on and speculate about
character, incident, and the overall meaning of the story, she
empowered her students to be responsive, thoughtful readers. But perhaps the most valuable effect of this type of lively,
child-centered interaction with literature and with others
through literature—beyond the pleasure it provides—are the
opportunities it offers children to use language for real
purposes and explicit functions. It may be that one result of
inviting children to immerse themselves in books is more
children who love to read—as does this child who, at age ten,
dashed off a poem that celebrates the joy of reading:

               Books

          Books,
         ·Books,
          Books,
          Neato books,
          Strong books,
          Short books, long books,
          Very expensive books,
          These are just a few.
          Action books,
          Tough books,
          Big, fat $4.50 books,
          250 dollar books,
          Adventure books,
          Old books,
          Don't forget good books.
          Last of all, best of all . . .
          Hardy Boy books!
                    Sean A. Seward

EXTENDING CHILDREN'S ENCOUNTERS WITH LITERATURE

When children are given many options for expressing their responses to literature, the quality of their response improves. In one long-range study of children's experiences with literature in a literature-based program that spanned grades K through Five, the development and improvement of literary response hinged on the interplay between verbal and nonverbal expressions of response during both private and public encounters with books.[40] The students' experiences with literature covered the gamut: spontaneous and planned dramatizations; large- and small-group discussions; handling books from the classroom library and sharing them with peers; unsolicited oral responses such as retelling a story, comments, and storytelling; and demonstrations of response through art and writing. Allowed a full range of meaningful options for exploring literature and sharing their responses to it, they were actively drawn into the reading process and expressed their awarenesses of the characteristics and themes they discovered in literature in individual and collaborative activities and projects that involved reading, writing, speaking, and listening.

One well-documented premise which supports the type of integration observed in these classrooms stems from the commonsense notion that learning to read and acquiring literacy skills in the areas of writing, listening, and speaking are in fact integrated processes that should involve children in actual language experiences which encourage them to seek and construct meaning. Like other tools, language needs practice, and language learning is more likely to be encouraged when, in contrast to always learning *about* reading and writing, for example, children spend a great deal of their time actually reading and writing. "Children's doing," one language arts educator has pointed out, "their active social experience, and their own thinking, create the occasions for becoming more perceptive readers and listeners, more eloquent speakers and writers."[41]

The Thematic or Topical Unit

For teachers of literature, then, one crucial task—and challenge—is to develop instructional plans that not only make students attentive to the characteristics of literature, but also encourage them to further develop and refine their responses to the literature they hear and read. One effective method of fostering children's active involvement in literature and of integrating literature with all types of content is the method of organizing various selections of literature around a general topic or a specific theme or issue that children explore individually or with their peers or teacher over a designated period of time.

Teachers of all subjects who are making the transition to more literature-based instruction particularly find the integrated topical unit a helpful way to organize instruction. Frequently, they cite the following reasons for endorsing topical and thematic units:

- Although a unit plan includes a clear structure, it also provides for flexibility and options.
- As students move through a unit they attend to characteristics and elements of literature and selected literacy skills.
- In a unit content is approached from various perspectives and points of view. Students can compare different types of literature as well as the different perspectives the literature presents, while the topics on which they focus can lead them into any curricular area.
- A unit is response-centered. It provides many opportunities for children to express their reactions to literature and the topics, issues, or themes which the literature illustrates.
- A unit is child-centered. The focus can evolve out of, or be geared to specific concerns and interests of children; the selections of literature and the activities that complement them can accommodate the various needs and abilities of one's students.
- A unit is based on teacher input. Planning and implementing a focus unit require creativity which in turn leads to ownership and a personal commitment to teaching.

A topical or thematic unit can serve many purposes. One purpose is to involve students actively in meaningful experiences with literature that focus on the issues, themes, or concepts which the literature reveals to them while they are improving their ability to read. Another purpose is to give students opportunities to reflect on the discoveries they make about human experience in literature, and to draw on these discoveries as they interact and communicate with language in order to develop skills that are essential to effective writing, speaking, and listening. Given this attention to the themes and issues that writers of any type of literature propose, as well as the emphasis placed on using language for real purposes, a topical or thematic unit makes it possible to integrate children's experiences with literature and language with any curricular subject.

The plan for a unit lays out a sequence of methods and strategies. It includes such elements as a listing of various types of literature for self-selected reading, small-group reading experiences and sessions that will involve the entire group, and a description of activities for independent work and group collaboration. A given unit plan might include questions to initiate and sustain discussion and to elicit inferential and evaluative responses; sequences for involving students in drama, drawing, maskmaking, or music that invite them to interpret character, situation, or theme, or the information gleaned from an informational book; a layout for activity centers where students listen to literature on tape, record literature, or make their own books; a description of writing activities that direct students to respond to literature in journals or to write original stories, poems, plays, or "how-to" or "all about" books. The unit plan might also include a course to follow when conducting brief lessons that lead to oral reading, a film version of a book or a writing activity, or introducing a specific reading skill, an author or illustrator, a type of literature, or a particularly effective passage, stanza, or paragraph from literature or from the student's own works.

Types of Integrated Units

The first step to building an effective unit is to choose a meaningful concept or topic around which the literature and the learning activities will revolve. In one unit this central idea might derive from the literature itself. In this case, a type of literature, such as poetry, historical fiction, or folktale variants, an element of literature, such as characterization, setting, language style, or mood, a particular structure, such as the journey, or an author or illustrator, might provide the focus. In another unit, the focus could be provided by a general or specific topic or theme (developing friendships, relationships with siblings, becoming a wise consumer, or dealing with peer pressure), or a social issue (prejudice, accepting human differences, caring for the environment, drug use and abuse, or the differences and similarities between communicable, degenerative, and chronic diseases).

Some teachers link a unit to specific content, objectives or skills in their prescribed courses of study. For example, LaCheryl Parks, a sixth grade teacher in inner-city Cleveland, is responsible for teaching varying weather and climate conditions as part of her district's social studies curriculum. She has broadened this topic to include a brief exploration of the environmental issues that she is also required to teach in relation to a lesson titled "The Earth Then and Now," which is one of the sequences found in the sixth grade science textbook, published by Harcourt Brace Jovanovich. This teacher now organizes the unit around various children's books including a picturebook version of a classic poem about the seasons (*January Brings the Snow* by Coleridge), informational picturebooks (*Hurricane Watch* by Branley; *Tornado!* by Adoff), a collection of Native American poetry on nature themes (*The Earth is Sore: Native Americans on Nature* by Amon), and a collection of regional stories based on traditional songs (*Hear the Wind Blow* by Sanders).

Other teachers correlate literature units with the types of reading skills prescribed by their district's objectives for reading. In relation to a unit titled "Facing Personal Conflict," Barbara Seward, a ninth grade language arts teacher, has her students contrast story structure, character motivation, and the element of conflict in a number of novels that deal with personal and social issues surrounding drug abuse, suicide, family stress, and relationships with authority figures. Her students read, discuss, and respond in their journals to *A Hero*

Ain't Nothin' But a Sandwich by Childress, *The Mock Revolt* by Vera and Bill Cleaver, *Slake's Limbo* by Holman, *The Chocolate War* by Cormier, *Killing Mr. Griffin* by Duncan, and other works of fiction. Also, poems on these topics are read aloud and discussed in large and small-group sessions. These include "First Kiss" by Holden, "Beaver Moon—The Suicide of a Friend" by Oliver, "Storm Warnings" by Rich, which can be found in *Going Over to Your Place* by Paul Janeczko and, in Silverstein's *Where the Sidewalk Ends,* "Listen to the Mustn'ts" and "Point of View."

Units which are designed to integrate health, literature, and the language arts should also allow children many opportunities to consider health topics and issues from the different perspectives that a wide variety of literature provides. In a three-week literature-based unit developed by Peg Smith, a first grade teacher, students explored many aspects of human emotions and their relation to self-concept. In addition to their experiences with nursery rhymes that dramatize the emotional ups and downs of a horde of eccentric characters, the children heard and read poetry (two examples are "Sulk" and "Wiggly Giggles"from *The Random House Book of Poetry for Children,* edited by Prelutsky), fantasy (*Leo, the Late Bloomer* by Kraus), realistic fiction (*So What?* by Cohen; *The Day Jimmy's Boa Ate the Wash* and *Jimmy's Boa Bounces Back* by Noble), and nonfiction (*It Looked Like Spilt Milk* by Shaw).

The nutrition unit which Peg Smith developed for third grade students focused on food sources, a balanced diet, the appeal and hazards of junk food, and the significance—and pleasure—of at least experiencing the tastes of a wide range of foods. Her students wrote and shared five-line poems (the formula and examples supplied by their teacher) before she introduced them to selections in *What's on Your Plate?,* a poetry collection by Norah Smaridge, which depicts the negative effects that junk food can have on the body. Peg Smith's students also participated in an oral presentation of *Jingle Jangle Jingle,* a Readers Theatre script that introduces children to food-related words and phrases, and the nutrition-related experiments in *Foodworks,* a lively, entertaining "how-to" manual published by the Ontario Science Centre, provided opportunities for some hands-on experiences with the nature and function of digestion and ethnic variations and customs that center on food and eating.

For Nancy Joyce, who designed a unit on grandparents for students in the primary grades, variety implies the need to expose students to literature that depicts the authentic experiences of people from various regional, ethnic, and racial groups. Included among the many books she found on the topic are *When I Was Young in the Mountains,* Cynthia Rylant's tribute to her Appalachian grandparents, *Tales of a Gambling Grandma,* Dayal Kaur Khalsa's story of an endearing relationship between a little girl and her Russian grandmother, *Benjie,* in which Lexau tells of a shy black child who forces himself to go out alone to look for his grandmother's lost earring, and *The Remembering Box* by Eth Clifford, which explores the customs and memories a young boy is introduced to by his Jewish grandmother.

In order to provide children with a rich learning experience, teachers and librarians should avoid the tendency to develop units that contain a random selection of literature. The literature should be chosen with specific purposes in mind. First and foremost, there is the need to find selections of literature that complement the various needs, concerns, interests, tastes, and abilities of the children the unit is intended to serve. In addition to this fundamental requirement, the literature should be thoughtfully chosen to foster an understanding of specific concepts, conditions, and experiences related to the unit's central theme. It should be kept in mind, as well, that one essential objective of a literature-based unit is to increase children's awareness of literature and of themselves as readers of literature. An awareness of the different ways in which well-written literature fathoms human experience should further influence the teacher's or librarian's choice of books.

Components of an Integrated Literature Unit

An effective literature-based unit lays out a clear and thoughtful route for both the adult and child to follow. The various components of a unit should fit into an overall structure, one that makes it possible for skills and insights to develop in a sequential and cumulative manner over time. Planning a good unit takes time, but it is time well spent, for the product will likely be a useful resource that, allowing for flexibility as well as meaningful variation on the unit's central theme, increases ownership and generates much enthusiasm on the part of both the adult and the children.

Although there is no standard formula for designing an effective literature-based unit, a typical unit includes several basic components out of which any number of activities and interactions can evolve:

- Whole-group experiences with literature
- Individualized experiences with self-selected literature
- Activities, including extended projects, that involve individuals, small groups, or pairs of children.

Whole-group Experiences with Literature

A spirit of collaboration should characterize a session in which a large group of children gathers to experience literature. At these times children can listen to good literature, share their responses, talk about specific aspects of an assigned selection, be introduced to different writers, illustrators, and literary types, consider examples of particularly effective writing and illustrating as well as the ideas and themes writers and illustrators reveal, and share their own writing. With the teacher or librarian as both a guide and a fellow reader, children should have opportunities to talk to one another about what the selection personally means to them, how it affects them, what it makes them think about, wonder about, and notice. Whole-group sessions are also invitations to look closely at specific characteristics and elements of different selections and types of literature.

The shape and tone of a whole-group session are influenced by the manner in which the adult sets the stage for the experience. This in an important moment since children need time to settle down and settle into the literature as they make the transition from previous activities to group encounters with literature. At times, the adult's comments will initiate conversation. In Dona Bolton's preschool classroom, for example, a brief unit on the subject of death was planned after the group's pet turtle had died. The children were anxious to talk about their feelings, the need for a proper burial for the turtle, and their ideas concerning what happens to a person or animal after death. A conversation about their pet set the unit into motion and led to an oral reading of *The Tenth Good Thing About Barney* by Viorst, and *The Dead Bird* by Brown.

Children also can be drawn into a group experience with literature through:

- An invitation to make predictions about the content or another element of the literature. Here, the adult shows the cover of the book, reads the title and the name of the author and illustrator, and elicits predictions about what might happen in the story, poem, play, or informational book and who might be involved. Later, predictions are either verified, extended, or revised based on textual evidence.
- A picture from a magazine, a famous painting, a film version of the book, a film related to the unit's central theme, or a sound filmstrip (Appendix II contains several guides to literature-related media). One teacher began a literature-based unit on safe living by having her fifth graders discuss a number of magazine illustrations that showed unsafe situations. Following the discussion, the students worked in small groups and developed brief skits that dramatized both the hazardous situations and ways to correct them.
- An invitation to conjecture about the situation a selection of literature may present. Using a "What if?" proposal as an opener, the adult asks the children to wonder about their involvement in a situation which is similar to the one the literature will reveal to them. In relation to *The Dead Bird,* for example, the adult might ask, "What if you and your friends were playing one day and you found a dead bird. What would you do?"
- A significant object. For example, in relation to *Doors,* a play by Suzan Zeder about divorce, the adult might introduce a model of a spaceship and encourage the children to describe a young person who likes to build models.
- An activity. For example, in a third grade unit on physical disabilities the students are prepared for *I'm Deaf and It's Okay*

by Aseltine, Mueller, and Trait, by acting out one of the scenes from the book before the teacher reads it aloud. To initiate a unit that explored various emotions, a first grade teacher used a poetry apron with several large pockets. Each pocket contained an item of interest and a related poem, and all of the poems focused on emotions. Each session began with individual children selecting a pocket and making predictions about the poem based on the object (a flashlight for "My Parents Think I'm Sleeping" by Prelutsky; a rubber worm for "I Wouldn't Be Afraid" by Viorst; a comb and brush for "A Spooky Sort of Shadow" by Prelutsky).

• A brainstorming session in which children are invited to express their spontaneous responses to key concepts which the unit will explore. To begin a three-week unit on the differences and similarities among people, seventh grade students responded to the word "prejudice." Their teacher recorded and posted the list, for she encouraged her students to use the vocabulary and concepts in the reading journals they kept as they reacted to *The Island on Bird Street* by Orlev, *The Slave Dancer* by Fox, *Black Out Loud: An Anthology of Modern Poems by Black Americans* edited by Adoff, and many other selections that explored the experiences of people from a variety of ethnic, racial, and social groups.

Question-asking is another strategy for initiating and sustaining interest in literature. However, questions need to be varied by giving equal attention to ones that emphasize factual recall and ones that are open-ended and can therefore foster critical and interpretive thinking. Also, when response to literature is synonymous with answering a deluge of questions, reading is likely to become a tedious chore. An effective technique for curbing an inordinate dependence on question-asking is to recast a question as a statement or comment. It's important to remember that questions or comments should assist comprehension, focus children's attention on significant elements in the literature, and serve as a guide to personal response and social interaction.

In *Focus Units in Literature*, Joy Moss has classified various kinds of questions according to the type of thinking they are meant to stimulate, the activity they are intended to promote, and the attention to literature that question-asking can nurture.[42] According to Moss, who field-tested her strategies, questions about literature center around seven basic, but overlapping categories:

- Questions that set the stage for experiences with literature. Such questions foster predictions and explore expectations. In the third-grade unit on nutrition that focused on the folktale motif of the magic cooking pot, Geri McGill initiated the unit by eliciting predictions and expectations with questions that pertained to the title and the cover illustration for *Strega Nona,* written and illustrated by Tomie dePaola. These she recorded for future reference as the students gradually gained further information about the story.
- Questions that ask for basic facts about a selection. Related to the "Dragons and Giants" chapter in *Frog and Toad Together* by Lobel, Mary Beth Fulks asked her students to recall the type of book Frog and Toad were reading, the things they feared, and specific words Lobel used to create a particular mood.
- Questions that involve children in literary analysis. Questions of this type encourage children to focus on the elements of language use and style, characterization, setting, plot development, conflicts, problems, mood, noticeable patterns, and the like. For example, Mary Beth Fulks prompted her students to consider how Frog and Toad change throughout the story by comparing the characters' emotional condition at the beginning and end of the tale.
- Questions that ask readers to draw inferences based on evidence in the text and illustrations. Beth Doan, in a unit designed for third or fourth graders, asked her students to delineate the central characters in *The Hundred Penny Box* by Mathis, by finding specific descriptions that help them to piece together portraits of Dew, Michael, and Michael's mother. Further, she pointed out specific dialogue and passages in *The Hundred Penny Box* in which meanings are implied rather than overtly stated. The students are invited to consider motivation, feeling, intention, and the thoughts behind the words the characters use.
- Questions that focus on techniques used by authors and illustrators. Mary Beth Fulks draws student attention to the illustrations in *There's a Nightmare in My Closet* by Mayer, by focusing on the emotions expressed in the pictures and the thoughts that underlie an expression ("Look at the little boy's face when he is hiding under the covers. What do you think he is thinking?" and "The little boy looks different when he

decides to get rid of the nightmare. What is he thinking now?").
In her unit on outcasts for students in the upper elementary
school grades, Donna Miller concludes an oral reading of
several poems (including "Eat-It-All Elaine" by Kaye Starbird,
"Father William" by Lewis Carroll, and "Harriet Tubman" by
Eloise Greenfield) with questions that pertain to the similarities and differences between the type of outcasts each poem
reveals. She then enriches this discussion with a viewing of
Shadows in the Street, a film that depicts the experiences of
adolescents who were forced to live in the streets. Her students
now compare the young people who appear in the film with the
outcasts they had previously met in various types of literature.

• Questions that help children recognize similarities and differences among various selections of literature. In Barbara Seward's unit which focuses on some of the problems and
conflicts adolescents face, she asked her students: "What do the
three stories we have read so far say about ways to cope with
personal problems?"

• Questions that encourage readers to relate literary situations
and themes to their own experiences. In relation to an incident
in "Giants and Dragons," the teacher asked: "Have you ever
said you weren't afraid when you really were?" About the
theme in *The Hundred Penny Box:* "Did you ever have a favorite
possession that you lost or one that was thrown away?" After
considering Davey's reactions to her father's death in *Tiger Eyes*
by Judy Blume: "If you could give advice to Davey what would
you say to her?"

Promoting Independent Reading

While meaningful whole-group encounters with literature
provide children with opportunities to develop a wide range
of skills and attitudes about reading, independent reading
experiences help them to extend and refine the skills and
attitudes they develop during collaborative interactions with
literature.[43] There are several standard practices for promoting independent reading in school, but the practices are
equally feasible and effective at home. In the first, often
called Sustained Silent Reading (S.S.R.), or Drop Everything
and Read (D.E.A.R.), a brief period of each school day is

reserved for private, self-selected reading. In this approach, everyone in the school, including teachers, administrators, and support staff, is involved in reading materials of his or her own choosing. Students are not evaluated concerning the materials they read, nor are they required to report what they read. S.S.R. is not a time to complete assignments, work on projects, or interact with others. The objective of S.S.R. is to give the entire school community a consistent opportunity to engage in pleasurable, individualized reading.

There is some controversy concerning the types of materials students should be allowed to read. In some schools, the period is used for free reading; students may select any type of appropriate material, from comics to classics. In other schools, student choice is restricted to standard types of literature (poetry, plays, short stories, novels, and so forth); the reading of magazines and newspapers is not allowed. Whether independent reading is encouraged in the home or at school, however, children's choices are influenced by the types of literature made available to them. They are more likely to choose books that are immediately accessible, ones they know about through formal booktalks as well as informal conversations about literature, and ones the significant adults in their lives are enthused about. At school, children will often opt to reread literature which the entire group has explored together. This tendency, particularly among young children, to choose literature they already know, reinforces the value of developing a lending library in the classroom that is stocked with multiple copies of the literature analyzed in whole-group sessions or introduced in visits to the school library.

The same principles apply at home. Children's tastes and appreciation for literature will develop when parents demonstrate an interest in their children's reading habits and interests by taking at least some time to find out about good books for children and young adults, regularly introducing books at home, visiting the public library with their children, occasionally buying copies of favorite books as well as new discoveries, and providing uninterrupted periods of time when the entire family reads. In many families this will mean cutting down on the amount of time spent watching television.

The effects of independent reading on children's achievement are well documented. In *The Read-Aloud Handbook,* Jim Trelease reports that many studies have shown that children who consistently engage in independent reading have much in their favor.[44] It has been demonstrated that these children, particularly the ones with learning disabilities, show a marked improvement in reading skills and significant changes in their attitudes toward the importance of both voluntary and assigned reading. Ongoing involvement in independent reading also is known to influence decision-making skills, self-discipline, and the development of reading interests. Independent reading is a practice that takes little time and energy to establish; it costs relatively little compared with the huge expense of buying into a basal program; it helps to improve skills; and it attracts children to literature of all types. It thus warrants the serious attention of anyone who is interested in supporting and nurturing young readers.

Encouraging Response Through Meaningful Activities

As all enthused readers know, a good work of literature that sparks a special interest is the type of literature that readers are willing to commit themselves to. This is the literature—poem, play, historical novel, fantasy, biography, nonfiction—that keeps us alert as we give ourselves over to the pleasurable task of piecing together a steady stream of obvious and subtle clues to meaning. This is also the type of literature that takes time to process because it warrants our full attention and a great deal of reflection. Such engagement with literature is not foreign to children. When a book causes intense interest, when its ideas and themes speak to children in a special way, they like to linger in the pleasure of the reading—through repeated readings, discussion, drama, choral reading, writing, art, and other expressive activities in which they can crystallize and share both private and collaborative interpretations of a given selection. Children's involvement in meaningful activities and projects should be an invitation to take a close look at particular selections of literature, experiment with different ways to express responses to ideas, concepts, situations, and interact with literature and with others in an effort to make sense of the experiences that writers and illustrators form with language and visual images. Involved in individual and group activities that are worthwhile, children use language for real purposes and tap into their creative energies.

While the demands of classroom life make it impossible to pause and reflect on each and every selection of literature that evokes a particularly meaningful response, children will more likely refine their reading skills and strategies, develop positive attitudes toward reading, grow in their awareness of the characteristics of different types of literature, and personally connect with the ideas and insights literature provides when they have at least occasional opportunities to engage in activities and projects that encourage them to closely examine literature that genuinely interests them.

Literature-related activities can cover a wide range of possibilities. At times, a brief, spontaneous choral reading of a poem about friendship, for example, or the natural environment will involve the entire group in oral interpretation. In some instances, individual students may be writing a journal entry in response to the teacher's invitation to predict an outcome, consider what might happen to a character five years after a story has ended, or retell an incident from a different point of view. At other times, small groups of children might be working collaboratively over an extended period of time to develop thematic or topical poetry anthologies that will include poems they have found as well as ones they themselves have planned, written, and revised. Related to a literature-based unit on consumer health, for example, small groups of first or second graders might prepare oral reports by first researching specific consumer issues in books such as *General Store* by Rachel Field, *Vitamins—What They Are, What They Do* by Judith Seixas, or, concerning the effects of television viewing on consumer choices, *The Problem with Pulcifer* by Florence Parry Heide. The possibilities for literature-related activities and projects are as limitless as the adult's and children's imaginations.

Linking Literature to Writing

Literature can serve as a model for student writers since it reveals what writers write about as well as how they write. Just as children learn about and frequently emulate the successful techniques of their favorite sports figures, they often model the content and techniques they discover in the literature they hear and read. One purpose of alerting children to literary elements such as setting, mood, language style, structure, rhetorical devices like simile, metaphor, and personification, and the sequence, format, and development of an informational author's presentation is to provide them with a foundation as writers by making them conscious of the techniques and strategies which professional authors use to shape an experience, entice readers into it, and sustain their interest. The topics and themes with which professional authors and illustrators concern themselves and the ways they go about writing and illustrating can inspire children. It's as though their knowledge of such things gives them permission to experiment with similar topics and techniques.

The tendency to model the literature they read and hear surfaces at all grade levels. Even before they can write in the conventional sense, young children will imitate the writing behaviors they have observed and invent words or use their drawings to communicate information or tell a story. For example, four-year-old Elizabeth invented a wordless book with color illustrations after she had been exposed to several books of this type in her preschool classroom. Titled *The Day,* Elizabeth's book, which includes a cover with the title and author's name, progresses from dawn to nighttime. When young children have not yet acquired the necessary writing skills, they can make their drawings and dictate captions to the teacher.

Older children who have been read to and who read on their own often make a conscious effort to borrow overt and subtle elements from the literature they know best. For example, Carrie, a student in a literature-based seventh grade classroom, makes good use of suspense and conflict in *Never Trust a Smiling Cat.* With simple illustrations, vivid sound effects—like those used in comic books—touches of wry humor, and an awareness of how to build suspense and incorporate elements of surprise, she tells of an ongoing battle between a dog and a cat that live in the Fuzzy household. Like other young readers, Carrie also modeled the parts of a book. She included a title page, a dedication, and the name of her invented publishing company, and she concludes with a note to the reader that reminds one of a publisher's advertisement: "Stay tuned for the next exciting Fuzzy story, *The Cat Strikes Back*."

Teachers, parents, and librarians can encourage children of all ages to read from a writer's perspective by drawing children's attention to the nature and function of professional authors, illustrators, and the works they create. They can do this by:

- Making children aware of the people who create and produce books. Regarding books, children are surrounded by polished products. This can give them the impression that literature is always in this ready-made condition. By focusing on the people who write, illustrate, and produce books, the adult paves the way to an awareness of the complex processes involved in putting a book together. Like all writers, professionals have choices to make; they move through a process that involves hard work and much planning and thinking and revising. There are a number of resources that can reveal these processes to children. *How a Book Is Made,* an informational picture book by Aliki, introduces young children to the entire bookmaking process: the author's initial idea, the illustrator's role, and the various people in a publishing company who are responsible for editing, typesetting, printing, binding, and marketing books. Aliki emphasizes both the creative and highly technical work that goes into book production. In *Books from Writer to Reader,* Howard Greenfeld lays out a similar course for older students.
- Making children aware of the parts of a book. When children are aware of the function of a cover, title/author/illustrator page, a dedication, the company that published the book, the description on a book jacket, and the biographical sketch(es) of the author and illustrator, they begin to sense something of the effort that goes into bookmaking. Point out the purpose of such features as a table of contents, chapter headings, the frequent

subheadings found in informational books, and an index. Often, children will use these elements in their own writing—once they know about them and are encouraged to incorporate them into the pieces they write.

- Presenting stories and anecdotes about writers and illustrators. This will further help to personalize the people behind the literature. The many volumes that comprise *Something About the Author* (Gale Research Co.) contain detailed information about authors and illustrators, including where they were born and raised, why they chose their career, where they received their training, the books they are currently working on, who inspired them, and what they like to read.

- Drawing attention to specific techniques and elements in both the text and illustrations. Focusing on particularly effective uses of language, color, texture, and visual impressions and expressions, the adult emphasizes the things writers and illustrators do to draw readers in and keep them alert. How does the writer begin the story, poem, or informational book? Why does the illustrator use that color or shape there? How does the writer reveal a change in a character's development? Why do you think the writer ended the poem that way? What do the illustrations reveal about these changes? Aware of techniques and methods, young writers often experiment in imitation of specific features in the books that interest them.

- Introducing children to a variety of books by the same author or illustrator. In this case, the objective is to trace an author's or illustrator's development over time. Discussions could center around consistencies and changes in terms of topics, themes, forms, and techniques, the type or types of literature the author has written and the artist has illustrated, and improvements. The message to children is that writers and artists grow, change, and frequently try their hands at different forms and types of literature. Such awarenesses can inspire children to experiment when they write.

There are basically two types of writing in integrated literature units. In the first type, students write about the literature they hear or read; writing is used as a means to express responses to literature. In the second type, they compose original pieces that are inspired by the selections they have discussed and analyzed in the classroom.

Many teachers use journals to encourage students to write openly and freely about literature. Typically, the journal is a spiral notebook that students receive the first day of school and throughout the year as a new journal is needed. According to its original purpose, the journal should be a place for students to freely express their thoughts and feelings about any aspect of the literature. When journals are first used, students will need some direction concerning what to write about and some encouragement about writing freely. Frequently, teachers will provide students with a specific assignment for journal writing. The assignment should serve to focus student attention and allow for a great deal of individual freedom. For example, after she and her fourth grade students had read *Julie of the Wolves* by Jean Craighead George, Carrie Goddard had her students use their journals to compose letters to the various characters in George's novel, which tells of an Eskimo girl's survival and her growing recognition of the value of her cultural heritage.

In some classrooms, teachers use the dialogue journal as a variation on the journal concept. As its name implies, a dialogue journal consists of an ongoing written correspondence between the teacher and the students as well as between the students themselves. In a dialogue journal that focuses on literature, writers exchange their responses to literature and share their opinions, questions, and concerns. The dialogue journal has been shown to be particularly beneficial to students with learning problems.[45] For all students, the journal can be a safe place to express thoughts and feelings, to exchange ideas and opinions, and to develop writings skills that derive from a need to communicate.

When writing original pieces students sometimes model particular forms and types of literature. Prior to writing, they are introduced to specific elements and characteristics of the literature they will model. In the primary grades, for example, many teachers do this with literature that contains rhythmic, repetitive language and a clearly defined structure. Whether prose or poetry, this is the type of literature which enhances familiarity, and, once children know the patterns and cadences, they have little trouble creating their own variations of the original. In *Chicken Soup with Rice,* for example, Sendak leads his readers through the cycle of a year in musical verses that celebrate the special joys of eating chicken soup in each of the months. In a collaborative writing project, the student and teacher could recreate the narrative with references to different kinds of food.

A similar approach can be taken with stories that contain an obvious structure and easily discernible elements. At any grade level, folktales, fables, legends, and myths can serve this purpose once students have a firm grasp of how these narratives work. In a unit titled "Disabilities/Abilities," designed for first grade students, Noreen Gambrill had decided to approach the topic with fairy tales and several modern fantasies. Using *The Ugly Duckling* and *The Steadfast Tin Soldier,* both by Andersen, *The Little Wood Duck* by Wildsmith, *Fish Is Fish* by Lionni, and several other tales, she set out to raise children's consciousness about some of the differences and similarities that characterize people of various ages. At the end of the unit the children invented a group story, dictated to the teacher, in the manner of the tales they had been hearing and discussing. In the upper grades, survival stories like *Tracker* by Gary Paulsen, which tells of a young man's intense response to his grandfather's ensuing death, and Streiber's *Wolf of Shadows,* a haunting futuristic novel that centers on the events following a nuclear holocaust, can be analyzed for structure and other elements before students construct stories in a similar fashion.

Different forms of poetry can be used for similar purposes. In this case, the poetry form serves as a formula which allows for individual creativity. In a third grade unit in which students explored different ways of coping with personal and social problems, Peg Smith used a five-line formula to encourage her students to give voice to life's problems. To prepare the students for writing, the teacher read aloud and then conducted a drama on *Alexander and the Terrible, Horrible, No Good, Very Bad Day* by Viorst. Their involvement in drama served as the lead to a brainstorming session about problems and ways of handling them, and poetry on the topic of problems was taken from *Red Is My Favorite Color* by

Phyllis Holloran. Once they had the necessary background, the students were introduced to the five-line formula:

> Formula for Simple Five-Line Poetry:
>
> Line 1: One-word title (noun)
>
> Line 2: Two words describing the noun (adjectives)
>
> Line 3: Three words expressing the action (verbs)
>
> Line 4: Four words expressing feelings (or a four-word phrase)
>
> Line 5: One-word synonym for title (with younger children the title may simply be repeated).

Carrie Goddard laid out a similar course in a two-week unit on emotions. She and her fourth-grade students explored several poetry forms, including the five-line stanza, haiku, and free verse. Together, they listed ideas for poems, prepared first drafts, and after sharing their drafts with peers and the teacher, revised their poems, and printed and illustrated the final versions. *A Celebration of Bees* by Barbara Esbensen describes many effective techniques for involving children in poetry writing and reading.

Original pieces of writing can take many forms as integrated units unfold at any grade level. In actual health-related units, original pieces have focused on the following topics:

- Family life unit in the primary grades: happiest or saddest memories associated with grandparents; tape-recorded interviews with grandparents; and writing letters and cards to an "adopted" grandparent in a local nursing home. (Examples of literature: *Grandpa Had a Windmill, Grandma Had a Churn* by Jackson; *When I Was Young in the Mountains* by Rylant; *Through Grandpa's Eyes* by MacLachlan; *Wilfrid Gordon McDonald Partridge* by Fox.)
- Unit on sibling relationships in the primary grades: brief scripts with action and dialogue that focus on a problem involving siblings and include a realistic resolution. (Examples of literature: *Arthur's Loose Tooth* and *Arthur's Pen Pal* by Hoban; *The Perfect Family* by Carlson; *Ups and Downs with Oink and Pearl* by Chorao.)

- Career unit in the fourth grade that includes exploration of careers in selected health areas: development of brief biographies of community members involved in health professions. (Examples of literature: *Charles Drew* by Bertol; *Clara Barton, Founder of the American Red Cross* by Boylston; *The Story of Johnny Appleseed* by Aliki; *Man of Molokai: The Life of Father Damien* by Roos.)
- Unit on relationship between mental, physical, and emotional health in the fifth grade: stories based on patterns in folktales; retelling folktales from the underdog's point of view. (Examples of literature: *Beauty and the Beast* by Harris; "The Three Princesses of Whiteland" by Lang; "The Three Brothers" by Lang; *East of the Sun and West of the Moon* by Asbjornsen and Moe.)
- Unit on personal and social responsibility in middle school grades: collaborative classroom newspaper that features characters and situations found in folktales that feature the theft of magical objects. (Examples of literature: *The Table, the Donkey, and the Stick* by Galdone; "Jack and the Northwest Wind" by Chase; *The Nose Tree* by Hutton.)

Effective writing experiences evolve out of a process approach to writing. Often, writing is taught as if the process contained two components: an assignment and a product. What students need to learn over time is that there are many steps and stages involved in writing pieces that they can not only be proud of, but which also communicate what they have in mind. Through teacher demonstrations and interactions with other writers, they can learn how to search for topics, organize their ideas, look for the best ways to begin, sustain, and end a piece, ask for feedback and assistance while they are involved in the actual process of composing, revise, edit, proofread, and prepare a final draft. In keeping with the current interest in children's writing development, there are hundreds of helpful resources, many of them based on actual classroom practice, which can help teachers develop a process approach to writing in their classrooms. In particular, see *The Art of Teaching Writing* by Calkins, *In the Middle* by Atwell, *Classroom Experiences* by Gordon, and *If You're Trying to Teach Kids How to Write, You've Gotta Have This Book* by Frank.

ADDRESSING CONTROVERSIAL HEALTH TOPICS
IN THE ELEMENTARY CLASSROOM

What a Teacher Needs

The education of a college president,
The executive ability of a financier,
The humility of a deacon,
The adaptability of a chameleon,
The hope of an optimist,
The courage of a hero,
The wisdom of a serpent,
The gentleness of a dove,
The patience of Job,
The grace of God, and
The persistence of the Devil.—*Anonymous*[46]

No subject places more emphasis on the teacher's own behavior and attitudes than health education.[47] This is no more evident than when an elementary teacher is confronted with an unexpected student question or even an anticipated unit about a controversial topic or issue. While sexuality education and death education are the two topics that most commonly result in public outcry, teachers can never afford to underestimate the significance of the great diversity in upbringing of their students. Consequently, the potential for controversy exists as a result of classroom activities. It is not unusual for elementary teachers in particular to be faced with situations that result in a continuum of controversy. The difficulty ranges from mild personal teacher embarrassment that results from being spotted by an elementary child in the grocery store in the company of a significant other, to the acting-out behavior of an obese fifth grader following a class discussion on nutritious snacks, to an HIV/AIDS education teacher in the State of New York, who said, "I believe my job is at risk due to the sensitivity of the subject matter I teach."[48] Whatever their degree of intensity, teachers must be prepared to cope with these situations in a manner that will result in the safest and best learning situation for all concerned. Although there are no easy or universal answers or cues for managing controversial health issues, it is abundantly clear that neither is it appropriate to ignore or pretend that such issues are not a valid part of today's health education.[49] While colleges and universities offer whole courses about such matters, it is our intent to provide some basic suggestions and parameters for coping with health-related controversial issues in the classroom, the school, and the community.

Classroom Issues

The pressures or lack of support that teachers feel when coping with controversial issues come from a variety of sources including the students, parents, community residents, agency representatives, administrators, or simply from the teacher's own accurate perceptions or interpretation of a negative response that may actually not exist.[50] Regardless of the source, teachers must maintain a strong commitment to enabling and empowering children to interact successfully with the world around them. It is critical for parents and concerned school-based practitioners to understand that they have little choice whether or not their children will be educated about certain issues, only how this education will occur. To this end, it is helpful to compare the impact of the informal or tacit education about these topics that goes on in a variety of contexts often unintentionally throughout the child's life, with the formal school-based treatments of these issues that are planned and implemented with careful attention to developmental needs and characteristics.[51]

While the informal learning is often much more consistently reinforced throughout the child's life, it may be biased or completely inaccurate. It should also be noted, that this informal learning may not occur in a developmentally appropriate fashion, and so may cause the child to be confused or frightened. On the other hand, formal school-based programs should be developmentally appropriate, incorporating language, learning strategies, and reinforcement of concepts in the safe and nurturing environment of the classroom. In this way, children can inquire and learn about potentially problematic content in the more controlled laboratory environment of the classroom facilitated by a skilled educator, rather than at the hands of someone less sensitive and knowledgeable, in a setting much less comfortable. Specifically, we have little control about whether our children will be educated about their sexuality. The informal process of such education begins at birth. We do, however, have choices about when and how we would prefer formal education to occur. Certainly, we would hope that all parents are doing timely, compassionate, and accurate sexuality education with their children, but given that these skills are not prerequisite criteria for bearing children, there is no guarantee that this is going on. For children who are not getting a firm foundation in the home, the alternative then becomes, do we want sexuality education to occur through the prolific media images or questionably informed peers, or do we want such supplemental education to be a part of universal and compulsory schooling?

A recent publication reinforces this notion in context of education for young children about AIDS and HIV infection. While we would all hope that this disease will soon be conquered and will not become a part of children's lives, for now we must honestly answer the question, why do young children need to know about HIV/AIDS? The following help provide a powerful rationale for helping children confront and manage diverse problematic issues in their lives:

- Children are naturally curious.
- Children may have anxieties about this disease being discussed by significant adults and the media.
- Some children may have parents, other family members, or friends with AIDS or HIV infection. These children will benefit from understanding and compassion from peers and teachers.
- Many communities, schools, and neighborhoods will be home to HIV-infected children and adults in the future.[52]

In this way, it is, and will continue to be common for such issues to come up in the classroom setting if the environment is comfortable and the teacher is approachable. The following resources are suggested that deal specifically with teacher concerns about AIDS and HIV curricula:

- The Centers for Disease Control—Atlanta, GA.
- *SIECUS Report.* Vol. 16, 6 (July/August 1988). "The AIDS Epidemic: Implications for the Sexuality Education of Our Youth," Debra W. Haffner.
- *"Does AIDS Hurt?" Educating Young Children About AIDS,* Marcia Quackenbush and Sylvia Villarreal. Network Publications, a division of ETR Associates, P. O. Box 1830, Santa Cruz, CA 95061-1830, (408) 438-4080.
- *What Kids Need to Know About AIDS: Resources and Life Skills Exercises for Educators K–6,* Planned Parenthood of Northeast Pennsylvania, 112 N. 13th Street, Allentown, PA 18102.

In addition to the content to be covered, inherent in the classroom process of coping with controversial issues are the characteristics and skills of the teacher who will be faced with student questions or formal instructional or curricular expectations. While spontaneous teachable moments can't be anticipated, school districts would be well served if teaching schedules would be arranged so that formal instructional programs about controversial issues could be taught by personnel who are qualified and capable. Such skills are not commonly developed in most teacher-training programs, and many individuals are uncomfortable and unwilling to deal with such issues with their students. If the district is not sensitive to this, and doesn't make arrangements for reticent teachers, the children either will not receive the very important instruction, or the teachers' discomfort will compromise any instruction that does get done. To this end, the following questions are provided to help clarify important teacher characteristics for teaching various controversial topics:

- Is the individual sincerely enthusiastic and comfortable enough to teach the topic?
- Is the individual knowledgeable and well-trained in the area?
- Does the teacher sincerely like and respect the student audience?
- Does the teacher have the skills necessary to work with the students?
- Is the instructor able to clarify her/his own values, teach

without imposing these values, and recognize and support differing value systems of students and their families?[53]

To respond to the demands of finding such an individual, many school districts look to school nurses or "experts" from outside the classroom environment. While this is often expedient, in the long run a skilled classroom teacher can provide more consistent reinforcement of the topics in a more stable context than can a guest. Further, is it our intent to convey to children that these issues require "special handling"? It is far superior to convey that such things are better taught in the context of the whole of the child's life.

Finally, it is critical that all teachers have the skills to respond effectively to the difficult questions that children pose. Even the most skilled and experienced teacher can be caught off guard, so the following general guidelines are offered:

- Listen carefully to the question.
- If the meaning behind the question is not clear, or to better assess the child's sophistication on the matter, reflect the question back to the child, using such comments as, "I wonder what you've heard about that" or "Do you have any idea what the answer might be?"
- Give a simple, honest, concise answer.
- Check back to see if the child understands your answer.
- If the child continues to be interested in the matter, offer further information or continue the discussion.[54]

Although there are no guarantees that all problems can be prevented at the classroom level, well-prepared teachers can effectively deliver controversial content or deal with the difficult questions that children ask. This is best accomplished not in isolation, but with the support of both the school district administration and the community-at-large.

School District and Community Issues

In the discussion in Chapter 2 of this book that focused on the comprehensive school health program, we were reminded that schools are agents of communities. To be effective, in-school programs must work in concert with parents, taxpayers, the media, agencies, etc., to solve the complex problems facing today's children. This is particularly true when dealing with potentially controversial content. While some school districts choose to develop an isolationist posture and engage in programs in a secret fashion waiting to see if there is any community response, it is far preferable to seek proactively the support of the community. "The most effective strategy for 'winning the battle' . . . is anticipation: an active, positive strategy, taking the initiative, being so well prepared, having achieved so much parent/community support in advance, that no real opposition develops."[55] Following is a list of steps to help school programmers avoid community opposition before it develops:

- Create a parent's support committee.
- Develop a community support network.
- Create a curriculum advising group that includes parents.
- Hold a PTA/parents-only meeting, spelling out:
  Curriculum materials
  Qualities, qualifications, and training of teachers
  Course schedules
  Written homework assignments
  Session/classes for parents
  Permission options for parents
  Parent-teacher complaint protocol
  Plans for reports to parents
  Post-semester critique
- Cultivate the media.
- Define parents' roles at public/school board meetings.[56]

When a school district has followed the appropriate steps in the context of its community in planning a program of controversial content, the mechanism is already in place should the ongoing program face difficulty. Again, the critical variables are planning and anticipation.

Summary

The road to effective programs to deal with controversial content is paved with the basics: strong public backing, wide support at the state and district levels, committed and concerned teachers, and developmentally appropriate practice for students.[57] The needs of today's children are so diverse and complex that we cannot afford to have reluctant teachers or a political battle between adults in power compromise the timely education that they desperately need. While it is not realistic to presume that school programs will please all taxpayers and that there will never be public outcry, planning is critical to insure that the education of children is not sacrificed in the process.

NOTES

1. Jim Trelease, *The Read-Aloud Handbook,* rev. ed. (New York: Philomel, 1985), p. 51.
2. These surveys include Richard C. Anderson, et al., *Becoming a Nation of Readers: The Report of the Commission on Reading* (Champaign, IL: The Center for the Study of Reading, 1985); John I. Goodlad, *A Place Called School* (New York: McGraw-Hill, 1984); Patrick Shannon, *Broken Promises* (Granby, MA: Bergin & Garvey, 1989); Kenneth Goodman, et al., *A Report Card on Basal Readers* (New York: Richard C. Owen, 1988); and Frank Smith, *Insult to Intelligence* (New York: Arbor, 1986).
3. Shannon, *Broken Promises,* p. 62.
4. Ibid., pp. xiii–xiv.
5. Ibid., p. 96.
6. Anderson, et al., *Becoming a Nation of Readers,* p. 35.
7. Regie Routman, *Transitions* (Portsmouth, NH: Heinemann, 1988), p. 24.
8. Ibid., p. 24.
9. Shannon, *Broken Promises,* p. 95.
10. Anderson, et al., *Becoming a Nation of Readers,* p. 35.
11. Ibid., p. 74.
12. Shannon, *Broken Promises,* p. 82.
13. Richard Allington, "If They Don't Read Much, How They Gonna Get Good?" *Journal of Reading* 21 (October 1977): 57–61.
14. Anderson, et al., *Becoming a Nation of Readers,* p. 76.
15. Ibid., p. 75.
16. The first two items are documented in Anderson, et al., *Becoming a Nation of Readers,* "Extending Literacy." The third item is found in Shannon, *Broken Promises,* p. 38; evidence for item four can be found in Routman, *Transitions,* Chaps. 2 and 5. Item five is supported by Anderson, et al., *Becoming a Nation of Readers,* "Extending Literacy." Relative to item six, see Janet Hickman, "A New Perspective on

Response to Literature: Research in an Elementary School Setting," *Research in the Teaching of English* 15 (December 1981): 343–54. Relative to item seven, see John I. Goodlad, *A Place Called School*, pp. 152ff.

17. Shannon, *Broken Promises*, p. 95.
18. Ibid., p. 96.
19. Ibid.
20. For a good description of reading as a constructive act, see Anderson, et al., *Becoming a Nation of Readers*, "What Is Reading?" and Louise Rosenblatt, "The Literary Transaction: Evocation and Response," *Theory into Practice* 21 (1982): 268–77.
21. Amy Anderson McClure, "Children's Responses to Poetry in a Supportive Literary Context" (Ph.D. dissertation, The Ohio State University, 1985).
22. Maureen and Hugh Crago, *Prelude to Literacy* (Carbondale, IL: Southern Illinois University Press, 1983); Dorothy Butler, *Cushla and Her Books* (Boston: The Horn Book, 1980).
23. Nancie Atwell, *In The Middle* (Upper Montclair, NJ: Boynton/Cook, 1987); Regie Routman, *Transitions* (Portsmouth, NH: Heinemann, 1988).
24. Routman, *Transitions*, p. 15.
25. Ibid., p. 13.
26. Gordon Wells, *The Meaning Makers* (Portsmouth, NH.: Heinemann, 1986.
27. In Atwell, *In the Middle*, p. 153.
28. G. Robert Carlsen, *Books and the Teenage Reader* (New York: Bantam, 1980), Chap. 4, "Subliterature."
29. A dominant attitude in Bruno Bettelheim and Karen Zalen, *On Learning to Read: The Child's Fascination with Meaning* (New York: Knopf, 1981).
30. A study conducted by Anthony L. Manna and Dona Greene Bolton. "Emerging Literacy in a Literature-Based Preschool Classroom," with support provided by a grant from Ohio Association for the Education of Young Children, 1987–1989.
31. Shannon, *Broken Promises*, Chap. 7, "Reading Instruction and Students' Independence."
32. Nancy L. Roser, "Research Currents: Relinking Literature and Literacy," *Language Arts* 64 (January 1987): 90–97.
33. Donald Fry, *Children Talk About Books* (Milton Keynes, England: Open University Press, 1985), p. 107.
34. Marilyn Cochran-Smith, *The Making of a Reader* (Norwood, NJ: Ablex, 1984); Harriet H. Ennis, "Learning to Respond to Literature (Part II): What Counts in the Classroom," *Children's Literature Association Quarterly* 12 (Summer 1987): 94–97.
35. Donald Fry, *Children Talk About Books*, p. 97.
36. Nancy Roser and Miriam Martinez, "Roles Adults Play in Preschoolers' Response to Literature," *Language Arts* 62 (September 1985): 485–90.

37. Ibid., p. 489.
38. Based on a strategy suggested by Bette Bosma, *Fairy Tales, Fables, Legends, and Myths* (New York: Teachers College Pess, 1987), p. 27.
39. Hickman, "A New Perspective on Response to Literature: Research in an Elementary School Setting"; Ennis, "Learning to Respond to Literature (Part II): What Counts in the Classroom."
40. Hickman, "A New Perspective on Response to Literature: Research in an Elementary School Setting," p. 347.
41. Beverly A. Busching and Sara W. Lundsteen, "Curriculum Models for Integrating the Language Arts," in Beverly A. Busching and Judith I. Schwartz, eds., *Integrating the Language Arts in the Elementary School* (Urbana, IL: National Council of Teachers of English, 1983), p. 3.
42. Joy F. Moss, *Focus Units in Literature: A Handbook for Elementary School Teachers* (Urbana, IL: National Council of Teachers of English, 1984), Chap. 3, "Guidelines for Questioning."
43. Daniel Fader, *The New Hooked on Books* (New York: Berkley, 1982).
44. Trelease, *The Read-Aloud Handbook,* Chap. 8, "Sustained Silent Reading: Reading-Aloud's Natural Partner."
45. Rebecca Waters, "Dialogue Journals: Communicating in the Remedial First Grade," *Ohio Reading Teacher* 22 (October 1987): 22.
46. Anonymous. *What a Teacher Needs.* In Jacqueline Manley, "Teacher Selection for Sex Education," *SIECUS Report* 15, 2 (Nov.–Dec. 1986): 11.
47. David Anspaugh, Gene Ezell, and Karen Nash Goodman, *Teaching Today's Health,* 2d ed. (Columbus: Merrill, 1987), p. 22.
48. *Risk and Responsibility: Teaching Sex Education in America's Schools Today* (New York: The Alan Guttmacher Institute, 1989), p. 6.
49. Anspaugh, et al., *Teaching Today's Health,* p. 23.
50. *Risk and Responsibility,* pp. 12–13.
51. Irving R. Dickman, *Winning the Battle for Sex Education* (New York: The Sex Information and Education Council of the U.S., 1982), p. 2.
52. Marcia Quackenbush and Sylvia Villarreal, *"Does AIDS Hurt?" Educating Young Children About AIDS* (Santa Cruz: Network Publications).
53. Manley, "Teacher Selection," pp. 10–11.
54. Quackenbush and Villarreal.
55. Dickman, *Winning the Battle,* p. 4.
56. Ibid.
57. *Risk and Responsibility,* p. 22.

CHILDREN'S BOOKS CITED IN CHAPTER 5
Books marked with a "bullet" (•) deal with multicultural experiences.

•Adoff, Arnold, ed. *Black Out Loud: An Anthology of Modern Poems by Black Americans.* Illus. Alvin Hollingsworth. Macmillan, 1969.

———. *Tornado! Poems.* Illus. Ronald Himler. Delacorte, 1977.

Aliki. *How a Book is Made.* Harper & Row, 1986.

———. *The Story of Johnny Appleseed.* Prentice-Hall, 1963.

Amon, Aline, ed. *The Earth Is Sore: Native Americans on Nature.* Atheneum, 1981.

Andersen, Hans Christian. *The Steadfast Tin Soldier.* Illus. Paul Galdone. Houghton Mifflin, 1979.

———. *The Ugly Duckling.* Trans. R. P. Keigwin. Illus. Adrienne Adams. Scribner's, 1965.

•Asbjornsen, Peter Christian and Jorgan E. Moe. *East of the Sun and West of the Moon.* Macmillan, 1966.

•———. *The Three Billy Goats Gruff.* Illus. Marcia Brown. Harcourt Brace Jovanovich, 1957.

Aseltine, Lorraine, et al. *I'm Deaf and It's Okay.* Whitman, 1986.

Bertol, Roland. *Charles Drew.* Illus. Jo Polseno. Crowell, 1970.

Blume, Judy. *Tiger Eyes.* Dell, 1981.

Boylston, Helen Dore. *Clara Barton, Founder of the American Red Cross.* Illus. Paula Hutchison. Random House, 1955.

Branley, Franklyn M. *Hurricane Watch.* Crowell, 1987.

Brown, Margaret Wise. *The Dead Bird.* Addison-Wesley, 1958.

•Bryan, Ashley. *The Dancing Granny.* Atheneum, 1977.

Carlson, Jan. *The Perfect Family.* Carolrhoda, 1985.

Chase, Richard. "Jack and the Northwest Wind." In *The Jack Tales.* Illus. Berkeley Williams, Jr. Houghton Mifflin, 1943.

•Childress, Alice. *A Hero Ain't Nothin' But a Sandwich.* Putnam, 1973.

Chorao, Kay. *Ups and Downs with Oink and Pearl.* Harper & Row, 1986.

Cleaver, Vera, and Cleaver, Bill. *The Mock Revolt.* Harper & Row, 1971.

•Clifford, Eth. *The Remembering Box.* Houghton Mifflin, 1985.

Cohen, Miriam. *So What?* Illus. Lillian Hoban. Greenwillow, 1982.

Coleridge, Sara. *January Brings the Snow.* Illus. Jenni Oliver. Dial, 1986.

Conly, Jane Leslie. *Racso and the Rats of NIMH.* Illus. Leonard Lubin. Harper & Row, 1986.

Cormier, Robert. *The Chocolate War.* Pantheon, 1974.

dePaola, Tomie. *Strega Nona.* Prentice-Hall, 1975.

Duncan, Lois. *Killing Mr. Griffin.* Little, Brown, 1978.

Field, Rachel. *General Store.* Illus. Giles Laroche. Little, Brown, 1988.

Fox, Mem. *Wilfrid Gordon McDonald Partridge.* Kane-Miller, 1989.

•Fox, Paula. *The Slave Dancer.* Illus. Eros Keith. Bradbury, 1973.

•George, Jean Craighead. *Julie of the Wolves.* Illus. John Schoenherr. Harper & Row, 1972.

Greenfeld, Howard. *Books from Writer to Reader.* Crown, 1976.

Gunther, John. *Death Be Not Proud.* Harper & Row, 1965.

Harris, Rosemary, reteller. *Beauty and the Beast.* Illus. Errol LeCain. Doubleday, 1979.

Heide, Florence Parry. *The Problem with Pulcifer.* Illus. Judy Glassner. Harper & Row, 1982.

Hermes, Patricia. *You Shouldn't Have to Say Goodbye.* Houghton Mifflin, 1982.

Hoban, Lillian. *Arthur's Loose Tooth.* Harper & Row, 1985.
———. *Arthur's Pen Pal.* Harper & Row, 1976.
Holman, Felice. *Slake's Limbo.* Scribner's, 1974.
Hutchins, Pat. *The Doorbell Rang.* Greenwillow, 1986.
Hutton, Warrick. *The Nose Tree.* Atheneum, 1981.
Jackson, Louis A. *Grandpa Had a Windmill, Grandma Had a Churn.* Parent's Magazine Press, 1977.
Janeczko, Paul, ed. *Going Over to Your Place.* Bradbury, 1987.
•Khalsa, Dayal Kaur. *Tales of a Gambling Grandma.* Crown, 1986.
Kraus, Robert. *Leo the Late Bloomer.* Illus. Jose Aruego. Harper & Row, 1973.
Lang, Andrew, ed. "The Three Brothers." In *The Yellow Fairy Book.* Dover, 1967.
———. "The Three Princesses of Whiteland." In *The Red Fairy Book.* Dover, 1966.
•Lester, Julius. *More Tales of Uncle Remus.* Illus. Jerry Pinkney. Dial, 1988.
•———. *The Tales of Uncle Remus.* Illus. Jerry Pinkney. Dial, 1987.
•Lexau, Joan. *Benjie.* Illus. Don Bolognese. Dial, 1964.
Lionni, Leo. *Fish Is Fish.* Pantheon, 1970.
Lobel, Arnold. *Frog and Toad Together.* Harper & Row, 1971.
MacLachlan, Patricia. *Through Grandpa's Eyes.* Harper & Row, 1979.
•Mathis, Sharon Bell. *The Hundred Penny Box.* Illus. Leo and Diane Dillon. Viking Kestrel, 1975.
Mayer, Mercer. *There's a Nightmare in My Closet.* Dial, 1968.
•McKissack, Patricia. *Flossie and the Fox.* Dial, 1986.
Noble, Trinka Hakes. *The Day Jimmy's Boa Ate the Wash.* Illus. Steven Kellogg. Dial, 1980.
Ontario Science Centre. *Foodworks.* Addison-Wesley, 1987.
•Orlev, Uri. *The Island on Bird Street.* Trans. Hillel Halkin. Houghton Mifflin, 1983.
Paulsen, Gary. *Tracker.* Bradbury, 1984.
Prelutsky, Jack, ed. *The Random House Book of Poetry for Children.* Random House, 1983.
Readers Theatre Script Service. *Jingle Jangle Jingle.* Readers Theatre Script Service, n.d.
Roos, Ann. *Man of Molokai: The Life of Father Damien.* Illus. Raymond Lufkin. Lippincott, 1943.
Rylant, Cynthia. *When I Was Young in the Mountains.* Illus. Diane Goode. Dutton, 1982.
Sanders, Scott. *Hear the Wind Blow.* Illus. Ponder Goembel. Bradbury, 1985.
Seixas, Judith. *Vitamins—What They Are, What They Do.* Illus. Tom Huffman. Greenwillow, 1986.
Sendak, Maurice. *Chicken Soup with Rice.* Harper & Row, 1962.
Shaw, Charles G. *It Looked Like Spilt Milk.* Harper & Row, 1947.
Silverstein, Shel. *Where the Sidewalk Ends.* Harper & Row, 1974.
Smaridge, Norah. *What's on Your Plate?* Abingdon, 1982.

Steinbeck, John. *The Red Pony.* Penguin, 1959.

Viorst, Judith. *Alexander and the Terrible, Horrible, No Good, Very Bad Day.* Illus. Ray Cruz. Atheneum, 1972.

——. *The Tenth Good Thing about Barney.* Illus. Erik Blegvad. Atheneum, 1971.

Wildsmith, Brian. *The Little Wood Duck.* Oxford University Press, 1987.

Wright, Betty. *The Day the TV Broke Down.* Raintree, 1980.

Zeder, Suzan. *Doors.* Anchorage Press, 1985.

——. *Other Doors.* Anchorage Press, 1987.

Zindel, Paul. *The Pigman.* Harper & Row, 1968.

6. Annotated Bibliography of Children's Literature for Health Awareness

Books marked with a bullet (•) deal with multicultural experiences.

A. GROWTH AND DEVELOPMENT

Body Parts

Adler, Irving, and Adler, Ruth. *Your Eyes.* John Day, 1962. 3–5. Structure of the eye and nature of sight.

Aliki. *My Five Senses.* Crowell, 1962. 1–3. Introduction to the senses and how they work.

———. *My Hands.* Crowell, 1962. 1–3. Nature and function of hands.

Allison, Linda. *Blood and Guts: A Working Guide to Your Own Insides.* Little, Brown, 1976. 4–6. Introduction to human anatomy.

Asimov, Isaac. *How Did We Find Out about Genes?* Illus. David Wool. Walker, 1983. 6-up. Heredity introduced in prose with diagrams.

Berger, Melvin. *Why I Cough, Sneeze, Shiver, Hiccup, and Yawn.* Illus. Holly Keller. Crowell, 1983. K–3. Introduction to reflex acts explaining why they occur.

Brown, Marc. *Arthur's Tooth.* Atlantic, 1986. Pres.–3. Losing baby teeth.

Brown, Marcia. *Touch Will Tell.* Watts, 1979. 1–4. Explores sense of touch and increases one's awareness.

Cooney, Nancy Evans. *The Wobbly Tooth.* Illus. Marylin Hafner. Putnam, 1978. K–2. Losing baby teeth.

Cosgrove, Margaret. *Your Muscles and Ways to Exercise Them.* Dodd, Mead, 1980. 5-up. Explains the body's muscle structure.

d'Arcier, Marima Faivre. *What Is Balance?* Illus. Volker Theinhardt. Viking Kestrel, 1986. Pres.–3. Explains what balance is.

Dinan, Carolyn. *Say Cheese!* Viking Kestrel, 1986. Pres.–3. Losing baby teeth.

Doss, Helen. *Your Skin Holds You In.* Illus. Christine Bondante. Messner, 1978. 3–6. Introduction to human skin, its properties, and its functions.

Freedman, Russell, and Morriss, James E. *The Brains of Animals and Man.* Holiday House, 1972. 4–6. How scientists explore the brain, their discoveries, and future research prospects.

Goldin, Augusta. *Straight Hair, Curly Hair.* Illus. Ed Emberley. Harper & Row, 1987 (Trophy paperback). 1–3. Simple explanation of the composition and characteristics of human hair.

Goode, Ruth. *Hands Up!* Illus. Anthony Kramer. Macmillan, 1984. 4–6. The various functions of hands described.

Gross, Ruth Belov. *A Book about Your Skeleton.* Illus. Deborah Robison. Hastings, 1979. 2–3. Introduction to skeletal system.

Gustafson, Anita. *Some Feet Have Noses.* Illus. April Peters Flory. Lothrop, Lee & Shepard, 1983. 3–7. Explores the range of foot forms and functions.

Hammond, Winifred G. *Riddle of Teeth.* Coward, 1971. 4–6. Formation and composition of teeth and how to care for them.

Hoban, Lillian. *Arthur's Loose Tooth.* Harper & Row, 1985. 1–3. Losing baby teeth.

Holzenthaler, Jean. *My Feet Do.* Photographs by George Ancona. Dutton, 1979. Pres.–2. Picturebook showing what feet can do.

Hvass, Ulrik. *How Do I Breathe?* Illus. Volker Theinhardt. Viking Kestrel, 1986. Pres.–3. Introduction to breathing.

———. *How My Body Moves.* Illus. Volker Theinhardt. Viking Kestrel, 1986. Pres.–3. Introduction to body motion.

———. *How My Heart Works.* Illus. Volker Theinhardt. Viking Kestrel, 1986. Pres.–3. Introduction to the heart's functions.

Isadora, Rachel. *I Hear I See.* Greenwillow, 1985. Pres.–2. Familiar objects to identify; simple words to repeat using the senses.

———. *I Touch.* Greenwillow, 1985. K. How familiar objects feel or react to touch.

Krishef, Robert K. *Our Wonderful Hands.* Illus. Allan R. Smith. Lerner, 1967. 4–6. Why humans have hands; how they function.

Lauber, Patricia. *What Big Teeth You Have.* Illus. Martha Weston. Crowell, 1986. 3–5. What animals' teeth can tell us.

LeSieg, Theo. *The Eye Book.* Illus. Roy McKie. Random House, 1986. Pres.–1. How the human eye works.

Liberty, Gene. *The First Book of the Human Senses.* Illus. Robert Tidd. Watts, 1961. 4–7. Explanation of the five basic senses as well as hunger, thirst, muscle sense, and balance.

Martin, Bill Jr., and Archambault, John. *Here Are My Hands.* Illus. Ted Rand. Holt, 1985. Pres.–3. Rhyming text used to teach body parts and their uses.

McCloskey, Robert. *One Morning in Maine.* Viking Kestrel, 1952. Pres.–3. The story of a child's search for her lost tooth.

Nerlove, Miriam. *Just One Tooth.* McElderry, 1989. Pres.–3. Coping with the loss of a tooth.

Parker, Steve. *Skeleton.* Photographs by Philip Dowell. Knopf, 1988. 4–6. Introduction to skeletons.

Perkins, Al. *Hand, Hand, Fingers, Thumb.* Illus. Eric Gurney. Random House, 1968. Pres.–1. Explanation of the uses of hands, fingers, and thumbs.

————. *The Ear Book.* Illus. William O'Brian. Random House, 1968. Pres.–K. Sounds of the world around us.

————. *The Nose Book.* Illus. Roy McKie. Random House, 1970. Pres.–K. Information about noses.

Pluckrose, Henry. *Hearing.* Photographs by Chris Fairclough. Watts, 1986. Pres.–3. Picturebook explaining the sense of hearing.

————. *Seeing.* Photographs by Chris Fairclough. Watts, 1986. Pres.–3. Picturebook explaining the sense of sight.

————. *Tasting.* Photographs by Chris Fairclough. Watts, 1986. Pres.–3. Picturebook explaining the sense of taste.

————. *Touching.* Photographs by Chris Fairclough. Watts, 1986. Pres.–3. Picturebook explaining the sense of touch.

Rahn, Joan Elma. *Ears, Hearing, and Balance.* Atheneum, 1984. 5-up. Discusses ears, hearing, and balance.

Ross, Pat. *Molly and the Slow Teeth.* Illus. Jerry Milord. Lothrop, Lee & Shepard, 1980. 1–3. Losing the first tooth.

Ruis, Maria, Parramon, J. M., and Puig, J. J. Five Senses Series. Barron's, 1985. K–3. Five separate books which explore the nature and functions of the five senses.

Scott, John M. *The Senses: Seeing, Hearing, Smelling, Tasting, Touching.* Illus. John E. Johnson. Parents, 1975. 4–6. Explains the physiological basis for and the functions of our senses.

Shorto, Russell, and Cwiklik, Robert. *Delmore's Brainstorm: The Workings of the Brain.* Illus. Matt Faulkner. Kipling, 1990. 4-up. Introduction to the workings of the human brain.

Showers, Paul. *Follow Your Nose.* Illus. Paul Galdone. Crowell, 1963. 1–3. Explanation of the sense of smell.

————. *How Many Teeth?* Crowell, 1962. 1–3. Explanation of the types of teeth.

————. *Look at Your Eyes.* Illus. Paul Galdone. Crowell, 1962. 1–3. Discusses the eye.

————. *Use Your Brain.* Illus. Rosalind Fry. Crowell, 1971. K–3. Explains the brain.

•————. *Your Skin and Mine.* Illus. Paul Galdone. Harper & Row, 1987 (Trophy paperback). 1–3. Explanation of the functions of skin.

Silverstein, Alvin, and Silverstein, Virginia B. *Cells: The Building Blocks of Life.* Prentice-Hall, 1969. 3–7. Introduction to cells.

————. *The Code of Life.* Illus. Kenneth Gosner. Atheneum, 1972. 5–8. How the genetic code operates.

————. *The Skin: Coverings and Linings of Living Things.* Illus. Lee J. Ames. Prentice-Hall, 1972. 4–6. Discussion of outer coverings of some animals and plants, with emphasis on human skin.

————. *The Story of Your Ear.* Illus. Susan Gaber. Coward, 1981. 5-up. Explains structure and function of the ear.

————. *The Story of Your Foot.* Illus. Greg Wenzel. Putnam, 1987. 7-up. Describes human feet, their properties, and their actions.

————. *The Story of Your Hand.* Illus. Greg Wenzel. Putnam, 1986. 4–6. Facts and folklore concerning the hand.

————. *World of the Brain.* Morrow, 1986. 7-up. Discusses the anatomy and functioning of the brain as well as brain research.

Simon, Seymour. *Finding Out with Your Senses.* McGraw, 1971. 4–6. Activity book with projects exploring the human senses.

Stone, A. Harris. *Science Projects That Make Sense.* Illus. Mel Furukawa. McCall, 1971. 3–5. Simple experiments exploring the five senses.

Thompson, Brenda, and Giesen, Rosemary. *Bones and Skeletons.* Lerner, 1984. K–3. Introduction to bones and skeletons.

Thomson, Ruth. *Look at Hair.* Photographs by Mike Galletly. Watts, 1988. 4–6. Overview of hair varieties and functions with list of facts about hair and hair experiments.

West, Colin. *The King's Toothache.* Illus. Anne Dalton. Lippincott, 1987. Pres.–2. Finding relief for the king's toothache.

White, Anne Terry, and Lietz, Gerald S. *Windows on the World.* Garrard, 1965. 4–6. Review of the functions of the five senses.

Winthrop, Elizabeth. *Shoes.* Illus. William Joyce. Harper & Row, 1986. Pres.–3. Survey of the many kinds of shoes worn in the world.

Zim, Herbert S. *Our Senses and How They Work.* Illus. Herschel Wartik. Morrow, 1956. 4–6. Introduction to the senses and the nervous system.

————. *Your Skin.* Illus. Jean Zallinger. Morrow, 1979. 4–6. Composition, uses, and layers of the skin and problems of dysfunction.

————. *Your Stomach and Digestive Tract.* Illus. René Martin. Morrow, 1973. 3–6. Introduction to digestion.

Body Systems

Baldwin, Dorothy, and Lister, Claire. *Your Senses.* Bookwright, 1984. 5-up. How the senses work.

Berger, Melvin. *Bionics.* Watts, 1978. 5–7. Introduction to the structure and system of plants and animals.

Branley, Franklyn M. *Oxygen Keeps You Alive.* Illus. Don Madden. Crowell, 1971. 2–3. How humans, plants, and fish use oxygen.

————. *Shivers and Goose Bumps.* Illus. True Kelley. Crowell, 1984. 3–6. How birds, humans, and other mammals keep their bodies and homes warm, on earth and in space.

Cosgrove, Margaret. *Your Muscles—And Ways to Exercise Them.* Dodd, Mead, 1980. 4–6. Composition and uses of muscles and how to keep them in shape.

d'Arcier, Marima Faivre. *What Is Balance?* Illus. Volker Theinhardt. Viking Kestrel, 1986. 1–3. Introduction to balance with experiments to perform.

Goldenson, Robert M. *All about the Human Mind.* Random House, 1963. 6–9. How the brain works; how personality develops.

Haines, Gail Kay. *Brain Power: Understanding Human Intelligence.* Watts, 1979. 6–9. Overview of the human brain and intelligence.

Hvass, Ulrik. *How Do I Breathe?* Illus. Volker Theinhardt. Viking Kestrel, 1986. 1–3. Explanation of breathing with experiments.

———. *How My Heart Works.* Illus. Volker Theinhardt. Viking Kestrel, 1986. 1–3. Explanation of how the heart works with experiments to perform.

———. *How My Body Moves.* Illus. Volker Theinhardt. Viking Kestrel, 1986. 1–3. Explanation of body motion with experiments.

Limburg, Peter R. *The Story of Your Heart.* Illus. Ellen G. Jacobs. Coward, 1979. 4–6. Functions and possible malfunctions of the human heart.

Rahn, Joan Elma. *Keeping Warm, Keeping Cool.* Atheneum, 1983. 6-up. How living things adapt to temperature changes to conserve heat in cold weather and lose it in hot weather.

Schneider, Leo. *Lifeline: The Story of Your Circulatory System.* Harcourt, 1958. 6–9. Introduction to the circulatory system.

Showers, Paul. *A Drop of Blood,* rev. ed. Illus. Don Madden. Crowell, 1989. K–4. Introduction to blood and its functions.

———. *Hear Your Heart.* Illus. Joseph Low. Harper & Row, 1987 (Trophy paperback). 1–3. Introduction to the heart and its functions.

———. *How You Talk.* Illus. Robert Galster. Crowell, 1966. 1–3. How speech sounds are produced with experiments.

———. *Use Your Brain.* Illus. Rosalind Fry. Crowell, 1971. 2–3. Structure and function of the brain and some other parts of the nervous system.

———. *What Happens to a Hamburger?* Illus. Anne Rockwell. Crowell, 1970. 1–3. Digestion in simple terms.

Silverstein, Alvin, and Silverstein, Virginia B. *Heart Disease.* Follett, 1976. 6–9. Overview of heart disease, its prevention and treatment.

———. *Heartbeats: Your Body, Your Heart.* Illus. Stella Ormai. Lippincott, 1983. 4–6. Explores the circulatory system and heart disease, emphasizing disease prevention through diet and exercise.

———. *The Digestive System.* Illus. Mel Erikson. Prentice-Hall, 1971. 4-up. Detailed discussion of the digestive system.

———. *The Respiratory System: How Living Creatures Breathe.* Illus. George Bakacs. Prentice-Hall, 1969. 4–6. Breathing of humans, plants, and animals outlined.

———. *The Skeletal System: Frameworks for Life.* Illus. Lee J. Ames. Prentice-Hall, 1972. 4–6. Skeletal structures of humans and animals.

———. *Wonders of Speech.* Morrow, 1988. 7-up. Survey of oral communication.

Simon, Seymour. *About Your Heart.* Illus. Angie Culfogienis. McGraw, 1974. 2–3. Introduction to the heart and its functions with simple projects.

Stafford, Patricia. *Your Two Brains.* Illus. Linda Tunney. Atheneum, 1986. 6-up. Introduction to the human brain and how it functions.

Weart, Edith L. *The Story of Your Blood.* Illus. Z. Onyshkewych. Coward, 1960. 4–6. Elementary introduction to the composition and uses of blood.

————. *The Story of Your Brain and Nerves.* Illus. Alan Tompkins. Coward, McCann, 1961. 5–7. Introduction to the human nervous system and its functions.

Zim, Herbert S. *Blood.* Illus. René Martin. Morrow, 1968. 4–6. Discussion of composition of blood, how the body uses it, and the variety of blood types.

————. *Bones.* Illus. René Martin. Morrow, 1969. 3–6. Parts and functions of the human skeleton with explanation of composition and formation of bones.

————. *Your Brain and How It Works.* Illus. René Martin. Morrow, 1972. 4–6. Growth and development of the human brain, parts, and functions with comparison to brains of other animals.

————. *Your Heart and How It Works.* Illus. Gustav Schrotter. Morrow, 1959. 4–6. Structure and function of heart and its role in the circulatory system.

Growth and Development

•Bryan, Ashley. *Lion and the Ostrich Chicks and Other African Folk Tales.* Macmillan, 1986. 3–5. An underdog triumphs in each of these amusing tales.

Conrad, Pam. *Staying Nine.* Illus. Mike Wimmer. Harper & Row, 1988. 2–4. Predicaments involved with growing older.

Hutchins, Pat. *Happy Birthday, Sam.* Greenwillow Books, 1978. Pres.–1. Small child's urge to be able to do more than he can.

McPhail, David. *Pig Pig Grows Up.* Dutton, 1980. 1–3. A pig grows up.

Miller, Jonathan, and Pelham, David. *The Human Body.* Illus. Harry Willock. Viking Kestrel, 1983. 6-up. Three-dimensional book about the human body.

————. *The Facts of Life.* Illus. Harry Willock. Viking Kestrel, 1984. 6-up. Three-dimensional book explaining the facts of life.

•Morimoto, Junko. *The Inch Boy.* Viking Kestrel, 1986. Pres.–3. Japanese folktale retold about growing up.

Patent, Dorothy Hinshaw. *Babies!* Holiday House, 1988. 1–4. Stages of human development from birth to age two.

Solotareff, Gregoire. *Don't Call Me Little Bunny.* Farrar, Straus & Giroux, 1988. Pres.–2. Growing up.

Takihara, Koji. *Rolli.* Picture Book Studio, 1989. Pres.–3. A story of growth and progress.

Williams, Susan. *Poppy's First Year.* Four Winds Press, 1989. Pres.–2. Description of the stages of a baby's first year.

Zolotow, Charlotte. *Someone New*. Illus. Erik Blegvad. Harper & Row, 1978. Pres.–3. Picturebook about a young child growing up.

The Human Body

ABC's of the Human Body: A Family Answer Book. Reader's Digest, 1987. 6-up. Encyclopedia-like volume that demystifies the functions and systems of the human body.

Asimov, Isaac. *The Human Body: Its Structure and Operation*. Houghton Mifflin, 1963. 6–9. Mature introduction to systems and parts of the human body.

Bell, Neill. *Only Human: Why We Are the Way We Are*. Illus. Sandy Clifford. Little, Brown, 1983. 6-up. Explains the human animal by way of games, clever text, and illustrations.

Brenner, Barbara. *Bodies*. Illus. George Ancona. Dutton, 1973. K–3. Qualities that make the animal world different from plants and manmade objects are discussed.

Bruun, Ruth Dowling, and Bruun, Bertel. *Human Body*. Illus. Patricia J. Wynne. Random House, 1982. 6-up. An atlas of the human body with easy reading-level text.

Cole, Joanna. *The Human Body: How We Evolved*. Illus. Walter Geoffney-Kessell and Juan Carlos Barberis. Morrow, 1987. 6-up. Traces the historical evolution of the human body.

Donner, Carol. *The Magic Anatomy Book*. Freeman, 1986. 4–6. Two children learn how the human body works by being transported into a live human body, using logic and intuition to escape.

Jackson, Gordon. *Medicine*. Illus. Chris Forsey and Jim Robins. Watts, 1984. 6-up. Discusses the structure and function of the human body.

Klein, Aaron E. *You and Your Body*. Illus. John Love. Doubleday, 1977. 3–6. Manual that emphasizes activities that can help young readers learn about the body.

Lauber, Patricia. *Your Body and How It Works*. Illus. Stephen Rogers Peck. Random House, 1962. 3–4. Explanation of the functions of the human body.

Rutland, Jonathan. *Human Body*. Watts, 1977. 4–7. Overview of the human body organized by various body systems.

Simon, Seymour. *Body Sense, Body Nonsense*. Illus. Dennis Kendrick. Harper & Row, 1981. 3–6. Are the twenty-one beliefs listed about the human body fact or fiction?

Whitefield, Phillip, and Whitefield, Ruth. *Why Do Our Bodies Stop Growing?* Viking Kestrel, 1988. 3-up. How the body works, in question-and-answer format.

Wilton, Ron. *How the Body Works*. Larousse, 1979. 4–7. Body parts, systems, and how they function.

Zim, Herbert S. *What's Inside Me?* Illus. Herschel Wartik. Morrow, 1952. 2–5. The functions of the human body explained.

B. EMOTIONAL AND MENTAL HEALTH

Grades K Through Three

Coping Behaviors

•Abells, Chana Byers. *The Children We Remember.* Greenwillow, 1986. All ages. Tells the story of Jewish children before, during, and after the Holocaust, with black-and-white photographs.

Aliki. *We Are Best Friends.* Greenwillow, 1982. Pres.–3. Friendship doesn't always end when a best friend moves away.

Asch, Frank. *Goodbye House.* Prentice-Hall, 1986. K–2. Fear of moving.

Aseltine, Lorraine. *First Grade Can Wait.* Illus. Virginia Wright-Frierson. Whitman, 1989. Pres.–2. Being held back because of immaturity.

Barbato, Juli. *From Bed to Bus.* Illus. Brian Schatell. Macmillan, 1985. K–3. Preparation for the first day of school.

Berenstain, Stan, and Berenstain, Jan. *The Berenstain Bears and Mama's New Job.* Random House, 1984. 1–3. Coping with change.

Blegvad, Lenore. *Rainy Day Kate.* Illus. Erik Blegvad. McElderry, 1988. Pres.–2. Coping with loneliness.

Boegehold, Betty. *You Can Say "No".* Illus. Carolyn Bracken. Golden, 1985. Pres.–4. How a child can handle potentially dangerous situations.

Brown, Laurene Krasny, and Brown, Marc. *Dinosaurs Divorce: A Guide for Changing Families.* Illus. Marc Brown. Little, Brown, 1986. Pres.–3. Dealing with divorce.

Brown, Marc. *Arthur's Baby.* Little, Brown, 1987. Pres.–3. Coping with a new baby.

Bulla, Clyde Robert. *The Cardboard Crown.* Illus. Michele Chessare. Crowell, 1984. 2–4. Making a new friend.

———. *The Chalk Box Kid.* Illus. Thomas B. Allen. Random House, 1987. 2–4. Coping with loneliness and change.

Burnett, Frances Hodgson. *The Secret Garden.* Illus. Ruth Sanderson. Knopf, 1988. K–6. Friendship developed between an unhappy girl and her invalid cousin.

•Cameron, Ann. *The Most Beautiful Place in the World.* Illus. Thomas B. Allen. Knopf, 1988. Pres.–3. A Guatemalan boy copes with abandonment and poverty and triumphs.

•———. *The Stories Julian Tells.* Illus. Ann Strugnell. Pantheon, 1981. K–3. Stories of family interaction and childhood mischief.

Carlson, Nancy. *Arnie and the Stolen Markers.* Viking Kestrel, 1987. 1–3. Coping with stress, confessing guilt.

Carrick, Carol. *Left Behind.* Illus. Donald Carrick. Clarion, 1988. K–3. Coping with being lost.

Castiglia, Julie. *Jill the Pill.* Illus. Steven Kellogg. McElderry/Atheneum, 1979. K–3. Deals with sibling rivalry.

Chapman, Carol. *Ig Lives in a Cave.* Illus. Bruce Degen. Dutton, 1979. K–3. Five short stories about a cave boy growing up.

Chorao, Kay. *Oink and Pearl.* Harper & Row, 1981. K–3. Acceptance of a younger sibling.

Christiansen, C. B. *My Mother's House, My Father's House.* Illus. Irene Trivas. Atheneum, 1989. K–3. Dealing with separated parents.

Cole, Joanna. *It's Too Noisy!* Illus. Kate Duke. Crowell, 1989. Pres.–3. Learning to deal with noise.

Cooney, Nancy Evans. *The Blanket That Had to Go.* Illus. Diane Dawson. Putnam, 1981. K–3. Overcoming fears, gaining security.

Delton, Judy. *The New Girl at School.* Illus. Lillian Hoban. Dutton, 1979. K–3. Adjusting to a new school.

Drescher, Joan. *My Mother's Getting Married.* Dial, 1986. Pres.–3. Dealing with family change.

Fair, Sylvia. *The Bedspread.* Morrow, 1982. K–3. Sibling rivalry.

Ferguson, Alane. *That New Pet!* Illus. Catherine Stock. Lothrop, Lee & Shepard, 1986. Pres.–2. Dealing with jealousy of a new baby.

Fox, Mem. *Wilfrid Gordon McDonald Partridge.* Illus. Julie Vivas. Kane/ Miller, 1985. Pres.–2. Understanding old age.

Freedman, Sally. *Devin's New Bed.* Illus. Robin Oz. Whitman, 1986. Pres.–1. Getting used to something new.

Giff, Patricia Reilly. *Today Was a Terrible Day.* Illus. Susanna Natti. Viking Kestrel, 1980. K–3. Dealing with stress.

Gordon, Shirley. *Happy Birthday, Crystal.* Illus. Edward Frascino. Harper & Row, 1981. K–3. Dealing with jealousy.

Gould, Deborah. *Aaron's Shirt.* Illus. Cheryl Harness. Bradbury, 1989. Pres.–1. Coping with change, growing.

Graham, Bob. *Bath Time for John.* Little, Brown, 1988. Pres.–1. A dog and a young boy discover bath time.

———. *Here Comes John.* Little, Brown, 1988. Pres.–1. A young boy almost eats something revolting.

———. *Here Comes Theo.* Little, Brown, 1988. Pres.–1. Features an overly enthusiastic dog.

———. *Where's Sarah?* Little, Brown, 1988. Pres.–1. Sibling relationships.

Green, Phyllis. *Ice River.* Illus. James Crowell. Addison-Wesley, 1975. K–3. Coping with feelings; with new father.

Grimm Brothers and Zwerger, Lisbeth. *Hansel and Gretel.* Picture Book Studio, 1989. Pres.–3. Folktale of childlike trust and innocence triumphing over wickedness.

Henkes, Kevin. *Two Under Par.* Greenwillow, 1987. 2–6. Coping with a stepfamily.

Hest, Amy. *The Purple Coat.* Illus. Amy Schwartz. Macmillan, 1986. 1–3. Learning to live within means.

•Hill, E. *Evan's Corner.* Holt, 1967. 1–2. A young child seeks a quiet space in his crowded home.

Hines, Anna Grossnickle. *They Really Like Me!* Greenwillow, 1989. Pres-2. Sibling rivalry between a young boy and his older sisters.

Hughes, Shirley. *Another Helping of Chips.* Lothrop, Lee & Shepard. 1987. 2–3. Dealing with friends.

Iverson, Genie. *I Want to Be Big.* Illus. David McPhail. Dutton, 1979. K–3. Coping with growing up.

Kleeberg, Irene C. *Latch-Key Kid.* Illus. Anne C. Green. Watts, 1985. 2–4. Advice for children who must be home alone.

Lakin, Patricia. *Oh, Brother!* Illus. Patience Brewster. Little, Brown, 1987. Pres.–3. Coping with a little brother.

Lasky, Kathryn. *Sea Swan.* Illus. Catherine Stock. Macmillan, 1988. 1–4. Coping with old age.

Leedy, Loreen. *Pingo the Plaid Panda.* Holiday House, 1989. Pres.–3. Coping with loneliness, making friends.

LeShan, Eda. *What's Going to Happen to Me?* Macmillan, 1978. 3-up. Coping with separation and divorce.

Leverich, Kathleen. *Best Enemies.* Illus. Susan Condie Lamb. Greenwillow, 1989. 1–3. Learning how to make friends.

Lionni, Leo. *Nicolas, Where Have You Been?* Knopf, 1987. Pres.–3. Learning how to get along with others, overcoming prejudice.

•Lloyd, Errol. *Nini at Carnival.* Crowell, 1979. K–3. Coping with stress.

MacLachlan, Patricia. *Mama One, Mama Two.* Illus. Ruth Lercher Bornstein. Harper & Row, 1982. K–3. Coping with depression.

Manes, Stephen. *Life Is No Fair.* Illus. Warren Miller. Dutton, 1985. 2–4. Coping with moving.

Martin, Rafe. *Foolish Rabbit's Big Mistake.* Illus. Ed Young. Putnam, 1985. K–3. How one's behavior influences another.

Milord, Sue. *Maggie and the Goodbye Gift.* Illus. Jerry Milord. Lothrop, Lee & Shepard, 1979. K–3. Coping with moving.

•Mohr, Nicholasa. *Going Home.* Dial, 1986. Pres.–3. Coming to terms with ethnic heritage.

Murrow, Liza Ketchum. *Good-bye, Sammy.* Illus. Gail Owens. Holiday House, 1989. Pres.–3. Coping with loss.

O'Brien, Anne Sibley. *Come Play with Us.* Holt, 1985. Pres.–2. Dealing with childhood problems.

————. *I Want That.* Holt, 1985. Pres.–2. Dealing with childhood problems.

————. *I'm Not Tired.* Holt, 1985. Pres.–2. Dealing with childhood problems.

————. *Where's My Truck?* Holt, 1985. Pres.–2. Dealing with childhood problems.

O'Donnell, Elizabeth Lee. *Maggie Doesn't Want to Move.* Illus. Amy Schwartz. Four Winds, 1987. Pres.–3. Coping with moving.

Pearson, Susan. *Saturday I Ran Away*. Illus. Susan Jeschke. Lippincott, 1981. K–3. Coping with family conflicts.

Prelutsky, Jack. *The New Kid on the Block*. Illus. James Stevenson. Greenwillow, 1984. K–4. Poetry about coping with everyday experiences.

Roberts, Willo Davis. *Eddie and the Fairy Godpuppy*. Illus. Leslie Morrill. Atheneum, 1984. 2–3. An orphan learns to cope.

Ross, Pat. *M and M and the Big Bag*. Illus. Marylin Hafner. Pantheon, 1981. 1–3. Handling stress.

Schuchman, Joan. *Two Places To Sleep*. Illus. Jim LaMarche. Carolrhoda Books, 1988. K–4. Coping with divorce.

Schwartz, Amy. *Annabelle Swift, Kindergartner*. Watts, 1988. Pres.–1. Coping with stress the first day of school.

Shyer, Marlene F. *Here I Am, an Only Child*. Illus. Donald Carrick. Scribner's, 1985. Pres.–3. Coping with being an only child.

Smith, Janice Lee. *The Show-and-Tell War: and Other Stories About Adam Joshua*. Illus. Dick Gackenbach. Harper & Row, 1988. 1–4. Coping with the frustrations of being a youngster.

Snyder, Zilpha Keatley. *Come On, Patsy*. Illus. Margot Zemach. Atheneum, 1982. Pres.–3. Dealing with peer pressure.

Stanek, Muriel. *All Alone After School*. Illus. Ruth Rosner. Whitman, 1985. 2–4. Coping with being left alone.

———. *My Little Foster Sister*. Whitman, 1981. 1–3. Adjusting to a new sibling, adoption.

Steig, William. *Spinky Sulks*. Farrar, 1988. Pres.–3. Coping with family problems.

Stevenson, James. *That Dreadful Day*. Greenwillow, 1985. Pres.–2. Coping with school.

Vigna, Judith. *Daddy's New Baby*. Whitman, 1982. Pres.–3. Adjusting to divorce, a new baby.

———. *Grandma Without Me*. Whitman, 1984. K–3. Dealing with feelings of loss, separation, and disorientation.

———. *She's Not My Real Mother*. Whitman, 1980. 1–3. Learning to accept stepparents.

Vincent, Gabrielle. *Feel Better, Ernest!* Greenwillow, 1988. Pres.–2. Coping with illness.

Waber, Bernard. *Ira Says Goodbye*. Houghton Mifflin, 1988. Pres.–3. Coping with the loss of a best friend.

———. *Ira Sleeps Over*. Houghton Mifflin, 1972. K–3. Growing up and becoming independent.

Wahl, Jan. *So Many Raccoons*. Illus. Beth Lee Weiner. Caedmon, 1985. K–3. Running away; family relationships.

Wells, Rosemary. *Hazel's Amazing Mother*. Dial, 1985. Pres.–2. Coping with stress; family relationships.

Wilhelm, Hans. *A New Home, A New Friend*. Random House, 1985. K–3. Coping with moving.

———. *More Bunny Trouble*. Scholastic, 1989. Pres.–3. Learning to be responsible to others.

Williams, Barbara. *So What If I'm a Sore Loser?* Illus. Linda Strauss Edwards. Harcourt Brace Jovanovich, 1981. K–3. Dealing with conflict.

Yaffe, Alan. *The Magic Meatballs.* Illus. Karen Born Andersen. Dial, 1979. K–3. Coping with family stress.

Zemach, Margot. *It Could Always Be Worse.* Scholastic, 1986. Pres.–4. Learning to cope with life's stresses.

Ziefert, Harriet. *I Won't Go to Bed!* Illus. Andrea Baruffi. Little, Brown, 1987. Pres.–3. Learning to cope with fears.

Responsibility to Self and Others

Andersen, Hans Christian. *The Ugly Duckling.* Illus. Robert Van Nutt. Knopf, 1986. Pres.–3. Classic tale of developing positive self-image.

•Andrews, Jan. *The Very Last First Time.* Illus. Ian Wallace. Atheneum, 1986. 1–4. A journey to self discovery.

•Autumn, White Deer. *Ceremony—In the Circle of Life.* Illus. Sanyan Tawa Wicasta. Carnival, 1982. K–4. Learning to accept oneself.

Barr, June. *The Three Little Kittens.* In *Plays Children Love,* Coleman A. Jennings and Aurand Harris, eds. St. Martins, 1988. K–3. Play about coping with everyday problems; learning to cooperate.

Baylor, Byrd. *Everybody Needs a Rock.* Macmillan, 1974. K–3. Special places can help us grow spiritually.

Bingham, Mindy. *Minou.* Illus. Itoko Maeno. Girls Clubs of America, 1985. K–3. Learning to become self sufficient.

Bingham, Mindy, and Paine, Penelope. *My Way Sally.* Illus. Itoko Maeno. Girls Clubs of America, 1986. K–3. Learning leadership skills.

Brown, Marc. *Arthur's Nose.* Little, Brown, 1976. Pres.–3. Learning to live with one's uniqueness.

———. *The True Francine.* Little, Brown, 1981. 1–3. Developing conflict-resolution skills.

Browne, Anthony. *Willy the Wimp.* Knopf, 1985. Pres.–2. Developing self-image.

Bryan, Ashley. "Tortoise, Hare, and the Sweet Potatoes." In *The Ox of the Wonderful Horns and Other African Folktales.* Atheneum, 1971. K–3. The slow tortoise outwits the trickster hare; self-image.

Cameron, Ann. *The Most Beautiful Place in the World.* Illus. Thomas B. Allen. Knopf, 1988. 1–3. Developing self-concept.

Caple, Kathy. *The Purse.* Houghton Mifflin, 1986. K–3. Growing up; accepting responsibility.

Carlson, Nancy. *Making the Team.* Carolrhoda, 1985. K–3. Discovering talents; developing self-concept.

Castle, Caroline, reteller. *The Hare and the Tortoise.* Illus. Peter Weevers. Dial, 1985. K–3. Developing self-concept.

Cleary, Beverly. *Janet's Thingamajigs.* Illus. Dyanne Disalvo-Ryan. Morrow, 1987. Pres.–1. Developing pride in growing up.

Cosgrove, Stephen. *Tee-Tee.* Illus. Robin James. Price/Stern/Sloan, 1983. Pres.–3. Finding oneself; developing independence.

Delton, Judy. *I Never Win!* Illus. Cathy Gilchrist. Carolrhoda, 1981. 1–3. Developing a self-concept.

dePaola, Tomie. *Oliver Button Is a Sissy.* Harcourt Brace Jovanovich, 1979. K–3. Learning to accept oneself.

Duvoisin, Roger. *The Importance of Crocus.* Knopf, 1981. 1–3. Learning to accept oneself.

Frank, Josette, selector. *Poems to Read to the Very Young.* Illus. Eloise Wilkin. Random House, 1982. Pres.–3. Selection of more than seventy poems about childhood experiences.

Gackenback, Dick. *Hattie, Tom, and the Chicken Witch.* Harper & Row, 1980. 1–3. A play about cooperation.

Hadithi, Mwenye. *Tricky Tortoise.* Illus. Adrienne Kennaway. Little, Brown, 1988. Pres.–3. A small creature triumphs over a large bully.

•Haller, Danita Ross. *Not Just Any Ring.* Illus. Deborah Kogan Ray. Knopf, 1982. 2–5. Developing a self-concept.

Heide, Florence Parry. *Time Flies!* Illus. Marylin Hafner. Holiday House, 1984. 2–5. Gaining self-confidence; dealing with a new sibling.

Hines, Anna Grossnickle. *Keep Your Old Hat.* Dutton, 1987. Pres.–1. Learning to cooperate with others.

Hoban, Tana. *Panda, Panda.* Greenwillow, 1986. Pres.–K. A board book about a day in the life of a panda.

Hoff, Syd. *Soft Skull Sam.* Harcourt Brace Jovanovich, 1981. K–3. Developing a self-concept.

Hoffman, Mary. *Nancy No-Size.* Illus. Jennifer Northway. Oxford, 1987. Pres.–3. Developing a sense of self.

Hurwitz, Johanna. *Russell Rides Again.* Illus. Lillian Hoban. Morrow, 1985. Pres.–1. Childhood experiences; developing a sense of self.

Johnston, Tony. *The Quilt Story.* Illus. Tomie dePaola. Putnam, 1985. K–3. Developing a sense of heritage; developing self-concept.

Kellogg, Steven. *Best Friends.* Dial, 1986. Pres.–3. Accepting responsibility for oneself.

Kline, Suzy. *Herbie Jones.* Illus. Richard Williams. Putnam, 1985. 2–5. Developing a sense of self.

————. *Ooops!* Illus. Dora Leder. Whitman, 1989. Pres.–2. Everyday childhood experiences; developing self-concept.

Lagercrantz, Rose, and Lagercrantz, Samuel. *Brave Little Pete of Geranium Street.* Jack Prelutsky, adapter. Illus. Eva Eriksson. Greenwillow, 1986. Pres.–3. Developing self-identity.

Lakin, Patricia. *Don't Touch My Room.* Illus. Patience Brewster. Little, Brown, 1985. Pres.–3. Getting along with siblings; developing sense of self.

•Lattimore, Deborah Nourse. *The Flame of Peace.* Harper & Row, 1987. 2–4. Learning cooperation; developing a positive self-image.

LeGuin, Ursula K. *A Visit from Dr. Katz.* Illus. Ann Barrow. Atheneum, 1988. Pres.–3. Friendship with pets.

Lewis, Rob. *Friska, the Sheep That Was Too Small.* Sunburst, 1989. Pres.–3. Developing self-concept; being the smallest.

Lindgren, Astrid. *I Want a Brother or Sister.* Trans. Barbara Lucas. Illus. Ilon Wikland. Harcourt Brace Jovanovich, 1981. 1–3. Accepting a new baby.

Lionni, Leo. *Cornelius.* Pantheon, 1983. Pres.–3. Accepting differences; self-image.

———. *It's Mine!* Knopf, 1986. Pres.–2. Learning to cooperate; childhood experiences.

Livermore, Elaine. *Looking for Henry.* Houghton Mifflin, 1988. Pres.–3. Learning to accept oneself.

Lopshire, Robert. *I Want To Be Somebody New!* Random House, 1986. K–3. Accepting oneself.

Maris, Ron. *I Wish I Could Fly.* Greenwillow, 1987. Pres.–1. Learning to accept oneself.

Martin, Judith. *Hands Off! Don't Touch!* In *Plays Children Love.* Coleman A. Jennings and Aurand Harris, eds. Doubleday, 1981. 2-up. Plays about learning respect for others.

McCarthy, Ruth. *Katie and the Smallest Bear.* Illus. Emilie Boon. Knopf, 1986. Pres.–1. Developing a friendship.

McCaslin, Nellie. *The Rabbit Who Wanted Red Wings.* Morton Grove, IL: Coach House Press, 1963. K–3. Play about developing a self-concept.

Moncure, Jane Belk. *Happy Healthkins.* Illus. Lois Axeman. Childrens Press, 1982. 2-up. How to be physically and emotionally happy.

Morel, Roselyne. *The Two Rabbits.* Illus. Doris Smith. Aladdin, 1988. K–3. Developing friendship; survival.

Newman, Alyse. *It's Me, Claudia!* Watts, 1981. K–3. Accepting oneself.

Parenteau, Shirley. *I'll Bet You Thought I Was Lost.* Illus. Lorna Tomei. Lothrop, Lee & Shepard, 1981. 1–3. Learning to solve problems.

Parks, Van Dyke, and Jones, Malcolm. *Jump! The Adventures of Brer Rabbit.* Adapted from folktales collected by Joel Chandler Harris. Illus. Barry Moser. Harcourt Brace Jovanovich, 1986. K–4. Developing self-concept.

Pinkwater, Daniel. *Bear's Picture.* Dutton, 1984. K–3. Developing individuality.

Piper, Watty. *The Little Engine That Could.* Illus. George and Doris Hauman. Platt, 1961. Pres.–2. Positive thinking, self-image, and persistence.

•Prusski, Jeffrey. *Bring Back the Deer.* Illus. Neil Waldman. Harcourt Brace Jovanovich, 1988. Pres.–3. Story of growth and coming of age.

Pryor, Bonnie. *Grandpa Bear.* Illus. Bruce Degen. Morrow, 1985. K–3. Developing self-concept; friendship.

Reit, Seymour V., Hooks, William H., and Boegehold, Betty D. *When Small Is Tall and Other Read-Together Tales.* Illus. Lynn Munsinger. Random House, 1985. Pres.–1. Developing a positive self-image.

Richardson, Jean. *Tall Inside.* Illus. Alice Englander. Putnam, 1988. 1–3. Developing a positive self-image.

Sadler, Marilyn. *It's Not Easy Being a Bunny.* Illus. Roger Bollen. Random House, 1983. K–3. Accepting oneself.

Schumacher, Claire. *King of the Zoo.* Morrow, 1985. K–3. A look at mischievous behavior.

Sharmat, Marjorie Weinman. *I'm Terrific.* Illus. Kay Chorao. Holiday House, 1977. K–3. Accepting oneself.

———. *My Mother Never Listens to Me.* Whitman, 1984. Pres.–3. Communicating with parents.

Sharmat, Marjorie, and Sharmat, Mitchell. *The Day I Was Born.* Illus. Diane Dawson. Dutton, 1980. K–3. Relationship between siblings.

Sheldon, Dyan. *I Forgot.* Illus. John Rogan. Aladdin, 1989. Pres.–2. Dealing with forgetfulness; developing self-concept.

Shreve, Susan. *The Flunking of Joshua T. Bates.* Illus. Diane de Groat. Knopf, 1984. 2–5. Developing relationships; self-image.

Solotareff, Grégoire. *Don't Call Me Little Bunny.* Farrar, Straus & Giroux, 1987. K–3. Developing a self-concept.

Swortzell, Lowell. *The Little Humpback Horse.* Anchorage, 1984. 3-up. Play about learning to have faith in one's self.

Thaler, Mike. *Hippo Lemonade.* Illus. Maxie Chambliss. Harper & Row, 1986. Pres.–3. Childhood experiences; developing self-esteem.

Ure, Jean. *Supermouse.* Illus. Ellen Eagle. Morrow, 1984. 2–5. Developing a self-concept in the shadow of a younger sister.

Watson, Wendy. *Lollipop.* Penguin, 1987. 1–3. Making choices.

Wilhelm, Hans. *Tyrone the Horrible.* Scholastic, 1988. Pres.–3. A bully copes with self-concept.

Williams, Barbara. *Donna Jean's Disaster.* Illus. Margot Apple. Whitman, 1986. 1–4. Growing self-esteem.

Williams, Vera B. *Something Special for Me.* Greenwillow, 1983. 1–3. Making choices; developing self-esteem.

•Yashima, Taro. *Crow Boy.* Viking, 1955. K–3. Developing self-esteem.

Zimelman, Nathan. *If I Were Strong Enough.* Illus. Diane Paterson. Abingdon, 1982. Pres.–3. Developing a self-concept.

Zolotow, Charlotte. *I Like to Be Little.* Illus. Erik Blegvad. Crowell, 1987. K–4. The joys of childhood; developing self-concept.

Emotions and Feelings

Alexander, Martha. *I'll Protect You From Jungle Beasts Maybe a Monster.* Dial, 1983. Pres.–K. Dealing with emotions.

Aliki. *Feelings.* Mulberry Books, 1986. K–3. Learning how to express feelings.

Allard, Harry. *Bumps in the Night.* Illus. James Marshall. Doubleday, 1979. K–3. Coping with fears.

•Andrews, Jan. *Very Last First Time.* Illus. Ian Wallace. Atheneum, 1986. Pres.–3. Dealing with fears.

Baker, Alan. *Benjamin's Dreadful Dream.* Lippincott, 1980. K–3. Having nightmares.

•Barrett, Joyce Durham. *Willie's Not the Hugging Kind.* Illus. Pat Cummings. Harper & Row, 1989. K–3. Dealing with feelings.

Berenstain, Stan, and Berenstain, Jan. *The Berenstain Bears in the Dark.* Random House, 1982. Pres.–3. Dealing with fears.

Bergström, Gunilla. *Is That a Monster, Alfie Atkins?* Trans. Robert Swindells. R & S Books, 1989. Pres.–3. Dealing with fears.

Billam, Rosemary. *Fuzzy Rabbit.* Illus. Vanessa Julian-Ottie. Random House, 1984. K–3. Coping with emotions; uniqueness.

Blegvad, Lenore. *Anna Banana and Me.* Illus. Erik Blegvad. McElderry, 1985. K–3. Friendship; dealing with fears.

Bonsall, Crosby. *Who's Afraid of the Dark?* Harper & Row, 1980. Pres.–2. Dealing with fear of the dark.

Brett, Jan. *Annie and the Wild Animals.* Houghton Mifflin, 1985. K–3. The meaning of friendship.

Bridwell, Norman. *Clifford and the Grouchy Neighbors.* Scholastic, 1985. Pres.–3. Coping with emotions.

Brierley, Louise. *The Singing Ringing Tree.* Holt, 1988. 1–2. Love overcomes selfishness and vanity.

Brown, Marc. *Arthur's Halloween.* Little, Brown, 1982. Pres.–3. Coping with fears.

Brown, Marc, and Brown, Laurene Krasny. *The Bionic Bunny Show.* Little, Brown, 1984. Pres.–3. The difference between fantasy and reality.

Browne, Anthony. *Gorilla.* Knopf, 1985. Pres.–2. Dealing with loneliness.

Carlson, Nancy. *Harriet's Recital.* Carolrhoda, 1987. Pres.–3. Dealing with emotions.

———. *Loudmouth George and the Sixth-Grade Bully.* Carolrhoda, 1985. Pres.–3. Learning to cope with successes and failures.

———. *The Talent Show.* Carolrhoda, 1985. Pres.–3. Dealing with different emotions.

Carrick, Carol. *Left Behind.* Illus. Donald Carrick. Clarion, 1988. Pres.–2. Dealing with fears; survival.

Caseley, Judith. *Molly Pink.* Greenwillow, 1985. 2–4. Family helps to work out fears.

Cazet, Denys. *Frosted Glass.* Bradbury, 1987. 1–3. Learning to express emotions.

Christelow, Eileen. *Henry and the Dragon.* Clarion, 1984. K–3. Dealing with fear of the dark.

Clapp, Patricia. *The Invisible Dragon.* Woodstock, IL: The Dramatic Publishing Co., 1972. 3-up. Play about giving of oneself.

Conrad, Pam. *I Don't Live Here!* Illus. Diane deGroat. Dutton, 1984. 2–5. Dealing with fears; learning to adjust to change.

Crowe, Robert L. *Tyler Toad and the Thunder.* Illus. Kay Chorao. Dutton, 1980. 1–3. Learning to cope with fears.

Deitz. *The Good Morning Grump.* Illus. Debbie Deinemann. Abingdon, 1982. Pres.–3. Dealing with emotions.

Delton, Judy. *A Birthday Bike for Brimhall.* Illus. June Leary. Carolrhoda, 1989. Pres.–3. Coping with emotions.

————. *I Never Win!* Illus. Cathy Gilchrist. Carolrhoda, 1989. Pres.–4. Dealing with emotions.

Dennis, Wesley. *Flip and the Cows.* Linnet Books, 1989. Pres.–3. Learning to deal with fears.

Denton, Kady MacDonald. *Granny Is a Darling.* McElderry, 1987. Pres.–3. Living with fear of the dark.

de Regniers, Beatrice Schenk. *The Way I Feel . . . Sometimes.* Illus. Susan Meddaugh. Clarion, 1988. K–4. Poems about the changing emotions of children.

Dragonwagon, Crescent. *Will It Be Okay?* Illus. Ben Shecter. Harper & Row, 1977. K–3. Coping with fears.

Eriksson, Eva. *One Short Week.* Carolrhoda, 1985. 2–4. Making friends; dealing with a new sibling.

Fujikawa, Gyo. *Fraidy Cat.* Grosset, 1982. Pres.–3. Living with fears.

Galbraith, Kathryn Osebold. *Katie Did!* Illus. Ted Ramsey. Atheneum, 1983. Pres.–1. Coping with a new sibling.

Greenberg, Barbara. *The Bravest Babysitter.* Illus. Diane Paterson. Dial, 1986. Pres.–3. Coping with fears.

•Grifalconi, Ann. *Darkness and the Butterfly.* Little, Brown, 1987. Pres.–3. Coping with fear of the dark.

Hague, Kathleen. *The Legend of the Veery Bird.* Illus. Michael Hague. Harcourt Brace Jovanovich, 1985. 2–4. Overcoming shyness.

•Hamilton, Virginia, reteller. "Little Eight John." In *The People Could Fly.* Illus. Leo and Diane Dillon. Knopf, 1985. 2-up. What is acceptable/ unacceptable behavior.

Harper, Anita. *What Feels Best?* Illus. Susan Hellard. Putnam, 1988. Pres.–2. Dealing with feelings.

Hawkins, Colin, and Hawkins, Jacqui. *Snap! Snap!* Illus. Colin Hawkins. Putnam, 1984. K–3. Dealing with bedtime fears.

Hayward, Linda. *I Had a Bad Dream: A Book About Nightmares.* Illus. Eugenie. Western, 1985. Pres.–2. Coping with fears.

Herman, Charlotte. *My Mother Didn't Kiss Me Goodnight.* Illus. Bruce Degen. Dutton, 1980. K–3. Discovering emotions.

Hill, Susan. *Go Away, Bad Dreams.* Illus. Vanessa Julian-Ottie. Random House, 1985. Pres.–2. Coping with fears.

Howe, James. *There's a Monster Under My Bed.* Illus. David Rose. Atheneum, 1987. Pres.–3. Coping with nighttime fears.

————. *When You Go to Kindergarten.* Photographs by Betsy Imershein. Knopf, 1986. Pres.–K. How to cope with the first day of school.

Jones, Rebecca C. *The Biggest, Meanest, Ugliest Dog in the Whole Wide World.* Illus. Wendy Watson. Macmillan, 1982. Pres.–3. How to make fears disappear.

Joosse, Barbara M. *Dinah's Mad, Bad Wishes.* Illus. Emily Arnold McCully. Harper & Row, 1989. Pres.–3. Coping with anger; emotions.

Kachenmeister, Cherryl. *On Monday When It Rained.* Photographs by Tom Berthiaume. Houghton Mifflin, 1989. K–3. A photo essay about childhood emotions.

Kraus, Robert. *Spider's First Day at School.* Scholastic, 1987. K–3. Coping with the first day of school.

Lester, Helen. *Pookins Gets Her Way.* Illus. Lynn Munsinger. Houghton Mifflin, 1987. 1–4. How to express emotions appropriately; learning cooperation.

•Lexau, Joan. *Benjie.* Illus. Don Bolognese. Dial, 1964. Pres.–2. Overcoming shyness.

Marks, Alan. *Nowhere to Be Found.* Picture Book Studio, 1989. K–3. Dealing with emotions.

Martin, Ann M. *Stage Fright.* Illus. Blanche Sims. Scholastic, 1986. Pres.–3. Coping with shyness.

Martin, Bill, Jr. and Archambault, John. *The Ghost-Eye Tree.* Illus. Ted Rand. Holt, 1985. 3–6. Facing fear of the dark.

Marzollo, Jean. *Cannonball Chris.* Illus. Blanche Sims. Random House, 1987. 1–3. Coping with fears.

•McKissack, Patricia C. *Flossie and the Fox.* Illus. Rachel Isadora. Dial, 1986. Pres.–4. Coping with fear.

Most, Bernard. *Boo!* Prentice-Hall, 1980. K–3. Learning to overcome fears.

Oakley, John. *Would You Be Scared?* Andre Deutsch, 1987. Pres.–1. Coping with childhood fears.

Osborn, Lois. *My Brother Is Afraid of Just About Everything.* Illus. Jennie Williams. Whitman, 1982. 1–3. Coping with fears.

Panek, Dennis. *Detective Whoo.* Bradbury, 1981. K–3. Coping with fear of the night.

Peet, Bill. *Cowardly Clyde.* Houghton Mifflin, 1979. K–3. Learning to overcome fear.

•Perrine, Mary. *Nannabah's Friend.* Illus. Leonard Weisgard. Houghton Mifflin, 1989. K–3. Coping with fear.

Prelutsky, Jack. *My Parents Think I'm Sleeping.* Illus. Yossi Abolafia. Greenwillow, 1985. Pres.–3. Coping with bedtime fears.

Preston, Edna Mitchell. *The Temper Tantrum Book.* Illus. Rainey Bennett. Penguin, 1976. Pres.–3. Dealing with emotions.

Ross, Dave. *Baby Hugs.* Crowell, 1987. All ages. Dealing with emotions.

Sabraw, John. *I Wouldn't Be Scared.* Orchard Books, 1989. Pres.–3. Conquering fears.

Saltzberg, Barney. *What to Say to Clara.* Atheneum, 1984. Pres.–3. Learning to overcome shyness.

Schlein, Miriam. *The Way Mothers Are.* Whitman, 1963. Pres.–2. Coping with fear of loss of love.

Sendak, Maurice. *Where the Wild Things Are.* Harper & Row, 1963. Pres.–3. Coping with fears, fantasies.

Sharmat, Marjorie Weinman. *Attila the Angry.* Illus. Lillian Hoban. Holiday House, 1985. K–3. Learning to control anger.

———. *Frizzy the Fearful.* Illus. John Wallner. Holiday House, 1983. K–3. Learning to question fears.

———. *Rollo and Juliet, Forever!* Illus. Marylin Hafner. Doubleday, 1981. 1–3. Friendships; dealing with many different emotions.

———. *Thornton the Worrier.* Illus. Kay Chorao. Holiday House, 1978. K–3. Dealing with worries.

Simon, Norma. *How Do I Feel?* Whitman, 1970. Pres.–3. Coping with emotions.

———. *I Am Not a Crybaby.* Illus. Helen Cogancherry. Whitman, 1989. 1–4. It's all right to express emotions.

———. *I Was So Mad.* Illus. Dora Leder. Whitman, 1974. K–2. Dealing with anger.

Smith, Wendy. *Think Hippo!* Carolrhoda, 1989. Pres.–3. Conquering fears.

Stanek, Muriel. *Who's Afraid of the Dark?* Illus. Helen Cogancherry. Whitman, 1980. K–3. Dealing with fear of the dark.

Stanton, Elizabeth, and Stanton, Henry. *Sometimes I Like To Cry.* Whitman, 1978. Pres.–2. Learning to express emotions.

Stevenson, James. *What's Under My Bed?* Greenwillow, 1983. Pres.–3. Dealing with fears of the nighttime.

Stokes, Jack. *Wiley and the Hairy Man.* Morton Grove, IL: Coach House Press, 1979. 3-up. Play about confronting fears.

Tompert, Ann. *Will You Come Back for Me?* Illus. Robin Kramer. Whitman, 1989. Pres.–K. Dealing with fears about the first day of school.

Turner, Ethel. *Walking to School.* Illus. Peter Gouldthorpe. Orchard Books, 1989. Pres. 2. Poem about fear of the first day of school.

Tyler, Linda Wagner. *Waiting for Mom.* Illus. Susan Davis. Viking Kestrel, 1987. Fear of being left behind.

Viorst, Judith. *I'll Fix Anthony.* Illus. Arnold Lobel. Harper & Row, 1969. K–4. Coping with sibling rivalry.

———. *The Good-bye Book.* Illus. Kay Chorao. Atheneum, 1988. Pres.–1. Learning to say good-bye; dealing with emotions.

Wagner, Jenny. *John Brown, Rose and the Midnight Cat.* Bradbury, 1978. K–3. Dealing with jealousy; cooperation.

Warren, Cathy. *Springtime Bears.* Illus. Pat Cummings. Lothrop, Lee & Shepard, 1987. Pres.–2. Family love.

Watson, Jane W. *Sometimes I Get Angry.* Illus. Irene Trivas. Crown, 1986. K–3. What can bring on a child's anger.

———. *Sometimes I'm Afraid.* Illus. Irene Trivas. Crown, 1986. K–3. Deals with childhood fears and their sources.

———. *Sometimes I'm Jealous.* Illus. Irene Trivas. Crown, 1986. K–3. Dealing with a new family member.

Wells, Rosemary. *Shy Charles.* Dial, 1988. Pres.–2. Coping with shyness.

———. *Timothy Goes to School.* Dial, 1981. K–3. Dealing with the first day of school; finding a friend.

Williams, Linda. *The Little Old Lady Who Was Not Afraid of Anything.* Illus. Megan Lloyd. Harper & Row, 1987. Pres.–2. A read-aloud rhyme about dealing with fears.

Willis, Jeanne. *The Monster Bed.* Illus. Susan Varley. Lothrop, Lee & Shepard, 1987. Pres.–3. Rhyme about nighttime fears.

Willoughby, Elaine Macmann. *Boris and the Monsters.* Illus. Lynn Munsinger. Houghton Mifflin, 1980. K–3. Coping with fear of the dark.

Winthrop, Elizabeth. *Belinda's Hurricane.* Illus. Wendy Watson. Dutton, 1984. 2–4. Coping with fears.
Zolotow, Charlotte. *The Hating Book.* Illus. Ben Shecter. Harper & Row, 1969. Pres.–3. Friendship; dealing with emotions.
———. *The Quarreling Book.* Illus. Arnold Lobel. Harper & Row, 1963. Pres.–3. Learning to cooperate.

Relationships

Adler, C. S. *Always and Forever Friends.* Clarion, 1988. Pres.–2. How to build friendships.
•Appiah, Sonia. *Amoko and Efua Bear.* Illus. Carol Easmon. Macmillan, 1989. Pres.–1. Relationship with a fantasy friend.
Barbato, Juli. *From Bed to Bus.* Illus. Brian Schatell. Macmillan, 1985. K–3. Preparing for the first day of school.
Berenstain, Stan, and Berenstain, Jan. *The Berenstain Bears and the Messy Room.* Random House, 1983. K–3. Learning how to cooperate.
Bottner, Barbara. *Mean Maxine.* Pantheon, 1980. K–3. Learning to get along with others.
Boyd, Lizi. *Bailey the Big Bully.* Viking Kestrel, 1989. Pres.–3. Learning to get along.
Bröger, Achim. *Francie's Paper Puppy.* Illus. Michele Sambin. Picture Book Studio USA, 1984. 2–4. Developing a friendship.
•Bryant, Sara. *The Burning Rice Fields.* Illus. Mamoru Funai. Holt, 1963. 1–4. Accepting responsibility for others.
Bunting, Eve. *Monkey in the Middle.* Illus. Lynn Munsinger. Harcourt Brace Jovanovich, 1984. Pres.–3. Friendship; coping with anger.
•Cameron, Ann. *The Stories Julian Tells.* Illus. Ann Strugnell. Pantheon, 1981. K–4. Six stories of life in loving family.
Carlson, Nancy. *Harriet Books.* Carolrhoda Books, 1989. Pres.–3. Learning to get along with others.
Carrick, Carol. *Left Behind.* Illus. Donald Carrick. Clarion, 1988. K–3. Coping with being lost.
Clements, Andrew, and Yoshi. *Big Al.* Picture Book Studio, 1989. Pres.–2. The meaning of true friendship.
Clifford, Eth. *I Hate Your Guts, Ben Brooster.* Houghton Mifflin, 1989. 3–7. Learning to get along with others.
Collins, Pat Lowery. *Tumble, Tumble, Tumbleweed.* Illus. Charles Robinson. Whitman, 1982. 1–3. Deals with the concept of friendship.
Coutant, Helen. *The Gift.* Illus. Vo-Dinh Mai. Knopf, 1983. K–4. Sharing and the nature of friendship.
Craig, Helen. *A Welcome for Annie.* Knopf, 1986. Pres.–2. Winning respect and friendship.
Cunningham, Julia. *A Mouse Called Junction.* Illus. Michael Hague. Pantheon, 1980. K–3. Survival; making a friend.

————. *Oaf.* Illus. Peter Sis. Knopf, 1986. 2–5. Innocence triumphs over evil; the value of support and friendship.

Cuyler, Margery. *Freckles and Willy: A Valentine's Day Story.* Illus. Marsha Wilborn. Holt, 1986. K–3. Developing a friendship.

Davis, Gibbs. *The Other Emily.* Illus. Linda Shute. Houghton Mifflin, 1984. Pres.–3. Coping with the first day of school; making a friend.

Delaney, Ned. *Bert and Barney.* Houghton Mifflin, 1979. K–3. The meaning of friendship.

Delton, Judy. *No Time for Christmas.* Illus. Anastasia Mitchell. Carolrhoda, 1989. Pres.–4. The meaning of friendship.

Edwards, Pat. *Little John and Plutie.* Houghton Mifflin, 1988. 3–7. Friendship and discovery of the world.

Edwards, Patricia. *Chester and Uncle Willoughby.* Illus. Diane Worfolk Allison. Little, Brown, 1987. 1–3. Friendship between a young and an old person.

Eriksson, Eva. *Jealousy.* Carolrhoda, 1985. Pres.–2. Making friends.

Feagles, Anita. *Casey—The Utterly Impossible Horse.* Illus. Dagmar Wilson. Linnet Books, 1989. 1–5. Developing a relationship.

Fleischman, Sid. *The Scarebird.* Illus. Peter Sis. Greenwillow, 1987. K–4. Developing a friendship.

Gackenbach, Dick. *Mr. Wink and His Shadow, Ned.* Harper & Row, 1983. 2–4. The value of a true friend.

Giff, Patricia Reilly. *The Beast in Ms. Rooney's Room.* Illus. Blanche Sims. Dell, 1985. 1–3. Friends' experiences.

————. *Fish Face.* Illus. Blanche Sims. 1–3. Dell, 1985. Friends' experiences.

————. *Lazy Lions, Lucky Lambs.* Illus. Blanche Sims. 1–3. Dell, 1985. Friends' experiences.

————. *Purple Climbing Days.* Illus. Blanche Sims. 1–3. Dell, 1985. Friends' experiences.

————. *Say Cheese.* Illus. Blanche Sims. 1–3. Dell, 1985. Friends' experiences.

————. *Snaggle Doodles.* Illus. Blanche Sims. Dell, 1985. 1–3. Friends' experiences.

————. *Valentine Star.* Illus. Blanche Sims. Dell, 1985. 1–3. Friends' experiences.

Greene, Constance. *Ask Anybody.* Viking Kestrel, 1983. 2–4. How to choose friends.

Gretz, Susanna. *Roger Takes Charge!* Dial, 1987. 1–3. Learning to cooperate.

Hale, Irina. *Brown Bear in a Brown Chair.* McElderry/Atheneum, 1983. 1–3. Friendship and caring.

Hayes, Geoffrey. *Patrick and Ted.* Four Winds/Macmillan, 1984. K–3. A story of friendship.

Hest, Amy. *The Best-ever Good-bye Party.* Illus. Dyanne Disalvo-Ryan. Morrow, 1989. K–3. When a best friend moves away.

Himmelman, John. *The Ups and Downs of Simpson Snail.* Dutton, 1989. Pres.–3. Story of friendship.

Hoban, Lillian. *Arthur's Funny Money.* Harper & Row, 1981. K–3. Learning cooperation and sharing.

Holmes, Barbara Ware. *Charlotte the Starlet.* Illus. John Himmelman. Harper & Row, 1988. 2–4. The meaning of true friendship.

Hopkins, Lee Bennett. *Best Friends.* Illus. James Watts. Harper & Row, 1986. 1–4. Poetry about friendships.

Hughes, Shirley. *Another Helping of Chips.* Lothrop, Lee & Shepard, 1987. 2–4. Relationships.

Joosse, Barbara M. *Better with Two.* Illus. Catherine Stock. Harper & Row, 1988. Pres.–2. Building a friendship with an older person.

Kamen, Gloria, reteller. *The Ringdoves.* Atheneum, 1988. Pres.–3. A story of true friendships.

King, Larry L. *Because of Lozo Brown.* Illus. Amy Schwartz. Viking Kestrel, 1982. Pres.–3. Making a new friend.

Komaiko, Leah. *Annie Bananie.* Illus. Laura Cornell. Harper & Row, 1987. K–3. A best friend moves away.

Le Gallienne, Eva, translator. *Hans Christian Andersen's The Snow Queen.* Illus. Arieh Zeldich. Harper & Row, 1985. 2–4. A fairy tale about friendship.

Lester, Helen. *Cora Copycat.* Dutton, 1979. K–3. Learning individuality.

Lillie, Patricia. *Jake and Rosie.* Greenwillow, 1988. Pres.–3. Being friends.

Lionni, Leo. *A Color of His Own.* Pantheon, 1976. Pres.–2. Fable about friendship and self-awareness.

———. *It's Mine!* Knopf, 1986. Pres.–1. A fable about peaceful co-existence.

———. *Six Crows.* Knopf, 1988. Pres.–2. Learning the art of compromise; value of relationships.

Luttrell, Ida. *Tillie and Mert.* Illus. Doug Cushman. Harper & Row, 1985. Pres.–2. The value of friendship.

Lyon, George Ella. *Together.* Illus. Vera Rosenberry. Orchard Books, 1989. Pres.–1. What true friendship is like.

Malone, Nola Langner. *A Home.* Bradbury Press, 1988. Pres.–2. Making new friends.

Marshall, Edward. *Fox in Love.* Illus. James Marshall. Dial, 1982. K–3. Three stories about the trials of friendship.

Marshall, James. *George and Martha Back in Town.* Houghton Mifflin, 1984. K–3. Tales of friendship.

———. *George and Martha Round and Round.* Houghton Mifflin, 1988. Pres.–3. Lessons in friendship.

———. *George and Martha Tons of Fun.* Houghton Mifflin, 1980. K–3. How true friendship persists.

McDonnell, Christine. *Lucky Charms & Birthday Wishes.* Illus. Diane deGroat. Viking Kestrel, 1984. 2–5. Making new friends.

Minarik, Else Holmelund. *Little Bear.* Illus. Maurice Sendak. Harper & Row, 1957. Pres.–3. Childhood experiences and relationships.

Myers, Bernice. *Not at Home?* Lothrop, Lee & Shepard, 1981. 1–3. Conflict in friendship.

Newton, Patricia Montgomery. *The Frog Who Drank the Waters of the World.* Atheneum, 1983. K–3. Learning cooperation.

Nobleman, Roberta. *Henry Mouse.* New Plays, 1968. K–3. Play about learning to communicate.

Orgel, Doris. *Starring Becky Suslow.* Illus. Carol Newsom. Viking Kestrel, 1989. 2–5. Friendships.

Ormerod, Jan. *The Story of Chicken Licken.* Lothrop, Lee & Shepard, 1985. Pres.–3. Picture play about cooperation among friends.

Pearson, Susan. *Saturday I Ran Away.* Illus. Susan Jeschke. Lippincott, 1981. K–3. Dealing with family conflicts.

Phillips, Joan. *My New Boy.* Illus. Lynn Munsinger. Random House, 1986. Pres.–3. Communicating with others.

Potter, David Lord. *Mine!* Houghton Mifflin, 1981. 1–3. Learning to cooperate.

Priestley, Dinah. *Hector the Bully.* Illus. Wendy Smith. Carolrhoda, 1989. Pres.–3. Forming a friendship.

Ross, Pat. *M and M and the Big Bag.* Illus. Marylin Hafner. Pantheon, 1981. 1–3. Handling stress.

———. *M and M and the Super Child Afternoon.* Illus. Marylin Hafner. Viking Kestrel, 1987. Pres.–3. Learning to share; friendship.

Rylant, Cynthia. *All I See.* Illus. Peter Catalanotto. Orchard Books, 1988. 1–3. Friendship between a child and an artist.

Sharmat, Marjorie Weinman. *Bartholomew the Bossy.* Illus. Normand Chartier. Macmillan, 1984. Pres.–3. Learning cooperation; meaning of friendship.

———. *Grumley the Grouch.* Illus. Kay Chorao. Holiday House, 1980. K–3. Learning to get along.

———. *Taking Care of Melvin.* Illus. Victoria Chess. Holiday House, 1980. K–3. Learning cooperation.

Siekkinen, Raija. *Mister King.* Illus. Hannu Taina. Carolrhoda, 1989. K–4. The value of caring for others.

Silverstein, Shel. *The Giving Tree.* Harper & Row, 1964. All ages. Looks at friendship, love, and sharing.

Smith, Janice Lee. *The Kid Next Door and Other Headaches: Stories About Adam Joshua.* Illus. Dick Gackenbach. Harper & Row, 1984. Pres.–3. Developing friendships.

———. *The Show-and-Tell War.* Illus. Dick Gackenbach. Harper & Row, 1988. 2–4. Five stories about friendships.

Smith, Jennifer. *Grover and the New Kid.* Illus. Tom Cooke. Random House, 1987. 1–3. Learning how to get along; making a friend.

•Steptoe, John. *Stevie.* Harper & Row, 1969. Pres.–3. Learning to share; making a friend.

Stevenson, James. *Oh No, It's Waylon's Birthday!* Greenwillow, 1989. K–3. A story of friendship.

Still, James. *The Velveteen Rabbit.* Available from Emmy Gifford Children's Theatre, 3504 Center St., Omaha, NE 68105. 2–4. Dramatic adaptation of Margery Williams's tale of love, caring, and responsibility.

Thaler, Mike. *It's Me, Hippo!* Illus. Maxie Chambliss. Harper & Row, 1983. 2–4. Four tales about friendships.

————. *Moonkey.* Illus. Giulio Maestro. Harper & Row, 1981. K–3. Learning the meaning of friendship.

•Tsutsui, Yoriko. *Anna's Secret Friend.* Illus. Akiko Hayashi. Viking Kestrel, 1987. Pres.–3. Making friends in a new home.

Udry, Janice May. *Let's Be Enemies.* Illus. Maurice Sendak. Harper & Row, 1988. Pres.–2. The meaning of true friendship.

Vincent, Gabrielle. *Feel Better, Ernest!* Greenwillow, 1989. Pres.–2. Helping a sick friend.

Weiss, Nicki. *Maude and Sally.* Greenwillow, 1983. K–3. Learning to share friends.

White, E. B. *Charlotte's Web.* Illus. Garth Williams. Harper & Row, 1952. 2–4. Friendship; the cycle of life.

Winthrop, Elizabeth. *Lizzie and Harold.* Illus. Martha Weston. Lothrop, Lee & Shepard, 1986. Pres.–3. Friendship with the opposite sex.

————. *The Best Friends Club.* Illus. Martha Weston. Lothrop, Lee & Shepard, 1989. Pres.–3. The tests of true friendship.

Wosmek, Frances. *A Brown Bird Singing.* Illus. Ted Lewin. Lothrop, Lee & Shepard, 1986. K–3. The meaning of family.

You and Me! San Diego, CA: Readers Theatre Script Service, no date. K–3. "The Duel" by Eugene Field, "Two Little Kittens," and "London Bridge" in readers-theatre format examine friendship and the meaning of relationships.

Zalben, Jane Breskin. *Oliver and Alison's Week.* Illus. Emily Arnold McCully. Farrar, Straus & Giroux, 1980. K–3. Stories about friendships.

Zolotow, Charlotte. *I Know a Lady.* Illus. James Stevenson. Greenwillow, 1984. K–3. Love, sharing, and the continuity of life.

————. *The New Friend.* Illus. Emily Arnold McCully. Crowell, 1981. 1–3. Friends deal with conflict.

Human Differences/Similarities

•Anno, Mitsumasa. *All in a Day.* Illus. ten international artists. Philomel, 1986. 1–5. The similarities and differences of all people.

•Battles, Edith. *What Does the Rooster Say, Yoshio?* Illus. Toni Horman. Whitman, 1978. K–3. Dealing with differences.

Blos, Joan W. *Old Henry.* Illus. Stephen Gammell. Scribner's, 1987. All ages. Accepting others' differences.

Browne, Anthony. *Willy the Champ.* Knopf, 1986. Pres.–3. Developing a self-concept.

Carlson, Nancy. *Loudmouth George and the New Neighbors.* Puffin Books, 1986. Pres.–3. Prejudices and preconceptions explored.

•Climo, Shirley. *The Egyptian Cinderella.* Illus. Ruth Heller. Crowell, 1989. Pres.–3. Accepting human differences.

•Esbensen, Barbara Juster, reteller. *The Star Maiden: An Ojibway Tale.* Illus. Helen K. Davie. Little, Brown, 1988. Pres.–3. Uniqueness; human differences.

Giff, Patricia Reilly. *Next Year I'll Be Special.* Illus. Marylin Hafner. Dutton, 1980. K–3. Dealing with emotions and changes.
•Greenfield, Eloise. *Rosa Parks.* Illus. Eric Marlow. Crowell, 1973. 2–4. Biography; accepting racial differences.
•Haseley, Dennis. *The Scared One.* Illus. Deborah Howland. Warne, 1983. K–3. Personal heritage; human differences.
Hazen, Barbara S. *The Me I See.* Illus. Ati Forberg. Abingdon, 1978. 1–2. Differences among people.
Lerner, Marguerite Rush. *Lefty: The Story of Left-Handedness.* Illus. Rov Andre. Lerner, 1960. K–5. Mental and emotional differences.
•Lewin, Hugh. *Jafta.* Illus. Lisa Kopper. Carolrhoda, 1989. Pres.–3. Human similarities and differences.
•———. *Jafta and the Wedding.* Illus. Lisa Kopper. Carolrhoda, 1983. Pres.–2. Accepting differences.
•———. *Jafta's Father.* Illus. Lisa Kopper. Carolrhoda, 1983. Pres.–2. Accepting differences.
•———. *Jafta's Mother.* Illus. Lisa Kopper. Carolrhoda, 1983. Pres.–2. Accepting differences.
Lewis, Rob. *Friska, the Sheep That Was Too Small.* Farrar, Straus & Giroux, 1988. Pres.–3. Being different.
Loeb, Robert H., Jr. *Meet the Real Pilgrims: Everyday Life on Plimoth Plantation in 1627.* Doubleday, 1979. 3–6. Human differences.
•May, Julian. *Why People Are Different Colors.* Illus. Symeon Shimin. Holiday House, 1971. 2–4. Superficial human differences.
•Meriwether, Louise. *Dona Ride the Bus on Monday.* Illus. David Scott Brown. Prentice-Hall, 1973. 3–5. Dealing with racial differences.
•Mohr, Nicholasa. *Felita.* Illus. Ray Cruz. Dial, 1979. 3–6. Dispels the stereotype of city families.
Simon, Norma. *Why Am I Different?* Whitman, 1976. K–2. Dealing with poor self-concept.
•Tobias, Tobi. *Arthur Mitchell.* Illus. Carole Byard. Crowell, 1975. 3–5. Biography; dealing with racial differences.
•Yashima, Taro. *Crow Boy.* Viking Kestrel, 1987. K–3. Human differences.

Grades Four Through Six

Relationship Between Physical Well-Being and Mental/Emotional Health

Aaseng, Nathan. *Winners Never Quit: Athletes Who Beat the Odds.* Lerner, 1980. 5–8. Athletes who conquered amazing odds.
Adler, C. S. *With Westie and the Tin Man.* Macmillan, 1985. 5–6. Finding a new friend; adjusting to a new life.
•Angell, Judie. *One-Way to Ansonia.* Bradbury, 1985. 5–6. Historical fiction about an immigrant family; nonconformity.

•Association for Childhood Education International. *And Everywhere, Children!* Greenwillow, 1979. 5-up. Collection about growing up in other lands.

Baehr, Patricia. *Louisa Eclipsed.* Morrow, 1988. 6-up. Dealing with adolescent changes.

Baldwin, Anne. *Sunflowers for Tina.* Four Winds Press, 1970. 5–8. Finding self-esteem; relationship with older person.

Benjamin, Carol Lea. *Nobody's Baby Now.* Berkley, 1986. 4–6. Finding self-esteem.

Berry, James R. *Kids on the Run.* Four Winds, 1978. 6-up. Firsthand accounts of seven teenage runaways.

Blue, Rose. *Nikki 108.* Illus. Ted Lewin. Watts, 1972. 5–8. Dealing with addiction; mental illness; finding identity.

Bosse, Malcolm J. *Cave Beyond Time.* Crowell, 1980. 5-up. Search for identity.

Brodeur, Ruth Wallace. *Callie's Way.* Atheneum, 1984. 4–6. Developing self-concept; relationship with older person.

Burns, Marilyn. *I Am Not a Short Adult: Getting Good at Being a Kid.* Illus. Martha Weston. Little, Brown, 1977. 5-up. Understanding personal and family characteristics.

Byars, Betsy. *The Cartoonist.* Illus. Richard Cuffari. Viking Kestrel, 1978. 5-up. Coping with family problems; finding your own space.

———. *The Glory Girl.* Viking Kestrel, 1983. 4–6. Discovering self-worth; dealing with family changes.

———. *The Pinballs.* Harper & Row, 1977. 5–7. Foster children learn to cope.

———. *The TV Kid.* Illus. Richard Cuffari. Viking Kestrel, 1976. 4–6. Dealing with emotions.

Carkeet, David. *The Silent Treatment.* Harper & Row, 1988. 6-up. Dealing with emotions.

Cassedy, Sylvia. *Behind the Attic Wall.* Crowell, 1983. 4–6. Learning to accept oneself.

———. *Lucie Babbidge's House.* Crowell, 1989. 4–7. Coping with being different; personal transformation.

———. *M. E. and Morton.* Harper & Row, 1987. 4–7. Accepting one's individuality.

Cheatham, K. Follis. *The Best Way Out.* Harcourt Brace Jovanovich, 1982. 5–8. Dealing with moving to a new school; growing up.

Christina, Mary Blount. *Growin' Pains.* Penguin, 1987. 4–6. Transforming oneself; dealing with emotions.

Christopher, Matt. *Football Fugitive.* Illus. Larry Johnson. Little, Brown, 1976. 4–6. Dealing with emotions.

Conford, Ellen. *The Revenge of the Incredible Dr. Rancid and His Youthful Assistant, Jeffrey.* Little, Brown, 1980. 5–7. The meaning of courage and friendship.

Conley, Pauline C. *The Code Breaker.* Anchorage Press, 1983. 5-up. Play about growing up; self-discovery.

DeClements, Barthe. *Nothing's Fair in Fifth Grade.* Viking Kestrel, 1981. 5-up. Dealing with self-image.

Dinner, Sherry H. *Nothing To Be Ashamed Of: Growing Up with Mental Illness in Your Family.* Children's Books, 1989. 5–8. Dealing with mental illness of a family member.

Easton, Patricia Harrison. *Summer's Chance.* Harcourt Brace Jovanovich, 1988. 6–8. Self awareness.

Eige, Lillian. *Cady.* Illus. Janet Wentworth. Harper & Row, 1987. 3–6. Developing self concept; the meaning of family.

Farrar, Susan Clement. *Samantha on Stage.* Illus. Ruth Sanderson. Dial, 1979. 4–6. The true meaning of friendship.

Fradin, Dennis Brindell. *Remarkable Children: Twenty Who Made History.* Little, Brown, 1987. 4–6. Children's accomplishments.

Gilbert, Sara. *Get Help: Solving the Problems in Your Life.* Morrow, 1989. 5–8. Getting help to cope with life's problems.

Greene, Constance. *Monday I Love You.* Harper & Row, 1988. 6-up. Developing a feeling of self-worth; changing one's life.

Greenwald, Sheila. *Give Us a Great Big Smile, Rosy Cole.* Little, Brown, 1981. 3-up. Developing a self-concept.

Hall, Lynn. *Mrs. Portree's Pony.* Scribner's, 1986. 4–6. Developing a relationship with an older person; coping with problems.

———. *Troublemaker.* Illus. Joseph Cellini. Follett, 1974. 6–9. Dealing with family alcoholism; developing self-esteem.

•Harris, Aurand. *Ming Lee and the Magic Tree.* In *Plays Children Love.* Coleman A. Jennings and Aurand Harris, editors. Doubleday, 1981. 5-up. Self-knowledge as the key to happiness.

Harris, Robie H. *Rosie's Double Dare.* Illus. Tony De Luna. Knopf, 1980. 4–6. Developing self-image.

Heide, Florence Parry. *Time Flies!* Illus. Marylin Hafner. Holiday House, 1984. 4–6. Developing self-concept.

Holl, Kristi D. *Cast a Single Shadow.* Atheneum, 1988. 3–6. Developing a sense of self-reliance.

Holmes, Barbara Ware. *Charlotte Shakespeare and Annie the Great.* Illus. John Himmelman. Harper & Row, 1989. 4–6. Self concept; the meaning of friendship.

Hunter, Mollie. *Cat, Herself.* Harper & Row, 1986. 6-up. Defying traditional women's roles; coming to maturity.

Hyde, Margaret O. *Is This Kid "Crazy"? Understanding Unusual Behavior.* Westminster, 1983. 6-up. Discusses mental health.

Janeczko, Paul. *Brickyard Summer.* Illus. Ken Rush. Orchard Books, 1989. 6-up. Poems of self-discovery.

Johnson, Julie Tallard. *Celebrate You!* Lerner, 1991. 5-up. Advice and activities for building self-esteem.

———. *Understanding Mental Illness: For Teens Who Care about Someone with Mental Illness.* Lerner, 1989. 6-up. Various types of mental illness; how to live with a mentally ill person.

Johnston, Ginny, and Cutchins, Judy. *Andy Bear: A Polar Bear Cub Grows up at the Zoo.* Illus. with photographs by Constance Noble. Morrow, 1985. 3–5. The process of growing up depicted; friendship.

Jukes, Mavis. *Getting Even.* Knopf, 1988. 4–6. Dealing with divorce; developing independence.

Kesselman, Wendy. *Becca.* Anchorage Press, 1988. 5-up. Play about emotional and mental life of a child.

Koste, Virginia Glasgow. *Scraps: The Ragtime Girl of Oz.* Morton Grove, IL: Coach House Press, 1987. 4-up. Play about self-esteem.

Latham, Jean Lee. *Carry On, Mr. Bowditch.* Illus. John O'Hara Cosgrove. Houghton Mifflin, 1955. 6-up. Overcoming personal odds to succeed.

Lawrence, Louise. *The Dram Road.* Harper, 1983. 5–8. The power of acceptance and love.

LeShan, Eda. *What Makes Me Feel This Way?* Macmillan, 1972. 5–8. Sorting out one's feelings.

•Levoy, Myron. *Alan and Naomi.* Harper & Row, 1977. 6–9. Developing self-concept; friendship.

Lingard, Joan. *Strangers in the House.* Lodestar, 1983. 6–8. Developing self-image; independence.

Luenn, Nancy. *The Ugly Princess.* Illus. David Wiesner. Little, Brown, 1981. 4–6. Accepting oneself.

Luhrmann, Winifred Bruce. *Only Brave Tomorrows.* Houghton Mifflin, 1989. 5–9. Finding strength; self-awareness.

Madison, Arnold. *Runaway Teens: An American Tragedy.* Elsevier/Nelson, 1979. 4–6. The dangers and hardships of running away; ways to get help.

•Malone, Mary. *Actor in Exile: The Life of Ira Aldridge.* Illus. Eros Keith. Crowell, 1969. 4–6. Biography; accepting racial differences.

Martens, Anne Coulter. *The Wizard of Oz.* Woodstock, IL: The Dramatic Publishing Co., 1963. 4-up. Play about finding inner strength; what matters in life.

Mazer, Norma Fox. *B, My Name Is Bunny.* Scholastic, 1987. 6–9. Dealing with envy; developing self-concept.

McFarland, Rhoda. *Coping Through Self-Esteem.* Rosen, 1988. 6-up. Informational book about developing self-esteem.

Miller, Kathryn Schultz. *Blue Horses.* Coach House Press, 1984. 5-up. Play about developing trust; self-confidence.

Miller, Kathryn Schultz; Miller, Barry; and Bowden, Bruce. *I Think I Can.* Pioneer, 1985. 4-up. Play about developing self-concept.

•Mohr, Nicholasa. *Going Home.* Dial, 1986. 4–6. Learning to accept self and others.

Morris, Winifred. *Dancer in the Mirror.* Atheneum, 1987. 4–6. Developing self-image.

Naylor, Phyllis Reynolds. *Night Cry.* Atheneum, 1984. 4–6. Finding courage; developing independence.

———. *One of the Third-Grade Thonkers.* Illus. Walter Gaffney-Kessell. Atheneum, 1987. 3–6. Dealing with peer pressure; developing self-concept.

———. *The Agony of Alice.* Atheneum, 1985. 3–6. Developing self-concept.

————. *The Keeper*. Atheneum, 1986. 4–6. Dealing with family mental illness.

Oppenheimer, Joan L. *A Clown Like Me*. Crowell, 1985. 4–6. Finding one's self-image.

Park, Barbara. *Buddies*. Knopf, 1985. 4–6. Choosing friends.

Pascal, Francine. *The Hand-Me-Down Kid*. Viking Kestrel, 1980. 4–6. Acceptance of self.

Patroon, Katherine. *The Great Gilly Hopkins*. Crowell, 1978. 5-up. Coping with being a foster child.

Paulsen, Gary. *Hatchet*. Bradbury, 1987. 6-up. Dealing with divorce; learning to survive alone.

Pfeffer, Susan Beth. *Dear Dad, Love Laurie*. Scholastic, 1989. 4–7. Developing self-concept; being a child of divorce.

Reading, J. P. *The Summer of Sassy Jo*. Houghton Mifflin, 1989. 5–9. Dealing with family alcoholism; accepting change.

Rodowsky, Colby. *The Gathering Room*. Farrar, Straus & Giroux, 1981. 4–6. Coping with fears; mental illness.

Rostkowski, Margaret L. *After the Dancing Days*. Harper & Row, 1986. 6–8. Friendship with an invalid; the human casualties of war.

Sachar, Louis. *There's a Boy in the Girls' Bathroom*. Knopf, 1987. 5–9. Learning to be independent; developing self-confidence.

Sachs, Marilyn. *The Bears' House*. Doubleday, 1971. 5-up. Coping with alcoholism.

Saltzberg, Barney. *What to Say to Clara*. Atheneum, 1984. 3–5. Dealing with shyness; developing sense of self.

Segel, Elizabeth, compiler. *Short Takes: A Short Story Collection for Young Readers*. Illus. Jos. A. Smith. Lothrop, Lee & Shepard, 1986. 5-up. Nine short stories of personal change.

Silsbee, Peter. *The Big Way Out*. Bradbury, 1984. 6–9. Coping with a mentally ill parent; family supportiveness.

Silverstein, Shel. *The Missing Piece Meets the Big O*. Harper & Row, 1981. 4–6. Developing self-concept.

Simon, Marcia L. *A Special Gift*. Harcourt Brace Jovanovich, 1978. 3–6. Sex roles; developing self-concept.

Smith, Doris Buchanan. *Last Was Lloyd*. Viking Kestrel, 1981. 4–6. Dealing with emotion; self-concept.

Snyder, Carol. *The Leftover Kid*. Putnam, 1986. 4–6. Cooperating with family; developing independence.

Springer, Nancy. *A Horse to Love*. Harper & Row, 1987. 4–6. Developing responsibility; independence.

Talbert, Marc. *Thin Ice*. Little, Brown, 1986. 4–6. Dealing with parents' separation.

Tolan, Stephanie S. *The Liberation of Tansy Warner*. Scribner's, 1980. 5–9. Dealing with abandonment; confronting feelings.

Urquhart, John; Grauer, Rita; and Picus, Paul. *Fool of the World*. Anchorage Press, 1986. 4-up. Play about believing in oneself.

Ustinov, Lev. *The City Without Love*. In *Russian Plays for Young Audiences*.

Miriam Morton, translator and editor. Rowayton, CT: New Plays Books, 1977. 4-up. Play about the meaning of love.
Vedral, Joyce L. *I Dare You: How to Get What You Want Out of Life.* Holt, 1983. 6-up. How to improve adolescent self-esteem.
•Voight, Cynthia. *Come a Stranger.* Atheneum, 1986. 6–8. Sensitive story about coming of age.
Walker, Stuart. *The Birthday of the Infanta.* In *Plays Children Love.* Coleman A. Jennings and Aurand Harris, eds. Doubleday, 1981. 5-up. Play about lack of love and compassion for others.
•Wallin, Luke. *Ceremony of the Panther.* Bradbury, 1987. 5–8. Emotional well-being; sense of heritage.
Winthrop, Elizabeth. *The Castle in the Attic.* Illus. Trina Schart Hyman. Holiday House, 1985. 3–6. Developing self-concept.
•Yep, Laurence. *Sea Glass.* Harper & Row, 1979. 5-up. Achieving self-understanding.

Relationships

•Adoff, Arnold. *All the Colors of the Race.* Illus. John Steptoe. Lothrop, Lee & Shepard, 1982. 3–7. Poems about human differences.
•*And Everywhere Children! An International Story Festival.* Sel. by the Literature Committee, Association for Childhood Education International. Greenwillow, 1979. 4–6. Anthology of tales about human differences.
•Arrick, Fran. *Chernowitz!* Bradbury, 1981. 6–9. Dealing with anti-Semitism.
Ashabranner, Brent. *People Who Make a Difference.* Illus. with photographs by Paul Conklin. Cobblehill Books, 1989. 5-up. Stories of people who have helped others.
Atkinson, Linda. *In Kindling Flame: the Story of Hannah Senesh, 1921–1944.* Lothrop, Lee & Shepard, 1985. 6-up. Story of heroism; fighting for human rights.
Barger, Gary W. *Life Is Not Fair.* Clarion, 1984. 4–6. Interracial friendship.
•Berssel, Henry. *Inook and the Sun.* Toronto, Ontario: Playwright's Co-op, 1973. 5-up. Play about responsibility to others; learning cooperation.
Bethancourt, T. Ernesto. *The Me Inside of Me.* Lerner, 1987. 5-up. Dealing with prejudice.
Brill, Michael. *The Masque of Beauty and the Beast.* Anchorage Press, 1979. 4-up. Play about finding inner beauty.
Byars, Betsy. *After the Goat Man.* Illus. Ronald Himler. Viking Kestrel, 1974. 4–6. Relationship with older person; dealing with emotions.
Carlson, Bernice Wells. *Let's Find the Big Idea.* Nashville, TN: Abingdon, 1982. 3-up. Collection of stories, playlets, and plays about interpersonal relationships.
•Chang, Heidi. *Elaine, Mary Lewis, and the Frogs.* Crown, 1988. 3–5. Dealing with stress of moving; finding a new friend.

Chase, Mary. *Mrs. McThing.* Dramatists Play Service, 1954. 4-up. Play about responsibility to others.

Christopher, Matt. *Baseball Pals.* Little, Brown, 1956. 4–6. How to be a leader; friendship.

•Cohen, Robert. *The Color of Man.* Illus. Ken Heyman. Random House, 1968. 5–8. Color differences in humans.

Corcoran, Barbara. *The Private War of Lillian Adams.* Atheneum, 1989. 3–6. Learning about human differences.

Danziger, Paula. *It's an Aardvark-Eat-Turtle World.* Delacorte, 1985. 4–8. Finding a family; learning to cope.

•Dolan, Edward F., Jr. *Anti-Semitism.* Watts, 1985. 4–6. Explains anti-Semitism.

Drimmer, Frederick. *The Elephant Man.* Putnam, 1985. 4–6. Learning to accept human deformities.

Eller, Scott. *Short Season.* Scholastic, 1985. 5–7. Developing relationships; maturing.

Falls, Gregory A. *The Forgotten Door.* Anchorage Press, 1985. 5-up. Play about accepting responsibility; cooperating with others.

———. *The Pushcart War.* Anchorage Press, 1983. 5–7. Play about resolving conflicts.

Fox, Paula. *The Village by the Sea.* Orchard Books, 1988. 4–8. Coping with envy; the power of love and forgiveness.

Gaines, Frederick. *The Legend of Sleepy Hollow.* University of Minnesota Press, 1975. 4-up. Play about accepting human differences.

Gardiner, Judy. *Come Back Soon.* Viking Kestrel, 1985. 4–6. Coping with family problems.

Glennon, William. *Beauty and the Beast.* Morton Grove, IL: Coach House Press, 1966. 4-up. Play about accepting others.

Golden, Joseph. *Johnny Moonbeam and the Silver Pony.* In *Plays for Young People.* William B. Birner, compiler. Anchorage Press, 1967. 5-up. Play about learning responsibility; gaining self-esteem.

Greenberg, Jan. *The Iceberg and Its Shadows.* Sunburst, 1989. 5–8. Dealing with cliques; developing friendships.

Hahn, Mary Downing. *December Stillness.* Clarion, 1988. 4–6. Developing social awareness.

•Hamilton, Virginia, reteller. "The People Could Fly." In *The People Could Fly.* Illus. Leo and Diane Dillon. Knopf, 1985. 3-up. Folktale about slavery and the desire for freedom.

•Harder, Eleanor, and Harder, Ray. *Rhumba Tiya: A Rain Forest Rumpelstiltskin.* New Plays, 1981. 4-up. Play about greed; dealing with emotions.

Harris, Aurand. *Ride a Blue Horse.* Anchorage Press, 1986. 5-up. Play about being different.

•———. *Steal Away Home.* Anchorage Press, 1972. 5-up. Play about racial freedom and justice.

———. *The Plain Princess.* Anchorage Press, 1955. 4-up. Play about learning to get along with others; being unselfish.

Hayes, Sheila. *You've Been Away All Summer.* Dutton, 1986. 5-up. Dealing with friendship; relationships.

Hermes, Patricia. *Friends Are Like That.* Harcourt Brace Jovanovich, 1984. 5–6. Friendship and loyalty are threatened.

•Hirschfelder, Arlene. *Happily May I Walk: American Indians and Alaska Natives Today.* Scribner's, 1986. 4-up. Informational book about the Indian peoples; accepting others.

Horvath, Polly. *An Occasional Cow.* Illus. Gioia Fiammenghi. Farrar, Straus & Giroux, 1989. 3–6. Learning to cope with life; coping with changes.

Hurwitz, Johanna. *The Hot and Cold Summer.* Morrow, 1984. 4–6. Dealing with the opposite sex; accepting others.

Hutton, Warwick, reteller. *Beauty and the Beast.* McElderry, 1985. 3–6. Recognizing inner beauty.

Korschunow, Irina. *The Foundling Fox.* James Skofield, translator. Illus. Reinhard Michl. Harper & Row, 1984. 3–6. The value of sharing; making a commitment.

Koste, Virginia Glasgow. *The Wonderful Wizard of Oz.* Coach House Press, 1987. 4-up. Play about finding courage; accepting one's own life; learning to care.

•Kraus, Joanna Halpert. *Mean to Be Free.* New Plays, 1967. 5-up. Play about two children who are led out of bondage to freedom.

•Linden, Barbara. *Tribe.* New Plays, 1970. 5-up. Play about accepting human differences.

Lindgren, Astrid. *Ronia, the Robber's Daughter.* Patricia Crampton, translator. Viking Kestrel, 1983. 5-up. The meaning of friendship.

Low, Alice. *The Macmillan Book of Greek Gods and Heroes.* Illus. Arvis Stewart. Macmillan, 1985. 4-up. Myths and legends about Greek gods and heroes retold. Some deal with personal relationships.

Lowry, Lois. *Anastasia, Ask Your Analyst.* Houghton Mifflin, 1984. 4–6. Coping with problems; seeking help.

Martin, Ann M. *Bummer Summer.* Holiday House, 1983. 4–6. Developing self-concept.

Martin, Patricia Miles. *Two Plays about Foolish People.* Putnam, 1972. 3–6. Plays about resolving conflict.

McGowen, Tom. *The Time of the Forest.* Houghton Mifflin, 1988. 3–6. Dealing with differences; resolving conflict.

•Mohr, Nicholasa. *Going Home.* Dial, 1986. 5–8. Explores cultural and sexual stereotyping.

•Newell, Martha Hill. *Phillis: A Life of Phillis Wheatley.* New Plays, 1981. 4-up. Biographical play about learning to accept oneself.

•O'Dell, Scott. *My Name Is Not Angelica.* Houghton Mifflin, 1989. 5–9. Accepting human differences.

Orlick, Terry. *The Cooperative Sports and Games Book.* Pantheon, 1978. 6-up. Collection of games based on cooperation, not competition.

———. *The Second Cooperative Sports and Games Book.* Pantheon, 1982. 4–6. More noncompetitive, noncombative games.

Pasnak, William. *Degrassi Junior High: Exit Stage Left.* Scholastic, 1987. 4–6. Developing relationships with the opposite sex.

Peavy, Linda, and Smith, Ursula. *Dreams Into Deeds: Nine Women Who Dared.* Scribner's, 1985. 4–6. Nine biographies of great women.

Peck, Robert Newton. *Soup.* Illus. Charles Gehm. Knopf, 1974. 4–6. The adventures of two friends.

――――. *Soup and Me.* Illus. Charles Lilly. Knopf, 1975. 4–6. Further adventures of two friends.

Pfeffer, Susan Beth. *Truth or Dare.* Scholastic, 1983. 5–up. Developing relationships.

Robinette, Joseph. *Charlotte's Web.* Woodstock, IL: The Dramatic Publishing Co., 1983. 3–up. Play exploring the meaning of friendship and responsibility.

Rylant, Cynthia. *A Fine White Dust.* Bradbury, 1986. 6–8. Search for self; search for God.

Sachar, Louis. *There's a Boy in the Girls' Bathroom.* Knopf, 1987. 4–6. Developing self-image; making friends.

•San Souci, Robert. *Song of Sedna.* Illus. Daniel San Souci. Doubleday, 1981. 4–6. Resolution of family problems.

•Sebestyen, Ouida. *Words by Heart.* Bantam, 1979. 4–6. Family; accepting differences.

Sendak, Philip. *In Grandpa's House.* Seymour Barofsky, translator and adaptor. Illus. Maurice Sendak. Harper & Row, 1985. 3–6. Family; maturing; satisfying needs.

Sender, Ruth Minsky. *To Life.* Macmillan, 1988. 4–6. The courage of holocaust victims.

Shwartz, Evgeny. *The Two Maples.* In *Russian Plays for Young Audiences.* Miriam Morton, translator and editor. Rowayton, CT: New Plays Books, 1977. 4-up. A play about love, kindness, and courage.

Smith, Doris Buchanan. *The First Hard Times.* Viking Kestrel, 1983. 5–7. Accepting a stepfather.

•Smith, K. *Skeeter.* Houghton Mifflin, 1981. 5–9. Acceptance of others; friendship.

•Springer, Nancy. *They're All Named Wildfire.* Atheneum, 1989. 4-up. The effects of prejudice and bigotry.

Strauss, Victoria. *Worldstone.* Four Winds, 1985. 5-up. Accepting human differences.

Townsend, John Rowe. *Cloudy-Bright.* Lippincott, 1984. 6-up. The meaning of true friendship.

Van Leeuwen, Jean. *More Tales of Amanda Pig.* Illus. Ann Schweninger. Dial, 1985. 3–6. Stories about family and friends.

Voigt, Cynthia. *The Runner.* Atheneum, 1985. 5–6. Learning the value of other people.

•Wagenheim, Kal. *Clemente!* Praeger, 1973. 4–8. Dealing with injustice.

•Winther, Barbara. *Listen to the Hodga.* In *Plays from Folktales of Africa and Asia.* Plays, Inc., 1976. 4-up. Plays about responsibility to others.

Zeder, Suzan. *Mother Hicks.* Anchorage Press, 1984. 5-up. Play about an orphan's growth to self-esteem.

Zolotow, Charlotte. *Everything Glistens and Everything Sings: New and Selected Poems.* Illus. Margot Tomes. Harcourt Brace Jovanovich, 1988. 3–6. Poems about friendship.

All Kinds of Friendships

Asher, Sandra Fenichel. *Just Like Jenny.* Delacorte, 1982. 5–7. Finding one's identity; friendship.

Avery, Helen P. *The Secret Garden.* Anchorage Press, 1986. 4-up. Play about self-realization, love, and friendship.

Burnett, Frances Hodgson. *The Secret Garden.* Adapted by James Howe. Illus. Thomas B. Allen. Random House, 1987. 4–6. Friendship grows; coping with infirmity.

Byars, Betsy. *The Cybil War.* Illus. Gail Owens. Viking Kestrel, 1981. 4–6. Friendships; first love.

Carris, Joan. *Rusty Timmons' First Million.* Illus. Kim Mulkey. Lippincott, 1985. 4–6. Learning about friendship and responsibility.

Cleary, Beverly. *Ralph S. Mouse.* Illus. Paul O. Zelinsky. Morrow, 1982. 4–6. The meaning of friendship.

Davis, Jenny. *Sex Education.* Orchard Books, 1988. 6-up. Dealing with love and loss.

Duder, Tessa. *In Lane Three, Alex Archer.* Houghton Mifflin, 1989. 5–9. Friendship; coping with the death of a friend.

Edwards, Pat. *Little John and Plutie.* Houghton Mifflin, 1988. 3–7. Learning about friendship and injustice.

Fisher, Lois I. *Rachel Vellars, How Could You?* Dodd, Mead, 1984. 3–6. Explores friendship.

Fox, Paula. *Portrait of Ivan.* Illus. Saul Lambert. Bradbury, 1969. 6–9. Making friends; developing identity.

Gardner, Sandra. *Street Gangs.* Photographs by Rebecca Lepkoff. Watts, 1983. 6-up. Why people join gangs; what gang life is like.

Giff, Patricia Reilly. *Left-Handed Shortstop.* Illus. Leslie Morrill. Delacorte, 1980. 4–6. Peer pressure; nonconformity.

Greenberg, Jan. *The Iceberg and Its Shadows.* Farrar, Straus & Giroux, 1980. 4–8. Discovering what true friendship is.

Greene, Carol. *The Jenny Summer.* Illus. Ellen Eagle. Harper & Row, 1988. 3–5. The frustrations and rewards of friendship.

Greene, Constance. *A Girl Called Al.* Illus. Byron Barton. Viking Kestrel, 1969. 4–6. Story of two friends.

———. *I Know You, Al.* Illus. Byron Barton. Viking Kestrel, 1975. 4–8. Entering adolescence.

———. *Your Old Pal, Al.* Viking Kestrel, 1979. 5–9. The making of a friendship.

———. *Al{exandra} the Great.* Viking Kestrel, 1982. 5–9. Adjusting to father's new family.

———. *Just Plain Al.* Viking Kestrel, 1986. 5–9. Adolescent problems.

Greenwald, Sheila. *Valentine Rosy.* Dell, 1986. 3–7. Rivalry among friends.

Hansen, Joyce. *The Gift-Giver.* Houghton/Clarion, 1980. 4–6. Withstanding peer pressure and family difficulties in the ghetto.

•———. *Yellow Bird and Me.* Clarion, 1986. 4–6. Developing new friendships.

Harris, Aurand. *Androcles and the Lion*. In *Plays Children Love*. Coleman A. Jennings and Aurand Harris, eds. Doubleday, 1981. 4-up. Play about friendship.

Haynes, Betsy. *Taffy Sinclair Strikes Again*. Bantam, 1984. 4–7. Learning the meaning of friendship.

Hermes, Patricia. *Friends Are Like That*. Harcourt Brace Jovanovich, 1984. 4–7. Struggling with cliques; friendship.

Hinton, S. E. *That Was Then, This Is Now*. Viking Kestrel, 1971. 6-up. Deals with delinquency; developing a sense of responsibility.

Keller, Beverly. *Desdemona—Twelve Going on Desperate*. Lothrop, Lee & Shepard, 1986. 4–6. Dealing with family and friends.

Lawlor, Laurie. *Addie's Dakota Winter*. Illus. Toby Gowing. Whitman, 1989. 2–6. Learning about friendship and courage.

Lipp, Frederick J. *Some Lose Their Way*. Atheneum, 1980. 6–8. Loneliness and finding friendship.

Mazer, Norma Fox. *Silver*. Children's Books, 1988. 6-up. Developing a positive self-concept; developing friendship.

McMullan, Kate. *Great Advice from Lila Fenwick*. Illus. Diane deGroat. Puffin Books, 1989. 5–9. Learning about the deeper meaning of friendship.

Ness, Evaline Michelow. *Sam, Bangs, and Moonshine*. Holt, Rinehart and Winston, 1966. 4–8. Living with the reality of one's life.

•Neville, Emily Cheney. *Garden of Broken Glass*. Delacorte, 1975. 6-up. Dealing with parental alcoholism; peer pressure.

Newton, Suzanne. *An End to Perfect*. Viking, 1984. 3–7. Peer relationships.

Park, Barbara. *Buddies*. Knopf, 1985. 5–8. Insights into friendship.

———. *The Kid in the Red Jacket*. Knopf, 1987. 3–6. Making friends with the opposite sex.

Pfeffer, Susan Beth. *Truth or Dare*. Four Winds, 1984. 5–8. Learning about friendship.

———. *Turning Thirteen*. Scholastic, 1988. 6–8. Friendship; making mature decisions.

Pryor, Bonnie. *The Plum Tree War*. Illus. Dora Leder. Morrow, 1989. 3–6. Getting along with others; coping.

Quin-Harkin, Janet. *Wanted: Date for Saturday Night*. Pacer/Putnam, 1985. 5–8. Coping with peer pressure.

Rockwell, Thomas. *How to Eat Fried Worms*. Delacorte, 1980. 4-up. Play about friends.

Roy, Ron. *Frankie Is Staying Back*. Illus. Walter Kessel. Clarion, 1981. 4–6. The ups and downs of friendship.

Shalant, Phyllis. *The Rock Star, the Rooster, and Me, the Reporter*. Illus. Charles Robinson. Dutton, 1989. 3–7. Learning about winning, losing, and friendship.

Shura, Mary Francis. *Chester*. Illus. Susan Swan. Dodd, 1980. 4–6. Being accepted; dealing with jealousy.

Springer, Nancy. *A Horse To Love*. Harper & Row, 1987. 4–6. Learning responsibility; importance of friendship.

Springstubb, Tricia. *Eunice Gottlieb and the Unwhitewashed Truth About Life*. Delacorte, 1987. 5–9. The meaning of friendship.

Strasser, Todd. *The Complete Computer Popularity Program*. Delacorte, 1984. 4–6. Making new friends.

Thesman, Jean. *Appointment with a Stranger*. Houghton Mifflin, 1989. 5–9. Gaining the acceptance of others; dealing with illness.

Wersba, Barbara. *Just Be Gorgeous*. Harper & Row, 1988. 6-up. Mental and emotional health; friendship with a gay person.

Winther, Barbara. *Pacca, the Little Bowman*. In *Plays from Folktales of Africa and Asia*. Plays, Inc., 1976. 4-up. Play about humility and friendship.

Coping With Stress

Agard, John, ed. *Life Doesn't Frighten Me at All*. Holt, 1989. 5-up. Grouped topically, these brief poems focus on concerns about family relationships, gender issues, self-esteem, individuality, and political issues.

Aldiss, Dorothy. *Nothing Is Impossible: The Story of Beatrix Potter*. Illus. Richard Cuffari. Atheneum, 1969. 3–6. Coping with loneliness.

Amoss, Berthe. *The Mockingbird Song*. Harper & Row, 1988. 3–5. Developing relationship with a new stepmother.

•Ashabranner, Brent. *Gavriel and Jemal: Two Boys of Jerusalem*. Photographs by Paul Conklin. Dodd, Mead, 1984. 3–6. Similarities and differences among people; social awareness.

Auch, Mary Jane. *Glass Slippers Give You Blisters*. Holiday House, 1989. 3–7. Discovering one's identity.

———. *Mom Is Dating Weird Wayne*. Holiday House, 1988. 4–7. Coping with new family member.

Baird, Thomas. *Where Time Ends*. Harper & Row, 1988. 6-up. Coping with stress; societal problems.

Bawden, Nina. *The Outside Child*. Lothrop, Lee & Shepard, 1989. 4–9. Discovering one's own identity.

Berger, Terry. *How Does It Feel When Your Parents Get Divorced?* Photographs by Miriam Shapiro. J. Messner, 1977. 4-up. Coping with divorce.

Bergreen, Gary. *Coping with Difficult Teachers*. Rosen, 1988. 6-up. Informational book on how to deal with problems.

Billington, Elizabeth T. *The Move*. Warne, 1984. 3–6. Accepting change.

Blume, Judy. *Superfudge*. Dutton, 1980. 4–6. Coping with family stress.

Boeckman, Charles. *Surviving Your Parents' Divorce*. Watts, 1980. 5-up. How to cope with divorce.

Bunting, Eve. *Is Anybody There?* Harper & Row, 1988. 4–7. Coping with being a latchkey child.

Byars, Betsy. *Good-bye, Chicken Little*. Harper & Row, 1979. 5-up. Coping with guilt after an accident.

———. *The TV Kid*. Illus. Richard Cuffari. Viking Kestrel, 1976. 4–7. Learning to live with reality.

Christopher, Matt. *Catch That Pass!* Illus. Harvey Kidder. Little, Brown, 1969. 4–6. Overcoming fears.

————. *Johnny Long Legs.* Illus. Harvey Kidder. Little, Brown, 1988. 3–6. Adjusting to new family members.

————. *Soccer Halfback.* Illus. Larry Johnson. Little, Brown, 1978. 4–6. Making one's own decisions.

————. *The Fox Steals Home.* Illus. Larry Johnson. Little, Brown, 1978. 4–6. Coping with moving.

————. *The Hit-Away Kid.* Illus. George Ulrich. Little, Brown, 1988. 3–5. Establishing personal values.

————. *Tight End.* Little, Brown, 1981. 4–6. Coping with prejudice.

Cleary, Beverly. *Dear Mr. Henshaw.* Illus. Paul O. Zelinsky. Morrow, 1983. 4–7. Coping with loneliness; divorce.

————. *Ramona and Her Mother.* Illus. Alan Tiegreen. Morrow, 1979. 4–6. Coping with family concerns.

————. *Ramona Quimby, Age 8.* Illus. Alan Tiegreen. Morrow, 1981. 4–6. Coping with family concerns.

Cleaver, Vera. *Belle Pruitt.* Harper & Row, 1988. 4–8. Coping with death of a family member.

Cohen, Barbara. *The Orphan Game.* Illus. Diane deGroat. Lothrop, Lee & Shepard, 1988. 3–6. Discovering the meaning of family and friendship.

Conford, Ellen. *If This Is Love, I'll Take Spaghetti.* Four Winds, 1983. 4–6. Nine short stories about adolescent concerns.

Conrad, Pam. *Prairie Songs.* Illus. Darry S. Zudeck. Harper & Row, 1985. 4–6. Coping with change at the turn of the century.

Cooper, Susan. *Seaward.* Atheneum, 1983. 4-up. Two adolescents pursue the meaning of life and death in a survival adventure.

Corcoran, Barbara. *I Am the Universe.* Atheneum, 1986. 4–8. Working through family problems and developing self-respect.

————. *The Sky Is Falling.* Atheneum, 1987. 3–7. Depression-era story about dealing with family problems and separation.

Danziger, Paula. *It's An Aardvark-Eat-Turtle World.* Delacorte, 1985. 4–6. Dealing with friendship; stress.

DeClements, Barthe. *Nothing's Fair in Fifth Grade.* Viking Kestrel, 1981. 4–6. Working through adolescent emotions.

————. *Sixth Grade Can Really Kill You.* Viking Kestrel, 1985. 5–7. Coping with family and school problems.

Duder, Tessa. *Jellybean.* Viking Kestrel, 1986. 4–6. Single-parent family problems.

Duffy, James. *The Doll Hospital.* Scholastic, 1989. 4–7. Coping with illness.

Dygard, Thomas J. *Halfback Tough.* Puffin Books, 1989. 5-up. Coping with a troubled past.

•Evans, Mari. *JD.* Illus. Jerry Pinckney. Doubleday, 1973. 4–7. Four short stories about coping with poverty.

Ewing, Kathryn. *Things Won't Be the Same.* Harcourt, 1980. 4–6. Coping with family crises.

Eyerly, Jeannette Hyde. *The Girl Inside.* Lippincott, 1968. 6-up. Coping with parents' deaths and depression.

Fleischman, Sid. *The Whipping Boy.* Illus. Peter Sis. Greenwillow, 1986. 3–5. Making friends and being loyal.

Glass, Stuart M. *A Divorce Dictionary: A Book for You and Your Children.* Illus. Bari Weissman. Little, Brown, 1980. 4–6. Explains divorce terminology to children.

Greenwald, Sheila. *Give Us a Great Big Smile, Rosy Cole.* Atlantic/Little, Brown, 1981. 4–6. Dealing with emotions.

———. *Rosy Cole's Great American Guilt Club.* Little, Brown, 1985. 3–5. Establishing values, making friends.

———. *Write On, Rosy! A Young Author in Crisis.* Little, Brown, 1988. 3–6. Discovering one's talents.

•Hamilton, Virginia. *Cousins.* Philomel, 1990. 4–6. With the support of her extended family, eleven-year-old Cammy copes with her cousin's accidental death.

Hermes, Patricia. *Kevin Corbett Eats Flies.* Harcourt Brace Jovanovich, 1986. 4–6. Learning to cope with loss.

Holl, Kristi D. *Hidden in the Fog.* Atheneum, 1989. 4–8. Coping with problems.

Holman, Felice. *Slake's Limbo.* Scribner's, 1974. 6-up. Coping with emotions; poverty.

Hotze, Sollace. *A Circle Unbroken.* Clarion, 1988. 4–6. Learning to adjust to change.

Howe, James. *Nighty-Nightmare.* Illus. Leslie Morrill. Atheneum, 1987. 4–6. Coping with nighttime fears.

Hughes, Langston. *The Dream Keeper and Other Poems.* Illus. Helen Sewell. Knopf, 1976. 3-up. Collection of sixty poems about hopes, dreams, the blues, and an imperfect world.

Hunter, Mollie. *Cat, Herself.* Harper & Row, 1986. 5–6. Learning to accept others.

Hurwitz, Johanna. *Aldo Applesauce.* Illus. John Wallner. Puffin Books, 1989. 3–7. Coping with moving.

Jones, Charlotte Foltz. *Only Child Clues for Coping.* Westminster, 1984. 4–6. Coping with being an only child.

Klein, Norma. *Confessions of an Only Child.* Illus. Richard Cuffari. Knopf, 1988. 3–6. Coping with death of a family member.

Knudson, R. R. *Rinehart Shouts.* Farrar, Straus & Giroux, 1987. 5-up. Overcoming fears.

Konigsburg, E. L. *Altogether, One at a Time.* Illus. Mercer Mayer, Gail E. Haley, Laurel Schindelman, and Gary Parker. Aladdin, 1989. 4–7. Four short stories about coping; growing up.

Kyte, Kathy S. *In Charge: A Complete Handbook for Kids with Working Parents.* Illus. Susan Detrich. Knopf, 1983. 5-up. Coping with being a latchkey child; developing independence.

LeShan, Eda. *When A Parent Is Very Sick.* Illus. Jacqueline Rogers. Little, Brown, 1986. 4–6. Coping with the illness of a parent.

Lindbergh, Anne. *The Worry Week.* Illus. Kathryn Hewett. Harcourt Brace Jovanovich, 1985. 4–6. How three sisters survive in the Maine wilderness.

Martin, Ann M. *Stage Fright.* Illus. Blanche Sims. Holiday House, 1984. 3–5. Learning to handle shyness.

Mazer, Harry. *The War on Villa Street: A Novel.* Delacorte, 1978. 6–8. Coping with abuse and parental alcoholism.

Mazer, Norma Fox. *A, My Name Is Ami.* Scholastic, 1986. 4–6. Developing self-awareness and sense of belonging.

McAfee, Annalena and Browne, A. *Visitors Who Came to Stay.* Illus. Anthony Browne. Viking Kestrel, 1985. 4–6. Dealing with emotions; new family members.

McDonnell, Christine. *Count Me In.* Viking Kestrel, 1986. 4–6. Dealing with new family members and adolescent changes.

———. *Lucky Charms & Birthday Wishes.* Illus. Diane deGroat. Viking Kestrel, 1984. 3–6. Coping with everyday obstacles and fears.

Miller, Judi. *Ghost in My Soup.* Bantam Books, 1985. 5–8. Developing friendships.

Miller, Madge. *OPQRS, Etc.* Anchorage Press, 1983. 5-up. Play about individuality.

Mills, Claudia. *What About Annie?* Walker, 1985. 3–6. Coping with joblessness during the Great Depression.

Moore, Emily. *Whose Side Are You On?* Farrar, Straus & Giroux, 1988. 3–7. Coping; developing friendships.

•Myers, Walter Dean. *It Ain't All for Nothin'.* Viking Kestrel, 1978. 6–8. Making moral decisions.

•Naidoo, Beverly. *Journey to Jo'Burg: A South African Story.* Illus. Eric Velasquez. Lippincott, 1986. 4–8. Dealing with human differences.

Norton, Andre and Miller, Phyllis. *Seven Spells to Sunday.* McElderry/ Atheneum, 1979. 4–6. Two children learning to work together and to cope with their problems.

O'Shaughnessy McKenna, Colleen. *Fourth Grade Is a Jinx.* Scholastic, 1989. 3–7. Coping with stress.

Park, Barbara. *The Kid in the Red Jacket.* Knopf, 1987. 4–6. Coping with moving; friendships.

Paterson, Katherine. *Come Sing, Jimmy Jo.* Dutton, 1985. 4–6. Dealing with family changes.

———. *The Great Gilly Hopkins.* Thomas Y. Crowell, 1978. 5–7. Coping with stress; being a foster child.

Pearson, Gayle. *The Coming Home Cafe.* Atheneum, 1987. 6–8. Developing self-concept, inner strength during the Great Depression.

Pfeffer, Susan Beth. *What Do You Do When Your Mouth Won't Open?* Illus. Lorna Tomei. Delacorte, 1981. 4–6. Fear of public speaking.

Pinkwater, Jill. *Buffalo Brenda.* Macmillan, 1989. 5–9. Finding one's individuality.

Potter, Marian. *Mark Makes His Move.* Morrow, 1986. 5-up. Overcoming fears and taking responsibility.

Reeder, Carolyn. *Shades of Gray.* Macmillan, 1989. 3–7. Learning to adjust to a new family.

Rinaldi, Ann. *The Last Silk Dress.* Holiday House, 1988. 5–6. Dealing with family secrets.

Rofes, Eric E., editor. *The Kids' Book of Divorce By, For and About Kids.* Greene, 1981. 6-up. Information for children about divorce.

Rogers, June Walker. *Heidi.* Woodstock, IL: Dramatic Publishing Co., 1969. 4. Play about the restorative power of love.

Rudolph, Wilma. *Wilma.* Signet Books, 1977. 6-up. Autobiography about overcoming handicaps.

Sachar, Louis. *There's a Boy in the Girls' Bathroom.* Knopf, 1987. 4–6. Coping; developing relationships.

Schneider, Hansjorg. *Robinson and Friday.* Ken and Barbi Rugg, translators. Carol Korty, editor. Bakers, 1980. 5-up. Play about physical survival and dealing with longings and fears.

Seale, Nancy. *The Little Princess, Sara Crewe.* Anchorage Press, 1982. 4-up. Play about coping with changes.

Shura, Mary Francis. *The Search for Grissi.* Illus. Ted Lewin. Dodd Mead, 1985. 3–5. Learning to accept others.

Smith, Alison. *Billy Boone.* Scribner's, 1989. 3–6. Deals with intergenerational support and stress, growth, and development.

Smith, Doris Buchanan. *Return to Bitter Creek.* Viking Kestrel, 1986. 3–7. Developing family relationships.

———. *Voyages.* Viking Kestrel, 1989. 5-up. Surviving illness.

Smith, Robert Kimmel. *Mostly Michael.* Illus. Katherine Coville. Delacorte, 1987. 3–6. Coping and growing up.

Snyder, Zilpha Keatley. *And Condors Danced.* Delacorte, 1988. 3–6. Dealing with loss.

•Soto, Gary. *Baseball in April and Other Stories.* Harcourt, 1990. 5–9. Contemporary Mexican American children deal with typical difficulties of growing up. Glossary of Spanish words provided.

•Speare, Elizabeth George. *The Sign of the Beaver.* Houghton Mifflin, 1983. 5–8. Living with differences; survival.

Springer, Nancy. *Not on a White Horse.* Atheneum, 1988. 5-up. Coping with an alcoholic parent; growing up.

Steele, Mary Q. *The First of the Penguins.* Greenwillow, 1985. 4–8. Developing friendship.

Stock, Gregory. *The Kids' Book of Questions.* Workman, 1988. 6-up. Presents questions children have about ethics, self-concept, family, and identity formation.

Sutton, Jane. *Me and the Weirdos.* Illus. Sandy Kossin. Houghton Mifflin, 1981. 4–6. Dealing with family individuality.

Talbot, Toby. *Dear Greta Garbo.* Putnam, 1978. 5–8. A young person searches for identity.

Turnbull, Ann. *Marco of the Winter Caves.* Clarion, 1984. 3–6. Tale of responsibility and survival.

Wallace, Bill. *Beauty.* Holiday House, 1988. 3–7. Story of growth, family love, and devotion to an animal.

Wright, Betty Ren. *The Ghost in the Window.* Holiday House, 1988. 6–8. Dealing with a troubled family.

•Zeder, Suzan. *Wiley and the Hairy Man.* Anchorage, 1978. 4-up. Play about dealing with fears.

Grades Seven and Up

Coping With Stress

Adler, C. S. *In Our House Scott Is My Brother.* Macmillan, 1980. 7-up. Coping with family stress.

――――. *The Magic of the Glits.* Illus. Ati Forberg. Macmillan, 1979. 6-up. Developing a friendship.

Brancato, Robin. *Winning.* Bantam, 1976. 7-up. Coping with injury.

Busselle, Rebecca. *Bathing Ugly.* Orchard Books, 1989. 7-up. Developing a self-concept.

Byars, Betsy. *The Night Swimmers.* Delacorte, 1980. 7-up. Sibling relationships; dealing with family crises.

Colman, Hila. *What's the Matter with the Dobsons?* Crown, 1980. 7-up. Solving family problems.

Conrad, Pam. *What I Did for Roman.* Harper, 1987. 7-up. Coping with emotional problems.

Crutcher, Chris. *The Crazy Horse Electric Game.* Greenwillow, 1987. 7-up. Coping with an injury.

Gauch, Patricia Lee. *Kate Alone.* Putnam, 1980. 7-up. Coping with emotions.

Gibbons, Kaye. *Ellen Foster.* Algonquin, 1987. 7-up. Coping with a family death; survival.

Green, Constance C. *Your Old Pal.* Viking Kestrel, 1979. 7-up. Coping with the strains of true friendship.

Greenwald, Dorothy. *Coping with Moving.* Rosen, 1987. 7-up. Learning to cope with change.

•Guy, Rosa. *And I Heard a Bird Sing.* Delacorte, 1987. 7-up. Coping with family problems.

•――――. *The Friends.* Holt, 1973. 7-up. Developing a friendship.

Hall, Lynn. *Just One Friend.* Collier, 1987. 7-up. Coping with loneliness; developing friendships.

Harris, Mark Jonathan. *With a Wave of the Wand.* Lothrop, 1980. 7-up. Dealing with divorce.

Hinton, S. E. *Tex.* Doubleday/Delacorte, 1979. 7-up. Learning to survive; dealing with family problems.

――――. *That Was Then, This Is Now.* Viking Kestrel, 1971. 7-up. Dealing with sibling problems.

――――. *The Outsiders.* Viking Kestrel, 1967. 7-up. Adolescent problems.

Holman, Felice. *Slake's Limbo.* Scribner's, 1974. 7-up. Learning to survive.

•Hotze, Sollace. *A Circle Unbroken.* Clarion, 1988. 7-up. Coping with differences; finding identity.

Jacoby, Alice. *My Mother's Boyfriend and Me.* Dial, 1987. 7-up. Coping with relationships.

Janeczko, Paul B., compiler. *Going Over to Your Place: Poems for Each Other.* Bradbury Press, 1987. 7-up. Poems about everyday love and loss.

Kerr, M. E. *Fell.* Harper, 1987. 7-up. Coping with relationships.

Klass, Sheila Solomon. *Page Four.* Scribner's, 1987. 7-up. Dealing with father's desertion.

Klein, Norma. *Older Men.* Dial, 1987. 7-up. Coping with family problems.

Koertge, Ron. *The Arizona Kid.* Little, Brown, 1988. 7-up. Dealing with homosexuality.

―――. *Where the Kissing Never Stops.* Little, Brown, 1986. 7-up. Dealing with sexuality.

Kolodny, Robert, Kolodny, Nancy J., and Bratter, Dr. Thomas. *Smart Choices: A Guide to Surviving at Home and in School, Dating and Sex, Dealing with Crises, Applying to Colleges, and More.* Little, Brown, 1986. 7-up. Addresses contemporary adolescent concerns.

Lackey, Mercedes. *Arrows of the Queen.* New American Library, 1987. 7-up. Developing a self-concept.

Langone, John. *Goodbye to Bedlam: Understanding Mental Illness and Retardation.* Little, Brown, 1974. 7-up. Explanation of mental retardation and mental illness.

―――. *Violence! Our Fastest-Growing Public Health Problem.* Little, Brown, 1984. 7-up. Study of violence in society.

LeVert, John. *The Flight of the Cassowary.* Little, Brown, 1986. 6-up. A boy questions his sanity.

•Levitt, Saul. *Jim Thorpe, All-American.* Anchorage, 1980. 6-up. Play about coping with differences, adversity.

Lyon, George Ella. *Borrowed Children.* Orchard Books, 1988. 5–7. Family love and acceptance during the Great Depression.

Mahy, Margaret. *Memory.* Mcmillan, 1988. 7-up. Dealing with death, disease; relationship with an older person.

McGuire, Paula. *Putting It Together: Teenagers Talk About Family Breakup.* Delacorte, 1987. 7-up. Coping with divorce.

Mearian, Judy Frank. *Someone Slightly Different.* Dial, 1980. 7-up. Solving family problems.

•Meyer, Carolyn. *Denny's Tapes.* McElderry, 1987. 7-up. Coping with family heritage.

Miles, Betty. *Maudie and Me and the Dirty Book.* Knopf, 1980. 7-up. Dealing with stress; censorship.

Miller, Kathryn Schultz. *Haunted Houses.* Coach House, 1987. 6-up. Play about learning to cope with problems.

Murray, Marguerite. *Like Seabirds Flying Home.* Atheneum, 1987. 7-up. Coping with family break-up.

Naylor, Phyllis Reynolds. *The Keeper.* Atheneum, 1986. 7-up. Dealing with parent's mental illness.

―――. *Unexpected Pleasures.* Putnam, 1987. 7-up. Relationship between younger and older persons.

Newton, Suzanne. *I Will Call It Georgie's Blues.* Viking Kestrel, 1983. 7-up. Dealing with emotional illness.

Nida, Patricia Cooney. *The Teenager's Survival Guide to Moving.* Collier, 1987. 7-up. Coping with change.

O'Neal, Zibby. *The Language of Goldfish.* Viking Kestrel, 1980. 6–8. Dealing with change; mental illness.

Osborne, Mary Pope. *Run, Run, as Fast as You Can.* Dial, 1982. 7-up. Dealing with family tragedy; friendships; new school.

Park, Barbara. *Buddies.* Knopf, 1985. 6-up. Relationships.

Pfeffer, Susan Beth. *The Year Without Michael.* Bantam, 1987. 7-up. Coping with the disappearance of a child.

Phipson, Joan. *Bianca.* McElderry, 1987. 7-up. Coping with disappearance of a child; being a runaway.

Pinkwater, Daniel M. *Alan Mendelsohn, The Boy from Mars.* Dutton, 1979. 7-up. Humorous story about coping, friendship.

Powledge, Fred. *You'll Survive.* Scribner's, 1986. 7-up. Coping with the problems of adolescence.

Rinaldi, Ann. *But in the Fall I'm Leaving.* Holiday House, 1985. 7-up. Coping with emotions; leaving home.

Roy, Ron. *I Am a Thief.* Dutton, 1982. 7-up. Coping with peer pressure.

Ryan, Mary C. *Who Says I Can't?* Little, Brown, 1988. 7-up. Developing identity; relationships.

Snyder, Carol. *Leave Me Alone, Ma.* Bantam, 1987. 7-up. Resolving family conflicts.

Sweeney, Joyce. *Right Behind the Rain.* Delacorte, 1987. 7-up. Coping with stress of success; adolescent problems.

Terris, Susan. *Nell's Quilt.* Farrar, Straus & Giroux, 1987. 7-up. Coping with stress.

Tolan, Stephanie S. *A Good Courage.* Morrow, 1988. 7–9. Coping with life in a cult; family relationships.

Vinke, Hermann (trans. Hedwig Pachter). *The Short Life of Sophie Scholl.* Harper & Row, 1984. 7-up. Courage and determination of a child who fought against the Nazis.

Voigt, Cynthia. *Dicey's Song.* Random House, 1982. 7-up. Coping with parent's mental illness.

———. *Izzy, Willy-Nilly.* Atheneum, 1986. 7-up. Coping after a disfiguring accident.

White, Ellen Emerson. *Life Without Friends.* Scholastic, 1987. 7-up. Learning to cope with loss.

Zeder, Suzan. *In a Room Somewhere.* Anchorage Press, 1988. 7-up. Play about coping with childhood memories.

Zindel, Paul. *The Pigman.* Harper, 1968. 7-up. Relationship with older person; coping with loss.

Developing a Personal Identity

Asher, Sandy. *Everything Is Not Enough.* Delacorte, 1987. 7-up. Developing goals; becoming independent.

Branscum, Robbie. *Johnny May Grows Up*. Illus. Bob Marstall. Harper & Row, 1987. 7-up. Story of growth and determination; coping with stress.

Cuyler, Margery. *The Trouble with Soap*. Unicorn/Dutton, 1982. 7-up. Developing friendships.

Davis, Jenny. *Sex Education*. Watts, 1988. 7-up. Dealing with sexuality.

Denson, Will. *Tinker Autumn*. Coach House, 1985. 6-up. Play about being outcast; developing self-identity.

Derby, Pat. *Goodbye Emily, Hello*. Farrar, Straus & Giroux, 1989. 7-up. Developing self-concept.

Deuker, Carl. *On the Devil's Court*. Little, Brown, 1989. 7-up. Coming to terms with feelings of inadequacy.

•Dorris, Michael. *A Yellow Raft in Blue Water*. Holt, 1987. 7-up. The search for identity.

Ferris, Jean. *Amen, Moses Gardenia*. Farrar, Straus & Giroux, 1985. 7-up. Dealing with depression.

Guernsey, Joann Bren. *Room to Breathe*. Clarion, 1986. 7-up. Asserting independence.

Hall, Lynn. *The Leaving*. Collier, 1988. 7-up. Moving away and gaining independence.

Hobbs, Will. *Changes in Latitudes*. Atheneum, 1988. 7-up. Dealing with family problems.

•Klass, David. *Breakaway Run*. Lodestar, 1987. 7-up. Adjusting to a new culture; facing personal loss.

Konigsburg, E. L. *Throwing Shadows*. Collier, 1988. 7-up. Five short stories about adolescents learning to cope.

•Kroeber, Theodora. *Ishi: Last of His Tribe*. Illus. Ruth Robbins. Parnassus, 1964. 7-up. Dealing with stress and racial differences.

Lowry, Lois. *Rabble Starkey*. Houghton Mifflin, 1987. 7-up. Dealing with mental illness; families; friendships.

Mahy, Margaret. *Memory*. McElderry, 1988. 7-up. Learning to take responsibility for oneself.

Mazer, Harry. *The Girl of His Dreams*. Crowell, 1987. 7-up. Coping with parental alcoholism; achieving maturity.

McIntyre, Vonda N. *Barbary*. Houghton Mifflin, 1986. 6-up. Making choices; developing self-concept.

Morris, Winifred. *Dancer in the Mirror*. Atheneum, 1987. 7-up. Accepting oneself.

Oldham, June. *Grow Up, Cupid*. Delacorte, 1987. 7-up. Developing adolescent relationships.

Park, Barbara. *Beanpole*. Knopf, 1983. 7-up. Developing a positive self-concept.

Peck, Richard. *Princess Ashley*. Delacorte, 1987. 7-up. Coping with peer pressure; developing a positive self-concept.

Peterson, P. J. *Good-Bye to Good Ol' Charlie*. Delacorte, 1987. 7-up. Making changes in one's life.

Rylant, Cynthia. *A Fine White Dust*. Bradbury, 1986. 5–8. Making choices; coping with family life and friendships.

Stolz, Mary. *Scarecrows and Their Child.* Illus. Amy Schwartz. Harper & Row, 1987. 7-up. Coping with adolescence; developing relationships.

Strasser, Todd. *Wildlife.* Delacorte, 1987. 7-up. Coping with responsibilities; fame.

•Thomas, Joyce Carol. *Journey.* Scholastic, 1988. 7-up. A journey from innocence to maturity.

Voigt, Cynthia. *Izzy, Willy-Nilly.* Atheneum, 1986. 6–9. Coping with an accident; peer pressure.

————. *The Runner.* Atheneum, 1985. 7-up. Changing relationships with parents and peers; developing self-image.

Wells, Rosemary. *Through the Hidden Door.* Dutton, 1987. 7-up. Developing friendship; self-image.

Interrelationships Among Physical, Mental/Emotional and Social Well-Being

Anderson, Mary. *Do You Call That a Dream Date?* Delacorte, 1987. 7-up. Developing values; making choices.

Anderson, Norman and Brown, Walter. *Rescue! True Stories of the Winners of the Young American Medal for Bravery.* Walker, 1983. 7-up. Twelve stories about responsibility to others.

Avi. *Romeo and Juliet—Together (and Alive!) at Last.* Orchard Books, 1987. 7-up. Dealing with shyness.

Baeher, Patricia. *Always Faithful.* New American Library, 1983. 7-up. Friendship; solving conflicts.

Blume, Judy. *Just as Long as We're Together.* Orchard Books, 1987. 7-up. The meaning of friendships.

Bonderoff, Jason. *Alan Alda: An Unauthorized Biography.* Signet, 1982. 7-up. Biography detailing surviving illness and achieving.

•Carew, Jan. *Children of the Sun.* Illus. Leo and Diane Dillon. Little, Brown, 1980. 5–8. The quest for personal values.

Cassedy, Sylvia. *Behind the Attic Wall.* Crowell, 1983. 7-up. Learning to love again; conquering loneliness.

•Childress, Alice. *When the Rattlesnake Sounds.* Coward, McCann, 1975. 6-up. Play about accepting differences in others.

Cohen, Barbara. *People Like Us.* Bantam, 1987. 7-up. Dealing with family conflicts.

Craig, Eleanor. *If We Could Hear the Grass Grow.* New American Library, 1985. 7-up. Dealing with emotionally disturbed children.

Crutcher, Chris. *The Crazy Horse Electric Game.* Greenwillow, 1987. 7-up. Coping with illness; finding dignity.

•Davis, Ossie. *Escape to Freedom.* Viking Kestrel, 1976. 6-up. Learning to accept differences.

•————. *Langston.* Delacorte, 1982. 7-up. Play about self-esteem; family relationships.

DeClements, Barthe, and Greimes, Christopher. *Double Trouble.* Viking Kestrel, 1987. 7-up. Twins handle the stress in their lives.
————. *How Do You Lose Those Ninth Grade Blues?* Viking Kestrel, 1983. 7-up. First love; adjusting to adolescence.
————. *I Never Asked You to Understand Me.* Viking Kestrel, 1987. 7-up. Coping with adolescent problems.
Ferguson, Alane. *Show Me the Evidence.* Bradbury, 1989. 7-up. Teen friendship is tested.
Girion, Barbara. *Like Everybody Else.* Scribner's, 1980. 7-up. A family learns to cope with problems.
•Gordon, Sheila. *Waiting for the Rain.* Orchard Books, 1987. 7-up. A friendship is challenged by apartheid.
•Henderson, Nancy. *Walk Together.* Julian Messner, 1972. 7-up. Plays about human rights and developing self-esteem.
•Humphrey, Kathryn Long. *Satchel Paige.* Watts, 1988. 7-up. Biography about the struggle against discrimination.
Killien, Christi. *All of the Above.* Houghton Mifflin, 1987. 7-up. Dealing with adolescent emotions.
•Kraus, Joanna Halpert. *The Ice Wolf.* New Plays, 1963. 6-up. Play about being different; developing love and tolerance.
Lipke, Jean C. *Loving.* Illus. Robert Fontaine and Patricia Bateman. Lerner, 1986. 7-up. How to maintain relationships that are caring and honest.
Mamlin, Gennadi. *Hey There—Hello!* In *Russian Plays for Young Audiences.* Miriam Morton, translator and editor. New Plays, 1977. 6-up. Play about dealing with personal conflicts.
Melwood, Mary. *Five Minutes to Morning.* In *Contemporary Theater.* Betty Jean Lifton, editor. New Plays, 1988. 6-up. Play about accepting responsibility to others.
•Meyer, Carolyn. *A Voice from Japan: An Outsider Looks In.* Harcourt Brace Jovanovich, 1988. 7-up. A personal view of another culture.
•————. *Voices of South Africa.* Harcourt Brace Jovanovich, 1988. 7-up. Personal account of racial discord in South Africa.
Pevsner, Stella. *Cute Is a Four-Letter Word.* Houghton Mifflin, 1980. 7-up. Developing a self-concept.
Phifer, Kate Gilbert. *Tall and Small.* Illus. Dennis Kendrick. Walker, 1987. 5–8. Dealing with physical differences.
•Scott, John Anthony. *Fanny Kemble's America.* Crowell, 1973. 7-up. Fighting for the rights of others.
Shyer, Marlene Fanta. *My Brother, the Thief.* Scribner's, 1980. 7-up. Coping with delinquency; family relations.
Smith, Anne Warren. *Sister in the Shadow.* Atheneum, 1986. 5–9. Sibling relations; developing a self-concept.
•Smith, Mary-Anne Tirone. *Lament for a Silver-eyed Woman.* Morrow, 1987. 7-up. The meaning of friendship.
Stanek, Lou Willett. *Megan's Beat.* Pacer Books/Putnam, 1983. 7-up. Developing values; defending the rights of others.
Stevens, Janice. *Take Back the Moment.* New American Library, 1983. 7-up. Dealing with juvenile crime; the meaning of friendship.

•Thomas, Janet. *Newcomer.* Anchorage Press, 1986. 6-up. Play dealing with peer pressure; accepting others.

White III, Josh, and Williams, Robert C. *The Land of Everywhere.* Coach House, 1986. 6-up. Play about learning to resolve conflict.

C. PERSONAL HEALTH

Grades K Through Three

Health Advisors

Barnett, Naomi. *I Know a Dentist.* Putnam, 1978. K–3. Tale of a first trip to the dentist.

Berenstain, Stan, and Berenstain, Jan. *The Berenstain Bears Visit the Dentist.* Random House, 1981. 1–3. Learning about what happens on a visit to the dentist.

DeSantis, Kenny. *A Dentist's Tools.* Photographs by Patricia A. Agre. Dodd, Mead, 1988. Pres.–1. Explains all the dentist's tools and their uses.

———. *A Doctor's Tools.* Photographs by Patricia A. Agre. Dodd, Mead, 1985. Pres.–1. Identifies common doctor's tools and their uses.

Krementz, Jill. *Taryn Goes to the Dentist.* Crown, 1986. Pres.–K. An eyewitness account of a first trip to the dentist.

Kuklin, Susan. *When I See My Doctor.* Bradbury, 1988. Pres.–1. What happens in a pediatric examination.

Linn, Margot. *A Trip to the Dentist.* Illus. Catherine Siracusa. Harper & Row, 1988. K–3. Why to visit the dentist and what happens there.

Rey, H. L. *Curious George Goes to the Dentist.* Houghton Mifflin, 1989. Pres.–2. What goes on in the examining room at the dentist.

Rockwell, Harlow. *My Dentist.* Macmillan, 1975. K–2. Informative book about a trip to the dentist.

———. *My Doctor.* Macmillan, 1973. Pres.–2. What to expect when you visit the doctor.

Roop, Peter, and Roop, Connie. *Stick Out Your Tongue!* Illus. Joan Hanson. Lerner, 1986. 1–4. Book of jokes about doctors and patients.

Wolfe, Bob, and Wolfe, Diane. *Emergency Room.* Carolrhoda, 1983. K–4. How an emergency room functions.

Health Care Practices

Allen, Marjorie N. *One, Two, Three—Ah-Choo!* Illus. Dick Gackenbach. Coward, 1980. K–3. Being allergic.

Brown, Marc. *Arthur's Eyes.* Little, Brown, 1979. K–3. Learning to live with glasses.
Goldin, Augusta. *Straight Hair, Curly Hair.* Illus. Ed Emberley. Crowell, 1966. 1–3. The nature, purpose, and care of hair.
Showers, Paul. *Sleep Is for Everyone.* Illus. Wendy Watson. Crowell, 1974. 1–3. What happens during sleep; because of lack of sleep.
Silverstein, Alvin, and Silverstein, Virginia R. *Itch, Sniffle, and Sneeze: All About Asthma, Hay Fever, and Other Allergies.* Illus. Ray Doty. Four Winds, 1978. 1–5. The facts about allergies.
Stanek, Muriel. *Left, Right, Left, Right!* Illus. Lucy Hawkinson. Whitman, 1969. K–2. What it is like to wear glasses.
Wise, William. *Fresh as a Daisy, Neat as a Pin.* Illus. Dora Leder. Parents, 1970. 1–3. The importance of cleanliness.

Physical Fitness

Asch, Frank, and Asch, Jan. *Running with Rachel.* Photographs by Jan Asch and Robert M. Buscow. Dial, 1979. 2–5. Informational book about running.
Briggs, Carole S. *Diving Is for Me.* Lerner, 1983. 2–5. Introduction to diving.
———. *Waterskiing Is for Me.* Lerner, 1986. 2–5. Introduction to waterskiing.
Carlson, Nancy. *Bunnies and Their Sports.* Viking Kestrel, 1987. Pres.–3. Physical fitness.
Carr, Rachel. *Be a Frog, a Bird or a Tree.* Doubleday, 1973. 1–3. Introduction to yoga.
Chappell, Annette Jo. *Skiing Is for Me.* Lerner, 1978. 2–5. Introduction to skiing.
Dickmeyer, Lowell A. *Baseball Is for Me.* Lerner, 1978. 2–5. Close look at team baseball.
———. *Basketball Is for Me.* Lerner, 1980. 2–5. Introduction to basketball.
———. *Football Is for Me.* Lerner, 1979. 2–5. The basics of football explained.
———. *Hockey Is for Me.* Lerner, 1978. 2–5. The basics of hockey explained.
———. *Ice Skating Is for Me.* Lerner, 1980. 2–5. Introduction to ice skating.
———. *Skateboarding Is for Me.* Lerner, 1978. 2–5. The basics of skateboarding explained.
———. *Track Is for Me.* Lerner, 1979. 2–5. Explains track and field.
Dickmeyer, Lowell A., and Chappell, Annette Jo. *Tennis Is for Me.* Lerner, 1978. 2–5. Explains the basics of tennis.
Hyden, Tom, and Anderson, Tim. *Rock Climbing Is for Me.* Lerner, 1984. 2–5. The basic techniques of rock climbing explained.

Isenberg, Barbara, and Wolf, Susan. *The Adventures of Albert, the Running Bear*. Illus. Dick Gackenbach. Houghton Mifflin, 1982. 2-up. Running in a marathon.

Kent, Jack. *Round Robin*. Prentice-Hall, 1982. K–3. Overeating problems.

Klein, Monica. *Backyard Basketball Superstar*. Illus. Nola Langer. Pantheon, 1981. 1–3. A girl wants to play basketball.

Knudson, R. R. *Babe Didrikson*. Illus. Ted Lewin. Viking Kestrel, 1985. 2–4. Biography of a woman athlete.

———. *Martina Navratilova: Tennis Power*. Illus. George Angelini. Viking Kestrel, 1986. 3–6. Biography of a tennis player.

Moncure, Jane Belk. *Healthkins Exercise!* Illus. Lois Axeman. Children's, 1982. 2–4. The importance of exercise.

———. *Healthkins Help*. Illus. Lois Axeman. Children's, 1982. 2–4. Exercises for physical fitness in rhyme.

Moran, Tom. *Canoeing Is for Me*. Lerner, 1984. 2–5. Equipment, techniques, and safety measures for canoeing.

———. *Roller Skating Is for Me*. Lerner, 1981. 2–5. The basic moves and safety skills for roller skating.

Phang, Ruth, and Roth, Susan. *We Build a Climber*. Atheneum, 1986. Pres.–2. Children build play equipment with a carpenter.

Preston-Mauks, Susan. *Field Hockey Is for Me*. Lerner, 1983. 2–5. The basics of field hockey are covered.

———. *Synchronized Swimming Is for Me*. Lerner, 1983. 2–5. Explains the sport of synchronized swimming.

Schultz, Sam. *101 Sports Jokes*. Illus. Joan Hanson. Lerner, 1983. 1–4. Book of jokes about sports.

•Scioscia, Mary. *Bicycle Rider*. Illus. Ed Young. Harper, 1983. 2–4. A story of courage and determination.

Terkel, Susan Neiburg. *Yoga Is for Me*. Lerner, 1982. 2–5. Breathing, stretching, and relaxing exercises.

Thomas, Art. *Archery Is for Me*. Lerner, 1981. 2–5. The equipment and technique for archery.

———. *Bicycling Is for Me*. Lerner, 1979. 2–5. Riding and caring for a ten-speed bicycle.

———. *Volleyball Is for Me*. Lerner, 1980. 2–5. The basics of volleyball explained.

———. *Wrestling Is for Me*. Lerner, 1979. 2–5. Rules, equipment, and preparation for wrestling.

Thomas, Art, and Storms, Laura. *Boxing Is for Me*. Lerner, 1982. 2–5. Basics of the sport of boxing.

Trier, Carola S. *Exercise: What It Is, What It Does*. Illus. Tom Hoffman. Greenwillow, 1982. K–3. The importance of exercise.

Washington, Rosemary G. *Cross-Country Skiing Is for Me*. Lerner, 1982. 2–5. The basics and equipment for this sport.

———. *Gymnastics Is for Me*. Lerner, 1979. 2–5. An overall view of balancing and tumbling skills.

Grades Four Through Six

Health Advisors

Ardley, Neil. *Health and Medicine.* Watts, 1982. 4–6. How health and medicine interrelate.

Arnold, Caroline. *Pain: What Is It? How Do We Deal With It?* Illus. Frank Schwarz. Morrow, 1986. 6-up. The many facets of experiencing pain.

Berger, Melvin. *Sports Medicine.* Crowell, 1982. 4-up. Describes the work of sports scientists; discusses career opportunities.

Betancourt, Jeanne. *Smile! How to Cope With Braces.* Illus. Mimi Harrison. Knopf, 1982. 5-up. Coping with physical and emotional discomforts associated with having braces.

Epstein, Sam, and Epstein, Beryl. *Dr. Beaumont and the Man with the Hole in His Stomach.* Illus. Joseph Scrofani. Coward, 1978. 3–6. The biography of a doctor and his pioneer work on digestion.

Fisher, Leonard Everett. *The Hospitals.* Holiday House, 1980. 6-up. The forerunners of modern hospitals discussed.

Fleischman, Paul. *Path of the Pale Horse.* Harper & Row, 1983. 6-up. Medical practices in early America, myths, and superstitions.

Herzig, Alison C., and Mali, Jane L. *A Season of Secrets.* Little, Brown, 1982. 5–8. Misconceptions and truths about epilepsy.

Holmes, Burnham. *Early Morning Rounds: A Portrait of a Hospital.* Four Winds, 1981. 5–8. The various areas of a hospital explained.

Howe, James. *A Night Without Stars.* Atheneum, 1983. 5–7. Open-heart surgery depicted and explained.

———. *The Hospital Book.* Crown, 1981. 4–6. What happens in a hospital.

Lightner, Alice M. *Doctor to the Galaxy.* Norton, 1965. 5-up. Novel about medical care in the future on a fictional planet.

Health Care Practices

Blume, Judy. *Blubber.* Bradbury, 1974. 4–6. Friendship with an obese classmate.

•Childress, Alice. *A Hero Ain't Nothin' But a Sandwich.* Coward, 1973. 4–6. Facing the reality of one's own drug addiction.

Cobb, Vicki. *Keeping Clean.* Illus. Marylin Hafner. Harper, 1989. 4–6. A history of products intended to promote cleanliness.

Curtis, Robert. *Medical Talk for Beginners.* Illus. William Jaber. Messner, 1976. 4–6. Dictionary of medical terms for children.

Doss, Helen. *Your Skin Holds You In.* Messner, 1978. 3–5. Basic structure and functions of skin.

Fritz, Jean. *Stonewall.* Illus. Stephen Gammell. Putnam, 1979. 5-up. Biography of Thomas Jackson; his views on health maintenance.

Hentoff, Nat. *Does This School Have Capital Punishment?* Delacorte, 1981. 6-up. Developing moral and ethical values; marijuana usage.

Herbst, Judith. *Bio Amazing: A Casebook of Unsolved Human Mysteries.* Atheneum, 1985. 5–6. Unexplained health phenomena.

Holland, Isabella. *Dinah and the Green Fat Kingdom.* Harper & Row, 1978. 5–7. A twelve-year-old plagued by a weight problem.

Kastner, Jonathan, and Kastner, Marianna. *Sleep: The Mysterious Third of Your Life.* Illus. Don Madden. Harcourt Brace Jovanovich, 1968. 4–6. The causes and needs for sleep.

McGrath, Judith. *Pretty Girl: A Guide to Looking Good, Naturally.* Illus. Frederic Marvin. Lothrop, Lee & Shepard, 1981. 5–9. Interrelationship between good grooming and personal beauty.

Phillips, Betty Lou. *Brush up on Hair Care.* Illus. Lois Johnson. Messner, 1982. 6–8. How to care for your hair.

Saunders, Rubie. *Franklin Watts Concise Guide to Good Grooming for Boys.* Watts, 1972. 5–7. A guide to grooming for boys.

Simon, Seymour. *Body Sense, Body Nonsense.* Illus. Dennis Kendrick. Lippincott, 1981. 4–6. Sense and nonsense about health and wellness.

Tchudi, Stephen. *The Burg-O-Rama Man.* Delacorte, 1983. 4–6. Cultural and social impact of fast food places on young people.

Ward, Brian R. *Body Maintenance.* Watts, 1983. 5–8. Descriptions of glands, hormones, and body organs and their functions.

———. *Health and Hygiene.* Watts, 1988. 6-up. Disease prevention discussed.

Physical Fitness

Aaseng, Nathan. *Baseball: It's Your Team.* Lerner, 1986. 4-up. Situations where the reader can solve problems from baseball history, with the facts of what really happened.

———. *Baseball: You Are the Manager.* Lerner, 1983. 4-up. Situations where the reader can play manager, with answers to the outcome of each choice.

———. *Basketball's Sharpshooters.* Lerner, 1983. 4-up. Biographies of some of basketball's greatest players.

———. *Basketball: You Are the Coach.* Lerner, 1983. 4-up. Second-guessing the coaches of some of America's top teams.

———. *Bruce Jenner: Decathlon Winner.* Lerner, 1979. 4-up. Biography of Bruce Jenner; explanation of what competition is like.

———. *Carl Lewis: Legend Chaser.* Lerner, 1985. 4–6. Biography of this Olympic track star.

———. *College Basketball: You Are the Coach.* Lerner, 1984. 4-up. Reader coaches some of the NCAA's top teams.

———. *College Football: You Are the Coach.* Lerner, 1984. 4-up. Readers decide how top college football teams will be coached.

———. *Comeback Stars of Pro Sports.* Lerner, 1983. 4-up. Stories of players who encountered setbacks and made it back to the top.

———. *Dwight Gooden: Strikeout King.* Lerner, 1988. 4-up. Biography of a pitcher who has had many ups and downs.

———. *Eric Heiden: Winner in Gold.* Lerner, 1980. 4-up. Highlights from Eric Heiden's life and career as speed skater.

———. *Football: It's Your Team.* Lerner, 1985. 4-up. The reader plays the role of team owner in ten situations.

———. *Football: You Are the Coach.* Lerner, 1983. 4-up. Readers coach some of the best games in football history.

———. *Hockey: You Are the Coach.* Lerner 1983. 4–6. The reader acts as coach of some of the major teams in the NHL.

———. *Steve Carlton: Baseball's Silent Strongman.* Lerner, 1984. 4–9. Biography of this famous Phillies' pitcher.

———. *Track's Magnificent Milers.* Lerner, 1981. 4-up. Biographies of ten famous milers in track.

———. *Winning Men of Tennis.* Lerner, 1981. 4-up. Profiles of eight outstanding tennis players.

———. *Winning Women of Tennis.* Lerner, 1981. 4-up. Profiles of eight important women on the international tennis scene.

———. *World-Class Marathoners.* Lerner, 1982. 4-up. Great moments in distance running detailed.

•Adoff, Arnold. *I Am the Running Girl.* Illus. Ronald Himler. Harper & Row, 1979. 4-up. The training experiences of a runner in verse.

Anderson, Dave. *The Story of Basketball.* Morrow, 1988. 5-up. Memorable moments and people in basketball history detailed.

Benjamin, Carol Lea. *Running Basics.* Photographs by M. Beth Brennan. Prentice-Hall, 1979. 4–7. Informational book on running.

Boyd, Brendan. *Hoops: Behind the Scenes with the Boston Celtics.* Photographs by Henry Horenstein. Little, Brown, 1988. 3–7. Goes through one year in the life of the Boston Celtics team.

Cebulash, Mel. *Ruth Marini: Dodger Ace.* Lerner, 1983. 4-up. A woman makes the roster of this major league team.

———. *Ruth Marini of the Dodgers.* Lerner, 1983. 4-up. The trials of a woman signed to play for the Dodgers.

———. *Ruth Marini: World Series Star.* Lerner, 1985. 4-up. A woman is the winning pitcher in the seventh game of the World Series.

Checki, Haney Erene, and Richards, Ruth. *Yoga for Children.* Illus. Betty Schilling. Bobbs-Merrill, 1973. 3–5. Simple yoga exercises for children explained.

Christopher, Matt. *Catcher With a Glass Arm.* Illus. Foster Caddell. Little, Brown, 1964. 4–6. Learning how to cope with adversity.

———. *Red-Hot Hightops.* Illus. Paul D. Mock. Little, Brown, 1987. 4–6. A sports mystery.

Church, Carol B. *Billie Jean King: Queen of the Courts.* Greenhaven, 1976. 4-up. Biography of this tennis star, her goals, and strategies.

Einstein, Charles, ed. *The Fireside Book of Baseball.* Simon & Schuster, 1987. 6-up. Pictures, cartoons, history, and poetry celebrating baseball.

Faulkner, Margaret. *I Skate.* Little, Brown, 1979. 4–6. Photoessay on ice skating.

Goodbody, Slim. *The Force Inside You.* Putnam, 1983. 4–6. Simple exercises for achieving physical fitness.

Hammond, Mildred. *Square Dancing Is for Me.* Lerner, 1983. 2–5. The basic steps and styles of square dancing.

Hawkins, Jim W. *Cheerleading Is for Me.* Lerner, 1981. 2–5. Demonstrates the basic movements involved in cheerleading.

Jones, Billy Millsaps. *Wonder Women of Sports.* Random House, 1981. 4–7. Twelve biographies of famous female sports figures.

Kalbfleisch, Susan. *Jump! The New Jump Rope Book.* Illus. Laurie McGugan. Morrow, 1987. 3–6. A step-by-step guide to sixty jumping exercises.

Killien, Christi. *Rusty Fertlanger, Lady's Man.* Houghton Mifflin, 1988. 5-up. Encountering the opposite sex in sports.

Knudson, R. R. *Zanballer.* Puffin, 1986. 5–8. Sexism in sports.

Krementz, Jill. *A Very Young Skater.* Knopf, 1979. 3–6. The life of a child who figure skates.

Leder, Jane Mersky. *Martina Navratilova.* Crestwood, 1985. 4–8. Biography of the tennis player.

Marzollo, Jean. *Soccer Sam.* Illus. Blanche Sims. Random House, 1987. 2–4. Tale of friendship and sports.

Monroe, Judy. *Steffi Graf.* Crestwood, 1986. 4–8. Biography of the German tennis player.

Morrison, Lillian, selector. *Rhythm Road: Poems to Move to.* Lothrop, Lee & Shepard, 1988. 4–7. Poems capturing the essence of motion.

———, compiler. *Sprints and Distances: Sports in Poetry and the Poetry in Sports.* Illus. Clare Ross and John Ross. Crowell, 1989. 5-up. Sports verses.

•———. *The Break Dance Kids: Poems of Sport, Motion and Locomotion.* Lothrop, Lee & Shepard, 1985. 3–5. Poetry about movement, sports.

Olsen, James T. *Billie Jean King, the Lady of the Court.* Creative Education, 1974. 4-up. Biography of King's rise to fame.

Reynolds, Robert E. *Lacrosse Is for Me.* Photographs by Ross R. Olney. Lerner, 1984. 2–5. Basic information on the sport.

Rosenthal, Bert. *Larry Bird, Cool Man on the Court.* Childrens, 1981. 3–6. Biography of the famous basketball player.

•Sorine, Stephanie. *At Every Turn! It's Ballet.* Photographs by Daniel S. Sorine. Knopf, 1981. 4–6. How dance movements are comparable to everyday motion.

Sullivan, George. *Better Soccer for Boys and Girls.* Dodd, Mead, 1978. 4–7. How the game is played.

———. *Better Softball for Boys and Girls.* Dodd, Mead, 1975. 4–7. Exercises and tips to improve one's softball game.

———. *Better Tennis for Boys and Girls.* Dodd, Mead, 1987. 4–6. How to improve one's tennis game.

———. *Center.* Illus. Don Madden. Harper & Row, 1988. 3–6. Tips on how to be a good center in basketball.

———. *Mary Lou Retton.* Messner, 1985. 4-up. Biography of the famous Olympic gymnast.

Thomas, Art. *Fencing Is for Me.* Lerner, 1982. 2–5. Fundamental fencing moves explained.

Tolle, Jean Bashor. *The Great Pete Penney.* McElderry, 1979. 4–6. The story of a female pitcher.

Walsh, John. *The First Book of Physical Fitness.* Watts, 1961. 4–6. Facts about how to keep fit.

Grades Seven and Up

Improving Personal Health Care

Godfrey, Martin. *Marijuana.* Illus. Peter Harper. Watts, 1987. 6-up. What the drug is, why people use it, and how it affects the body.

Graebner, Laurel. *Are You Dying for a Drink? Teenagers and Alcohol Abuse.* Messner, 1985. 7-up. The rise of alcoholism among teens.

Hollander, Phyllis. *100 Greatest Women in Sports.* Grosset & Dunlap, 1976. 7-up. Short biographies on 100 famous sports women.

•Hollander, Phyllis, and Hollander, Zander, eds. *Winners Under Twenty-One.* Random House, 1982. 7-up. Famous sports personalities who achieved status under the age of twenty-one.

Klass, David. *A Different Season.* Lodestar, 1988. 7-up. A female on the varsity baseball team.

Lee, Mary Price. *The Team That Runs Your Hospital.* Westminster, 1980. 5–8. Behind-the-scenes look at how hospitals work.

Matthews, Dee; Zullo, Allan; and Nash, Bruce. *The You Can Do It! Kids Diet.* Holt, 1985. 6-up. Following a sensible diet.

Pownall, Mark. *Inhalants.* Illus. Peter Harper. Watts, 1987. 6-up. How inhalants affect the user, and sources of help.

Sanchez, Gail Jones, and Gerbino, Mary. *Overeating: Let's Talk about It.* Illus. Lucy Miskiewicz. Dillon, 1986. 6-up. How to maintain a healthy weight.

Stepney, Rob. *Alcohol.* Illus. Peter Harper. Watts, 1987. 6-up. Introduction to alcohol, why people drink it, its effects on the body, and how to get help.

Strasser, Todd. *Angel Dust Blues.* Coward, 1979. 7-up. The story of a user of this drug.

•Wallin, Luke. *Ceremony of the Panther.* Bradbury, 1987. 7-up. A teen is treated for drug and alcohol abuse.

Ward, Brian R. *Smoking and Health.* Watts, 1986. 6-up. The effects of tobacco on the body and how to give up the habit.

Washington, Rosemary G. *Mary Lou Retton: Power Gymnast.* Lerner, 1985. 4–9. Biography of this Olympic gymnast.

Woods, Geraldine, and Woods, Harold. *Cocaine.* Watts, 1985. 6-up. Where cocaine comes from and how it affects the user.

Personal Health Care Habits

Abrams, Joy. *Look Good, Feel Good, through Yoga, Grooming, Nutrition.* Holt, 1978. 6–9. Natural beauty habits explained.

Carlson, Dale, and Fitzgibbon, Dan. *Manners That Matter: For People Under 21.* Dutton, 1983. 5-up. Handbook of proper etiquette.

Claypool, Jane, and Nelson, Cheryl Diane. *Food Trips and Traps: Coping with Eating Disorders.* Watts, 1983. 6–9. Overview of eating disorders.

Dolan, Edward F., Jr. *Drugs in Sports.* Watts, 1986. 6-up. The kinds of drugs used in sports and their effects on the body and mind.

Fodor, R. V., and Taylor, G. J. *Growing Strong.* Sterling, 1980. 6–9. Muscle-building exercises are described.

Gelinas, Paul J. *Coping with Weight Problems.* Rosen, 1983. 6-up. Why people use food to solve their problems; how to confront eating problems.

Giles, Frank. *Toughen Up: A Boy's Guide to Better Physical Fitness.* Putnam, 1963. 6–8. Introduction to boy's physical fitness.

Jacobs, Helen Hull. *Better Physical Fitness for Girls.* Dodd, Mead, 1964. 6–8. Exercises and shaping-up activities for girls.

Knudson, R. R., and Swenson, May. *American Sports Poems.* Orchard Books, 1988. 5-up. A collection of sports poetry.

Laklan, Carli. *Golden Girls: True Stories of Olympic Women Stars.* McGraw, 1980. 7-up. Biographies of famous women Olympic athletes.

Lyttle, Richard B. *The Complete Beginner's Guide to Physical Fitness.* Doubleday, 1978. 6–9. The fun and satisfaction of achieving physical fitness.

Parks-McKay, Jane. *The Make-Over: A Teen's Guide to Looking and Feeling Beautiful.* Illus. Betty de Araujo. Morrow, 1985. 6-up. Hygiene, grooming, nutrition, exercising, and behavior to make you feel better about yourself.

Silverstein, Alvin, and Silverstein, Virginia B. *Sleep and Dreams.* Lippincott, 1974. 7–10. Why we need sleep; theories about dreams.

———. *So You're Getting Braces: A Guide to Orthodontics.* Illus. Barbara Remington. Lippincott, 1978. 5–9. The function of and reasons for braces.

Sorensen, Robert. *Shadow of the Past: True Life Sports Stories.* Bluejeans Books, 1978. 7-up. Biographies of seven famous athletes with troubled pasts.

Sullivan, George. *Better Gymnastics for Girls.* Dodd, Mead, 1977. 5–9. Brief history of the sport, description of the events.

Sweetgall, Robert, Rippe, James, and Katch, Frank. *Fitness Walking.* Illus. Frederick Bush. Putnam, 1985. 6-up. Advice on walking programs; tips on diet; explanation of the cardiovascular system.

Ward, Brian R. *Body Maintenance.* Watts, 1983. 6-up. How the body's systems work, with special attention to glands and hormones.

Ward, Hiley H. *Feeling Good about Myself.* Westminster, 1983. 7-up. Teens discuss how they cope with problems, pressures, and stress.

D. FAMILY LIFE AND HEALTH

Grades K Through Three

Reproduction and Birth

Ancona, George. *It's a Baby!* Scribner's, 1976. K–3. Documents growth and development of a child from birth to one year.

Andry, Andrew, and Schepp, Steven. *How Babies Are Made*. Illus. Blake Hampton. Little, Brown, 1984. Pres.–3. Discusses reproduction.

Banish, Roslyn. *Let Me Tell You About My Baby*. Harper, 1988. Pres.–1. Experiences of an older sibling through gestation and birth.

Cole, Joanna. *How You Were Born*. Illus. with photographs by Hella Hammid and others. Morrow, 1984. Pres.–2. The growth of a fetus, birth process, and baby's first life experiences.

DeSchweinitz, Karl. *Growing Up: How We Become Alive, Are Born, and Grow*. Macmillan, 1968. 1–3. Animal mating, human reproduction, and growing up explained.

Dragonwagon, Crescent. *Wind Rose*. Illus. Ronald Himler. Harper, 1976. Pres.–2. Reproduction, pregnancy, and birth with the aid of a midwife explained.

Ets, Marie Hall. *The Story of a Baby*. Viking Kestrel, 1967. K–3. The story of reproduction.

Fagerström, Grethe, and Hansson, Gunella. *Our New Baby*. Illus. Gunella Hansson. Barron's. K–3. Siblings' parents explain reproduction and childbirth to them to prepare them for a new baby.

Freedman, Russell. *Getting Born*. Holiday House, 1978. K–3. How animals are reproduced.

Girard, Linda. *You Were Born on Your Very First Birthday*. Whitman, 1983. Pres.–3. Introduction to pregnancy and birth.

Gordon, Sol, Gordon, Judith, and Cohen, Judith. *Did the Sun Shine Before You Were Born? A Sex Education Primer*. Illus. Vivien Cohen. The Third Press/Odarkai Books, 1974. Pres.–3. Relates birth to the cycle of life, in the family and in the universe.

Gruenberg, Sidonie M. *The Wonderful Story of How You Were Born*. Illus. Hildegard Woodward. Doubleday, 1962. 1–4. Presentation of the facts of life.

Kitzinger, Sheila. *Being Born*. Illus. with photographs by Lennart Nilsson. Grosset & Dunlap, 1986. 2–5. Informational book on childbirth.

Lasky, Kathryn. *A Baby for Max*. Photographs by Christopher G. Knight. Scribner's, 1984. Pres.–1. A sibling copes with the birth of a new baby.

Mayle, Peter. *"Where Did I Come From?"* Illus. Arthur Robins. Lyle Stuart, 1973. K–3. Humor used to explain the facts of life.

Meeks, Esther, and Bagwell, Elizabeth. *How Life Begins*. Follett, 1969. 1–4.

The beginning of life in plants and animals and the growth processes explained.

Power, Jules. *How Life Begins: The Exciting Story of Human and Animal Birth.* Illus. Barry Geller. Simon and Schuster, 1965. 2–4. The story of reproduction in animals and humans.

Selsam, Millicent. *All About Eggs.* Illus. Stephenie Fleischer. Addison-Wesley, 1980. Pres.–3. Eggs and the creatures that grow from them.

————. *Egg to Chick.* Illus. Barbara Wolff. Harper & Row, 1970. Pres.–3. Reproduction, gestation, and birth of creatures from eggs.

Sheffield, Margaret. *Before You Were Born.* Illus. Sheila Bewley. Knopf, 1984. Pres.–3. How a baby develops in the womb.

————. *Where Do Babies Come From?* Illus. Sheila Bewley. Knopf, 1973. 2–5. Questions and answers about the beginnings of life.

Showers, Paul. *A Baby Starts to Grow.* Illus. Rosalind Fry. Harper & Row, 1987. Pres.–3. Development of a human embryo.

Showers, Paul, and Showers, Kay. *Before You Were a Baby.* Illus. Ingrid Fetz. Crowell, 1968. 2–3. The gestation period explained.

Stein, Lara Bonnett. *Making Babies.* Illus. with photographs by Doris Penney. Walker, 1974. 1–3. Deals with touchy questions about reproduction and birth.

Relationships With Siblings

Alexander, Martha. *Nobody Asked Me If I Wanted a Baby Sister.* Dial, 1971. Pres.–2. Coping with a new sibling.

Ancona, George. *It's a Baby.* Dutton, 1979. K–3. The first year of a child's life.

Andry, Andrew C., and Schepp, Steven. *How Babies Are Made.* Little, Brown, 1984. Pres.–3. Process of reproduction in flowers, animals, and humans.

Banish, Roslyn. *Let Me Tell You About My Baby.* Harper & Row, 1988. Pres.–K. The ups and downs of having a new baby in the house.

Berenstain, Stan, and Berenstain, Jan. *The Berenstain Bears Get in a Fight.* Random House, 1982. K–3. Everyone argues, once in a while.

Blume, Judy. *The Pain and the Great One.* Illus. Irene Trivas. Bradbury, 1984. Pres.–3. Siblings tell their sides of an event.

Brandenberg, Franz. *I Wish I Was Sick, Too!* Illus. Aliki. Puffin, 1978. Pres.–3. Illness is not as glamorous as it seems.

Brenner, Barbara. *Nicky's Sister.* Illus. John E. Johnson. Knopf, 1966. K–3. Dealing with a baby sibling.

Brown, Marc. *Arthur's Baby.* Little, Brown, 1987. Pres.–3. Dealing with a new baby.

Burningham, John. *The Baby.* Harper & Row, 1975. Pres.–1. Learning to accept a new baby.

Caseley, Judith. *Silly Baby.* Greenwillow, 1988. Pres.–2. Learning to accept a new sibling.

Chorao, Kay. *George Told Kate.* Dutton, 1987. Pres.–K. Siblings learn to get along.

Cole, Joanna. *How You Were Born.* Morrow, 1984. Pres.–3. Reproduction, birth, and the first year of life detailed.

———. *The New Baby at Your House.* Photographs by Hella Hammid. Morrow, 1985. Pres.–3. Preparing for a new sibling.

Crowley, Arthur. *Bonzo Beaver.* Illus. Annie Gusman. Houghton Mifflin, 1980. 1–3. Getting along with a sibling.

Cuyler, Margery. *Shadow's Baby.* Illus. Ellen Weiss. Clarion, 1989. Pres.–1. Family love and the arrival of a new baby.

deBagniers, Beatrice. *Picture Book Theater.* Clarion, 1982. 1–3. Two plays about relationships with siblings.

Delton, Judy. *Angel's Mother's Baby.* Illus. Margot Apple. Houghton Mifflin, 1989. 2–5. Dealing with a new father and a new sibling.

de Lynam, Alicia Garcia. *It's Mine!* Dial, 1988. Pres.–2. Sibling relationships shown in a wordless book.

Douglass, Barbara. *Good as New.* Illus. Patience Brewster. Lothrop, Lee & Shepard, 1982. Pres.–2. Conflict between two siblings over a possession.

Dragonwagon, Crescent. *I Hate My Sister Maggie.* Illus. Leslie Morrill. Macmillan, 1989. Pres.–3. Sibling rivalry; new baby.

Edelman, Elaine. *I Love My Baby Sister (Most of the Time).* Illus. Wendy Watson. Lothrop, Lee & Shepard, 1984. Pres.–1. The joys and trials of a new baby.

Foreman, Michael. *Ben's Baby.* Harper & Row, 1987. K–3. A new baby arrives.

Freedman, Florence B., reteller. *Brothers: A Hebrew Legend.* Illus. Robert Andrew Parker. Harper & Row, 1985. 2–4. Ancient tale of brotherly love and friendship.

Galbraith, Kathryn Osebold. *Katie Did!* Illus. Ted Ramsey. McElderry, 1982. Pres.–1. Dealing with new sibling; less attention.

Goble, Paul. *Her Seven Brothers.* Bradbury, 1988. 2–4. Indian legend of eight siblings who form the Big Dipper.

•Greenfield, Eloise. *She Come Bringing Me That Little Baby Girl.* Illus. John Steptoe. Lippincott, 1974. K–3. Acceptance of a new sibling.

Grimm, Jakob, and Grimm, Wilhelm. Wanda Gag, reteller. *Wanda Gag's The Six Swans.* Illus. Margot Tomes. Coward, McCann, 1982. 2–5. A princess rescues her brothers from an evil spell.

•Havill, Juanita. *Jamaica Tag-Along.* Illus. Anne Sibley O'Brien. Houghton Mifflin, 1989. K–3. Lesson in getting along with siblings.

Hazen, Barbara. *Gorilla Wants To Be the Baby.* Atheneum, 1978. K–3. Living with a new baby.

Henkes, Kevin. *Margaret and Taylor.* Greenwillow, 1983. 1–4. Siblings attempt to coexist.

Hines, Anna Grossnickle. *Big Like Me.* Greenwillow, 1989. Pres.–3. A brother helps his new little sibling.

Hoban, Russell. *A Baby Sister for Frances.* Harper & Row, 1964. K–3. Getting along with a new sibling.

Hughes, Shirley. *Angel Mae: A Tale of Trotter Street.* Lothrop, Lee &

Shepard, 1989. Pres.–2. A new baby is born; her sister learns to cope with a new family member.

Hutchins, Pat. *Where's the Baby?* Greenwillow, 1988. Pres.–3. Grandma praises the new baby as he disrupts the entire household.

Iwasaki, Chihiro. *A New Baby Is Coming to My House.* McGraw-Hill, 1972. K–3. A sibling imagines what her new brother will be like.

Jarrell, Mary. *The Knee-Baby.* Illus. Symeon Shimin. Michael Di Capua Books, 1988. Pres-3. A wise mother handles sibling jealousy.

Johnston, Johanna. *The Great Gravity Cat.* Illus. Melissa Bay Mathis. Linnet Books, 1989. 1–5. Dealing with a sense of displacement after the birth of a new baby.

•Keats, Ezra Jack. *Peter's Chair.* Harper & Row, 1967. K–3. Dealing with the birth of a new baby.

Keller, Holly. *Maxine in the Middle.* Greenwillow, 1989. Pres.–3. Dealing with being the middle chid.

Kismaric, Carole, adaptor. *The Rumor of Pavel and Paali.* Illus. Charles Mikolaycak. Harper & Row, 1988. 1–3. A story of a good and an evil twin.

Knox-Wagner, Elaine. *The Oldest Kid.* Whitman, 1981. K–3. Sibling hierarchy in one family.

Kraus, Robert. *Where Are You Going, Little Mouse?* Illus. Jose Aruego and Ariane Dewey. Greenwillow, 1986. K–3. A mouse runs away from home.

Lasky, Kathryn. *A Baby for Max.* Macmillan, 1987. Pres.–2. How a sibling comes to accept his new sister.

Lindgren, Astrid. *I Want a Brother or Sister.* Eric Bibb, translator. Illus. Ilon Wikland. Farrar, Straus & Giroux, 1987. Pres.–2. Dealing with the attention focused on a new sibling.

•Louie, Ai-Ling, reteller. *Yeh-Shen: A Cinderella Story from China.* Illus. Ed Young. Putnam, 1982. 2–6. A persistent adolescent discovers a way to save herself from the influence of her abusive stepmother and stepsisters.

Lowry, Lois. *All About Sam.* Houghton Mifflin, 1988. 1–5. A younger sibling tells his story.

Margolis, Richard J. *Secrets of a Small Brother.* Illus. Donald Carrick. Macmillan, 1984. 1–4. The relationship between two brothers in verse, explained by the younger brother.

———. *Secrets of a Small World.* Illus. Donald Carrick. Macmillan, 1984. 1–4. Poetry about siblings; childhood experiences.

Martin, Jr., Bill, and Archambault, John. *The Ghost-eye Tree.* Illus. Ted Rand. Holt, 1985. K–3. Sibling cooperation.

McCully, Emily Arnold. *New Baby.* Harper, 1988. Pres.–1. A young mouse deals with a new sibling.

McPhail, David. *Sisters.* Harcourt Brace Jovanovich, 1984. K–3. Picture-book about sisters.

———. *The Story of James.* Dutton, 1989. Pres.–3. The trials of being an older brother.

Minarik, Elsa Holmelund. *No Fighting, No Biting!* Illus. Maurice Sendak. Harper, 1978. Pres.–2. Siblings learn to cooperate.

My Little Foster Sister. Illus. Judith Cheng. Whitman, 1981. Pres.–2. Story of adjustment to a new foster sister.

Naylor, Phyllis Reynolds. *All Because I'm Older.* Illus. Leslie Morrill. Atheneum, 1981. 1–4. Two brothers learn to get along.

Nillsson, Lennart. *How Was I Born?* Delacorte, 1975. Pres.–3. Explains human reproduction and birth.

Ormerod, Jan. *101 Things To Do With a Baby.* Lothrop, Lee & Shepard, 1984. Pres.–2. What to do with a new baby.

Pryor, Bonnie. *Vinegar Pancakes and Vanishing Cream.* Illus. Gail Owens. Morrow, 1987. 2–5. The predicaments of family life.

Ra, Carol F., compiler. *Trot, Trot to Boston: Play Rhymes for Baby.* Illus. Catherine Stock. Lothrop, Lee & Shepard, 1987. Pres.–K. Rhymes to use with very young children.

Rocklin, Joanne. *Dear Baby.* Illus. Eileen McKeating. Macmillan, 1988. K–3. A sister writes letters to her unborn sibling.

Rogers, Fred. *The New Baby.* Photographs by Jim Judkis. Putnam, 1985. Pres.–K. Introduction to coping with a new baby.

Root, Phyllis. *Moon Tiger.* Illus. Ed Young. Holt, 1985. 2–4. A child fantasizes an escape from her younger brother.

Ruffins, Reynold. *My Brother Never Feeds the Cat.* Scribner's, 1979. 1–3. A sibling complains about taking all the responsibilities.

Russo, Marisabina. *Waiting for Hannah.* Greenwillow, 1989. Pres.–2. A mother describes expecting a child to her other child.

Samuels, Barbara. *Faye and Dolores.* Bradbury, 1985. 1–4. Daily activities of two sisters.

San Souci, David D. *The Talking Eggs.* Illus. Jerry Pinckney. Dial, 1989. Pres.–3. A folktale about two sisters of opposite disposition.

•Scott, Ann Herbert. *On Mother's Lap.* McGraw-Hill, 1972. Pres.–K. A child discovers there is room for both him and his new sibling.

Sendak, Maurice. *Outside Over There.* Harper & Row, 1981. K–3. What would it be like not to have to take care of your younger sibling?

Showers, Paul, and Showers, Kay Sperry. *Before You Were a Baby.* Harper & Row, 1968. K–3. Facts about human conception, gestation, and birth.

Silverman, Maida. *Anna and the Seven Swans.* Illus. David Small. Morrow, 1984. 1–4. Folktale about child rescuing her sibling from a wicked witch.

Smith, Peter. *Jenny's Baby Brother.* Illus. Bob Graham. Viking Kestrel, 1984. K–2. Getting to know a younger sibling.

Smith, Wendy. *Twice Mice.* Carolrhoda, 1989. Pres.–2. Getting along with new twin siblings.

Steptoe, John. *Baby Says.* Lothrop, Lee & Shepard, 1988. Pres.–2. An older brother's loving actions toward his new sibling.

———. *Mufaro's Beautiful Daughters: An African Tale.* Lothrop, Lee & Shepard, 1987. K–3. A conflict between two dissimilar siblings.

———. *Stevie.* Harper & Row, 1969. K–3. Getting along with a younger child.

Stevenson, James. *Worse Than Willy!* Greenwillow, 1984. K–4. Grandfather helps grandchild cope with a new baby.

•Swortzell, Lowell. *The Chinese Cinderella.* In *Plays Children Love, Vol. II.* Coleman A. Jennings and Aurand Harris, eds. St. Martin's, 1988. 3-up. A play about sibling rivalry and kindness.

Thomas, Iolette. *Janine and the New Baby.* Illus. Jennifer Northway. Andre Deutsch, 1987. Pres.–1. A child prepares for a new sibling.

Titherington, Jeanne. *A Place for Ben.* Greenwillow, 1987. K–3. Sharing with a sibling.

Vigna, Judith. *Daddy's New Baby.* Whitman, 1982. Pres.–3. Getting along with a half sister.

Viorst, Judith. *I'll Fix Anthony.* Illus. Arnold Lobel. Harper & Row, 1969. K–5. Ideas for getting even with an older sibling.

Walter, Mildred Pitts. *My Mama Needs Me.* Illus. Pat Cummings. Lothrop, Lee & Shepard, 1983. Pres.–2. Finding a place in the family when a new sibling arrives.

Weiss, Nicki. *Chuckie.* Greenwillow, 1982. Pres.–1. Building a relationship with a new sibling.

Wells, Rosemary. *Noisy Nora.* Dial, 1973. Pres.–2. Getting parents' attention after the arrival of a new baby.

———. *Peabody.* Dial, 1983. K–3. A favorite old toy is replaced by a new doll; coping with a new arrival in the family.

Wilhelm, Hans. *Let's Be Friends Again!* Crown, 1986. K–3. Learning to forgive the carelessness of a younger sibling.

Williams, Barbara. *Jeremy Isn't Hungry.* Illus. Martha Alexander. Dutton, 1989. Pres.–1. Attempting to take care of a baby brother.

Wolde, Gunilla. *Betsy's Baby Brother.* Random House, 1982. Pres.–K. Taking care of a new baby.

Ziefert, Harriet. *Chocolate Mud and Cake.* Illus. Karen Gundersheimer. Harper & Row, 1988. Pres.–1. Two siblings play together at their grandparents' house.

———. *Me Too! Me Too!* Illus. Karen Gundersheimer. Harper & Row, 1988. Pres.–1. Two children play together on a rainy day.

———. *So Hungry!* Illus. Carol Nicklaus. Random House, 1987. Pres.–1. An account of sibling competition.

Zolotow, Charlotte. *Big Brother.* Illus. Mary Chalmers. Harper & Row, 1966. Pres.–3. A little sister is teased by her big brother.

———. *Big Sister and Little Sister.* Harper & Row, 1966. 2–4. How siblings share and get along.

———. *Timothy Too!* Illus. Ruth Robbins. Houghton Mifflin, 1985. Pres.–3. Little and big brother find a way to get along.

Grandparents

•Addy, Sharon Hart. *A Visit With Great-Grandma.* Whitman, 1989. 1–3. A child's relationship with her great-grandmother.

Aliki. *The Two of Them.* Greenwillow, 1979. Pres.–1. Story about the relationship between a child and her grandfather.

Anderson, Lena. *Stina.* Greenwillow, 1989. K–3. Relationship between a child and her grandfather.

•Bennett, Olivia. *A Family in Brazil.* Photographs by Liba Taylor. Lerner, 1986. 1–4. The relationships in a southern Brazilian family; their interests; their occupations.

Berenstain, Stan, and Berenstain, Jan. *The Berenstain Bears and the Week at Grandma's.* Random House, 1986. Pres.–2. Two siblings' relationship with their grandparents.

•Bunting, Eve. *The Happy Funeral.* Illus. Vo-Dinh Mai. Harper & Row, 1982. 2–5. A Chinese-American girl grieves over her grandfather's death.

Burningham, John. *Granpa.* Crown, 1985. Pres.–2. Situations between a grandfather and his granddaughter explored.

Caseley, Judith. *When Grandpa Came to Stay.* Greenwillow, 1986. Pres.–3. A family copes with the grandmother's death.

•Daly, Niki. *Not So Fast Songololo.* Atheneum, 1986. Pres.–3. A South African boy's shopping trip with his grandmother.

dePaola, Tomie. *Now One Foot, Now the Other.* Putnam, 1981. K–3. A child deals with his grandfather's illness.

•——. *Watch Out for the Chicken Feet in Your Soup.* Prentice-Hall, 1974. Pres.–3. A friend likes his friend's grandmother.

Delton, Judy, and Tucker, Dorothy. *My Grandma's in a Nursing Home.* Illus. Charles Robinson. Whitman, 1986. 2–5. A child accepts his grandmother's resettlement in a nursing home.

Donnelly, Elfie. *So Long, Grandpa.* Anthea Bell, translator. Crown, 1981. 4–7. The relationship between a boy and his dying grandfather.

Dorros, Arthur. *Abuela.* Illus. Eliza Kleven. Dutton, 1991. Pres.–3. Rosalba and her *abuela* (Spanish for grandmother) have an unforgettable adventure in New York City where they live.

Douglass, Barbara. *Good as New.* Illus. Patience Brewster. Lothrop, Lee & Shepard, 1982. K–3. A grandfather fixes his grandchild's teddy bear.

Egger, Bettina. *Marianne's Grandmother.* Illus. Sita Jucker. Dutton, 1988. Pres.–2. A girl's memories of her grandmother ease the pain of her death.

•Flournoy, Valerie. *The Patchwork Quilt.* Illus. Jerry Pinkney. Dial, 1985. 2–4. Relationships and memories that emerge during the making of a quilt by a grandmother.

Gantschev, Ivan. *The Train to Grandma's.* Picture Book Studio, 1989. Pres.–2. Two children take their first train ride to their grandmother's.

Gelfand, Marilyn. *My Great Grandpa Joe.* Photographs by Rosmarie Hausherr. Four Winds Press, 1986. 1–3. A look at old age through the perspective of a child.

Goldman, Susan. *Grandma Is Somebody Special.* Whitman, 1976. Pres.–2. The relationship between a child and her grandmother.

•Greenfield, Eloise. *Grandpa's Face.* Illus. Floyd Cooper. Philomel, 1988. 1–3. Relationship between a child and her grandfather.

Griffith, Helen V. *Georgia Music.* Illus. James Stevenson. Greenwillow,

1986. Pres.–3. A girl becomes close to her grandfather through their shared affection for the countryside and music.

──────. *Granddaddy's Place*. Illus. James Stevenson. Greenwillow, 1987. 1–4. A girl spends her first summer with her grandfather in the country.

Henkes, Kevin. *Grandpa and Bo*. Greenwillow, 1986. Pres.–3. A child visits his grandfather's alone.

Hest, Amy. *The Crack of Dawn Walkers*. Illus. Amy Schwartz. Macmillan, 1984. Pres.–3. A girl takes early morning walks with her grandfather.

Hines, Anna Grossnickle. *Grandma Gets Grumpy*. Clarion, 1988. Pres.–2. There are limits to even a loving relative's patience.

Honeycutt, Natalie. *The All New Jonah Twist*. Bradbury, 1986. 2–4. A child learns he doesn't have to be just like his older brother.

Hoopes, Lyn Littlefield. *Half a Button*. Illus. Trish Parcell Watts. Harper, 1989. Pres.–2. A child spends an afternoon with his grandfather.

Hurd, Edith Thacher. *I Dance in My Red Pajamas*. Illus. Emily Arnold McCully. Harper & Row, 1982. K–3. A child's relationship with her grandparents.

Keller, Holly. *The Best Present*. Greenwillow, 1989. K–4. A child visits her grandmother in the hospital.

Kibbey, Marsha. *My Grammy*. Illus. Karen Ritz. Carolrhoda, 1988. 1–3. A grandmother with Alzheimer's disease moves in with her family.

Lasky, Kathryn. *I Have Four Names for My Grandfather*. Photographs by Christopher Knight. Little, Brown, 1976. Pres.–3. The relationship of a boy with his grandfather in photographs.

──────. *Sea Swan*. Illus. Catherine Stock. Macmillan, 1988. Pres.–2. A pampered grandmother learns to take care of herself.

Levinson, Riki. *I Go With My Family to Grandma's*. Dutton, 1986. Pres.–3. Five turn-of-the-century families visit grandmother.

MacLachlan, Patricia. *Journey*. Delacorte, 1991. 4–7. With the help of his loving grandparents, eleven-year-old Journey learns to accept his troubled mother's abandonment of him and his older sister.

McCully, Emily Arnold. *The Grandma Mix-up*. Harper & Row, 1988. Pres.–3. Two very different grandmothers care for their grandchild.

•McKenna, Nancy Durrell. *A Zulu Family*. Lerner, 1986. 1–4. Photoessay about a relocated Zulu family.

•Montaufier, Poupa. *One Summer at Grandmother's House*. Tobi Tobias, translator. Carolrhoda, 1985. 2–5. The author recalls a summer spent with her grandmother.

Moore, Elaine. *Grandma's House*. Illus. Elise Primavera. Lothrop, Lee & Shepard, 1985. 1–3. Recollections of summer visits with a grandmother.

──────. *Grandma's Promise*. Illus. Elise Primavera. Lothrop, Lee & Shepard, 1988. Pres.–2. A grandmother visits with her grandchild in the winter.

Pearson, Susan. *Happy Birthday, Grampie*. Illus. Ronald Himler. Dial, 1987. K–3. A family visits their blind grandfather on his birthday.

Pomerantz, Charlotte. *Timothy Tall Feather*. Illus. Catherine Stock. Greenwillow, 1986. K–3. A child and his grandfather talk and dream about Indians.

Root, Phyllis, and Marron, Carol A. *Gretchen's Grandma.* Illus. Deborah Kogan Ray. Carnival/Raintree, 1983. K–3. A child and her German grandmother spend a day together.

Roth, Susan L. *We'll Ride Elephants Through Brooklyn.* Farrar, Straus & Giroux, 1989. Pres.–2. A celebration when grandfather gets better.

Rylant, Cynthia. *When I Was Young in the Mountains.* Illus. Diane Goode. Dutton, 1982. K–3. A child's remembrances of life in the Appalachian mountains.

Scheffler, Ursel. *A Walk in the Rain.* Illus. Ulises Wensell. Putnam, 1986. Pres.–3. A child and her grandmother go out in the rain.

Schertle, Alice. *William and Grandpa.* Illus. Lydia Dabcovich. Lothrop, Lee & Shepard, 1989. Pres.–3. A boy spends the day with his grandfather, finding much in common.

Stevenson, James. *Could Be Worse!* Greenwillow, 1977. K–3. Two children hear Grandpa recount some of his adventures.

―――. *Will You Please Feed Our Cat?* Greenwillow, 1987. Pres.–3. Grandpa recounts the trouble he and his brother had taking care of neighbors' animals.

Titherington, Jeanne. *Where Are You Going, Emma?* Greenwillow, 1988. K–3. A child is relieved to be reunited with her grandfather.

Ward, Sally G. *Punky Spends the Day.* Dutton, 1989. Pres.–1. Three stories of a child's adventures when she spends time with her grandparents.

•Williams, Vera B. *Music, Music for Everyone.* Greenwillow, 1984. Pres.–3. Raising money to help a sick grandparent.

Ziefert, Harriet. *With Love from Grandma.* Illus. Deborah Kogan Ray. Viking Kestrel, 1989. Pres.–3. Grandma comes for a visit and brings a surprise as well as a present.

Divorce, Single-Parent Families, Foster Families

Bawden, Nina. *The Finding.* Lothrop, Lee & Shepard, 1985. 2–6. A mystery story about the adoption of a child.

Berger, Terry. *How Does It Feel When Your Parents Get Divorced?* Messner, 1977. 2–5. How to survive your parents' divorce.

Boegehold, Betty. *Daddy Doesn't Live Here Anymore: A Book About Divorce.* Illus. Deborah Borgo. Western, 1985. Pres.–2. A child's feelings about her parents' divorce.

Bulla, Clyde Robert. *Open the Door and See All the People.* Crowell, 1972. 2–5. A story about the loss of a home and adoption.

Bunin, Catherine and Bunin, Sherry. *Is That Your Sister?* Pantheon Books, 1976. K–3. Dealing with being adopted.

Caines, Jeanette. *Abby.* Harper & Row, 1973. Pres.–3. The family of an adopted child from the child's point of view.

―――. *Daddy.* Illus. Ronald Himler. Harper & Row, 1977. Pres.–3. The experiences of a child of divorce.

Dragonwagon, Crescent. *Always, Always.* Illus. Arieh Zeldich. Macmillan, 1984. Pres.–3. A child is still loved after a divorce.

————. *Diana, Maybe.* Illus. Deborah Kogan Ray. Macmillan, 1987. K–5. A child deals with a new second marriage family.

Fassler, David, Lash, Michele, and Ives, Sally B. *Changing Families.* Waterfront Books, 1988. Pres.–5. Living in stepfamilies.

First, Julia. *I, Rebekah, Take You, The Lawrences.* Watts, 1981. 3–7. Learning to deal with adoption.

Girard, Linda Walvoord. *Adoption Is for Always.* Illus. Judith Friedman. Whitman, 1986. 1–5. Beginning to understand adoption.

————. *At Daddy's on Saturdays.* Illus. Judith Friedman. Whitman, 1987. K–3. Story of a divorce from the child's point of view.

Goff, Beth. *Where Is Daddy? The Story of a Divorce.* Illus. Susan Perl. Beacon Press, 1969. Pres.–K. The story of one divorce.

Gordon, Shirley. *The Boy Who Wanted a Family.* Harper & Row, 1980. 1–4. The trials of a child about to be adopted; coping with adoption.

Krementz, Jill. *How It Feels When Parents Divorce.* Knopf, 1984. 2–6. Children tell how they were affected by their parents' divorces.

MacLachlan, Patricia. *Mama One, Mama Two.* Illus. Ruth Bornstein. Harper & Row, 1982. K–4. The relationship between a foster mother and child.

McAfee, Annalena. *The Visitors Who Came to Stay.* Illus. Anthony Browne. Viking Kestrel, 1985. 2–4. Insight into changing family relationships.

Miles, Miska. *Aaron's Door.* Atlantic-Little, Brown, 1977. K–4. Adjusting to an adoptive home.

Myers, Walter Dean. *Me, Mop, and the Moondance Kid.* Delacorte, 1988. 3–5. The trials of adopted and unadopted children.

Roy, Ron. *Breakfast with My Father.* Illus. Troy Howell. Houghton Mifflin, 1980. K–3. A child deals with his parents' separation.

Schuchman, Joan. *Two Places To Sleep.* Illus. Jim La Marche. Carolrhoda, 1986. 1–4. A story of a divorced family.

Simon, Norma. *I Wish I Had My Father.* Illus. Arieh Zeldich. Whitman, 1983. 1–3. Single parenthood discussed.

Sobol, Harriet Langsam. *My Other-Mother, My Other-Father.* Photographs by Patricia Agre. Macmillan, 1979. K–4. What it means to be a stepchild.

Stanek, Muriel. *I Won't Go Without a Father.* Whitman, 1972. 2–4. Dealing with being in a single-parent household.

————. *My Little Foster Sister.* Whitman, 1981. Pres.–3. A child rejects the foster child her parents bring into the home.

Stein, Sara Bonnett. *On Divorce.* Photographs by Erika Stone. Walker, 1979. K–3. Deals with the subject of divorce.

————. *The Adopted One: An Open Family Book for Parents and Children Together.* Walker, 1979. Pres.–3. Brings out special needs of adopted children.

Vigna, Judith. *Grandma Without Me.* Whitman, 1984. Pres.–3. A boy is separated from his beloved grandmother by a divorce.

————. *Mommy and Me by Ourselves Again.* Whitman, 1987. Pres.–3. Dealing with being in a single-parent home.

Wasson, Valentina. *The Chosen Baby.* Illus. Glo Coalson. Lippincott, 1977. K–3. The story of a couple's experiences with adoption.

All Kinds of Families

•Alexander, Sue. *Nadia the Willful.* Illus. Lloyd Bloom. Pantheon, 1983. K–3. Cherishing memories of a deceased loved one.

Allison, Diane Worfolk. *In Window Eight, the Moon is Late.* Little, Brown, 1988. Pres.–3. Poetry expressing the experiences of a large extended family.

Asch, Frank. *Just Like Daddy.* Prentice, 1981. 1–3. Tale of a father-son relationship.

Bauer, Caroline Feller. *My Mom Travels a Lot.* Illus. Nancy Winslow Parker. Warne, 1981. Pres.–3. The good and bad things about a traveling mother.

Brisson, Pat. *Your Best Friend, Kate.* Illus. Rick Brown. Bradbury, 1989. Pres.–3. Story of a family's travels.

Brown, Marc. *Arthur's Baby.* Little, Brown, 1988. Pres.–2. Getting along with a new sibling.

Browne, Anthony. *Piggybook.* Knopf, 1986. Pres.–3. What happens in a household where the mother is not appreciated.

•Bunin, Catherine, and Bunin, Sherry. *Is That Your Sister? A True Story of Adoption.* Pantheon, 1976. K–3. A white family adopts two black sisters.

•Caines, Jeanette. *Daddy.* Illus. Ronald Himler. Harper & Row, 1977. Pres.–2. Story of a separated family.

•———. *Just Us Women.* Illus. Pat Cummings. Harper & Row, 1982. K–3. A trip with a beloved aunt is detailed.

Carlson, Nancy. *Louanne Pig in the Perfect Family.* Penguin, 1986. Pres.–3. An only child sees the benefits and down side to a big family.

———. *The Perfect Family.* Carolrhoda, 1985. K–3. How another kind of family lives.

Conrad, Pam. *The Tub People.* Illus. Richard Egielski. Harper & Row, 1985. Pres.–3. A family is separated and joyfully reunited.

Cooney, Barbara. *Island Boy.* Viking Kestrel, 1988. Pres.–2. A loving family is described.

d'Aulaire, Ingri and d'Aulaire, Edgar Parin. *Abraham Lincoln.* Doubleday, 1957. 3-up. A focus on Lincoln's family life.

Delton, Judy. *My Mom Hates Me in January.* Whitman, 1977. 1–3. A mother can be cranky and still love you.

———. *My Uncle Nikos.* Illus. Marc Simont. Crowell, 1983. 1–4. A girl's relationship with her loving uncle.

•Domanska, Janina. *Busy Monday Morning.* Greenwillow, 1985. Pres.–2. Polish folksong about father and son who work together daily.

Drescher, Joan. *Your Family, My Family.* Walker, 1980. K–3. Portrays the many kinds of families.

•Fife, Dale. *Rosa's Special Garden.* Whitman, 1985. Pres.–2. Story about a loving Hispanic family.

Florian, Douglas. *A Summer Day.* Greenwillow, 1988. Pres.–3. Tells about a family outing into the country.

Foreman, Michael. *The Angel and the Wild Animal.* Atheneum, 1989. Pres.–2. The trials of being a parent.

•Freedman, Florence. B., reteller. *Brothers: A Hebrew Legend.* Illus. Robert Andrew Parker. Harper & Row, 1985. K–4. Retelling of a Hebrew legend about two loving brothers.

Goffstein, M. B. *Our Snowman.* Harper/Charlotte Zolotow, 1986. K–3. A child and her father create two snowmen.

Hall, Donald. *Ox-Cart Man.* Illus. Barbara Cooney. Viking Kestrel, 1979. Pres.–3. A family of nineteenth-century rural New England.

Harvey, Brett. *Cassie's Journey.* Illus. Deborah Kogan Ray. Holiday House, 1988. Pres.–4. A family's journey to California in the 1860s.

———. *Immigrant Girl.* Illus. Deborah Kogan Ray. Holiday House, 1987. 2–4. A family moves from their Russian village to New York City in 1910.

Hendershot, Judith. *In Coal Country.* Illus. Thomas B. Allen. Knopf, 1987. K–4. Life in a mining town in the 1930s.

Henry, Joanne Landers. *Log Cabin in the Woods: A True Story About a Pioneer Boy.* Illus. Joyce Audy Zarins. Four Winds, 1988. 3–4. An account of a family in the Indiana woods of 1832.

Hertz, Ole, translator. *Tobias Goes Ice Fishing.* Carolrhoda, 1984. K–3. Portrait of daily family life in a small settlement in Greenland.

Hest, Amy. *The Mommy Exchange.* Illus. Dyanne DiSalvo-Ryan. Four Winds, 1988. Pres.–2. Two children switch homes only to discover there's no place like their own homes.

Hewett, Joan. *Rosalie.* Illus. Donald Carrick. Lothrop, Lee & Shepard, 1987. K–3. A dog is old and deaf, but still an important family member.

Hines, Anne Grossnickle. *Daddy Makes the Best Spaghetti.* Clarion, 1987. K–3. Coping with working parents.

Hofer, Angelika, and Ziesler, Gunter. Picture Book, 1988. Pres.–3. The lives of a pride of lions.

Hoopes, Lyn Littlefield. *Daddy's Coming Home.* Illus. Bruce Degan. Harper & Row, 1984. Pres.–2. A child and his mother watch for father to come home.

Hurd, Edith Thatcher. *The Mother Owl.* Illus. Clement Hurd. Little, Brown, 1974. 2-up. A year in the life of a mother screech owl.

•Jenness, Aylette. *Families: A Celebration of Diversity, Commitment, and Love.* Photographs by the author. Houghton Mifflin, 1990. 3–5. A photo essay that includes portraits of nuclear, one-parent, multigenerational, gay and lesbian, adoptive, and foster families in communities throughout the U.S.A. A Notable Children's Trade Book in the Field of Social Studies.

•Jenness, Aylette, and Rivers, Alice. *In Two Worlds: A Yup'ik Eskimo Family.* Photographs by Aylette Jenness. Houghton Mifflin, 1985. 5–9.

A unique way of life revealed. A Notable Children's Trade Book in the Field of Social Studies.

•Johnson, Angela. *Tell Me a Story, Mama.* Illus. David Soman. Orchard Books/Franklin Watts, 1989. Pres.–1. A mother shares her personal history with her child.

Johnston, Tony. *Yonder.* Illus. Lloyd Bloom. Dial, 1988. Pres.–3. A nineteenth-century farm family's life.

Joosse, Barbara M. *Dinah's Mad, Bad Wishes.* Illus. Emily Arnold McCully. Harper & Row, 1989. Pres.–3. Ups and downs of child-parent relationships.

Jukes, Mavis. *Like Jake and Me.* Illus. Lloyd Bloom. Knopf, 1984. 1–4. A new family adjusts to each other.

———. *No One Is Going to Nashville.* Illus. Lloyd Bloom. Knopf, 1983. 1–4. The story of a family of father, stepmother, and child who see each other on weekends.

Kent, Jack. *Joey Runs Away.* Prentice-Hall, 1985. K–3. A young kangaroo runs away from home but discovers that's where he belongs.

Kroll, Steven. *Happy Father's Day.* Illus. Marylin Hafner. Holiday House, 1988. Pres.–3. Father's day in a loving family.

Lampert, Emily. *A Little Touch of Monster.* Illus. Victoria Chess. Little, Brown, 1986. Pres.–3. A child gets his own way for a day.

Lasker, Joe. *Mothers Can Do Anything.* Whitman, 1972. K–3. The many kinds of jobs that mothers do.

Laurie, Rona. *Children's Plays from Beatrix Potter.* Warne, 1980. 1–3. Six short plays based on Potter's original stories; family situations.

Le Tord, Bijou. *Joseph and Nellie.* Bradbury, 1986. K–3. A day in the life of a fishing family; each spouse's responsibilities.

•Lewin, Hugh. *Jafta—The Journey.* Illus. Lisa Kopper. Carolrhoda, 1984. K–3. A child journeys to the city to visit his father.

Livingston, Myra Cohn, selector. *Poems for Fathers.* Illus. Robert Casilla. Holiday House, 1989. K–3. Collection of poetry about fathers.

———. *Poems for Mothers.* Illus. Deborah Kogan Ray. Holiday House, 1988. Pres.–3. Collection of poetry about mothers.

Long, Earlene. *Gone Fishing.* Illus. Richard Brown. Houghton Mifflin, 1984. Pres.–1. A child spends the day fishing with his father.

MacLachlan, Patricia. *The Sick Day.* Illus. William Pène duBois. Pantheon, 1979. K–3. A father takes care of his sick child.

Martin, Ann M. *Ten Kids, No Pets.* Holiday House, 1988. 2–4. The experience of living in a large, suppportive family.

Mattingley, Christobel. *The Angel with a Mouth-Organ.* Illus. Astra Lacis. Holiday House, 1986. Pres.–3. A mother tells her children about the family's separation during World War II.

McCaslin, Nellie. *Little Snow Girl.* Coach House, 1963. K–3. Play about a couple who lose and regain their child through love.

McCloskey, Robert. *Blueberries for Sal.* Viking Kestrel, 1948. Pres.–3. Two children hunt for blueberries with their mothers.

McCurdy, Michael. *Hannah's Farm: The Seasons on an Early American*

Homestead. Holiday House, 1988. 1–4. The experiences of living on a farm with an extended family.

McPhail, David. *Farm Morning*. Harcourt Brace Jovanovich, 1985. Pres.–2. A father and daughter work together on the family farm.

Messenger, Norman. *Annabel's House*. Orchard Books, 1989. K-up. A child's life in an Edwardian house.

Miller, Edna. *Mousekins Woodland Birthday*. Prentice-Hall, 1974. K–3. The early life of a mouse; how animal mothers raise their children.

Mitchell, Joyce Slayton. *My Mommy Makes Money*. Illus. True Kelley. Little, Brown, 1984. Pres.–3. A story of working mothers.

Monjo, F. N. *Grand Papa and Ellen Aroon, Being an Account of Some of the Happy Times Spent Together by Thomas Jefferson and His Favorite Granddaughter*. Illus. Richard Cuffari. Holt, 1974. 2–4. A granddaughter's feelings about her grandfather.

———. *Poor Richard in France*. Illus. Brinton Turkle. Holt, 1973. 2–4. Ben Franklin's visit to France with his grandsons, from their point of view.

Musil, Rosemary G. *Five Little Peppers*. Anchorage Press, 1940. 2–4. Poor people can better themselves; rich have an obligation to help others.

Newton, Laura. *Me and My Aunts*. Illus. Robin Oz. Whitman, 1986. 2–5. A child's relationship with her aunts.

Ormerod, Jan. *Dad's Back*. Lothrop, Lee & Shepard, 1985. Pres.–2. Experiences of a father with his young child.

———. *Messy Baby*. Lothrop, Lee & Shepard, 1985. Pres.–2. A father's experiences with his young child.

———. *Reading*. Lothrop, Lee & Shepard, 1985. Pres.–2. A father reads to his very young child.

———. *Sleeping*. Lothrop, Lee & Shepard, 1985. Pres.–2. A father's experiences with his toddler.

Osborn, Lois. *My Dad Is Really Something*. Whitman, 1983. 1–3. A child's feelings about his father.

Parker, Kristy. *My Dad the Magnificent*. Illus. Lillian Hoban. Dutton, 1987. Pres.–2. A child spends Saturdays with his father.

Purdy, Carol. *Least of All*. Illus. Tim Arnold. McElderry, 1987. K–3. A young girl learns to read from the family Bible and can contribute now to her family.

Ray, Deborah Kogan. *Fog Drift Morning*. Harper & Row, 1983. K–3. A child describes a morning walk with her mother.

•Reisner, Joanne. *Hannah's Alaska*. Illus. Julie Downing. Carnival Press Books, 1983. K–3. Common episodes in the life of an Alaskan family.

Robins, Joan. *Addie Runs Away*. Illus. Sue Truesdell. Harper & Row, 1989. Pres.–2. Coping with leaving family and going to camp.

Roth, Susan L., and Phang, Ruth. *Patchwork Tales*. Atheneum, 1984. Pres.–2. Story of patches that make up a family memory quilt.

Rylant, Cynthia. *Birthday Presents*. Illus. Suçie Stevenson. Orchard Books, 1987. Pres.–1. Family history and memories of a child's first five birthdays.

———. *Henry and Mudge and the Forever Sea*. Illus. Suçie Stevenson.

Bradbury, 1989. 1–3. Henry, his father, and dog Mudge spend a day at the beach.

————. *The Relatives Came*. Illus. Stephen Gammell. Bradbury, 1985. K–3. The relatives arrive and stay for an extended visit.

Segal, Lore. *Tell Me a Trudy*. Illus. Rosemary Wells. Sunburst, 1989. Pres.–3. Stories of a loving family.

Sharmat, Marjorie Weinman. *Hooray for Father's Day!* Illus. John Wallner. Holiday House, 1987. Pres.–3. Two siblings compete for their father's attention on Father's Day.

Showers, Paul. *Me and My Family Tree*. Illus. Don Madden. Crowell, 1978. 2–4. Simple explanation of genealogy.

Simon, Norma. *Nobody's Perfect, Not Even My Mother*. Whitman, 1981. K–3. Helping parents and children deal with imperfect behavior.

•Smith, Miriam. *Kimi and the Watermelon*. Illus. David Armitage. Puffin, 1989. Pres.–3. How our lives are bound to nature and our loved ones.

•Stanek, Muriel. *I Speak English for My Mom*. Whitman, 1989. 2–5. A child who is bilingual takes responsibility for translating for her mother.

Steig, William. *Brave Irene*. Farrar, Straus & Giroux, 1986. K–3. A child braves a storm to deliver a gown to her sick mother.

————. *Sylvester and the Magic Pebble*. Windmill, 1969. K–3. A child is separated and then reunited with his family.

Stevenson, James. *Grandpa's Great City Tour*. Greenwillow, 1983. Pres.–2. A trip through the city with grandfather.

•Surat, Michele Maria. *Angel Child, Dragon Child*. Illus. Vo-Dinh Mai. Carnival/Raintree, 1983. K–3. A Vietnamese child makes friends in America.

Thiele, Colin. *Farmer Schulz's Ducks*. Illus. Mary Milton. Harper & Row, 1988. Pres.–2. A family finds a way to keep the traffic from bothering their ducks.

Thomas, Ianthe. *Willie Blows a Mean Horn*. Illus. Ann Toulmin-Rothe. Harper & Row, 1981. K–3. A son hopes to grow up and be a musician like his father.

Tyler, Linda Wagner. *When Daddy Comes Home*. Illus. Susan Davis. Viking Kestrel, 1986. Pres.–3. A hippo child longs to spend time with his busy father.

Viorst, Judith. *The Good-Bye Book*. Illus. Kay Chorao. Atheneum, 1988. Pres.–K. Learning to cope with family separation.

Weiss, Nicki. *A Family Story*. Greenwillow, 1987. Pres.–3. A story of loving sisters through the generations.

•Williams, Vera B. *"More, More, More," Said the Baby: 3 Love Stories*. Greenwillow, 1990. Pres.–1. A simple text and radiant pictures depict loving relationships. Caldecott Honor Book.

•————. *Music, Music for Everyone*. Greenwillow, 1984. K–3. Story of a loving family and caring neighborhood.

————. *Stringbean's Trip to the Shining Sea*. Illus. by author and Jennifer Williams. Greenwillow, 1988. 1–4. Two brothers send home messages from their trip from Kansas to the Pacific.

Yamashita, Haruo. *Mice at the Beach*. Illus. Kazuo Iwamura. Morrow, 1987. K–3. A loving mouse family goes to the beach for a picnic.

Ziefert, Harriet. *Sarah's Questions.* Illus. Susan Bonners. Lothrop, Lee & Shepard, 1986. K–3. A child questions her mother about the world.

Zolotow, Charlotte. *Something is Going to Happen.* Illus. Catherine Stock. Harper & Row, 1988. Pres.–3. The members of a family awake to find that snow has fallen overnight.

————. *The Poodle Who Barked at the Wind.* Illus. June Otani. Harper & Row, 1987. K–3. Story of a family and its dog.

Families the World Over*

•Ashby, Gwynneth. *A Family in South Korea.* Lerner, 1987. 2–5. A child's life in the Republic of Korea.

•Bennett, Olivia. *A Family in Brazil.* Photographs by Liba Taylor. Lerner, 1986. 2–5. A young girl's family life in Brazil.

•Browne, Rollo. *A Family in Australia.* Lerner, 1986. 2–5. A child's family and social life in Australia.

•Elkin, Judith. *A Family in Japan.* Lerner, 1986. 2–5. Family life in a small town near Tokyo.

•Griffin, Michael. *A Family in Kenya.* Lerner, 1988. 2–5. A young girl's farm and family life in Kenya.

•Hubley, John, and Hubley, Penny. *A Family in Italy.* Lerner, 1986. 2–5. A small child's family life in a city near Florence.

ᵉHumphrey, Sally. *A Family in Liberia.* Lerner, 1986. 2–5. Village and family life for a child in Liberia.

•McKenna, Nancy Durrell. *A Family in Hong Kong.* Lerner, 1987. 2–5. A small boy's school and family life in Hong Kong.

•Moran, Tom. *A Family in Mexico.* Lerner, 1987. 2–5. A young girl's family and social life in Mexico.

•St. John, Jetty. *A Family in Bolivia.* Lerner, 1986. 2–5. A child wants to learn his father's trade of boat building in Bolivia.

•————. *A Family in England.* Lerner, 1988. 2–5. A young boy's family and social life in England.

•————. *A Family in Hungary.* Lerner, 1988. 2–5. A young girl's family life in Budapest.

•————. *A Family in Norway.* Lerner, 1988. 2–5. A young girl's family life in a fishing village in Norway.

•————. *A Family in Peru.* Lerner, 1986. 2–5. A child's family and school life in the Andean mountains.

•Stewart, Judy. *A Family in Sudan.* Lerner, 1988. 2–5. A child's family life and work life in the Sudan.

•Taylor, Allegra. *A Kibbutz in Israel.* Photographs by Nancy Durrell McKenna. Lerner, 1987. 2–5. A boy's life on a kibbutz in Israel.

---

*All the books listed in this section are from the *Families the World Over* series published by Lerner, 1986–1988.

•Thomson, Ruth, and Thomson, Neil. *A Family in Thailand.* Lerner, 1988. 2–5. A young girl's work, school, and family life in Thailand.

Gender Issues

•Adoff, Arnold. *I Am the Running Girl.* Illus. Ronald Himler. Harper & Row, 1979. 2–6. A poem about a young woman who is a runner.

Alda, Arlene. *Sonya's Mommy Works.* Messner, 1982. K–3. A story about a caring, responsible family where both parents work.

Babbitt, Natalie. *Phoebe's Revolt.* Farrar, Straus & Giroux, 1968. 2–5. A young girl revolts against feminine clothing, searching for her own style.

Bauer, Caroline Feller. *My Mom Travels a Lot.* Illus. Nancy Winslow Parker. Warne, 1981. K–3. A child tells about the ups and downs of having a traveling working mother.

Berenstain, Stan, and Berenstain, Jan. *He Bear, She Bear.* Random House, 1977. Pres.–2. Occupations pictured and discussed that can be chosen by men or women.

Blaine, Marge. *The Terrible Thing That Happened at Our House.* Illus. John C. Wallner. Parents' Magazine Press, 1975. K–4. A child resents her mother resuming her career, wanting the old life back.

Brenner, Barbara. *A Year in the Life of Rosie Bernard.* Harper & Row, 1971. 3–6. A child is left to live with her grandparents during the Depression, learning much from the experience.

•Caines, Jeanette. *Just Us Women.* Illus. Pat Cummings. Harper & Row, 1982. K–4. A child and her aunt take a trip together.

•Clifton, Lucille. *Don't You Remember?* Illus. Evaline Ness. Dutton, 1973. K–3. Family division of labor, in order to get things done.

Delton, Judy. *My Mother Lost Her Job Today.* Illus. Irene Trivas. Whitman, 1980. K–3. A child comforts her mother after she loses her job.

Gauch, Patricia Lee. *This Time, Tempe Wick?* Illus. Margot Tomes. Coward, McCann, 1974. 2–4. A child defies soldiers to protect her family and possessions during the Revolutionary War.

Grahame, Kenneth. *The Reluctant Dragon.* Illus. E. H. Shepard. Holiday House, 1953. 2–4. A boy makes friends with a peace-loving dragon.

Isadora, Rachel. *Max.* Macmillan, 1976. K–3. A boy joins his sister's dance class, finding he enjoys it as much as sports.

Klein, Norma. *Girls Can Be Anything.* Dutton, 1973. Pres.–3. Equality for employment; self-esteem for women in the workplace.

Larche, Douglas. *Father Gander Nursery Rhymes: The Equal Rhymes Amendment.* Illus. Carolyn Blattel. Girls Clubs of America, 1986. K–4. Nursery rhymes rewritten without gender or age bias.

Lurie, Allison, reteller. *Clever Gretchen and Other Forgotten Folktales.* Illus. Margot Tomes. Crowell, 1980. 2–6. Tales about assertive women told in a humorous way.

MacLachlan, Patricia. *The Sick Day.* Illus. William Pène du Bois. Pantheon,

1979. Pres.–3. A child and her father spend time together when she is ill and mother is at work.

Martin, Bill, Jr. and Archambault, John. *White Dynamite and Curly Kidd.* Illus. Ted Rand. Holt, 1986. Pres.–3. A girl shares a day at the rodeo with her bronco-busting father.

Minard, Rosemary, ed. *Womenfolk and Fairy Tales.* Illus. Suzanna Klein. Houghton Mifflin, 1975. 2-up. Fairy tales in which women are the central characters, exhibiting courage, intelligence, and integrity.

Mitchell, Joyce Slayton. *My Mommy Makes Money.* Illus. True Kelley. Little, Brown, 1984. Pres.–3. The various occupations mothers might hold.

•Phelps, Ethel J. *The Maid of the North: Feminist Folk Tales from Around the World.* Holt, 1981. 2–6. Tales in which women draw on their courage and honesty to outwit their rivals.

•Sorine, Stephanie Riva. *At Every Turn! It's Ballet.* Photographs by Daniel S. Sorine. Knopf, 1981. 2–4. Everyday movements compared with movements in ballet. Both boys and girls appear in photographs.

Waber, Bernard. *Ira Sleeps Over.* Houghton Mifflin, 1972. K–3. A child forgets to bring his beloved teddy bear on a sleepover.

Wandro, Mark, and Blank, Joanie. *My Daddy Is a Nurse.* Illus. Irene Trivas. Addison-Wesley, 1981. K–3. Dispels notions about gender-role careers.

Waxman, Stephanie. *What Is a Girl? What Is a Boy?* Harper & Row, 1989. Pres.–2. Discusses issues relating to sexuality.

Zolotow, Charlotte. *William's Doll.* Illus. William Pène du Bois. Harper, 1972. Pres.–4. Why it's alright for boys to have dolls.

Grades Four Through Six

Gender Issues

Adler, C. S. *The Magic of the Glits.* Illus. Ati Forberg. Macmillan, 1979. 4–7. A child invents imaginary creatures to entertain his young charge.

Ancona, George. *And What Do You Do?* Dutton, 1976. 3–5. Tells about the careers of twenty-one people.

Asbjornsen, P. C. *The Squire's Bride.* Illus. Marcia Sewell. Atheneum, 1975. 2–5. A young woman outwits the old man who wants her to marry him.

Burch, Robert. *Queenie Peavy.* Illus. Jerry Lazare. Viking, 1966. 4–6. A child copes with her father in prison; child deals with her tendencies to gravitate toward boy's interests.

Byars, Betsy. *The Midnight Fox.* Illus. Ann Grifalconi. Viking, 1968. 5–8. A child spends the summer on a farm away from his parents and gains independence.

Cleary, Beverly. *Ramona the Brave.* Illus. Alan Tiegreen. Morrow, 1975.

3–5. Two latchkey children deal with being alone; Ramona and her father's relationship is detailed.

Cleaver, Vera. *Hazel Rye.* Lippincott, 1983. 4–7. A child manages to overcome her father's destructive overprotectiveness.

Cleaver, Vera, and Cleaver, Bill. *Lady Ellen Grae.* Illus. Ellen Raskin. Lippincott, 1968. 4–7. A willful child manages to learn to be "ladylike."

———. *Where the Lilies Bloom.* Illus. Jim Spanfeller. Lippincott, 1969. 4–7. An Appalachian child cares for the family after the death of their father, which they have trouble accepting.

Coerr, Eleanor. *Jane Goodall.* Putnam, 1976. 5-up. A biography of the famous ethnologist who pioneered work on chimpanzee behavior.

Dalgliesh, Alice. *The Courage of Sarah Noble.* Illus. Leonard Weisgard. Scribner's, 1954. 2–5. A girl and her father travel into the wilderness in 1707.

Fitzhugh, Louise. *Harriet the Spy.* Harper & Row, 1964. 4–6. The observations of family and community life of a girl who wants to be a spy.

Foote, Patricia. *Girls Can Be Anything They Want.* Messner, 1980. 4–8. Careers for women are not limited.

•Greene, Bette. *Philip Hall Likes Me: I Reckon Maybe.* Illus. Charles Lilly. Dial, 1974. 4–6. A young, ambitious girl competes with her male friend.

Herzig, Alison, and Mali, Jane. *Oh Boy! Babies!* Photographs by Katrina Thomas. Little, Brown, 1980. 5–8. An all-male school offers a course on baby care to fifth and sixth graders.

•Howard, Moses. *The Ostrich Chase.* Illus. Barbara Seuling. Holt, Rinehart, 1974. 5–7. A young woman violates tribal tradition by learning to hunt and build fires, and saves lives because of it.

Klein, Norma. *Mom, the Wolf Man and Me.* Pantheon, 1972. 5–8. A child and her working mother share an open relationship.

Kyte, Kathleen. *In Charge: A Complete Handbook for Kids with Working Parents.* Knopf, 1983. 5–8. Ideas and advice for young people whose parents work outside the house.

Larrick, Nancy, and Merriam, Eve., eds. *Male and Female Under 18.* Avon, 1973. 3–6. Children eight to eighteen comment about their sex roles in poetry and narrative.

Levitin, Sonia. *Alan and Naomi.* Harper & Row, 1977. 5–8. A story of the attempts of a young boy to help his female friend recover from the Holocaust.

Malt, Christopher. *The Year Mom Won the Pennant.* Little, Brown, 1968. 3–5. An exploration of gender roles.

McKinley, Robin. *The Blue Sword.* Greenwillow, 1982. 6-up. A fantasy-adventure where women are warriors in a mythical empire.

•O'Dell, Scott. *Island of the Blue Dolphins.* Houghton Mifflin, 1960. 5–8. A young Native American girl survives alone on an island for many years.

Paterson, Katherine. *Bridge to Terabithia.* Crowell, 1977. 4–6. A story of a friendship between a girl and boy and his coming to terms with her death.

•Riordan, James. *The Woman in the Moon and Other Tales of Forgotten*

Heroines. Dial, 1985. 4–6. Oppressed female characters discover their power.

Speare, Elizabeth George. *The Witch of Blackbird Pond.* Houghton Mifflin, 1958. 6–8. An orphaned teen goes to live with her Puritan relatives and must adjust to a new culture and way of life.

Reproduction and Human Sexuality

Alexander, Lloyd. The Prydain Series. Includes *The Book of Three* (Holt, 1964); *The Black Cauldron* (Holt, 1965); *Taran Wanderer* (Holt, 1967); and *The High King* (Holt, 1968). 4–6. Blends Welsh legend and mythology in the tale of an assistant pig keeper who becomes a hero.

Bargar, Gary. *What Happened to Mr. Forster?* Houghton Mifflin, 1983. 5–8. How a class copes when their homosexual teacher is fired.

Barth, Edna. *Cupid and Psyche: A Love Story.* Illus. Ati Forberg. Houghton Mifflin, 1976. 5-up. Retelling of the Greek myth dealing with human sexuality.

Caveney, Sylvia. *Inside Mom: An Illustrated Account of Conception, Pregnancy and Childbirth.* St. Martin's, 1977. 4–8. Illustrated book about the stages of birth.

Cole, Joanna. *Asking About Sex and Growing Up: A Question and Answer Book.* Illus. Alan Tiegreen. Morrow, 1988. 4–7. Presentation of factual information about sex and maturity.

Day, Beth, and Liley, Margaret. *The Secret World of the Baby.* Illus. Lennart Nilsson and others. 6–8. Random House, 1968. The growth and movements of the embryo.

Fischer-Nagel, Heiderose, and Fischer-Nagel, Andreas. *A Kitten Is Born.* Andrea Mernan, translator. Putnam, 1983. 4–6. Cats from conception through kittens.

Forrai, Maria. *A Look at Birth.* Lerner, 1978. 4-up. The stages of pregnancy and birth process in text and photographs.

Gale, Jay. *A Young Man's Guide to Sex.* Illus. Scott E. Carroll. Holt, 1984. 6-up. Explanation of sex and sexuality for young men.

Gruenberg, Sidonce Matsner. *The Wonderful Story of How You Were Born.* Illus. Symeon Shimin. Doubleday, 1970, rev. ed. 3–5. Relates reproduction to the animal kingdom.

Harris, Rosemary, reteller. *Beauty and the Beast.* Illus. Errol Le Cain. Doubleday, 1979. 4–6. Finding the inner beauty of another is the root of love.

Hodges, Margaret. *Persephone and the Springtime: Myths of the World.* Illus. Arvis Stewart. Little, Brown, 1973. 2–4. A retelling of the origins of springtime.

Hunter, Mollie. *A Stranger Came Ashore.* Harper & Row, 1975. 4–7. Fantasy in which a seal takes human form and lures a young girl to his underground palace.

Johnson, Eric. W. *People, Love, Sex, and Families: Answers to Questions*

Preteens Ask. Illus. David Wool. Walker, 1985. 5–8. Questions and answers about human reproduction.

————. *Sex: Telling It Straight.* Lippincott, 1979. 5–8. A straightforward account of what sex is about.

McDermott, Gerald. *Daughter of Earth: A Roman Myth.* Delacorte, 1984. 2-up. Retelling of myth of Ceres and her daughter who is abducted and allowed to return to Earth only briefly each year.

Mintz, Thomas, and Miller, Lorelie. *Threshold: Straightforward Answers to Teenagers' Questions about Sex.* Walker, 1978. 5–8. Direct questions about sex and straightforward answers.

Nourse, Alan. *Menstruation: Just Plain Talk.* Walker, 1980. 5–9. How the female body functions.

Phelps, Ethel, selector. *The Maid of the North: Feminist Folktales from Around the World.* Holt, 1977. 4–8. Stories of determined women who have taken control of their lives.

Rench, Janice E. *Teen Sexuality: Decisions and Choices.* Lerner, 1988. 6-up. Information for teens on choices and consequences of decisions about their own sexuality.

Rogasky, Barbara, reteller. *Rapunzel.* Illus. Trina Schart Hyman. Holiday House, 1982. 3–7. An adolescent comes of age and learns to assert herself; developing a relationship with a young man.

Rylant, Cynthia. *A Couple of Kooks and Other Stories.* Orchard, 1990. 6–9. Compromise, a fulfillment, and heartache abound in these charming tales of love gained and lost.

Ward, Brian R. *Birth and Growth.* Franklin Watts, 1983. 4–8. A textbook-like approach to reproduction, birth, and growth.

Yolen, Jane, ed. *Favorite Folktales from Around the World.* Pantheon, 1986. All ages. A large collection of folktales which are grouped by topic; contains tales about sexuality.

Divorce, Single-Parent Families, Foster Families

Adler, C. S. *If You Need Me.* Macmillan, 1988. 4–8. A young girl learns about changing relationships.

Berger, Fredericka. *Nuisance.* Morrow, 1983. 5–9. A child's feelings about herself, her parents' divorce, and mother's remarriage change as she changes.

Blume, Judy. *It's Not the End of the World.* Bradbury, 1972. 4–7. A child faces her parents' divorce.

Carrick, Carol. *What a Wimp!* Illus. Donald Carrick. Clarion, 1983. 3–5. A divorce separates a family; child coping with new home and school.

Cone, Molly. *The Amazing Memory of Harvey Bean.* Illus. Robert MacLean. Houghton Mifflin, 1980. 3–6. Coping with separation of parents.

Corcoran, Barbara. *A Row of Tigers.* Illus. Allan Eitzen. Atheneum, 1969. 5–7. Two people with problems form a bond; running away from problems does not solve them.

Craven, Linda. *Stepfamilies: New Patterns of Harmony.* Messner, 1982. 6-up. Problems and solutions for when families merge.

Friedrich, Liz. *Divorce.* Gloucester Press, 1988. 4-up. Reasons, statistics, effects on children, and ways to cope with divorce.

•Girard, Linda Walvoord. *We Adopted You, Benjamin Koo.* Illus. Linda Shute. Whitman, 1989. 2–6. A nine-year-old Korean orphan relates his life story.

Gordon, Shirley. *The Boy Who Wanted a Family.* Illus. Charles Robinson. Harper & Row, 1980. 2–5. A foster child may finally be adopted.

Graeber, Charlotte Towner. *The Thing in Kat's Attic.* Illus. Emily Arnold McCully. Dutton, 1984. 3–6. A family copes after a divorce.

Hansen, Joyce. *The Gift-Giver.* Clarion, 1980. 4–6. Story about a child nonconformist who is a foster child.

Herman, Charlotte. *What Happened to Heather Hopkowitz?* Dutton, 1981. 4–8. A child wishes to follow Orthodox Jewish traditions, despite her parent's wishes; book explains those traditions.

Holl, Kristi. *Just Like a Real Family.* Atheneum, 1983. 4–7. A foster grandfather takes in a lonely girl and her mother.

Hughes, Dean. *Family Pose.* Atheneum, 1989. 3–7. A foster child makes a family with a group of strangers.

Hurwitz, Johanna. *DeDe Takes Charge!* Illus. Diane de Groat. Morrow, 1984. 4–7. A child decides to help her mother rebuild her life after a divorce.

Jukes, Mavis. *Like Jake and Me.* Illus. Lloyd Bloom. Knopf, 1984. 2–5. A child's relationship with his new stepfather.

Kaplan, Leslie S. *Coping with Stepfamilies.* Rosen, 1986. 5-up. Background information on developing new family relationships.

•Kraus, Joanna Halpert. *Kimchi Kid.* New Plays, 1988. 4-up. Play detailing the experiences of an American-Asian adoptee.

Krementz, Jill. *How It Feels to Be Adopted.* Knopf, 1982. 4–9. Nineteen young people from ages eight to sixteen voice their feelings on being adopted.

———. *How It Feels When Parents Divorce.* Knopf, 1984. 4–9. Children tell about divorce in their own words.

Kuklin, Susan. *Mine for a Year.* Coward, 1984. 4–6. A child develops a close relationship with a seeing-eye dog in training.

LeShan, Eda. *What's Going to Happen to Me?* Aladdin, 1986. 3–7. The stages of a divorce explained.

Love, Sandra. *Crossing Over.* Lothrop, Lee & Shepard, 1981. 3–6. A child goes to live for a year with her father, not nearly so easy-going as her mother.

MacLachlan, Patricia. *Sarah, Plain and Tall.* Trophy, 1987. 3–6. A mail-order bride comes to live with a pioneer family.

McAfee, Annalena. *The Visitors Who Came to Stay.* Illus. Anthony Browne. Viking Kestrel, 1985. 3–5. A child adjusts to his father's girlfriend and her son.

Mearian, Judy Frank. *Someone Slightly Different.* Dial, 1980. 6-up. A child copes with divorce; grandmother moves in and makes the house a home.

Mills, Claudia. *Boardwalk with Hotel.* Macmillan, 1985. 4–6. A story of adoption and sibling rivalry.

Morgenroth, Barbara. *Will the Real Renie Lake Please Stand Up?* Atheneum, 1981. 5-up. A child searches for her identity while coping with her parents' divorce.

Orgel, Doris. *Midnight Soup and a Witch's Hat.* Illus. Carol Newsom. Viking Kestrel, 1988. 4–6. A child learns to share her father with a stepsister.

Park, Barbara. *Don't Make Me Smile.* Knopf, 1981. 5–7. A child reacts to his parents' divorce with anger, sadness, and humor.

Pursell, Margaret Sanford. *A Look at Adoption.* Photographs by Maria S. Forrai. Lerner, 1977. 3–6. An informative look at adoption for children.

Rinaldi, Ann. *But in the Fall I'm Leaving.* Holiday, 1985. 4–6. The effects of divorce, family relations, life in a small town, and people's responsibility toward each other.

Rosenberg, Maxine B. *Being Adopted.* Photographs by George Ancona. Lothrop, Lee & Shepard, 1984. 4–6. Personal narratives about children's adoption experiences.

———. *Growing Up Adopted.* Bradbury, 1989. 4–8. Fourteen adoptees speak candidly about how adoption has affected their lives.

Rylant, Cynthia. *A Kindness.* Orchard Books, 1988. 6-up. A boy's attachment to his single-parent mother is badly shaken when she becomes pregnant by a unnamed man and he must face his own possessiveness of her.

Schuchman, Joan. *Two Places To Sleep.* Illus. Jim LaMarche. Carolrhoda, 1989. 1–4. The story of a divorced child.

Scott, Elaine. *Adoption.* Watts, 1980. 4-up. The aspects of adoption explained.

Simons, Wendy. *Harper's Mother.* Prentice-Hall, 1980. 4–6. Examines today's mores and life styles; relationship between a single parent and her daughter.

Smith, Doris Buchanan. *The First Hard Times.* Viking Kestrel, 1983. 4–6. A girl comes to accept her new stepfather.

•Sobol, Harriet. *We Don't Look Like Our Mom and Dad.* Illus. Patricia Agre. Coward McCann, 1984. 4–6. The adoption experience from the children's perspective.

Sommer, Susan. *And I'm Stuck with Joseph.* Illus. Ivan Moon. Herald Press, 1984. 4–7. A child adjusts to her new adoptive brother.

Talbert, Marc. *Thin Ice.* Little, Brown, 1986. 3–7. A child deals with divorce and school problems.

•Walter, Mildred Pitts. *Because We Are.* Lothrop, Lee & Shepard, 1983. 6-up. A child rebels during divorce.

Zeder, Suzan. *Step on a Crack.* In *Plays Children Love.* Coleman A. Jennings and Aurand Harris, eds. Doubleday, 1981. 4-up. Play about a child who adjusts to a new mother and learns to accept herself.

All Kinds of Families

Addy, Sharon Hart. *A Visit with Great-Grandma.* Illus. Lydia Halverson. Whitman, 1989. 1–4. A child visits her great grandmother and bakes a treat with her.

Adoff, Arnold. *Today We Are Brother and Sister.* Illus. Glo Coalson. Lothrop, Lee & Shepard, 1981. All ages. A brother and sister who always argue spend a day together, united by their surroundings.

Aiken, Joan. *Winterthing.* Samuel French, 1972. 6-up. Play about family life and what one needs to make a family work.

•Ammon, Richard. *Growing Up Amish.* Atheneum, 1989. 3–7. A year in the life of an Amish child.

•Ashabranner, Brent. *Children of the Maya: A Guatemalan Indian Odyssey.* Photographs by Paul Conklin. Dodd, Mead, 1986. 5–8. The story of Guatemalan refugees who have relocated to Florida.

Auch, Mary Jane. *Cry Uncle!* Holiday House, 1987. 4–6. A family copes with a crisis with love and understanding.

———. *Pick of the Litter.* Holiday House, 1989. 4–6. An only child learns to cope when mother has quadruplets.

Bates, Betty. *The Great Male Conspiracy.* Holiday House, 1986. 3–7. The men in a child's life seem to be letting her down until she sees another side of them.

Beatty, Patricia. *The Coach That Never Came.* Morrow, 1985. 5-up. A child visiting his grandmother becomes involved with the history of his family.

•Bennett, Olivia. *A Family in Egypt.* Lerner, 1985. 3–6. Daily family life in a small village in Egypt is depicted.

Blume, Judy. *Superfudge.* Bradbury, 1980. 3–5. Family life as seen by the eleven-year-old son.

Boyd, Candy Dawson. *Circle of Gold.* Scholastic-Apple, 1984. 3–5. A twin's effort to win her mother's love leads her to understand her mother's life.

Brosius, Peter C. and Staffa, Rosanna. *A Family Album.* Improvisational Theatre Project, Mark Taper Forum, 135 N. Grand Ave., Los Angeles, CA 90012. A play about family frustrations.

•Browne, Rollo. *An Aboriginal Family.* Photographs by Chris Fairclough. Lerner, 1985. K–5. Family life in a small Aboriginal tribe.

Burch, Robert. *King Kong and Other Poets.* Viking Kestrel, 1986. 4–6. A child escapes her troubled family life by writing poetry.

Byars, Betsy. *Beans on the Roof.* Illus. Melodye Rosales. Delacorte, 1989. 4–6. Family members come to appreciate each other.

———. *The Night Swimmers.* Illus. Troy Howell. Delacorte, 1980. 5–7. A child raises her two younger brothers with the help of television, in the absence of her father, a singer.

Carris, Joan. *Hedgehogs in the Closet.* Illus. Carol Newsom. Lippincott, 1988. 5–8. A family from Ohio moves to a London suburb.

Cassedy, Sylvia. *Behind the Attic Wall.* Crowell/Harper, 1983. 4–6. A child comes to love living with her two great-aunts.

Clark, Ann Nolan. *To Stand Against the Wind.* Viking Kestrel, 1978. 5–7. A child writes his memories of Vietnam before and during the war.

Cleary, Beverly. *Ramona and Her Father.* Illus. Alan Tiegreen. Morrow, 1977. 3–6. Ramona tries to help earn money when her father loses his job.

———. *Ramona Forever.* Illus. Alan Tiegreen. Morrow, 1984. 3–7. Ramona and her sister decide to care for themselves to unburden their family.

Cleaver, Vera. *Sweetly Sings the Donkey.* Lippincott, 1985. 5-up. A family falls apart after it moves to claim a small inheritance.

•Clifford, Eth. *The Remembering Box.* Illus. Donna Diamond. Houghton Mifflin, 1985. 3–6. A loving relationship between a child and his grandmother.

Clifton, Lucille. *Sonora Beautiful.* Illus. Michael Garland. Dutton, 1981. 5–8. A young girl discovers through her family the real meaning of beautiful.

Colman, Hila. *Rich and Famous Like My Mom.* Crown, 1988. 4–6. A child changes her attitude toward the homeless after meeting a bag lady.

DeClements, Barthe, and Greimes, Christopher. *Double Trouble.* Viking Kestrel, 1987. 4–6. Telepathic adventures of separated twins.

•de Trevino, Elizabeth Borton. *El Guero: A True Adventure Story.* Illus. Leslie W. Bowman. Farrar, Straus & Giroux, 1989. 3–7. A well-to-do family goes into political exile and must survive in a new life.

•Dunn, Marylois, with Mayhar, Ardath. *The Absolutely Perfect Horse.* Harper & Row, 1983. 4–6. A family adjusts to a new home, an adopted Vietnamese brother, and a new baby.

Ellis, Sarah. *A Family Project.* McElderry, 1988. 4–7. The changes a new baby brings to a family.

Farber, Norma. *How Does It Feel To Be Old?* Illus. Trina Schart Hyman. Dutton, 1979. 4–7. A grandmother discusses her life.

Fine, Anne. *The Granny Project.* Farrar, Straus & Giroux, 1983. 4–6. Four British children fight the idea of sending their grandmother to a nursing home.

Fox, Paula. *One-Eyed Cat.* Bradbury/Macmillan, 1984. 4-up. A child develops a sense of responsibility by caring for a cat he wounded.

———. *The Village by the Sea.* Orchard Books, 1988. 5–7. A child stays with her aunt and uncle during her father's bypass surgery.

Gaeddert, LouAnn. *The Kid with the Red Suspenders.* Illus. Mary Beth Schwark. Dutton, 1983. 3–5. A child deals with an overprotective mother and problems at school.

Gardiner, John Reynolds. *Stone Fox.* Illus. Marcia Sewall. Crowell, 1980. 3–6. A child takes care of his ailing grandfather.

Gilbert, Sara. *Trouble at Home.* Lothrop, Lee & Shepard, 1981. 5–8. Discusses troubled family situations, such as sibling rivalry, teen suicide, and child abuse as well as techniques for survival.

Goffstein, Brooke. *Our Prairie Home: A Picture Album.* Harper & Row, 1988. All ages. A story of one family's life on the prairie.

•Gonzalez, Gloria. *Gaucho.* Knopf, 1977. 5–7. A child wants to earn enough money to send his mother to San Juan.

Graebner, Charlotte Towner. *Fudge.* Illus. Cheryl Harness. Lothrop, Lee & Shepard, 1987. 3–7. A child learns about the responsibility of taking care of a pet.

Greenberg, Keith Elliot. *Erik Is Homeless.* Illustrated with photographs. Lerner, 1992. 4-up. Photographic essay about nine-year-old Erik and his mother, who are homeless in New York City.

Greene, Constance. *Ask Anybody.* Viking Kestrel, 1983. 4–6. A story about a divorced couple living in the same home and two unlikely friends.

•Greenfield, Eloise. *Grandmama's Joy.* Illus. Carole Byard. Philomel, 1980. 4–6. A loving relationship between grandmother and grandchild.

Greenwald, Sheila. *Alvin Webster's Surprise Plan for Success (and How It Failed).* Little, Brown, 1987. 3–5. A gifted child learns how to fail and to cope with a new family member.

Griffith, Helen V. *Georgia Music.* Illus. James Stevenson. Greenwillow, 1986. 2–4. A child soothes her ailing grandfather's homesickness with music from his home.

Hachfeld, Rainer. *Mugnog.* In *Political Plays for Children.* Jack Zipes, editor and translator. St. Louis, MO: Telos Press, 1976. 5-up. A play about a brother and sister fighting for their rights.

Halvorson, Marilyn. *Cowboys Don't Cry.* Delacorte, 1985. 6-up. A boy and his father work out their troubles on a ranch.

•Hamilton, Virginia. *Willie Bea and the Time the Martians Landed.* Greenwillow, 1983. 4–6. An Ohio family is terrified during Orson Welles's radio broadcast, "War of the Worlds."

Harris, Mark Jonathan. *Come the Morning.* Bradbury, 1989. 5–9. A single parent family copes with moving; a child sees his father realistically.

Harvey, Brett. *My Prairie Year: Based on the Diary of Elenore Plaisted.* Illus. Deborah Kogan Ray. Holiday House, 1986. 2–4. A child reflects on her family's first year on the Dakota prairie.

Hautzig, Esther. *A Gift for Mama.* Illus. Donna Diamond. Viking Kestrel, 1981. 4–6. A child purchases a Mother's Day gift for her mother.

———. *The Endless Steppe: Growing up in Siberia.* Crowell, 1968. 6-up. A mother and her children are forced to labor in Siberia for five years.

Haynes, Betsy. *The Great Mom Swap.* Bantam, 1986. 4–6. Two children trade mothers, learning to appreciate their own families.

Herman, Charlotte. *Our Snowman Had Olive Eyes.* Puffin, 1989. 3–7. A child shares her life with her grandmother.

Herzig, Alison Crafin, and Mali, Jane Lawrence. *Oh Boy! Babies!* Photographs by Katrina Thomas. Little, Brown, 1980. 5–8. Fifth and sixth-grade boys learn to care for infants.

Hest, Amy. *Where in the World Is the Perfect Family?* Clarion, 1989. 4–7. Coping with a new sibling; coping with moving.

•Jacobsen, Peter Otto, and Kristensen, Preben Sejer. *A Family in the U.S.S.R.* Watts, 1986. 3–5. Daily family life in Leningrad. Other countries in this series include China, Iceland, Ireland, and Japan.

Joseph, Lynn. *A Wave in Her Pocket: Stories from Trinidad.* Illus. Brian Pinkney. Clarion, 1991. 2–5. In the cadence of Island speech, Tantie tells six of her intriguing stories to Amber and her cousins.

•Kherdian, David. *Root River Run.* Illus. Nonny Hogrogian. Carolrhoda, 1984. 5-up. Problems of a first-generation American child.

Kinsey-Warnock, Natalie. *The Canada Geese Quilt.* Illus. Leslie W. Bowman. Cobblehill Books, 1989. 4–6. A child of the 1940s copes with a new baby and an ailing grandmother.

Klein, Robin. *Halfway across the Galaxy and Turn Left.* Viking Kestrel, 1986. 5-up. A futuristic family portrayed.

LeShan, Eda. *When a Parent Is Very Sick.* Little, Brown, 1986. 3–7. Handling the strains brought on a family by a very ill parent.

Levitin, Sonia. *Silver Days.* Atheneum, 1989. 5-up. A family fleeing Nazi Germany comes to America and attempts to settle.

Linden, Saphira Barbara. *Sunsong.* New Plays, 1976. 4-up. Play about a family in conflict.

Little, Jean. *Lost and Found.* Illus. Leoung O'Young. Viking Kestrel, 1986. 3–6. A child finds a lost dog and a new friend.

•Lord, Bette Bao. *In the Year of the Boar and Jackie Robinson.* Illus. Marc Simont. Harper & Row, 1984. 2–5. A Chinese girl adjusts to life in Brooklyn and her new school with the help of sports.

Lowry, Lois. *All About Sam.* Illus. Diane de Groat, Houghton Mifflin, 1988. 3–5. A younger brother reports on the exploits of his sister and family.

———. *Anastasia Has the Answers.* Houghton Mifflin, 1986. 5–7. Anastasia deals with adolescence.

———. *Anastasia Krupnik.* Houghton Mifflin, 1979. 4–6. A child learns to cope with new sibling and adolescent feelings.

———. *Us and Uncle Fraud.* Houghton Mifflin, 1984. 6–8. A story of family love.

Mann, Peggy. *My Dad Lives in a Downtown Hotel.* Doubleday, 1973. 4–6. A child copes with parental separation.

•Mark, Michael. *Toba.* Illus. Neil Waldman. Bradbury/Macmillan, 1984. 4–6. Jewish family life portrayed in nine short stories.

Marshak, Samuel, reteller. *The Month-Brothers: A Slavik Tale.* Thomas P. Whitney, translator. Illus. Diane Stanley. Morrow, 1983. 3–7. A child is aided by the month-brothers in her attempt to pacify a greedy stepmother and stepsister.

Martin, Ann M. *Bummer Summer.* Holiday House, 1983. 4–6. A child adjusts to a new family while at camp.

Martin, Judith. *Ma and the Kids.* In *Plays Children Love,* Coleman A. Jennings and Aurand Harris, eds. Doubleday, 1981. 3-up. An indulgent mother learns how to deal with her demanding children.

•Mathis, Sharon Bell. *Sidewalk Story.* Avon, 1981. 2–6. A child tries to help her best friend's family keep their home.

•———. *The Hundred-Penny Box.* Illus. Leo and Diane Dillon. Viking Kestrel, 1975. 3–5. Each penny in the box symbolizes an aunt's memory to be shared with her great-great-nephew.

•McHugh, Elisabet. *Raising a Mother Isn't Easy.* Greenwillow, 1983. 4–6. The open relationship between a single parent and her adopted Korean daughter.

Mills, Claudia. *The Secret Carousel.* Four Winds, 1983. 5–7. An orphaned child adjusts to life with her grandparents.

Milton, Joyce. *Save the Loonies.* Four Winds, 1983. 4–6. Families that look perfect from the outside aren't always that way.

Moeri, Louise. *First the Egg.* Dutton, 1982. 4–6. Two classmates care for an egg as though it were an infant in a class project.

•Mohr, Nicholasa. *Felita*. Illus. Ray Cruz. 3–6. A child must move to a new neighborhood.

Morgan, Alison. *Paul's Kite*. Atheneum, 1982. 4–6. A child goes to live with his mother in London, and she doesn't want to be his mother.

•Naidoo, Beverley. *Journey to Jo'burg: A South African Story*. Illus. Eric Velasquez. Harper & Row, 1988. 4–7. Two children become aware of apartheid when they travel to the city to fetch their mother.

Naylor, Phyllis. *Getting Along in Your Family*. Abingdon, 1976. 4–7. How to cope with family life and living.

•Nixon, Joan Lowery. *The Gift*. Illus. Andrew Glass. Macmillan, 1983. 3–7. The relationship between a child and his Irish great-grandfather who tells him folktales.

Noble, Iris. *Emmeline and Her Daughters: The Pankhurst Suffragettes*. Messner, 1971. 6-up. The story of a mother and daughters who championed the cause of women's rights in Victorian times.

Olsen, Violet. *View from the Pighouse Roof*. Atheneum, 1987. 4–7. A short story about changing family relationships on an Iowa farm during the Depression.

•Orlev, Uri. *The Island on Bird St*. Hillel Halkin, translator. Houghton Mifflin, 1984. 5-up. A child survives alone in the Warsaw Ghetto waiting for his father's return from concentration camp.

Palmisciano, Diane. *Garden Partners*. Atheneum, 1989. 4-up. A child and her grandmother plant, tend, and harvest a garden together.

Parker, Kristy. *My Dad the Magnificent*. Illus. Lillian Hoban. Dutton, 1987. 4–6. A child comes to appreciate his father.

Paterson, Katherine. *Park's Quest*. Dutton, 1988. 5–9. A child and his grandfather share guilt and grief after his father's death.

Peck, Robert Newton. *Spanish Hoof*. Knopf, 1985. 4–6. A child must face hard decisions during the Depression.

Pellowski, Anne. *Willow Wind Farm: Betsy's Story*. Illus. Wendy Watson. Philomel, 1981. 3–7. A year in the family life of a young girl from a midwestern farm family.

———. *Winding Valley Farm: Annie's Story*. Illus. Wendy Watson. Philomel, 1982. 4–6. A child's life on a Wisconsin farm in the early 1900s.

Potter, Marian. *A Chance Wild Apple*. Morrow, 1982. 4–6. The story of two children's struggles to subsist during the 1930s.

Rocklin, Joanne. *Dear Baby*. Illus. Eileen McKeating. Macmillan, 1988. 3–7. The changes in a family when a baby is expected.

•Rogers, Jean. *Goodbye, My Island*. Illus. Rie Muñoz. Greenwillow, 1983. 3–7. An Eskimo community's story of survival in a new home.

•Rosenberg, Maxine B. *Living in Two Worlds*. Photographs by George Ancona. Lothrop, Lee & Shepard, 1986. 1–4. A biracial marriage and the story of the child of the marriage.

Rüdstrom, Lennart. *A Family*. Illus. Carl Larsson. Putnam, 1980. 4–6. The story of the Swedish family of turn-of-the-century painter Carl Larsson.

Russo, Marisabina. *Why Do Grown-ups Have All the Fun?* Greenwillow, 1987. All ages. A child imagines her parents having a marvelous time during a typical evening at home.

Rylant, Cynthia. *A Blue-Eyed Daisy*. Bradbury, 1985. 5–7. A young girl works out her relationship with her troubled father.

•Sadler, Catherine Edwards. *Two Chinese Families*. Photographs by Alan Sadler. Atheneum, 1981. 5-up. The lifestyles of two Chinese families described.

Say, Allen. *The Lost Lake*. Houghton Mifflin, 1989. 4–8. A father shares his boyhood experiences with his son.

•Sebestyen, Ouida. *Words by Heart*. Little, Brown, 1979. 5–8. The only black family in a 1910 Texas community finds a way to survive.

Shura, Mary Frances. *The Josie Gambit*. Dodd, Mead, 1986. 5–8. A child has a tense stay with his grandmother, thanks to a chess opponent.

———. *The Sunday Doll*. Dodd, Mead, 1988. 5-up. A child learns to cope with problems at home during a visit with her aunt.

Slote, Alfred. *Moving In*. Trophy, 1989. 3–6. Two children try to sabotage their father's relationship with a business associate.

Smith, Doris Buchanan. *Return to Bitter Creek*. Viking Kestrel, 1986. 4–6. A family in Appalachia learns the meaning of grief and acceptance.

———. *Tough Chauncey*. Puffin, 1986. 4–6. A child learns to survive when sent to live with his brutal, abusive grandparents.

Smith, Robert Kimmel. *The War with Grandpa*. Illus. Richard Lauter. Delacorte, 1984. 3–5. A child declares war when his grandfather moves into his room.

Snyder, Zilpha Keatley. *Blair's Nightmare*. Atheneum, 1984. 4–7. A family unites when coping with danger presented by escaped convicts.

•Streich, Corrine, selector. *Grandparents' Houses*. Illus. Lillian Hoban. All ages. Greenwillow, 1984. Poetry from many cultures about the universality of family life.

Talbert, Marc. *Toby*. Dial, 1987. 4–6. A child deals with having parents who are mentally deficient with courage and strength.

•Taylor, Mildred. *Let the Circle Be Unbroken*. Dial, 1981. 4-up. A family deals with the Depression in Mississippi, united by love.

•———. *Roll of Thunder, Hear My Cry*. Dial, 1976. 5-up. A family refuses to give in to threats by their white neighbors.

•———. *The Gold Cadillac*. Illus. Michael Hays. Dial, 1987. 4–6. A loving black family deals with ignorance and prejudice while traveling from Ohio to Mississippi.

•Taylor, Sydney. *All-of-a-Kind Family*. Illus. Helen John. Dell, 1951. 3–6. Jewish family life in New York City.

Terry, Megan. *Family Talk*. Omaha Magic Theatre, 1417 Farnam St., Omaha, NE 68102. 5-up. Play about how a family can establish good interpersonal communication.

Thrasher, Crystal. *End of a Dark Road*. Atheneum, 1982. 4–6. A Depression-era child tells about her home and school life.

•Turnbull, Ann. *Maroo of the Winter Caves*. Clarion, 1984. 6-up. A story of an Ice Age family very similar to those in our times.

Turner, Ann. *Grasshopper Summer*. Macmillan, 1989. 3–7. A relocated farm family copes with the destruction of their crops.

•Uchida, Yoshiko. *The Best Bad Thing.* McElderry/Atheneum, 1983. 4–6. A Japanese-American family copes during the 1930s.

Voigt, Cynthia. *Homecoming.* Atheneum, 1981. 5-up. A child keeps her younger brothers and sister in tow alone against the world.

•Walter, Mildred Pitts. *Have a Happy.* Illus. Carole Byard. Lothrop, Lee & Shepard, 1989. 3–6. A family's sad circumstances change for the better during a holiday season.

•Watkins, Yoko Kawashima. *So Far from the Bamboo Grove.* Lothrop, Lee & Shepard, 1986. 4-up. A child tells of her family's escape from Korea to Japan at the end of World War II.

White, Ruth. *Sweet Creek Holler.* Farrar, Straus & Giroux, 1988. 6–8. An Appalachian family triumphs despite gossip and poverty in the 1950s.

•Wolf, Bernard. *In This Proud Land: The Story of a Mexican American Family.* Harper & Row, 1988. 4–6. Story of a family living in Texas.

Wright, Betty Ren. *Ghosts Beneath Our Feet.* Holiday, 1984. 3–7. Four people trying to become a family.

Cycle of Life

Atkin, Flora. *Grampo/Scampo.* New Plays, 1981. 4-up. Play about a family dealing with a grandparent who comes to live with them.

Bendick, Jeanne. *How Heredity Works: Why Living Things Are as They Are.* Parents, 1975. 3–5. Introduction to heredity in plants, animals, and people.

Dunbar, Robert E. *Heredity.* Watts, 1978. 4–9. Introduction to history of heredity.

Engdahl, Sylvia Louise, and Roberson, Rick. *Tool for Tomorrow.* Atheneum, 1979. 5–8. Recent studies and discoveries in genetics.

Fleischman, Paul. *The Borning Room.* Charlotte Zolotow/Harper Collins, 1991. 6-up. As Georgina lies dying in the room where she was born in 1851, she recalls her childhood on the Ohio frontier and contemplates the cycle of life and death.

•Flournoy, Valerie. *The Patchwork Quilt.* Illus. Jerry Pinckney. Dial, 1985. 2–5. A family stitches memories into a quilt and cares for an ailing grandmother.

The Four Musicians. San Diego, CA: Readers Theatre Script Service, P.O. Box 178333, San Diego, CA 92117. 5-up. Play about four aging animals off to seek their fortune in the city.

•Jennings, Coleman. *The Honorable Urashima Taro.* Woodstock, IL: The Dramatic Publishing Co., 1972. 4-up. Play about youth versus old age.

Khalsa, Dayal Kaur. *Tales of a Gambling Grandma.* Clarkson N. Potter, 1986. 2–5. A portrait of a young child's relationship with her offbeat Russian-born grandmother.

Martin, Judith. *Dandelion.* In *Plays Children Love, Vol. II.* Coleman A. Jennings and Aurand Harris, eds. St. Martin's, 1988. 4-up. A play about evolution, the life cycle, and culture.

McCaslin, Nellie. *Who Laughs Last?* In *Plays Children Love, Vol. II.* Coleman A. Jennings and Aurand Harris, eds. St. Martin's, 1988. 3-up. A play about old age and responsibility.

Miller, Kathryn Schultz. *The Shining Moment.* Anchorage Press, 1989. 5-up. Play about a grandfather who passes on memories to his grandson.

Adolescence

Bacon, Katharine Jay. *Pip and Emma.* McElderry, 1986. 4–7. A time of trial and maturity for a child spending the summer with grandmother.

Bates, Betty. *That's What T.J. Says.* Holiday House, 1989. 4–6. Two social misfits gain confidence after becoming friends.

Berger, Gilda. *PMS: Premenstrual Syndrome.* Watts, 1984. 5-up. Informational book on premenstrual syndrome.

Betancourt, Jeanne. *Dear Diary.* Avon Books, 1983. 5-up. Through her diary, a girl talks about the physical and emotional changes she is undergoing.

Bulla, Clyde Robert. *Charlie's House.* Illus. Arthur Dorros. Crowell/Harper & Row, 1983. 4–6. A child's role in eighteenth-century England and New World America.

Bush, Max. *Thirteen Bells of Boglewood.* Anchorage Press, 1986. 5-up. Play about rites of passage for a young boy into a larger universe.

Byars, Betsy. *The Burning Questions of Bingo Brown.* Viking, 1988. 4–6. A young boy goes through adolescent changes.

Chambers, Aidan. *The Present Takers.* Harper & Row, 1983. 5-up. A child must turn to her schoolmates for the solution to a problem.

Clarke, Barbara. *Conquering PreMenstrual Syndrome.* Franklin Press, 1987. 5-up. How to cope with premenstrual syndrome.

Cleaver, Vera, and Cleaver, Bill. *Trial Valley.* Lippincott, 1977. 5-up. An Appalachian orphan cares for her siblings and a new child.

Davis, Jenny. *Sex Education.* Orchard Books, 1988. 6-up. A young girl experiences love and loss with determination to go on.

Dobson, James. *Preparing for Adolescence.* Bantam, 1984. 6-up. A minister offers help to preteens on aspects of the adolescent experience.

Elgin, Kathleen, and Osterritter, John F. *Twenty-Eight Days.* McKay, 1973. 5–7. An informational book about the menstrual cycle and reproductive organs.

•Fritz, Jean. *Homesick: My Own Story.* Illus. Margot Tomes. Putnam, 1982. 5–7. A child grows up in China in the 1920s.

Gardner-Loulan, Joann, Lopez, Bonnie, and Quackenbush, Marcia. *Period.* Illus. Marcia Quackenbush. Volcano, 1981. 5–8. Facts and feelings about menstruation.

Gerber, Merrill Joan. *I'd Rather Think About Robby.* Harper & Row, 1989. 4–7. Adolescent relationships.

Greenberg, Jan. *Bye, Bye, Miss American Pie.* Farrar, Straus & Giroux, 1985. 6-up. A young girl learns to take control of her life.

Greene, Constance C. *Al's Blind Date*. Viking Kestrel, 1989. 5-up. Coping with the first date.

•Hall, Lynn. *Danza*. Aladdin, 1989. 3–7. A young boy learns responsibility and finds himself.

Holl, Kristi D. *No Strings Attached*. Atheneum, 1988. 3–7. Learning to deal with family life and older persons.

•Kral, Brian. *East of the Sun, West of the Moon*. Anchorage Press, 1987. 4-up. Play about a young girl who battles evil to save a young man from a curse.

Kurtzan, Harvey, and Preiss, Byron. *Nuts #1*. Bantam, 1985. 5–8. Adolescent life and problems presented humorously.

———. *Nuts #2*. Bantam, 1985. 5–8. Satirical parodies on adolescent life.

Lowry, Lois. *Rabble Starkey*. Houghton Mifflin, 1987. 5-up. An Appalachian child goes through many changes in sixth grade.

Ludwig, Volcker, and Lucker, Reiner. *Man Oh Man*. Jack Zipes, translator. In *Political Plays for Children*. Telos Press, 1976. 6-up. Play about a woman who marries a man of different social standards and the family's adjustment to a new life.

MacLachlan, Patricia. *Cassie Binegar*. Harper & Row, 1982. 4–6. A child learns to accept herself and her own world.

———. *The Facts and Fictions of Minna Pratt*. Harper & Row, 1988. 3–7. A child attempts to solve her own problems and finds independence.

McDonnell, Christine. *Count Me In*. Viking Kestrel, 1986. 5–9. A young girl copes with a new baby and finds a place in her family.

Mills, Claudia. *After Fifth Grade, the World!* Macmillan, 1989. 3–7. A child sets out to reform her teacher and her parents.

Mofid, Bijan. *The Butterfly*. Don Iaffon, translator. Anchorage Press, 1974. 6-up. Play about a butterfly who learns to consider others before herself.

Naylor, Phyllis Reynolds. *Alice in Rapture, Sort of*. Atheneum, 1989. 3–7. Dealing with the first romance.

Newton, Suzanne. *A Place Between*. Viking Kestrel, 1986. 5–9. A young girl copes with moving to a new town and gains maturity.

Noble, Iris. *Susan B. Anthony*. Messner, 1975. 6-up. The story of the crusader for women's rights.

Park, Barbara. *The Kid in the Red Jacket*. Knopf, 1987. 3–6. A child copes with moving to a new town and making new friends.

Pierce, Meredith Ann. *Birth of the Firebringer*. Four Winds, 1986. 3–6. A young unicorn comes of age.

Pople, Maureen. *The Other Side of the Family*. Holt, 1988. 5–8. A child learns about her family's history while staying with relatives in Australia during World War II.

•Riordan, James. *The Woman in the Moon and Other Tales of Forgotten Heroines*. Illus. Angela Barrett. Dial, 1985. 4-up. Tales featuring females who are bold, strong, and clever.

Rylant, Cynthia. *A Blue-Eyed Daisy*. Bradbury, 1985. 4-up. A young girl develops an understanding relationship with her father.

Sachs, Marilyn. *Almost Fifteen*. Dutton, 1987. 4–6. A young girl deals with new interests and relationships during early adolescence.

Selden, Bernice. *The Mill Girls: Lucy Larcom, Harriet Hanson Robinson and*

Sarah G. Bagley. Atheneum, 1983. 6-up. Three women who went to work during the Industrial Revolution and how work impacted on their lives.

Storch, Marcia, with Carmichael, Carrie. *How to Relieve Cramps and Other Menstrual Problems.* Workman, 1982. 5-up. An informational guide about menstruation with an exercise program.

Thomas, Jane Resh. *The Princess in the Pigpen.* Clarion, 1989. 3–7. A seventeenth-century princess is transported to an Iowa farm in the twentieth century and finds a way to return to her own world.

•Winther, Barbara. *The Princess Who Was Hidden from the World.* In *Plays from Folktales of Africa and Asia.* Boston: Plays, Inc., 1976. 4-up. Play about a father who learns to let go; the disadvantages of being sheltered from the world.

Yolen, Jane. *Dragon's Blood.* Delacorte, 1982. 6–8. A young boy and girl gain independence and maturity.

Relationships with Siblings

Adler, C. S. *Get Lost, Little Brother.* Clarion, 1983. 5–8. A young boy wins the respect and friendship of his older brothers.

———. *Split Sisters.* Macmillan, 1986. 4–8. Two sisters deal with their parent's separation.

Aliki. *Welcome, Little Baby.* Greenwillow, 1987. All ages. Dealing with the arrival of a new child in the family.

Arnold, Eric, and Loeb, Jeffrey, editors. *I'm Telling! Kids Talk About Brothers and Sisters.* Illus. G. Brian Karas. Little, Brown, 1987. 4–6. Children speak out about sibling relationships.

Auch, Mary Jane. *Pick of the Litter.* Holiday House, 1988. 3–7. A child must deal with family changes after the birth of quadruplets.

Blume, Judy. *The Pain and the Great One.* Illus. Irene Trivas. Bradbury, 1984. 4–6. A brother and sister tell about their rivalry with each other.

Bulla, Clyde. *Keep Running, Allen!* Crowell, 1978. 3–6. A child discovers the beauty of nature when older siblings reject him.

Chamberlain, Marisha. (Louisa May Alcott's) *Little Women.* Children's Theatre Company and School, 2400 3rd Avenue, South, Minneapolis, MN 55404. 4-up. Play based on the book chronicling the lives of four young sisters during the Civil War.

Fisher, Lois I. *Arianna and Me.* Dodd, Mead, 1986. 5–7. A twelve-year-old deals with adolescent problems.

Grimm, Jakob, and Grimm, Wilhelm. *The Seven Ravens.* Elizabeth D. Crawford, translator. Illus. Lisbeth Zwerger. Morrow, 1981. 2–5. A maiden rescues her seven brothers from a spell.

Hest, Amy. *Getting Rid of Krista.* Illus. Jacqueline Rogers. Morrow, 1988. 2–5. A child deals with the return of her college-age sister.

Kaye, Geraldine. *The Day After Yesterday.* Illus. Glenys Ambrus. Andre Deutsch, 1981. 4-up. A girl rescues her sister who has been sold into slavery in Hong Kong.

Landis, James David. *The Sisters Impossible.* Knopf, 1979. 4–6. Two sisters learn to cooperate while reversing roles.

Lively, Penelope. *Fanny's Sister.* Illus. Anita Lobel. Dutton, 1980. 4–6. A child deals with a new sibling.

Lord, Athena V. *Today's Special: Z.A.P. and Zoe.* Illus. Jean Jenkins. Macmillan, 1984. 2–5. Two Greek-American siblings growing up in New York in the late 1930s.

Martin, Ann M. *Me and Katie (the Pest).* Holiday House, 1985. 4–6. An older sibling learns to adjust to life with her gifted sister.

•McDonald, Joyce. *Mail-Order Kid.* Putnam, 1988. 4–6. A child develops a relationship with his newly adopted Korean brother.

•McHugh, Elisabet. *Karen's Sister.* Greenwillow, 1983. 5–7. A girl welcomes her new Korean sister.

McKenna, Colleen O'Shaughnessy. *Too Many Murphys.* Scholastic, 1988. 3–7. The eldest child learns to deal with her younger siblings.

Naylor, Phyllis Reynolds and Reynolds, Lura Schield. *Maudie in the Middle.* Illus. Judith Gwyn Brown. Atheneum, 1988. 2–6. A young farm girl copes with being the middle child.

Nelson, Theresa. *And One for All.* Orchard Books, 1989. 6–8. Letters home from a brother in Vietnam to his younger sister.

Orgel, Doris. *My War with Mrs. Galloway.* Illus. Carol Newsom. Viking Kestrel, 1985. 4–6. Two feuding sisters make up.

Park, Barbara. *Operation: Dump the Chump.* Knopf, 1982. 3–6. An older brother plans to get rid of his annoying sibling.

Pascal, Francine. *The Hand-Me-Down Kid.* Viking Kestrel, 1980. 4–6. An assertiveness training manual for the youngest in the family.

Ransom, Candice F. *My Sister, the Meanie.* Scholastic, 1988. 4–8. The ups and downs of sisterhood.

———. *My Sister, the Traitor.* Scholastic, 1989. 4–8. An older sibling with a job makes her sister feel left out.

Rocklin, Joanne. *Dear Baby.* Illus. Eileen McKeating. Harper & Row, 1988. 3–7. A child writes letters to her unborn sibling expressing her feelings.

Ross, Monica Long. *Wilma's Revenge.* Anchorage Press, 1989. 4-up. Play about a girl's struggles with her older brother who is a bully.

Spinelli, Jerry. *Who Put That Hair in My Toothbrush?* Little, Brown, 1984. 4–7. Two siblings are at war.

•Steptoe, John. *Mufaro's Beautiful Daughters.* Lothrop, Lee & Shepard, 1987. 4–6. African folktale about the relationship between two very dissimilar sisters.

Stevenson, Sucie. *Do I Have To Take Violet?* Dodd, Mead, 1987. 4–6. Can a sibling have a good time with a baby sister?

•Wilson, Johnniece Marshall. *Oh, Brother.* Scholastic, 1988. 3–7. The rivalry between two brothers who can't get along.

Grades Seven and Up

Human Sexuality

Aho, Jennifer S., and Petras, John J. *Learning about Sex: A Guide for Children and Their Parents.* Holt, 1978. 7–8. An informative guide on sex for parents and children with suggestions for its use.

Balis, Andrea. *What Are You Using?* Dial, 1981. 6-up. An objective discussion of various birth control methods.

Bell, Ruth, and other coauthors. *Changing Bodies, Changing Lives.* Random House, 1988. 7-up. A sex guide for young adults.

Benson, Michael D.. *Coping with Birth Control.* Rosen, 1988. 7-up. Explains the physical changes in adolescence and birth control methods.

Blume, Judy. *Forever.* Bradbury, 1975. 7-up. A rapidly progressing romance between two young adults—will it last?

Bode, Janet. *Kids Having Kids: The Unwed Teenage Parent.* Watts, 1980. 7-up. Teen sexuality and pregnancy through time and around the world.

Bowe-Gutman, Sonia. *Teen Pregnancy.* Illus. Donald Stewart. Lerner, 1987. 7-up. How to avoid pregnancy and options if you are pregnant.

Carlson, Dale. *Loving Sex for Both Sexes.* Watts, 1979. 7-up. The psychology and physiology of teen sex and its responsibilities.

Cole, William, ed. *A Book of Love Poems.* Viking, 1965. 5-up. Poems exploring sexuality and relationships.

Comfort, Alex, and Comfort, Jane. *Facts of Love: Living, Loving, and Growing Up.* Crown, 1980. 6-up. An open, honest look at sex.

Dunning, Stephen, et al., eds. *Reflections on a Gift of Watermelon Pickle . . . and Other Modern Verse.* Lothrop, Lee & Shepard, 1967. 5–9. A collection of poems including some about love.

Ewy, Donna, and Ewy, Rodger. *Teen Pregnancy: The Challenges We Faced, the Choices We Made.* Illus. Linda Gerrard Ely. New American Library, 1985. 7-up. Explains all aspects of pregnancy through methods of childbirth.

Eyerly, Jeannette. *Someone to Love Me.* Lippincott, 1987. 7-up. A young girl deals with pregnancy and responsibility.

Francke, Linda Bird. *The Ambivalence of Abortion.* Random House, 1978. 7-up. Feelings of adults and teens, male and female, about abortion.

Garden, Nancy. *Annie on My Mind.* Farrar, Straus & Giroux, 1982. 7-up. Two young girls deal with their love and their families' and friends' feelings about it.

Gilbert, Sara. *Feeling Good: A Book About You and Your Body.* Four Winds, 1978. 6–9. Body changes occurring during adolescence.

Gordon, Ruth. *Under All Silences, Shades of Love.* Harper & Row, 1987. 6-up. Love poems from classical to present times.

Gordon, Sol. *Facts About Sex for Today's Youth.* Illus. Vivien Cohen. Ed.-U. Press, 1987. 7-up. Facts about reproduction and sexuality.

Hamilton, Eleanor. *Sex with Love: A Guide for Young People.* Beacon, 1978. 7-up. An explanation of human sexuality.

Hanckel, Francis, and Cunningham, John. *A Way of Life, A Way of Love.* Lothrop, Lee & Shepard, 1979. 7-up. Differing points of view on human sexuality.

Head, Ann. *Mr. and Mrs. Bo Jo Jones.* Putnam, 1967. 7-up. A 16-year-old couple expecting a child cope with parents and personal problems.

Heron, Ann, ed. *One Teenager in 10: Writings by Gay and Lesbian Youth.* Alyson, 1983. 7-up. Letters from gay teens about their problems.

Hettlinger, Richard. *Growing up with Sex.* Seabury, 1971. 7-up. A liberal Christian perspective of human sexuality.

Hodges, Margaret. *The Gorgon's Head.* Illus. Charles Mikolaycak. Little, Brown, 1972. 4–8. Perseus saves a maiden from a sea monster and is made king.

Holbrook, Sabra. *Fighting Back: The Struggle for Gay Rights.* Lodestar Books, 1987. 7-up. Historical look at gay rights and attitudes toward homosexuality.

Holland, Isabelle. *The Man Without a Face.* Harper/Lippincott, 1972. 7-up. The many facets of love.

Homes, A. M. *Jack.* Macmillan, 1989. 7-up. A young adult deals with his father's homosexuality.

Janeczko, Paul, selector. *Going Over to Your Place.* Bradbury, 1987. 7-up. Poetry about relationships and loss.

Kaplan, Helen Singer. *Making Sense of Sex.* Illus. David Passalacqua. Simon & Schuster, 1979. 6-up. Explicit information about love and sex.

Kelly, Gary F. *Learning about Sex: The Contemporary Guide for Young Adults,* 3d ed. Barron's, 1986. 7-up. Understanding sexuality and sexual concerns.

Langone, John. *Like, Love, Lust: A View of Sex and Sexuality.* Little, Brown, 1980. 7-up. Facts to make informed decisions about sex.

Levy, Elizabeth. *Come Out Smiling.* Delacorte, 1981. 6–8. A young adult copes with the fact that her camp counselor is gay.

Mazer, Harry. *The Girl of His Dreams.* Harper/Crowell, 1987. 7-up. The realities of falling in love.

McCoy, Kathy, and Wibbelsman, Charles. *The Teenage Body Book.* Simon & Schuster, 1983. 7-up. Honest answers about changing bodies and emotions.

McGuire, Paula. *It Won't Happen to Me; Teenagers Talk About Pregnancy.* Delacorte, 1983. 7-up. Contraception, life choices, and sexual decision-making discussed.

Meyer, Carolyn. *Elliot & Win.* McElderry, 1986. 7-up. Adolescent life-styles, choices, and values.

Mintz, Thomas, and Mintz, Lorelle Miller. *Threshold. Straightforward Answers to Teenagers' Questions About Sex.* Illus. Loretta Mintz. Walker, 1978. 7-up. Questions and answers about puberty, sex, pregnancy, birth, and contraception.

Pascal, Francine. *My First Love and Other Disasters.* Viking Kestrel, 1979. 7-up. A teen sets out to get the man of her dreams.

Pomeroy, Wardell B. *Boys and Sex.* Delacorte, 1968. 6–8. Advice for teenage boys about sex.

Rich, Adrienne. *The Dream of a Common Language: Poems 1974–1977.* Norton, 1978. 5–8. Poems exploring sexuality and relationships.

Richards, Arlene Kramer, and Willis, Irene. *Under 18 and Pregnant: What to Do If You or Someone You Know Is.* Lothrop, Lee & Shepard, 1983. 7-up. Information for teens on pregnancy and single parenting.

Richardson, I. M. *The Adventures of Eros and Psyche.* Illus. Robert Baxter. Troll, 1983. 4–7. How Psyche proves her love for Eros.

Rinaldi, Ann. *The Good Side of My Heart.* Holiday House, 1987. 7up. A teen finds she is dating a homosexual and grapples with the fact.

Spinelli, Jerry. *Jason and Marceline.* Little, Brown, 1986. 7-up. A teen attempts to have a relationship with the opposite sex.

Terkel, Susan Neiburg. *Abortion; Facing the Issues.* Watts, 1988. 7-up. An examination of the abortion issue through history.

Topalian, Elyse. *Margaret Sanger.* Watts, 1984. 7-up. Biography of the woman who pioneered the birth control movement in the U.S.

Voss, Jacqueline, and Gale, Jay. *A Young Woman's Guide to Sex.* Holt & Co., 1987. 7-up. Guide to sex and sexuality for young women.

Wangerlin, Walter J. *The Book of the Dun Cow.* Harper & Row, 1978. 5–8. A rooster's domain is threatened; story of love between the rooster and his bride.

Warren Lindsay, Jeanne. *Parents, Pregnant Teens and the Adoption Option.* Morning Glory Press, 1989. 6-up. Advice for the parents of pregnant teenagers.

Witt, Reni L. and Michael, Jeannine Masterson. *Mom, I'm Pregnant.* Stein and Day, 1982. 6-up. Options available to pregnant teens.

Family Life

Adler, Carole. *The Cat That Was Left Behind.* Clarion, 1981. 4-up. Parallel between a foster child and a stray cat; foster child begins to accept warmth of new foster family as he tames and cares for the cat.

Adler, C. S. *Split Sisters.* Macmillan, 1986. 5–8. A child tries to keep her parents from separating and changing her and her sister's lives.

Ancona, George. *Growing Older.* Dutton, 1978. 6-up. Remembrances of elderly Americans.

Angell, Judie. *What's Best for You.* Bradbury, 1981. 6-up. The effects of divorce on an adolescent and on the other family members.

Bethancourt, T. Ernesto. *T.H.U.M.B.B.* Holiday House, 1983. 7-up. Two friends form a band to march in the St. Patrick's Day parade.

Block, Francesca Lia. *Weetzie Bat.* Harper & Row, 1988. 7-up. A teen from a broken home and a young gay friend make a home.

Byars, Betsy. *The Pinballs.* Harper & Row, 1977. 5-up. Three neglected or abused children are placed in a foster home.

Calvert, Patricia. *Yesterday's Daughter.* Scribner's, 1986. 7-up. A mother comes back to attempt to establish a relationship with her teenage daughter, abandoned by her at birth.

Carter, Alden R. *Wart, Son of Toad.* Pacer, 1986. 6–8. A boy and his widowed father learn to communicate.

Carter, Peter. *Bury the Dead.* Farrar, Straus & Giroux, 1987. 7-up. A long-gone relative causes chaos in an East Berlin family when he returns.

Clements, Bruce. *Anywhere Else But Here.* Farrar, Straus & Giroux, 1980. 6–9. A teen's problems dealing with a single parent and many unscrupulous adults who enter her family's life.

Cohen, Shari. *Coping with Being Adopted.* Rosen, 1988. 6-up. Explains that feelings and frustrations of teens are normal; deals with adoption.

Collura, Mary-Ellen Lang. *Winners.* Dial, 1986. 6-up. A foster child tries to fit in when he goes to live with his grandfather.

Colman, Hila. *Weekend Sisters.* Morrow, 1985. 7-up. Coping with a father's remarriage and a stepsister.

Conrad, Pam. *Holding Me Here.* Harper & Row, 1986. 7-up. A child interferes during her parents' divorce.

Cookson, Catherine. *Lanky Jones.* Lothrop, Lee & Shepard, 1981. 6-up. A story of the complexity of family life.

Cresswell, Helen. *Dear Shrink.* Macmillan, 1982. 6-up. Three children are sent to foster homes when their nanny dies while their parents are on a trip.

Danziger, Paula. *Remember Me to Harold Square.* Delacorte, 1988. 6–8. Three children see New York with their parents.

———. *The Divorce Express.* Delacorte, 1982. 7-up. A child spends part of each week with her divorced parents.

•Dunlop, Beverley. *The Poetry Girl.* Houghton Mifflin, 1989. 5–9. A family moves twice and deals with the father's attempted suicide.

Eige, Lillian. *Cady.* Illus. Janet Wentworth. Harper & Row, 1987. 6–8. A child passed around all his life pieces together his past.

Fleischman, Paul. *Rear-View Mirrors.* Harper & Row, 1986. 7-up. A child goes east to live with her father and recounts the past year.

Forman, James D. *Cry Havoc.* Scribner's, 1988. 7-up. A father realizes how he has manipulated his problem daughter and begins to rebuild their relationship.

Fox, Paula. *The Moonlight Man.* Bradbury, 1986. 7-up. A child spends a month with her father and must deal with his drinking and her own feelings about him.

Froehlich, Margaret Walden. *Reasons To Stay.* Houghton Mifflin, 1986. 6-up. The problems of the eldest child in a single-parent family.

Gardner, Richard. *The Boys and Girls Book about Divorce.* Bantam, 1974. 5–9. How to cope with parents' marital problems.

•Gay, Kathlyn. *The Rainbow Effect: Interracial Families.* Watts, 1987. 7-up. The problems of a child in an interracial family in America; children tell their own stories.

•Gilson, Jamie. *Hello, My Name Is Scrambled Eggs.* Illus. John Wallner. Lothrop, Lee & Shepard, 1985. 5–8. A child tries to Americanize a Vietnamese visitor to his family.

•Greenfield, Eloise, and Little, Lessie Jones, with Jones, Pattie Ridley. *Childtimes: A Three-Generation Memoir.* Illus. Jerry Pinckney. Crowell,

1979. 7-up. Black women from three generations reminisce about their childhoods.

•———. *Grandpa's Face.* Illus. Floyd Cooper. Philomel, 1988. 7-up. A child learns to understand her grandfather.

Guest, Elissa Haden. *Over the Moon.* Morrow, 1986. 7-up. A child learns to deal with life after the death of her parents.

Hales, Dianne. *The Family.* Chelsea House, 1988. 6-up. An informational book about the family and its future.

•Hamilton, Dorothy. *Winter Caboose.* Illus. James Converse. Herald, 1983. 5-up. A child decides whether to welcome his wayward father.

Hinton, S. E. *Rumble Fish.* Delacorte, 1975. 7-up. A child deals with the death of his brother after a robbery the brother committed.

Howker, Janni. *Badger on the Barge and Other Stories.* Greenwillow, 1985. 7-up. Stories about relationships between young people and old.

———. *The Nature of the Beast.* Greenwillow, 1985. 7-up. A child deals with the effects of a strike in his British mill town.

Hurwitz, Johanna. *DeDe Takes Charge!* Illus. Diane de Groat. Morrow, 1984. 5-up. A child helps her mother deal with the father's abandonment of the family.

Hyde, Margaret O. *Foster Care and Adoption.* Watts, 1982. 6-up. Examines the problem of unwanted children.

•Jenness, Aylette, and Rivers, Alice. *In Two Worlds: A Yup'ik Eskimo Family.* Houghton Mifflin, 1989. 5–9. A photodocumentary of a modern-day Eskimo family.

Jensen, Kathryn. *Pocket Change.* Macmillan, 1989. 7-up. A child's father has post-traumatic syndrome due to service in Vietnam.

Johnston, Norma. *The Potter's Wheel.* Morrow, 1988. 7-up. A child deals with her mother's abandonment of the family.

Jones, Adrienne. *Street Family.* Harper & Row, 1987. 7-up. A group of homeless people in a big city form a family.

Klass, Sheila Solomon. *The Bennington Stitch.* Scribner's, 1985. 7-up. A mother and daughter learn to cooperate.

Klein, David, and Klein, Marymae E. *Your Parents and Your Self.* Scribner's, 1986. 7-up. Discusses the biological and psychological bonds between parents and children.

Klein, Norma. *Breaking Up.* Avon, 1980. 6-up. A teenager's feelings when parents divorce.

Konigsburg, E. L. *Journey to an 800 Number.* Atheneum, 1982. 7-up. A child of divorce learns what things in life are really valuable.

Kosof, Anna. *Why Me? Coping with Family Illness.* Watts, 1986. 6-up. Young people who are coping with a chronic or fatal disease and how it affects their lives.

Krementz, Jill. *How It Feels to Be Adopted.* Knopf, 1982. 4–9. Interviews with children on their experiences with adoption.

Landis, J. D. *Daddy's Girl.* Morrow, 1984. 7-up. Should a child keep to herself a secret she doesn't understand?

Levitin, Sonia. *A Season for Unicorns*. Atheneum, 1986. 5–9. A child learns she is not responsible for her parents' flaws.

Lindard, Joan. *Strangers in the House*. Lodestar Books, 1981. 5–9. A child adjusts to new stepsiblings and a new parent.

Lutz, Norma Jean. *Good-bye, Beedee*. Cook, 1986. 6–8. A child moves to the city with her father and his new wife and tries to adjust.

Lyon, George Ella. *Borrowed Children*. Orchard Books, 1988. 5–7. A child learns responsibility during the Depression in Kentucky.

Lysander, Per, and Osten, Suzanne. *Medea's Children*. Ann-Charlotte Harvey, translator. New Plays, 1985. 7-up. Play about children dealing with divorce in two different times.

MacLachlan, Patricia. *The Facts and Fictions of Minna Pratt*. Harper & Row, 1988. 6–8. A child with an eccentric family learns about the truth.

Major, Kevin. *Dear Bruce Springsteen*. Delacorte, 1988. 7-up. A child's letters to his idol reflect his feelings about his parents' separation and other teen problems.

Martin, Ann. *Bummer Summer*. Holiday House, 1983. 7-up. A child comes to accept her new family during summer camp.

Mazer, Norma Fox. *After the Rain*. Morrow, 1987. 7-up. A child develops a loving relationship with her difficult grandfather.

———. *Downtown*. Morrow, 1984. 7-up. A child comes to accept his fugitive parents.

———. *Three Sisters*. Scholastic, 1986. 7-up. Relationships among three sisters.

McGraw, Eloise. *Hideaway*. Atheneum, 1983. 6–8. A child copes with a new family and a relationship with a new babysitter.

McHugh, Elisabet. *Karen and Vicki*. Greenwillow Books, 1984. 6–8. A child tries to organize her family for a school project.

———. *Raising a Mother Isn't Easy*. Greenwillow, 1983. 7-up. An adopted Korean child tries to find a mate for her mother.

McKenna, Colleen O'Shaughnessy. *Too Many Murphys*. Scholastic, 1988. 3–7. A child with pesky siblings longs to be an only child.

Melwood, Mary. *The Tingalary Bird*. Rowayton, CT: New Plays, 1969. 6-up. Play about the relationship between two elderly people.

Miller, Sandy. *Freddie the Thirteenth*. New American Library, 1985. 6–8. A child with thirteen brothers and sisters pretends to be one of two siblings and is found out.

Mills, Claudia. *All the Living*. Macmillan, 1983. 7-up. Two children learn to cope with death and feelings of inadequacy.

Murrow, Liza Ketchum. *Fire in the Heart*. Holiday House, 1989. 7-up. A child attempts to find out about her deceased mother.

•Myers, Walter Dean. *Won't Know Till I Get There*. Viking Kestrel, 1982. 6-up. A child learns to accept a foster brother.

Naylor, Phyllis Reynolds. *The Solomon System*. Atheneum, 1983. 5–9. Two brothers cope with their parents' divorce.

Newton, Suzanne. *A Place Between*. Viking Kestrel, 1986. 7-up. A child tries to cling to youth when facing adolescence.

————. *I Will Call It Georgie's Blues.* Viking Kestrel, 1983. 7-up. Tenuous relationships in a small-town preacher's family.

Nixon, Joan Lowery. *And Maggie Makes Three.* Harcourt, 1986. 6–8. A child copes with meeting her father's new wife.

————. *Maggie, Too.* Harcourt, 1985. 6–9. The comfort of a grandparent when things go wrong in the family.

O'Neal, Zibby. *In Summer Light.* Viking Kestrel, 1985. 7-up. A child finds her own talents.

Osborne, Mary Pope. *Love Always, Blue.* Dutton, 1984. 6–8. A child copes with her parents' separation and father's illness.

Pascal, Francine. *Hangin' Out with Cici.* Viking Kestrel, 1977. 7-up. A conflict between a girl and her mother.

Paterson, Katherine. *Jacob I Have Loved.* Harper & Row, 1980. 6–9. Rivalry between two very different sisters.

————. *The Great Gilly Hopkins.* Crowell, 1978. 5–9. A child wreaks havoc in her third foster family.

Paulsen, Gary. *The Winter Room.* Orchard Books, 1989. 6–9. Two brothers grow up while listening to their uncle's stories of his past.

Pearson, Gayle. *Fish Friday.* Atheneum, 1986. 5–9. Story of a girl's problems when her mother leaves the family to study art in New York.

Pfeffer, Susan Beth. *The Year without Michael.* Bantam, 1987. 7-up. A year in the life of a family whose son has disappeared from his sister's perspective.

Powledge, Fred. *So You're Adopted.* Scribner's, 1982. 6-up. Attitudes, experiences, and questions of adopted children.

Putterman, Ron. *To Find My Son.* Avon, 1981. 7-up. Story of a single-parent adoption.

Rabinowitz, Ann. *Bethie.* Macmillan, 1989. 7-up. The things a child learns during a divorce.

Roberts, Willo Davis. *Megan's Island.* Atheneum, 1988. 6–9. A child searches her past for a secret.

Robinson, Barbara. *My Brother Louis Measures Worms.* Harper & Row, 1988. 5–8. Ten stories about a family, friends, relatives, and their problems.

•Ron-Feder, Galila. *To Myself.* Linda Stern Zisquit, translator. Illus. Irwin Rosenhouse. Adama Books, 1987. 5–8. A child keeps a diary about living in Israel as a foster child.

Rosofsky, Iris. *Miriam.* Harper & Row, 1988. 7-up. A child finds her place in an Orthodox Jewish family.

Rudstrom, Lennart. *A Family.* Illus. Carl Larsson. G. P. Putnam's Sons, 1980. 7-up. An artist uses his family as the basis for his work as an artist.

Sachs, Marilyn. *Just Like a Friend.* Dutton, 1989. 5–9. A family crisis helps a girl to understand herself and her mother.

Silverstein, Alvin, and Silverstein, Virginia B. *Aging.* Watts, 1979. 6–9. An explanation of the aging process.

Smith, Doris Buchanan. *Tough Chauncey.* Viking Penguin, 1986. 5–8. A child learns what toughness really is.

Smucker, Barbara. *Amish Adventure.* Herald Press, 1983. 5–7. The contrast between urban life and Amish family life.

Snyder, Anne. *First Step.* Holt, 1975. 7-up. A child copes with her divorced mother's alcoholism.

Sommer, Sarah. *And I'm Stuck with Joseph.* Illus. Ivan Moon. Herald Press, 1983. 5–8. A child copes with an adoptive brother.

Springstubb, Tricia. *Which Way to the Nearest Wilderness?* Little, Brown, 1984. 7-up. A child wishes to escape family problems.

Stone, Bruce. *Half Nelson, Full Nelson.* Harper & Row, 1985. 5–8. A child attempts to cope with his parents' separation.

Streich, Corrine, compiler. *Grandparents' Houses: Poems about Grandparents.* Illus. Lillian Hoban. Greenwillow, 1984. 7-up. Poems about relationships between children and their grandparents.

Swindells, Robert. *Brother in the Land.* Holiday House, 1989. 7-up. A brother and sister struggle to survive after a nuclear war.

•Thomas, Joyce Carol. *The Golden Pasture.* Scholastic, 1986. 7-up. A child learns to communicate with his emotionally distant father.

Tolan, Stephanie S. *The Great Skinner Enterprise.* Four Winds, 1986. 6–8. A family attempts to run a business together.

———. *The Great Skinner Homestead.* Four Winds, 1988. 6–8. A family decides to live without modern conveniences.

———. *The Great Skinner Strike.* New American Library, 1985. 6–8. A mother strikes against her family.

Van Raven, Pieter. *The Great Man's Secret.* Scribner's, 1987. 7-up. A handicapped writer attempts to confront his past.

Voigt, Cynthia. *A Solitary Blue.* Atheneum, 1983. 7-up. A child's mother who abandoned him attempts to come back into his life.

———. *Building Blocks.* Atheneum, 1984. 5–7. A child is transported back in time to his father's childhood in the 1930s.

———. *Homecoming.* Macmillan, 1981. 7-up. Three abandoned children travel to their grandmother's in hopes of making a home with her.

———. *Seventeen Against the Dealer.* Atheneum, 1989. 7-up. A young woman struggles to have a better life and finds herself.

———. *Sons from Afar.* Atheneum, 1987. 7-up. Brothers search for the father who deserted them as infants.

———. *Tree by Leaf.* Atheneum, 1988. 6-up. A twelve-year-old accepts the history of her family.

Wallace-Brodeur, Ruth. *Steps in Time.* McElderry, 1986. 7-up. A child's growing relationship with her grandmother during a summer in Maine.

Wersba, Barbara. *Run Softly, Go Fast.* Atheneum, 1970. 7-up. A young man attempts to reconcile his poor relationship with his father.

•Wilkinson, Brenda. *Ludell and Willie.* Harper & Row, 1977. 6-up. A young black girl struggles with an ailing grandparent and with problems at school and at work.

Williams, Barbara. *Mitzi's Honeymoon with Nana Potts.* Illus. Emily Arnold McCully. Dell, 1983. 6–8. A child learns to get along with new stepbrothers.

Wolitzer, Hilma. *Toby Lived Here*. Farrar, Straus & Giroux, 1978. 6–9. A child learns to get along in a foster home after her mother is sent to a mental institution.

Wolkoff, Judie. *Where the Elf King Sings*. Bradbury, 1980. 6-up. A child deals with her father's problems of alcoholism and post-traumatic syndrome.

Zeder, Suzan. *Doors*. Anchorage Press, 1985. 5-up. Play about a child who uses fantasy to escape his parents' separation.

————. *Other Doors*. Anchorage, 1981. 5-up. Play about a child living with one parent, resenting his father's girlfriend.

————. *The Play Called Noah's Flood*. Anchorage Press, 1984. 6-up. Play about medieval times in which a son wants to join the army against his father's wishes.

Adolescence

Allan, Mabel Esther. *The Mills Down Below*. Dodd, Mead, 1981. 6-up. A child must make decisions during the summer of 1914 about women's suffrage and family loyalty.

Bell, Ruth. *Changing Bodies, Changing Lives*. Random House, 1987. 7-up. Discussions of teen sexuality focused on physical and emotional changes that occur during adolescence.

Blume, Judy. *Just as Long as We're Together*. Orchard Books, 1987. 5–8. Explores the customs, lifestyles, and mores of preteen girls.

Cohen, Shari. *Coping with Failure*. Rosen, 1988. 6-up. Deals with fear of failure, success, and developing a positive attitude about oneself.

Cross, Gillian. *Chartbreaker*. Holiday House, 1987. 7-up. Story of a British rock star and her feelings of rage.

Eagan, Andrea Boroff. *Why Am I So Miserable If These Are the Best Years of My Life?* Avon, 1988. 6-up. Discusses knowing your body, feeling good about yourself, making your own decisions, and talking about your feelings with others.

Ethridge, Kenneth E. *Toothpick*. Holiday House, 1989. 7-up. A child deals with teasing over a friendship with a terminally ill girl.

Foley, June. *Love by Any Other Name*. Delacorte, 1983. 6–8. Story of a first love.

Fox, Paula. *Blowfish Live in the Sea*. Bradbury, 1970. 6-up. Siblings deal with an alcoholic father and with their own relationship.

Gallo, Donald R., ed. *Sixteen: Short Stories by Outstanding Writers for Young Adults*. Delacorte, 1984. 7-up. Collection of short stories concerned with friendship, family, school, and love.

————. *Visions: Nineteen Short Stories by Outstanding Writers for Young Adults*. Delacorte, 1987. 7-up. Short stories of adolescence and discovery.

Gardner-Loulan, Joann, Lopez, Bonnie, and Quackenbush, Marcia. *Period*. Illus. Marcia Quackenbush. My Mama's Press, 1979. 6–8. A book on menstruation.

Greenberg, Jan. *Exercises of the Heart*. Farrar, Straus & Giroux, 1986. 7-up. A child copes with her mother's stroke and her friend's problems with an alcoholic mother.

Guernsey, JoAnn Bren. *Five Summers*. Clarion, 1983. 7-up. The events are detailed in five summers of a girls' life, including parental cancer, first love, and physical and emotional changes.

Hall, Lynn. *The Solitary*. Scribner's, 1986. 7-up. A woman copes with a tragic past and attempts to reconcile with her mother and begin her own business.

————. *Where Have All the Tigers Gone?* Scribner's, 1987. 7-up. A woman reminisces about her adolescent years and the changes life has brought her.

Hawley, Richard. *Shining Still*. Farrar, Straus & Giroux, 1989. 7-up. Two teens discover real love and must deal with their feelings.

Hunter, Mollie. *Hold On to Love*. Harper & Row, 1983. 7-up. A young woman seeks independence and a writing career.

Khomsky, Pavel. *Hey There—Hello!* In *Russian Plays for Young Audiences*. Miriam Morton, translator and editor. New Plays Books, 1977. 6-up. Explores psychological and emotional changes during adolescence.

Killien, Christi. *Rusty Fertlanger, Lady's Man*. Houghton Mifflin, 1988. 6–8. A boy faces losing to a girl opponent in his first wrestling match.

Kropp, Lloyd. *Greencastle*. Freundlich, 1987. 7-up. Difficulties faced by an awkward high school student in the 1950s.

Lambert, Beth. *The Riddle Machine*. In *Contemporary Children's Theatre*. Betty Jean Lifton, editor. Avon, 1974. 6-up. Play about a group of children who rebel against a robot and strike out for individuality.

Leslie, F. Andrew, adaptor. *Paul Zindel's The Pigman*. Dramatists Plays Service, 1975. 6-up. Two adolescents have a relationship with an older man that changes their lives.

Lieberman, Douglas L. *Starman Jones*. In *Contemporary Children's Theater*. Betty Jean Lifton, editor. Avon, 1974. 6-up. Play about a stowaway on a spaceship who proves his worth and takes his place as ship astrologer.

Lyon, George Ella. *Borrowed Children*. Orchard Books, 1988. 7-up. A Depression-era story of a child's discovery of her mother's past and the family's present.

————. *Red Rover, Red Rover*. Orchard Books, 1989. 6–9. A child deals with her mother's grief over the death of her grandfather.

Madaras, Lynda, and Saavedra, Dane. *The What's Happening to My Body? Book for Boys*. Newmarket Press, 1988. 6-up. Information on physical and emotional changes boys go through during puberty.

————. *The What's Happening to My Body? Book for Girls*. Newmarket Press, 1988. 6-up. Information on the physical and emotional changes occurring during puberty.

Mahoney, Ellen Voelckers. *Now You've Got Your Period*. Rosen, 1988. 6-up. Information on menstruation, reproduction, and physical and emotional changes during puberty.

•Miklowitz, Gloria D. *The War between the Classes*. Dell, 1986. 6-up. The rocky relationship between adolescents from two very different backgrounds.

Nourse, Alan E. *Menstruation: Just Plain Talk.* Watts, 1987. 6-up. Explains the physiological and emotional changes undergone by the female body at this time.

Powledge, Fred. *You'll Survive!* Scribner's, 1986. 6–8. Advice for adolescents with problems from an array of experts.

Rostkowski, Margaret I. *After the Dancing Days.* Harper & Row, 1988. 5–9. A girl goes to work at a veteran's hospital during World War I, despite her mother's insistence that she avoid it.

Rylant, Cynthia. *Waiting to Waltz.* Illus. Stephen Gammell. Bradbury, 1984. 6–8. Poetry about a girl growing up.

Sachs, Elizabeth-Ann. *Where Are You, Cow Patty?* Atheneum, 1984. 6–8. Explores the experiences of the beginning of adolescence.

Sachs, Marilyn. *Fourteen.* Dutton, 1983. 6-up. Tells of a teen's first fulfilling romance.

Simon, Nissa. *Don't Worry, You're Normal.* Harper & Row, 1982. 7-up. Guide to self-health for teens.

•Smith, Rukshana. *Sumitra's Story.* Coward, 1983. 7-up. Problems of race, changing mores, family, and role of women are issues for an East Indian girl.

Steiner, Barbara. *Tessa.* Morrow, 1988. 7-up. A child deals with divorce and choosing between parents in the 1940s.

Thompson, Julian F. *Goofbang Value Daze.* Scholastic, 1989. 6-up. A view of teenage life in the future.

Vedral, Joyce L. *I Dare You.* Holt, 1984. 6-up. Suggestions to improve teens' self-esteem.

Voigt, Cynthia. *A Solitary Blue.* Atheneum, 1983. 7-up. Ten years of a boy's life depicted.

Weiman, Eiveen. *Which Way Courage.* Atheneum, 1981. 5–9. An Amish girl decides she wants a different life for herself.

Wersba, Barbara. *Beautiful Losers.* Harper & Row, 1988. 7-up. A budding writer tries living with an older man.

Weston, Carol. *Girltalk About Guys: Real Questions, Real Answers.* Harper & Row, 1988. 7-up. Answers to questions all girls ask, from friendship to serious dating.

Social/Cultural Forces That Influence Health Behavior

Benedict, Helen. *Safe, Strong, and Streetwise.* Little, Brown, 1987. 7-up. How to protect oneself from sexual assault.

Brancato, Robin Fidler. *Blinded by the Light.* Knopf, 1978. 6-up. Contemporary look at religious cults and mind control.

Branscum, Robbie. *Johnny May Grows Up.* Illus. Bob Marstall. Harper & Row, 1987. 4–7. A child deals with adolescent problems and grows to meet the world around her.

Bridgers, Sue Ellen. *Permanent Connections.* Harper & Row, 1987. 7-up. A young adult deals with drugs, alcohol, and school problems.

Chomet, Julian. *Cocaine and Crack.* Illus. Peter Harper. Watts, 1987. 7-up.

Information on where crack and cocaine come from and their effects on the body.

Colman, Hila. *Accident*. Morrow, 1980. 7-up. A motorcycle accident leaves one teen paralyzed and one unharmed to live with guilt.

Dolmetsch, Paul, and Mauricette, Gail, eds. *Teens Talk about Alcohol and Alcoholism*. Doubleday, 1987. 7-up. Young people's stories about how alcoholism affects their lives, families, and friends.

Eagles, Douglas A. *Nutritional Diseases*. Watts, 1987. 6-up. Discusses diseases related to nutrition.

Ferris, Jean. *Looking for Home*. Farrar, Straus & Giroux, 1988. 7-up. A teen deals with pregnancy without family help.

Goldberg, Moses. *The Analysis of Mineral #4*. Anchorage Press, 1982. 6-up. Play about a high school chemistry student and her life.

Graczyk, Ed. *Runaway*. Anchorage Press, 1977. 5-up. Play about a runaway who finds a family among others like him.

Greenberg, Jan. *The Pig-Out Blues*. Farrar, Straus & Giroux, 1982. 7-up. A realization that a girl must take control of her own life and her weight problem.

Hawkes, Nigel. *AIDS*. Illus. Hayward Associates. Gloucester, 1987. 6-up. General information about AIDS including current treatment programs.

Holland, Isabelle. *Heads You Win, Tails I Lose*. Lippincott, 1973. 6-up. A teen with weight problems also deals with her mother's alcoholism and parents' arguments.

Kerr, M. E. *Night Kites*. Harper & Row, 1986. 7-up. A boy learns his older brother has AIDS and must deal with his brother and the family.

Kuklin, Susan. *Fighting Back: What Some People Are Doing About AIDS*. Putnam, 1989. 7-up. Chronicles nine months spent with a team of volunteers working with AIDS patients in New York City.

Langone, John. *Bombed, Buzzed, Smashed . . . Or Sober: A Book About Alcohol*. Little, Brown, 1976. 7-up. Summarizes the various theories on alcohol use and abuse for young people.

Lee, Essie E. *Breaking the Connection: How Young People Achieve Drug-Free Lives*. Messner, 1988. 6-up. Eight first-person accounts of substance abuser's lifestyles are detailed.

•Liss, Howard. *The Lawrence Taylor Story*. Enslow, 1987. 7-up. Describes the linebacker's career and his comeback after drug abuse problems.

Magorian, Michelle. *Back Home*. Harper & Row, 1984. 7-up. A child tries to readjust to her family after returning to postwar England from the United States.

•Mathis, Sharon Bell. *Teacup Full of Roses*. Viking Kestrel, 1972. 6-up. Devastating effects of drug abuse on an entire family.

McCoy, Kathy, and Wibbelsman, Charles. *The New Teenage Body Book*. The Body Press, 1987. 7-up. Resource for teen health questions, including section on AIDS.

Metos, Thomas H. *Communicable Diseases*. Watts, 1987. 5-up. How diseases such as the cold are spread.

Mohun, Janet. *Drugs, Steroids and Sports*. Watts, 1988. 6-up. Explains steroid abuse and side effects.

•Myers, Walter Dean. *Motown and Didi: A Love Story.* Viking Kestrel, 1984. 7-up. A girl deals with her mother's mental deterioration and brother's drug addiction.

Nourse, Alan E. *Birth Control.* Watts, 1988. 7-up. Factual presentation of the array of birth control methods available today.

O'Dell, Scott. *Kathleen, Please Come Home.* Houghton Mifflin, 1978. 7-up. Deals with abuse of drugs, runaways, and values.

Perl, Lila. *Fat Glenda's Summer Romance.* Clarion, n.d. 6-up. An overweight teen has her first crush and first summer job.

Rench, Janice E. *Teen Sexuality: Decisions and Choices.* Lerner, 1988. 6-up. Covers date rape, pornography, and peeping, among the usual questions about teen sexuality.

Reynolds, Pamela. *Will the Real Monday Please Stand Up.* Lothrop, Lee & Shepard, 1975. 6-up. A teen deals with her brother's addiction and arrest for marijuana possession.

Shaw, Diana. *Make the Most of a Good Thing: You!: What You Need to Know about Exercise, Diet, Stress, Sexuality, Relationships & More.* Atlantic, 1986. 5–8. Advice about coping with adolescent problems and confusion.

Silverstein, Alvin, and Silverstein, Virginia B. *Heart Disease.* Follett, 1976. 6–9. Introduction to cardiovascular disease, prevention, and treatment.

Snyder, Anne. *My Name Is Davy—I'm an Alcoholic.* Holt, 1977. 6-up. Dealing with alcoholism and peer pressure.

Sonnett, Sherry. *Smoking.* Watts, 1988. 5–6. The history of smoking and its side effects.

Sterling, Pamela. *Scrapbooks.* Muny/Student Theatre Project, 4219 Laclede St., St. Louis, MO 63108. 6-up. Play about struggles of two girls who are unwed mothers.

Trivers, James. *I Can Stop Any Time I Want.* Prentice-Hall, 1974. 7-up. Story of a teen who sells drugs to support his own habit.

E. NUTRITION

Grades K Through Three

Personal and Ethnic Variations in Foods

Alcott, Louisa May. *An Old-Fashioned Thanksgiving.* Illus. Michael McCurdy. Holiday House, 1989. 3–7. The children of a family decide to prepare a holiday meal by themselves, with disastrous results.

Boujon, Claude. *Bon Appétit, Mr. Rabbit!* McElderry, 1987. K–4. A rabbit learns that his own diet is best for his health.

Brown, Marc, and Krensky, Stephen. *Perfect Pigs: An Introduction to Manners.* Little, Brown, 1983. Pres.–3. A first guide to manners.

Burningham, John. *Avocado Baby.* Harper & Row, 1982. Pres.–1. A child becomes brave and strong, thanks to eating avocados.

Cobb, Vicki. *Feeding Yourself.* Illus. Marilyn Hafner. Lippincott, 1989. K–3. The story of eating implements.

Demarest, Chris L. *No Peas for Nellie.* Macmillan, 1988. Pres.–2. Story about a child's disliking for peas.

•Friedman, Ina R. *How My Parents Learned to Eat.* Illus. Allen Say. Houghton Mifflin, 1984. K–3. A Japanese-American girl tells the story of her parents' courtship.

Gibbons, Gail. *Thanksgiving Day.* Holiday House, 1989. K–3. Origins and traditions of Thanksgiving.

Hoban, Russell. *Bread and Jam for Frances.* Harper & Row, 1964. K–3. A child learns that you can have too much of a good thing.

Joly-Berbesson, Fanny, and Boucher, Brigitte. *Marceau Bonappétit.* Illus. Agnes Mathieu. Carolrhoda, 1989. Pres.–3. Not every family eats the same kinds of things.

•Kessel, Joyce K. *Squanto and the First Thanksgiving.* Illus. Lisa Donze. Carolrhoda, 1983. K–3. Explains the history of the first Thanksgiving.

Kroll, Steven. *Oh, What a Thanksgiving!* Illus. S. D. Schindler. Scholastic, 1988. K 3. A child imagines celebrating the holiday in 1620.

Morris, Ann. *Bread, Bread, Bread.* Photographs by Ken Heyman. Lothrop, Lee & Shepard, 1989. Pres.–2. All about bread.

Sharmat, Mitchell. *Gregory, the Terrible Eater.* Illus. Jose Aruego and Ariane Dewey. Four Winds, 1980. K–3. Explains the diet of a goat and the need to eat the proper foods.

Snow, Pegeen. *Eat Your Peas, Louise.* Children's, 1985. Pres.–2. A child refuses to eat her peas.

Turner, Dorothy. *Bread.* Illus. John Yates. Carolrhoda, 1989. 1–4. Breads eaten all around the world.

———. *Milk.* Illus. John Yates. Carolrhoda, 1989. 1–4. The kinds of milk people drink around the world and recipes with milk.

Watanabe, Shigeo. *What a Good Lunch!* Illus. Yasuo Ohtomo. Philomel, 1980. 1–3. A bear's messy attempts to eat lunch.

Food Sources

•Arnot, Kathleen, ed. "Temba's Monkey Friends." In *Tales of Temba: Traditional African Stories.* Illus. Tom Feelings. Walck, 1967. 1–4. The origins of certain foods are explained.

Barrett, Judi. *Cloudy With a Chance of Meatballs.* Macmillan, 1978. Pres.–3. Living in a town where food comes down from the sky.

Brown, Marcia. *Stone Soup.* Scribner's, 1947. K–3. Three soldiers trick villagers into thinking they are making soup out of stones.

Cobb, Vicki. *The Trip of a Drip.* Illus. Elliot Kreloff. Little, Brown, 1986. 2–4. Account of our drinking water and some magic tricks.

Fradin, Dennis B. *Farming.* Childrens Press, 1983. 1–4. Introduction to farming.

Gibbons, Gail. *The Milk Makers.* Macmillan, 1985. 1–3. Where and how we get our milk.

———. *The Seasons of Arnold's Apple Tree.* Harcourt Brace Jovanovich, 1984. K–2. The importance of an apple tree to a child through the four seasons.

Ginsburg, Mirra. *The Magic Stove.* Illus. Linda Heller. Coward, McCann, 1983. K–3. A king steals the magic stove from a poor man and his wife but a rooster recovers it for them.

Hall, Donald. *Ox-Cart Man.* Illus. Barbara Cooney. Viking Kestrel, 1979. K–3. A story of nineteenth-century New England life.

Horwitz, Joshua. *Nightmarkets: Bringing Food to a City.* Harper & Row, 1986. K–2. How food is delivered and distributed to a big city during the night.

McCloskey, Robert. *Blueberries for Sal.* Penguin, 1976. Pres.–1. A child and a bear are each picking blueberries with their mother.

McGovern, Ann, reteller. *Stone Soup.* Illus. Winslow Pinney Pels. Scholastic, 1986. K–3. Retelling of the classic folktale where a greedy old woman is tricked into making a soup for a traveler.

Mitgutsch, Ali; Reidel, Marlene; Fuchshuber, Annegert; and Högner, Franz. *From Blossom to Honey.* Carolrhoda, 1981. Pres.–3. Explains how honey is produced and manufactured.

———. *From Cacao Bean to Chocolate.* Carolrhoda, 1981. 1–3. An introduction to making chocolate.

———. *From Grain to Bread.* Carolrhoda, 1981. Pres.–3. Explains the process of refining grain into flour for bread.

———. *From Grass to Butter.* Carolrhoda, 1981. Pres.–3. Explains what happens to grass after the cow digests it.

———. *From Lemon to Lemonade.* Carolrhoda, 1981. Pres.–3. How lemons can be made into lemonade.

———. *From Milk to Ice Cream.* Carolrhoda, 1981. Pres.–3. How milk is used to make ice cream.

Patent, Dorothy. *A Picture Book of Cows.* Holiday House, 1982. 2–4. An introduction to all kinds of cattle.

Rockwell, Anne. *Apples and Pumpkins.* Illus. Lizzy Rockwell. Macmillan, 1989. Pres.–2. A child's visit to a farm to pick apples and a pumpkin for Halloween.

Schnieper, Claudia. *An Apple Tree Through the Year.* Photographs by Othmar Baumli. Carolrhoda, 1989. 2–5. The yearly cycle of a single apple tree explained in simple scientific details.

Selsam, Millicent E. *More Potatoes!* Illus. Ben Shecter. Harper & Row, 1972. 1–3. A child and her classmates visit farm and market to learn more about potatoes.

———. *Popcorn.* Photographs by Jerome Wexler. Morrow, 1976. 2–5. The history of popcorn and the life cycle of the plant.

Smith, E. Boyd. *The Farm Book*. Houghton Mifflin, 1982. 2–5. The activities associated with farm life.

Titherton, Jeanne. *Pumpkin Pumpkin*. Greenwillow, 1986. K–3. A child watches her pumpkin seed grow into a pumpkin, harvests its seeds, and plants more pumpkin seeds the following year.

Turner, Dorothy. *Eggs*. Illus. John Yates. Carolrhoda, 1989. 1–4. Explains the development and production of eggs and how to tell if they are good.

———. *Potatoes*. Illus. John Yates. Carolrhoda, 1989. 1–4. The history, use, and production of potatoes and how to grow them.

Wykeham, Nicholas. *Farm Machines*. Raintree, 1979. 2–4. Pictures and descriptions of farm machinery.

Zemach, Harve. *Nail Soup*. Illus. Margot Zemach. Follett, 1964. K–3. An old man tricks an old woman into feeding him, pretending to make soup from a nail.

Food Identification, Nutrition, and Health

Alborough, Jez. *Running Bear*. Knopf, 1986. Pres.–3. A polar bear attempts to lose weight with disastrous results.

•Aliki. *Corn Is Maize: The Gift of the Indians*. Harper & Row, 1976. 2–4. The origins, growth, and uses of corn.

Barab, Seymour. *Little Red Riding Hood*. Boosey & Hawkes, 1965. 2-up. Play about a wolf who is turned off his desire for sweets by Red Riding Hood and Grandmother.

Burningham, John. *The Shopping Basket*. Crowell, 1980. 1–3. A young child's imagined experiences on the way to and from the store.

Carle, Eric. *My Very First Book of Food*. Crowell, 1986. Pres.–K. A mix-and-match book with foods at the bottom of each page and corresponding animal associations at the top.

Carrick, Donald. *Milk*. Greenwillow, 1985. K–2. Follows milk from farm to the grocery store.

dePaola, Tomie. *Pancakes for Breakfast*. Harcourt Brace Jovanovich, 1978. Pres.–2. The attempts of a woman to make pancakes and the recipe.

———. *Strega Nona*. Prentice-Hall, 1975. Pres.–3. Big Anthony meddles with Strega Nona's magic pasta pot with disastrous results.

Domanska, Janina. *The Turnip*. Macmillan, 1969. K–3. Grandparents and animals pull a giant turnip out of the ground.

Eberts, Marjorie, and Gisler, Margaret. *Pancakes, Crackers, and Pizza: A Book about Shapes*. Illus. Stephen Hayes. Childrens, 1984. Pres.–2. An exploration of round, square, and triangular foods.

Ehlert, Lois. *Eating the Alphabet: Fruits and Vegetables from A to Z*. Harcourt Brace Jovanovich, 1989. Pres.–2. Upper and lowercase letters taught using fruits and vegetables from around the world.

Joly-Berbesson, Fanny. *Marceau Bonappétit*. Illus. Agnes Mathieu. Carolrhoda, 1989. Pres.–3. A mouse learns that he needs a balanced diet.

Kellogg, Cynthia. *Corn—What It Is, What It Does*. Illus. Tom Huffman. Greenwillow, 1989. 1–4. History, growth, and uses of corn.

Kimmelman, Leslie. *Frannie's Fruits.* Illus. Petra Mathers. Harper & Row, 1989. Pres.–3. Story of a family that operates a fruit and vegetable stand together.

Lerner, Sharon. *I Like Vegetables.* Lerner, 1967. 3–6. Histories of common and uncommon vegetables.

McMillan, Bruce. *Growing Colors.* Lothrop, Lee & Shepard, 1988. Pres.–2. Close-up photographs of fruits and vegetables showing how they grow.

Modesitt, Jeanne. *Vegetable Soup.* Illus. Robin Spowart. Macmillan, 1988. Pres.–1. Children make vegetable soup from neighbors' donations.

Roffey, Maureen. *Mealtime.* Four Winds Press, 1989. Pres.–K. What makes a child ready for mealtime.

Rogow, Zack. *Oranges.* Illus. Mary Szilagyi. Orchard Books, 1988. Pres.–1. Oranges, from tree to table.

Root, Phyllis. *Soup for Supper.* Harper & Row, 1986. Pres.–3. A woman gets her vegetables back from a near-sighted giant who stole them.

Sendak, Maurice. *Chicken Soup with Rice.* Harper & Row. 1962. Pres.–3. A poem about the times when chicken soup is best to eat.

Sobol, Harriet L. *A Book of Vegetables.* Photographs by Patricia A. Agre. Dodd, Mead, 1985. 1–3. Information about common vegetables and their growth cycles.

Steele, Mary Q. *Anna's Garden Songs.* Illus. Lena Anderson. Greenwillow, 1989. K–3. About the love and appreciation a garden nurtures.

Stock, Catherine. *Alexander's Midnight Snack.* Clarion, 1988. Pres.–1. An elephant overeats on his midnight snacking binge, a snack for every letter of the alphabet.

Westcott, Nadine Bernard. *The Giant Vegetable Garden.* Little, Brown, 1981. Pres.–3. Giant vegetables threaten a town.

Zeifert, Harriet. *Munchety Munch.* Viking Kestrel, 1984. Pres.–2. A board book that explains the sounds different foods make.

Unhealthy Eating Habits

Balian, Lorna. *The Sweet Touch.* Abingdon, 1976. K–5. A child with a sweet tooth is cured.

Berenstain, Stan, and Berenstain, Jan. *The Berenstain Bears and Too Much Junk Food.* Random House, 1985. Pres.–2. Mama Bear decides to change the eating habits of her family.

Hoberman, Mary Ann. *The Cozy Book.* Illus. Tony Chen. Viking Kestrel, 1982. Pres.–3. A poem cataloguing things that make children feel cozy, including some foods.

Seixas, Judith S. *Junk Food—What It Is, What It Does.* Illus. Tom Huffman, 1984. Greenwillow, 1984. 2–5. An account of foods that contain high calories and low nutrition.

Smith, Robert K. *Chocolate Fever.* Dell, 1978. 1–5. How a boy who is crazy for chocolate moderates his craving.

Yorinks, Arthur. *Company's Coming.* Illus. David Small. Crown, 1988.

Pres.–3. Mother welcomes creatures from another planet that is over-populated.

Snacks

Barbour, Karen. *Little Nino's Pizzeria*. Harcourt Brace Jovanovich, 1987. Pres.–3. Coping with the changes in a favorite restaurant.

dePaola, Tomie. *The Popcorn Book*. Holiday House, 1978. 1–3. Interesting facts about popcorn.

Douglass, Barbara. *The Chocolate Chip Cookie Contest*. Lothrop, Lee & Shepard, 1985. K–3. Two boys try to win a prize in a chocolate chip cookie contest; includes recipe.

Galdone, Paul. *The Gingerbread Boy*. Houghton Mifflin, 1983. K–3. The gingerbread boy tries to outrun everyone to escape being eaten.

Hearn, Michael Patrick, selector. *The Chocolate Book: A Sampler for Boys and Girls*. Illus. Anthony Chen, Janet D'Amato, Diane Dawson, Richard Egielski, June Goldsborough, James Marshall, and Sallie Potterton. Caedmon, 1983. K–3. Stories and recipes related to chocolate.

Hest, Amy. *The Midnight Eaters*. Illus. Karen Gundersheimer. Four Winds, 1989. K–3. A girl and her grandmother have a midnight snack and discuss death and aging.

Hutchins, Pat. *The Doorbell Rang*. Greenwillow, 1986. Pres.–3. The doorbell keeps ringing, bringing guests to eat the cookies made for a family.

Selsam, Millicent E. *Popcorn*. Illus. Jerome Wexler. Morrow, 1976. 2–5. The difference between popcorn and other varieties of corn.

Fanciful Food Stories

Adler, David A. *The Purple Turkey and Other Thanksgiving Riddles*. Illus. Marylin Hafner. Holiday House. 1986. K–3. A book of sixty riddles.

Asbjornsen, P. Chr., and Moe, Jorgen. *The Runaway Pancake*. Joan Tate, translator. Illus. Otto Svend. S. Larousse, 1980. 1–3. A new version of the folktale about the runaway pancake trying to save his life.

•Bang, Betsy. *The Old Woman and the Rice Thief*. Illus. Molly Bang. Greenwillow, 1978. K–3. An old woman cleverly catches a thief who has been stealing her rice.

Bond, Michael. *Paddington at the Zoo*. Illus. David McKee. Putnam, 1985. K–3. How Paddington's sandwiches disappear at the zoo.

Calhoun, Mary. *The Hungry Leprechaun*. Illus. Roger Duvoisin. Morrow, 1962. K–3. A young boy orders a leprechaun to turn soup into gold, to no avail.

Carle, Eric. *Catch the Ball!* Philomel, 1982. Pres.–K. Introduces some concepts to young children, among them various fruits.

Collins, Trish. *Grinkles: A Keen Halloween Story.* Watts, 1981. K–3. A witch sets out to find a grinkle to fix a spell, not knowing what one is.

Day, Alexandra. *Frank and Ernest.* Scholastic, 1988. K–3. Two animals take over a diner.

Degen, Bruce. *Jamberry.* Harper & Row, 1989. Pres.–1. A book of rhymes about berries.

•dePaola, Tomie. *Fin McCoul.* Holiday House, 1981. K–3. A giant is tricked into eating bread with a surprise inside.

Forest, Heather, reteller. *The Baker's Dozen.* Illus. Susan Gaber. Harcourt Brace Jovanovich, 1988. Pres.–3. Fame makes a baker greedy.

Galdone, Paul. *Little Red Hen.* Houghton Mifflin, 1973. Pres-2. An industrious hen teaches her friends a lesson.

Gantschev, Ivan. *RumpRump.* Picture Book Studio USA, 1984. 1–4. A bear endlessly searches for food.

•Goble, Paul. *Iktomi and the Berries.* Orchard Books, 1989. Pres.–4. A Sioux Indian trickster tries to pick berries growing in the river, just for him.

Gurney, Nancy, and Gurney, Eric. *The King, the Mice and the Cheese.* Beginner Books, Inc., 1965. K–3. How can a kingdom rid itself of cats brought in to rid the kingdom of mice?

Lester, Alison. *Rosie Sips Spiders.* Houghton Mifflin, 1989. Pres.–2. A book about children's favorite foods, some unique.

Levine, Abby, reteller. *Too Much Mush!* Illus. Kathy Parkinson. Whitman, 1989. Pres.–2. An enchanted pot doesn't stop cooking mush, which floods a village.

Manning, Paul. *Cook.* Illus. Nicola Bayley. Macmillan, 1988. Pres.–1. Two squirrels attempt to cook a chocolate cake.

Seuss, Dr. *Green Eggs and Ham.* Random House, 1960. Pres.–1. Can you eat green eggs and ham?

Stevenson, James Walker. *If I Owned a Candy Factory.* Greenwillow, 1989. K–3. What one child would do if he owned a candy factory.

Preparing and Sharing Food; Cookbooks

Brimner, Larry Dane. *Country Bear's Good Neighbor.* Illus. Ruth T. Councell. Orchard Books, 1988. Pres.–2. A bear repays a girl's kindnesses with a treat.

De Brunhoff, Laurent. *Babar Learns to Cook.* Random House, 1979. Pres.–2. Babar's children create some unusual foods and havoc when a chef comes to visit.

Devlin, Wende, and Devlin, Harry. *Cranberry Halloween.* Illus. Harry Devlin. Four Winds, 1982. K–3. A Halloween story which includes two recipes for cranberry desserts that children can make.

Dobrin, Arnold. *Peter Rabbit's Nature Foods Cookbook.* Warne, 1977. 2-up. Simple nutritional recipes paired with illustrations from Beatrix Potter's books.

Hayes, Phyllis. *Food Fun.* Illus. Irene Trivas. Watts, 1981. 2–5. Simple recipes with art-and-craft activities using food.

Mandry, Kathy, and Toto, Joe. *How to Make Elephant Bread.* Pantheon, 1971. Pres.–3. Fifteen snacks for young children to make.

Martin, Liz. *Making Chocolate Chip Cookies.* Viking Kestrel, 1986. Pres.–3. How to make chocolate chip cookies with illustrations.

———. *Making Muffins.* Viking Kestrel, 1986. Pres.–3. How to make pizza, with illustrations.

———. *Making Pizza.* Viking Kestrel, 1986. Pres.–3. How to make muffins, with illustrations.

———. *Making Pretzels.* Viking Kestrel, 1986. Pres.–3. How to make pretzels, with illustrations.

Moore, Eva. *The Seabury Cookbook for Boys and Girls.* Illus. Talivaldis Stubis. Seabury Press, 1971. 3–6. Includes recipes and safety tips.

Parents' Nursery School. *Kids Are Natural Cooks: Child-tested Recipes for Home and School Using Natural Foods.* Illus. Lady McCrady. Houghton Mifflin, 1974. 2–4. Recipes using natural foods, with variations and encouraging experimentation.

Rockwell, Anne. *The Mother Goose Cookie-Candy Book.* Random House, 1983. Pres.–3. Nursery tale characters show how children and parents can make desserts together.

Watson, N. Cameron. *The Little Pigs' First Cookbook.* Little, Brown, 1987. Pres.–3. A day in the life of the three pigs, complete with cooking meals.

Young, Ruth. *Starring Francine and Dave.* Orchard Books, 1988. K–3. Three plays about preparing and sharing food.

Ziefert, Harriet. *So Hungry!* Illus. Carol Nicklaus. Random House, 1987. 1–3. A contest to find, prepare, and eat an after-school snack.

Grades Four Through Six

Food Sources; Food Customs

Aliki. *A Medieval Feast.* Crowell/Harper, 1983. 4–6. Description of a day-long medieval feast and pageantry accompanying the meal.

•Anderson, Joan. *The First Thanksgiving Feast.* Photographs by George Ancona. Clarion, 1984. 3–6. Dramatized account of the first Thanksgiving, recreating seventeenth-century life in Plymouth.

Baldwin, Margaret. *Thanksgiving: A First Book.* Watts, 1983. 3–7. History of Thanksgiving, including projects and recipes.

Bellville, Cheryl Walsh. *Farming Today—Yesterday's Way.* Carolrhoda, 1984. 3–5. Story of a farm that uses yesterday's methods today.

Cobb, Vicki. *The Scoop on Ice Cream.* Illus. G. Brian Karas. Little, Brown, 1986. 2–5. Ice cream, from cow to freezer, including recipes.

Demuth, Patricia. *Joel: Growing Up a Farm Man.* Dodd, Mead, 1982. 4–7. The story of a young farmer and his work.

•Fichter, George S. *How the Plains Indians Lived.* Illus. Alexander Farquharson. McKay, 1980. 4–8. Information on twenty Native American tribes which includes the foods they eat.

Fischer, Robert. *Hot Dog!* Illus. Steve Gregg. Messner, 1980. 4–6. The origin, history, and composition of the hot dog.

Gibbons, Gail. *The Milk Makers.* Macmillan, 1985. 3–4. The story of the manufacture of milk.

Giblin, James Cross. *Milk: The Fight for Purity.* Crowell, 1986. 3–7. The production of milk with explanation of its purification process.

•Gifford, Douglas. *Warriors, Gods and Spirits from Central and South American Mythology.* Illus. John Sibbick. Schocken, 1983. 4–8. Tales included that explain the origin of salt and of honey.

Hautzig, Esther. *Holiday Treats.* Illus. Yaroslava. Macmillan, 1983. 3–6. How various holidays are celebrated with recipes that children can prepare.

Hearn, Michael Patrick, selector. *The Chocolate Book: A Sampler for Boys and Girls.* Illus. Anthony Chen, et al. Caedmon, 1983. 3–5. Lore, poetry, stories, and recipes about chocolate.

Horwitz, Joshua. *Night Markets: Bringing Food to a City.* Harper & Row, 1984. 3–6. Operation of markets that supply food to a large city.

Johnson, Sylvia A. *Apple Trees.* Lerner, 1983. 5–8. The story of the apple tree, seed, and fruit formation.

Lasky, Kathryn. *Sugaring Time.* Photographs by Christopher G. Knight. Macmillan, 1963. All ages. How a Vermont family gathers sap for maple syrup.

Livingston, Myra Cohn. *Thanksgiving Poems.* Illus. Stephen Gammell. Holiday House, 1985. 3–6. Collection of Thanksgiving poetry from past and present.

Loeper, John J. *Mr. Marley's Main Street Confectionery.* Atheneum, 1979. 5–8. History of candy, ice cream, and other sweets.

Marston, Hope Irvin. *Machines on the Farm.* Dodd, Mead, 1982. 3–5. Photo album of farm machinery with explanations of its uses.

McDermott, Gerald. *Daughter of Earth.* Delacorte, 1984. 2–6. A tale explaining the origins of the seasons and crops.

McMillan, Bruce. *Apples, How They Grow.* Houghton Mifflin, 1979. 2–7. Explains the life cycle and uses of the apple with photographs.

•Patterson, Geoffrey. *All About Bread.* Deutsch, 1985. 3–6. A history of bread.

Penner, Lucille Recht. *The Thanksgiving Book.* Hastings, 1986. 5-up. Explains Thanksgiving and harvest festivals from ancient times to the present, including recipes and games.

Rahn, Joan Elma. *Plants that Changed History.* Atheneum, 1982. 3–7. The stories of five plants and their impact on history and on people's lives.

Rice, Karen. *Does Candy Grow on Trees?* Illus. Sharon Adler Cohen. Walker, 1984. 3–5. The facts about ingredients for candy and a list of candy factories that can be visited.

Sancha, Sheila. *The Luttrell Village: Country Life in the Middle Ages.* Crowell/Harper, 1983. 2–6. A year in a Lincolnshire village, plowing and sowing through harvesting.

Schaeffer, Elizabeth. *Dandelion, Pokeweed, and Goosefoot; How the Early Settlers Used Plants for Food, Medicine, and in the Home*. Illus. Grambs Miller. Young Scott Books, 1979. 4-up. How wild plants were used by early settlers in North America.

Scott, Jack Denton. *The Book of the Pig*. Putnam, 1981. 3–5. Information about the pig, including its habits, intelligence, and various breeds.

Scuro, Vincent. *Wonders of Cattle*. Dodd, Mead, 1980. 4–8. Information on cattle breeds, their history, and the industry.

Preparing and Sharing Food; Cookbooks

Anderson, Gretchen, compiler. *The Louisa May Alcott Cookbook*. Illus. Karen Milone. Little, Brown, 1985. 4–6. Recipes from *Little Men* and *Little Women* adapted for modern kitchens with excerpts from the novels.

Bayley, Monica. *The Wonderful Wizard of Oz Cook Book*. Illus. W. W. Denslow. Macmillan, 1981. 5–9. Recipes organized by foods representing colors associated with places in the land of Oz.

Boxer, Arabella. *The Wind in the Willows Country Cookbook*. Illus. Ernest Shepard. Scribner's, 1983. 5–9. English and Cornish recipes that Toad and Mole would admire.

•Chung, Okwha, and Monroe, Judy. *Cooking the Korean Way*. Lerner, 1988. 5-up. Explanation of Korean cuisine, including recipes.

Ellison, Virginia. *The Pooh Cook Book*. Illus. Ernest H. Shepard. Dutton, 1969. 4–6. Recipes out of the *Winnie-the-Pooh* books.

•Hayward, Ruth Ann, and Warner, Margaret Brink. *What's Cooking? Favorite Recipes from Around the World*. Little, Brown, 1981. 4–6. Teens share favorite recipes reflecting their ethnic origins.

John, Sue. *The How-To Cookbook*. Illus. Nick Hardcastle, Carolyn Bull, and Judith Escreet. Philomel, 1982. 4–8. Variety of recipes that teach basic cooking and baking techniques.

•Kaufman, Cheryl. *Cooking the Caribbean Way*. Lerner, 1988. 5-up. A book of Caribbean recipes.

Krementz, Jill. *The Fun of Cooking*. Knopf, 1985. 5-up. Nineteen children share their favorite recipes.

•Montgomery, Bertha, and Chapman, Constance. *Cooking the African Way*. Lerner, 1988. 5-up. Recipes from East and West Africa.

•Moore, Eva. *The Great Banana Cookbook for Boys and Girls*. Illus. Susan Russo. Clarion, 1983. 2–6. Recipes for cooking with bananas.

•Parnell, Helga. *Cooking the German Way*. Lerner, 1988. 5-up. Recipes for the traditional foods of Germany.

•Purdy, Susan. *Christmas Cooking Around the World*. Watts, 1983. 5-up. Recipes for Christmastime treats from around the world with sketches.

Stein, Sara Bonnett. *Kids' Kitchen Takeover*. Workman, 1975. 4-up. Nutritious recipes and easy directions for making them.

Fanciful Food Poems and Stories

Agree, Rose H., collector. *How to Eat a Poem and Other Morsels; Food Poems for Children.* Pantheon, 1967. 3–5. Variety of poems on food, eating, and table manners.

Cole, William, selector. *Poem Stew.* Illus. Karen Weinhaus. Lippincott, 1981. 4–6. Fifty-seven poems about manners, food choices, and the effects of eating various foods.

Dewey, Ariane. *Febold Feboldson.* Greenwillow, 1984. K–6. An inventive farmer makes popcorn balls by mistake.

Pinkwater, Daniel. *Fat Men from Space.* Dodd, Mead, 1977. 3–5. Spacemen try to rid Earth of its junk food.

Roop, Peter, and Roop, Connie. *Out to Lunch! Jokes about Food.* Illus. Joan Hanson. Lerner, 1984. 3–6. A book of jokes about food.

Westcott, Nadine Bernard. *Peanut Butter and Jelly.* Dutton, 1988. 4–7. A verse about the concoction of a giant sandwich.

•Yolen, Jane, ed. "Rich Man, Poor Man." In *Favorite Folktales from Around the World.* Pantheon, 1986. 3-up. An African tale of justice.

Personal and Ethnic Variations in Foods

•Bacon, Josephine. *Cooking the Israeli Way.* Lerner, 1986. 3–7. Menus from Israel as well as information about its people, food, customs, religion, and culture.

•Drucker, Malka. *Shabbat: A Peaceful Island.* Holiday House, 1983. 4–6. The origins, rituals and customs of Shabbat as well as recipes.

•———. *Sukkot: A Time to Rejoice.* Holiday House, 1982. 4–6. History, customs, and meaning of this Jewish holiday season, including recipes.

•Fritz, Jean. *George Washington's Breakfast.* Coward, McCann and Geoghegan, 1969. 4-up. Facts about the first president's food preferences.

•LaFarque, Françoise. *French Food and Drink.* Bookwright Press, 1987. 4-up. Photos, diagrams, safety notes, and recipes from different regions of France.

•Riedman, Sarah R. *Food for People.* Harper & Row, 1976. 4–6. How the world is fed.

•Warner, Margaret Brink, and Hayward, Ruth Ann. *What's Cooking? Favorite Recipes from Around the World.* Little, Brown, 1981. 3–7. Thirty-six teens from different ethnic backgrounds tell their favorite family recipes.

•Watson, Tom, and Watson, Jenny. *Breakfast.* Childrens Press, 1983. 4–6. Breakfast from many lands described.

Effects of a Poor Diet

Anderson, Mary. *Tune In Tomorrow.* Avon, 1985. 5-up. An overweight child deals with her problem.

Fine, John Christopher. *The Hunger Road.* Atheneum, 1987. 5-up. Examines hunger crises in many countries around the world, with special focus on social and natural causes of hunger.

Holland, Isabelle. *Dinah and the Green Fat Kingdom.* Harper & Row, 1988. 3–7. A child deals with her weight problem by fantasizing.

Manes, Stephen. *Slim Down Camp.* Houghton Mifflin, 1981. 4–6. A child goes to a camp for losing weight.

Smith, Robert Kimmel. *Jelly Belly.* Illus. Bob Jones. Delacorte, 1981. 4–6. A child is sent to a camp for dieters for two months.

Nutrition and Health; Nutrients

Berger, Melvin, and Berger, Gilda. *The New Food Book: Nutrition, Diet, Consumer Tips, and Foods of the Future.* Illus. Byron Barton. Harper & Row, 1978. 6–8. Today's food, food sources, and the future developments proposed for food.

Cobb, Vicki. *More Science Experiments You Can Eat.* Illus. Giulio Maestro. Lippincott, 1979. 4–6. Scientific processes that cause changes in food, with experiments students can try.

Epstein, Sam, and Epstein, Beryl. *Bugs for Dinner?* Illus. Walter Gaffney-Kessell. Macmillan, 1989. 1–5. The food-seeking habits of squirrels, birds, bees, ants, spiders, and other creatures.

Fodor, R. V. *The Science of Nutrition.* Morrow, 1979. 4–6. What the components of a basic diet are and what poor nutrition does to the body.

Gilbert, Sara. *Fat Free: Common Sense for Young Weight Worriers.* Macmillan, 1975. 6–9. Information about fat and its storage in the body, and what foods contain fats.

———. *You Are What You Eat: A Commonsense Guide to the Modern American Diet.* Macmillan, 1977. 5–8. Introduction to food, nutrition, and the world's food crisis.

Jones, Hettie. *How to Eat Your ABC's: A Book about Vitamins.* Illus. Judy Glasser. Four Winds, 1976. 4–7. The nature of various nutrients and their food sources.

Newton, Lesley. *Meatballs and Molecules: The Science behind Food.* Black, 1984. 4–7. How various kinds of food affect the body.

Simon, Seymour. *About the Foods You Eat.* Illus. Dennis Kendrick. McGraw-Hill, 1979. 2–5. Traces food from the time it is eaten and through the body.

Ward, Brian R. *Food and Digestion.* Watts, 1982. 4-up. An introduction to the digestive system.

Food Choices; Types of Foods

Adler, Irving. *Food.* Illus. Peggy Adler. Harper & Row, 1977. 3–5. Information about food, including its many uses and problems of cultivating certain foods.

•Ancona, George. *Bananas: From Manolo to Margie*. Houghton Mifflin, 1982. 4–7. The story of bananas, from those involved in their growth and production.

Cuyler, Margery. *The All-Around Pumpkin Book*. Illus. Corbett Jones. Holt, 1980. 3–6. How to grow and use pumpkins, and lore surrounding them.

Earle, Olive L., and Kantor, Michael. *Nuts*. Morrow, 1975. 3–5. Descriptions of various kinds of nuts.

Fenton, Carroll Lane, and Kitchen, Hermine B. *Plants We Live On*. Harper & Row, 1971. 4–7. Discusses some of the plants we eat.

Gemming, Elizabeth. *The Cranberry Book*. Coward-McCann, 1983. 4–6. Cranberries—where and how they are grown and how to use them.

•Hughes, Meredith, and Hughes, E. Thomas. *The Great Potato Book*. Illus. G. Brian Karas. Macmillan, 1986. 3–7. History, uses, and folklore of the potato, including recipes.

Johnson, Hannah Lyons. *From Apple Seed to Applesauce*. Lothrop, Lee & Shepard, 1977. 3–5. Information about apples, from growth to uses.

Johnson, Sylvia A. *Potatoes*. Photographs by Maraharu. Lerner, 1984. 4–7. Information about potatoes and where and how they grow.

Penner, Lucille Recht. *The Honey Book*. Hastings, 1980. 5–7. Introduction to honey and some recipes for its use.

Pringle, Laurence. *Wild Foods; A Beginners Guide to Identifying, Harvesting and Cooking Safe and Tasty Plants from the Outdoors*. Illus. Paul Breeden. Four Winds, 1978. 5-up. Finding, cooking, and eating parts of some plants which can be found in the United States.

Schnieper, Claudia. *An Apple Tree Through the Year*. Photographs by Othmar Baumli. Carolrhoda, 1988. 2–5. Takes an apple tree through its yearly cycle.

Selsam, Millicent E. *Eat the Fruit, Plant the Seed*. Morrow, 1980. 2–5. Introduction to different fruits and their cultivation.

Sobol, Harriet Langsam. *A Book of Vegetables*. Photographs by Patricia A. Agre. Dodd, Mead, 1984. 3–5. How fourteen different vegetables grow.

Woodside, Dave. *What Makes Popcorn Pop?* Illus. Kay Woon. Atheneum, 1980. 3–6. The lore, myths, and legend of popcorn.

Grades Seven and Up

Nutrition and Health; Nutrients

Berger, Melvin, and Berger, Gilda. *The New Food Book: Nutrition, Diet, Consumer Tips, and Foods of the Future*. Illus. Byron Barton. Crowell, 1978. 6–8. Present food sources, nature of today's food, and future food developments.

Burns, Marilyn. *Good for Me: All about Food in 32 Bites*. Illus. Sandy Clifford. Little, Brown, 1978. 6–8. Discusses nutrition and digestion.
Erlanger, Ellen. *Eating Disorders*. Lerner, 1988. 6-up. Questions and answers about eating disorders.
Nourse, Alan E. *Vitamins*. Watts, 1977. 6–9. History of vitamin research, their nature, effects, and sources.
Perl, Lila. *Eating the Vegetarian Way: Good Food from the Earth*. Morrow, 1980. 5–9. The history of vegetarianism and sample diets.
Wrightson, Patricia. *Moon Dark*. Illus. Noela Young. McElderry, 1988. 6–9. A problem of food and space is solved between fighting wild creatures.

Food Choices; Types of Food

Brown, Elizabeth Burton. *Vegetables: An Illustrated History with Recipes*. Illus. Marisabina Russo. Prentice-Hall, 1981. 6–9. History of the growing and eating of vegetables.
Gethers, Judy. *The Sandwich Book*. Vintage, 1988. 6-up. A collection of sandwich recipes.
Johnson, Sylvia A. *Rice*. Illus. Noboru Moriya. Lerner, 1986. 4–8. Description of how rice is grown and harvested.
Rahn, Joan Elma. *Plants That Changed History*. Atheneum, 1982. 6–9. Five episodes where plants changed history are explained.
Tchudi, Stephen N. *Soda Poppery: The History of Soft Drinks in America*. Scribner's, 1986. 6-up. The cultural, economic, nutritional, and international aspects of manufacturing soda.

Food Sources; Food Customs; World Food Problems

•Burns, Marilyn. *The Hanukkah Book*. Illus. Martha Weston. Four Winds, 1981. 3–7. The spirit of Hanukkah and how it is celebrated; contains recipes and comparison to Christmas holiday.
Hawkes, Nigel. *Food and Farming*. Watts, 1982. 4–7. How energy is used to produce food in the United States.
Kushner, Jill Menkes. *The Farming Industry*. Watts, 1984. 6–8. Modern farming and its technology.
Loeper, John J. *Mr. Marley's Min Street Confectionery*. Atheneum, 1979. 4–7. An account of an old-time candy shop and how candy came to America.
•Perl, Lila. *The Global Food Shortage*. Morrow, 1976. 7-up. Which peoples are hungry and why.
Pizer, Vernon. *Eat the Grapes Downward: An Uninhibited Romp through the*

Surprising World of Food. Dodd, Mead, 1983. 6–9. A collection of myths and beliefs about food.

•Pringle, Laurence. *Our Hungry Earth.* Macmillan, 1976. 7-up. Introduction to food shortages and how to rectify them.

•Ritchie, Carson I. A. *Food in Civilization: How History Has Been Affected by Human Tastes.* Beaufort, 1981. 3–7. Theory that the quest for food has determined world history.

•Versfeld, Ruth. *Why Are People Hungry?* Gloucester, 1988. 5–7. An account of the world hunger problem and its implications for the future.

Preparing and Sharing Food; Cookbooks

Cosman, Madeleine Pelner. *Medieval Holidays and Festivals: A Calendar of Celebrations.* Scribner's, 1981. 6-up. Customs and celebrations through the medieval calendar year with recipes.

John, Sue. *The Time to Eat Cookbook.* Illus. Elizabeth Wood and Nick Hardcastle. Philomel, 1982. 5–8. Recipes for meals from simple to the complex with focus on nutritional balance.

Walker, Barbara M. *The Little House Cookbook: Frontier Foods from Laura Ingalls Wilder's Classic Stories.* Illus. Garth Williams. Harper & Row, 1979. 4–7. Recipes from the times of the pioneers with historical information and anecdotes.

Weight Control; Eating Disorders

Erlanger, Ellen. *Eating Disorders: A Question and Answer Book About Anorexia Nervosa and Bulimia.* Lerner, 1987. 6–9. Explains the two eating disorders and the emotional and psychological motivations behind them.

Gilbert, Sue. *Fat Free: Common Sense for Young Weight Worriers.* Macmillan, 1972. 6–9. Acceptable guidelines for deciding whether you are overweight.

Hautzig, Deborah. *Second Star to the Right.* Greenwillow, 1981. 6-up. The story of a teen with anorexia nervosa.

Kolodny, Nancy J. *When Food's a Foe: How to Confront and Conquer Eating Disorders.* Little, Brown, 1987. 6-up. Causes and effects of bulimia and anorexia nervosa with questionnaires, checklists, and exercises.

Rendell, Ruth. *Heartstones.* Harper & Row, 1987. 7-up. A victim of anorexia causes terrible family problems.

Sachs, Marilyn. *The Fat Girl.* Dutton, 1984. 6-up. A boy is attracted to a grossly overweight girl in his class and decides to transform her.

Wersba, Barbara. *Love Is the Crooked Thing.* Harper & Row, 1987. 7-up. An overweight teen's love affair with a man twice her age and her beginnings as a writer.

F. DISEASE PREVENTION AND CONTROL

Grades K Through Three

Types of Diseases

De Angeli, Marguerite. *The Door in the Wall.* Doubleday, 1969. 3–6. A disabled child's journey toward self-realization in thirteenth-century England.

Delton, Judy. *I'll Never Love Anything Ever Again.* Illus. Rodney Pate. Whitman, 1985. K–3. A young boy has to part with his pet because of allergies.

Emmert, Michelle. *I'm the Big Sister Now.* Illus. Gail Owens. Whitman, 1989. 2–6. A child writes about life with her older sister who has cerebral palsy.

Fassler, Joan. *Howie Helps Himself.* Whitman, 1975. 1–3. A child who has cerebral palsy overcomes feelings of frustration and triumphs.

Gretz, Susanna, and Sage, Alison. *Teddy Bears Cure a Cold.* Illus. Susanna Gretz. Four Winds, 1985. Pres.-2. Taking advantage of a bad situation where friends are helping out.

Lerner, Margaret Rush. *Dear Little Mumps Child.* Illus. George Overlie. Lerner, 1983. K–5. Details the causes and remedies for mumps.

———. *Peter Gets the Chickenpox.* Illus. George Overlie. Lerner, 1959. K–5. Causes and remedies for chicken pox.

Litchfield, Ada B. *A Button in Her Ear.* Illus. Eleanor Mill. Whitman, 1976. 1–3. Introduction to hearing problems and some correctional devices.

Little, Jean. *Mine for Keeps.* Little, Brown, 1962. 3–6. A child with cerebral palsy copes with fear of returning home after being in a special school for several years.

MacLachlan, Patricia. *Through Grandpa's Eyes.* Illus. Deborah Ray. Harper & Row, 1980. Pres.-1. A child's blind grandfather teaches him to "see" in other ways.

Ominsky, Elaine, *Jon O: A Special Boy.* Photographs by Dennis Simonetti. Prentice-Hall, 1977. Pres.-2. The life of a child with Down's Syndrome.

Payne, Sherry Neuwirth. *A Contest.* Illus. Jeff Kyle. Carolrhoda, 1988. 1–4. A child with cerebral palsy has his first year at a public school.

Silverstein, Alvin, and Silverstein, Virginia. *Itch, Sniffle, and Sneeze.* Illus. Roy Doty. Four Winds, 1978. 3–5. Information about allergies.

———. *Runaway Sugar: All About Diabetes.* Illus. Harriet Barton. Lippincott, 1981. 3–6. Detailed explanation of diabetes and overview of care.

Swenson, Judy Harris, and Kunz, Roxane Brown. *Cancer: The Whispered Word.* Dillon, 1986. 3–5. Answers to questions children ask about cancer.

Tyler, Linda Wagner. *The Sick-in-Bed Birthday.* Illus. Susan Davis. Viking Kestrel, 1988. Pres.-2. A child's experiences with chicken pox.

Vigna, Judith. *I Wish Daddy Didn't Drink So Much.* Whitman, 1988. 1–4.
A child learns ways to deal with her father's alcoholism.

Coping with Diseases

Adams, Barbara. *Like It Is: Facts and Feelings about Handicaps from Kids Who
Know.* Illus. James Stanfield. Walker, 1979. 3–6. Photographs and
descriptions of various disabilities.
Baldwin, Anne Norris. *A Little Time.* Viking Kestrel, 1978. 3–5. A child
learns to deal with her younger brother's Down's Syndrome.
Fassler, Joan. *Howie Helps Himself.* Illus. Joe Lasker. Whitman, 1975. 2–4.
A child adjusts to having cerebral palsy and using his wheelchair.
Landau, Elaine. *We Have AIDS.* Watts, 1990. 5-up. Nine first-person
stories of young people who have developed AIDS from a variety of
causes.
Litchfield, Ada B. *Making Room for Uncle Joe.* Whitman, 1985. 2–4. A child
adjusts to the arrival of his uncle who has Down's Syndrome and will live
with his family.
Mack, Nancy. *Tracy.* Photographs by Heinz Kluetmeier. Children's Press,
1976. Pres.-3. Examines the life of a handicapped person.
Martin, Patricia Miles. *Thomas Alva Edison.* Illus. Fermin Rocker. Putnam,
1971. K–3. A biography of this inventor, who was deaf.
Roy, Ron. *Where's Buddy?* Illus. Troy Howell. Houghton Mifflin, 1982.
3–5. A child must take care of his diabetic brother.
Sullivan, Mary Beth, and Bourke, Linda, with Regan, Susan. *A Show of
Hands: Say It in Sign Language.* Illus. Linda Bourke. Addison-Wesley,
1980. 1–5. Describes sign language and its use and those who use it.
Wolf, Bernard. *Anna's Silent World.* Lippincott, 1977. K–4. Describes the
training and equipment needed to help a deaf child talk, write, and read.
————. *Connie's New Eyes.* Lippincott, 1976. 4-up. Photoessay about a
blind woman and her guide dog.

Disease Prevention

Burnstein, John. *Slim Goodbody: What Can Go Wrong and How to Be Strong.*
McGraw-Hill, 1978. 2–5. Introduction to common illnesses and injuries
and how to prevent them.
Epstein, Sherie S. *Penny the Medicine Maker: The Story of Penicillin.* Illus.
Mark Springer. Lerner, 1960. K–5. History, nature, and production of
penicillin.
Veglahn, Nancy. *The Mysterious Rays: Marie Curie's World.* Illus. Victor
Juhasz. Coward, 1977. History of the research that led to the tracing and
isolation of radium.

Grades Four Through Six

Types of Diseases

Burns, Sheila L. *Cancer: Understanding It.* Messner, 1982. 4–6. Introduction to the disease, its characteristics, and methods of prevention and treatment.

Connelly, John P., and Berlow, Leonard. *You're Too Sweet: A Guide for the Young Diabetic.* Astor-Honor, 1969. 4–6. A nine-year-old boy's perspective on treatment and causes of diabetes.

Frank, Julia. *Alzheimer's Disease: The Silent Epidemic.* Lerner, 1985. 5-up. Follows one patient's mental and physical deterioration from this disease.

Haines, Gail Kay. *Cancer.* Watts, 1980. 4–7. Explores cancer by looking at the case histories of five patients.

Kurland, Morton. *Coping with AIDS: Facts and Fears.* Rosen, 1988. 6-up. Focuses on sexual transmission, homosexuality, and safe sex techniques.

Landau, Elaine. *Alzheimer's Disease.* Watts, 1987. 5-up. Discusses the disease, its effects on family members, and offers suggestions for coping and care.

Lerner, Ethan A. *Understanding AIDS.* Illus. Mark Wilken. Lerner, 1987. 3–6. How to treat those who have AIDS or who carry the virus.

Neimark, Anne E. *Damien, the Leper Priest.* Morrow, 1980. 4–6. Biography of the priest who served Hawaii's lepers.

Nourse, Alan E. *Lumps, Bumps and Rashes: A Look at Kids' Diseases.* Watts, 1976. 5–7. Discusses common childhood diseases and infections.

———. *Viruses.* Watts, 1983. 5–7. Traces the research on viruses from Jenner's and Pasteur's breakthrough research to current efforts.

Oleksy, Walter. *The Black Plague.* Watts, 1982. 6-up. The nature, causes, and effects of the disease on the history of mankind.

Patent, Dorothy Hinshaw. *Germs!* Holiday House, 1983. 4–6. Explains what germs are, how they attack the body, and how the body defends itself against them.

Riedman, Sarah R. *Diabetes.* Watts, 1980. 4-up. A description of diabetes and its diagnosis, what insulin is and how it works, and past and current research.

Silverstein, Alvin, and Silverstein, Virginia B. *Cancer.* Illus. Andrew Antal. John Day, 1977. 5–7. Introduction to cancerous cells, how they function, and current status of cancer prevention and treatment.

———. *The Sugar Disease: Diabetes.* Lippincott, 1980. 3–6. Discusses symptoms, history, diagnosis, and treatment of diabetes as well as the future of current research.

Tiger, Steven. *Arthritis.* Illus. Michael Reingold. Messner, 1986. 4–8. Defines arthritis, how it affects the body, its treatment, and current research.

Disease Prevention

Aaseng, Nathan. *The Inventors: Nobel Prizes in Chemistry, Physics, and Medicine.* Lerner, 1988. 5-up. Discusses eight inventions and their inventors.

Asimov, Isaac. *How Did We Find Out about Germs?* Illus. David Wool. Walker, 1974. 4–6. Knowledge about germs, including historical and current information on viruses and vaccines.

Berger, Melvin. *Disease Detectives.* Crowell, 1978. 4–6. How scientists worked to solve the riddle of Legionnaires' disease.

Cohen, Daniel. *Vaccination and You.* Illus. Haris Petie. Messner, 1969. 3–6. The history of immunization from Jenner's time to now.

Crofford, Emily. *Healing Warrior.* Illus. Steve Michaels. Carolrhoda, 1989. 3–6. Biography of the woman who found a treatment for polio.

Donahue, Parnell, and Capellaro, Helen. *Germs Make Me Sick: A Health Handbook for Kids.* Illus. Kelly Oechsli. Knopf, 1975. 4–6. A humorous guide to the viral illnesses children may encounter.

Jacobs, Francine. *Breakthrough: The True Story of Penicillin.* Dodd, Mead, 1988. 6-up. How penicillin was discovered by Fleming and researched by others.

Nourse, Alan E. *Your Immune System.* Watts, 1982. 4–6. Discussion of our defenses against disease and what occurs when they break down.

———. *Viruses.* Watts, 1976. 5–7. Account beginning with Jenner and Pasteur and tracing the research on viruses to the present.

Selsam, Millicent E. *Plants That Heal.* Illus. Kathleen Elgin. Morrow, 1959. 4–6. History of the usage of plants to heal.

Silverstein, Alvin, and Silverstein, Virginia B. *Glasses and Contact Lenses.* Lippincott, 1989. 6-up. Explains the structure of the eye, how vision works, and how glasses and contact lenses correct vision problems.

———. *The World of Bionics.* Methuen, 1979. 5–7. Overview of the use of artificial organs.

Coping with Disease; Lifestyle Choices

Adler, C. S. *Eddie's Blue-Winged Dragon.* Putnam, 1988. 4–6. A child's support systems for mainstreaming with cerebral palsy.

Arnold, Caroline. *Pain: What Is It? How Do We Deal with It?* Morrow, 1986. 3–7. Where pain comes from and how to measure pain, get relief, and prevent pain.

Blume, Judy. *Deenie.* Bradbury, 1974. 5–7. A child learns to cope with wearing a spinal brace.

Carter, Alden R. *Sheila's Dying.* Putnam, 1987. 7-up. A teen learns to cope with his girlfriend's terminal cancer.

•Coerr, Eleanor. *Sadako and the Thousand Paper Cranes.* Illus. Ronald Himler. Putnam, 1977. 3–5. Story of a Japanese child who dies of leukemia developed from radiation sickness from the bombing of Hiroshima.

Connelly, John P., and Berlow, Leonard. *You're Too Sweet: A Guide for the Young Diabetic.* Astor-Honor, 1969. 4–6. A child's perspective on the causes and treatment of diabetes.

Corcoran, Barbara B. *A Dance to Still Music.* Illus. Charles Robinson. Atheneum, 1974. 4–8. A fourteen-year-old girl refuses to accept her deafness.

————. *I Am the Universe.* Atheneum, 1986. 5-up. A child copes with her mother's cancer and other family problems, finding out who she really is.

De Angeli, Marguerite. *The Door in the Wall.* Doubleday, 1969. 5-up. Play about a disabled child's struggle for survival in plague-stricken thirteenth-century England.

Gould, Marilyn. *The Twelfth of June.* Lippincott, 1986. 5-up. A child finds she is not as handicapped by her cerebral palsy as those trying to cope with her disease.

Graber, Richard. *Doc.* Harper & Row, 1986. 5-up. A child refuses to recognize his grandfather's problems with Alzheimer's disease.

Greenberg, Jan. *No Dragons to Slay.* Farrar, Straus & Giroux, 1983. 6-up. A popular high school student finds out he has malignant cancer and learns to cope.

Hermes, Patricia. *What If They Knew?* Harcourt Brace Jovanovich, 1980. 4–6. An epileptic boy moves in with his grandparents.

Herzig, Alison Cragin, and Mali, Jane Lawrence. *A Season of Secrets.* Little, Brown, 1982. 4–6. A child discovers her little brother has epilepsy and forces her family to deal with it.

Howard, Ellen. *Circle of Giving.* Atheneum, 1984. 5–7. Two girls meet another girl with cerebral palsy in the 1920s.

Hyland, Betty. *The Girl with the Crazy Brother.* Watts, 1987. 4–6. A girl learns to deal with her brother's schizophrenia.

Jones, Rebecca C. *Madeline and the Great (Old) Escape Artist.* Dutton, 1983. 4–6. A child tries to escape the fact that she has epilepsy by running away.

Jordan, Marykate. *Losing Uncle Tim.* Illus. Judith Friedman. Whitman, 1989. 2–6. A child deals with the fact that his uncle is dying of AIDS.

Kipnis, Lynne, and Adler, Susan. *You Can't Catch Diabetes from a Friend.* Photographs by Richard Benkof. Triad, 1979. 2–6. The lives of four children with diabetes reveal the facts about the disease.

Knowles, Anne. *Under the Shadow.* Harper & Row, 1983. 5–8. Relationship between a teen and a boy who has muscular dystrophy.

L'Engle, Madeleine. *A Ring of Endless Light.* Farrar, Straus & Giroux, 1980. 5-up. A child learns to deal with life and death during a summer with her dying grandfather.

Little, Jean. *Mine for Keeps.* Illus. Lewis Parker. Little, Brown, 1962. 4–7. A child faces life in the world after five years in a home for the handicapped.

————. *Spring Begins in March.* Illus. Lewis Parker. Little, Brown, 1966. 4–6. A sequel to *Mine for Keeps,* focusing on the handicapped child's younger sister.

Rabe, Berniece. *Margaret's Moves.* Illus. Julie Downing. Dutton, 1987. 3–6. A child with spina bifida struggles to make her dreams come true despite her illness.

Radley, Gail. *CF in His Corner.* Four Winds, 1984. 6-up. A child faces the fact that his younger brother has cystic fibrosis and attempts to make his mother face the fact.

Roy, Ron. *Where's Buddy?* Illus. Troy Howell. Clarion, 1982. 3–6. A child in danger copes with his diabetes bravely.

Rubin, Robert. *Lou Gehrig: Courageous Star.* Putnam, 1979. 6-up. Biography of a famous baseball player stricken with a mysterious disease.

Sachs, Elizabeth-Ann. *Just Like Always.* Atheneum, 1982. 4–8. The growing friendship between two girls who have scoliosis.

Schlee, Ann. *Ask Me No Questions.* Holt, 1982. 4–6. A story of provincialism in small towns in Victorian England during a cholera outbreak.

Singer, Marilyn. *It Can't Hurt Forever.* Illus. Leigh Grant. Harper & Row, 1978. 5–7. A child's experiences as a heart patient.

Slote, Alfred. *Hang Tough, Paul Mather.* Lippincott, 1973. 5–7. A sports story about a boy's struggle against leukemia.

Sorensen, Candace, adaptor. *The Martian Chronicles.* Dramatic Publishing, 1985. 5-up. In one episode of this play, A chicken pox epidemic brought to Mars by earth people destroys the entire population.

Southall, Ivan. *Let the Balloon Go.* St. Martin's, 1968. 4-up. How a cerebral palsied child gains independence.

Tapp, Kathy Kennedy. *Smoke from the Chimney.* Atheneum, 1986. 5-up. A child fantasizes another world to escape her father's alcoholism, but finally confronts the realities of his illness.

Way, Brian. *On Trial.* Baker's Plays, 1977. 4-up. Play about an epidemic in an African village and the search for a healing herb.

Wright, Betty Ren. *The Summer of Mrs. MacGregor.* Holiday House, 1986. 6–9. A child deals with being jealous of her sister who has a heart problem.

Young, Helen. *What Difference Does It Make, Danny?* Illus. Quentin Blake. Dutton, 1980. 4–6. The story of a nine-year-old child with epilepsy.

Grades Seven and Up

Types of Diseases

Brown, Fern. *Hereditary Diseases.* Watts, 1987. 5-up. Causes, symptoms, and treatment of inheritable diseases are discussed.

Hyde, Margaret O. and Forsyth, Elizabeth H. *AIDS: What Does It Mean to You?* Walker, 1987. 7-up. Information on the nature and causes of AIDS and its physiological and psychological effects.

———. *VD: The Silent Epidemic.* McGraw-Hill, 1973. 5–9. Types of venereal disease, treatment, prevention, and symptoms.

Johnson, Eric W. *VD.* Lippincott, 1978. 5–9. Informational publication about venereal disease.

Knight, David C. *Viruses: Life's Smallest Enemies.* Illus. Christine Kettner. Morrow, 1981. 6–9. Description of the nature and effects of viruses on humans.

•Kuklin, Susan. *Fighting Back: What Some People Are Doing About AIDS.* Putnam, 1989. 8-up. Poignant testimonials.

Nourse, Alan E. *AIDS.* Watts, 1986. 6-up. Describes the origins, symptoms, and characteristics of AIDS, and chronicles the search for a cure.

———. *Herpes.* Watts, 1985. 7-up. Characteristics and prevention of genital herpes.

Riedman, Sarah R. *Diabetes.* Watts, 1980. 5–9. Causes and effects of diabetes are explained.

Silverstein, Alvin, and Silverstein, Virginia. *AIDS: Deadly Threat.* Enslow, 1986. 6–9. Introduction to the causes and prevention of AIDS, with a discussion of research being done towards a cure.

———. *Diabetes: The Sugar Disease.* Lippincott, 1979. 6–8. Information about diabetes for nondiabetics.

———. *Epilepsy.* Lippincott, 1975. 5-up. Explains fears and misunderstandings of epilepsy in the past and current treatments.

Warren, C. *Understanding and Preventing AIDS.* Childrens Press, 1988. 7-up. The social, personal, and emotional issues associated with AIDS are described through studies and illustrations.

Disease Prevention

Berger, Melvin. *Disease Detectives.* Crowell, 1978. 5–9. Information about the work of the Centers for Disease Control in Atlanta.

Brindze, Ruth. *Look How Many People Wear Glasses: The Romance of Lenses.* Atheneum, 1975. 6–9. History, composition, uses, and limits of eyeglasses.

Colman, Warren. *Understanding and Preventing AIDS.* Childrens Press, 1988. 7-up. Information intended to warn of the dangers and dispel irrational fears associated with AIDS.

deSaint Phalle, Niki. *AIDS: You Can't Catch It Holding Hands.* Lapis Press, 1986. 7-up. Information on homosexuality, intravenous drug abuse, and safe sex, in the form of a mother's letter to her son.

Freese, Arthur S. *The Bionic People Are Here.* McGraw-Hill, 1979. 6–9. Discusses restoration of limbs and organs through artificial parts.

Gleasner, Diana C. *Breakthrough: Women in Science.* Walker, 1983. 6-up. Stories of six women who have successfully pursued careers in science.

Jacobs, Francine. *Breakthrough, the True Story of Penicillin.* Dodd, Mead, 1985. 6-up. History and pioneers in the discovery and uses of penicillin.

Kavaler, Lucy. *Cold against Disease: The Wonders of Cold.* John Day, 1971. 6–9. The ways in which cold helps in medicine.

Keller, Mollie. *Marie Curie.* Watts, 1982. 7-up. Biography of the woman who discovered radium and the difficulties she experienced in pursuit of her career.

Kelley, Alberta. *Lenses, Spectacles, Eyeglasses, and Contacts: The Story of Vision Aids.* Nelson, 1979. 6–9. Account of past, present, and future aids for human vision.
Kettlekamp, Larry. *The Healing Arts.* Morrow, 1978. 6–8. Healing techniques, both conventional and unconventional, are described.
McCoy, J. J. *The Cancer Lady: Maud Slye and Her Heredity Studies.* Thomas Nelson, 1977. 6-up. Description of the work of Maud Slye in cancer research.
Nolen, William A. *Spare Parts for the Human Body.* Random House, 1971. 6–9. Discussion of recent developments in organ replacement.
Nourse, Alan E. *Viruses.* Watts, 1983. 6-up. Describes complexity of viruses, difficulty of isolating them, common and uncommon diseases, and vaccines.
———. *Your Immune System.* Watts, 1982. 6-up. Tells how the body's immune system works and describes current research in immunology.
Selsam, Millicent. *Plants That Heal.* Illus. Kathleen Elgin. Morrow, 1959. 6–9. Describes medicines made from plants that are in use today.
Silverstein, Alvin, and Silverstein, Virginia. *Cancer: Can It Be Stopped?* Lippincott, 1987. 7-up. The origins of cancer, what kinds exist, and current treatments.
———. *So You're Getting Braces: A Guide to Orthodontics.* Lippincott, 1978. 6–9. An introduction to braces.
Skurzynski, Gloria. *Bionic Parts for People.* Four Winds, 1978. 6–8. Explains artificial organs and replacements.

Coping with Disease; Lifestyle Choices

Atkin, Flora. *Hold That Tiger.* New Plays, 1986. 6-up. Play that chronicles the experiences of a family struck by polio.
Bosse, Malcolm. *Captives of Time.* Doubleday, 1987. 7-up. A brother and sister travel to the city to escape the plague in medieval times.
Butler, Beverly. *Maggie by My Side.* Dodd, Mead, 1987. 6-up. A blind girl's story of training a new guide dog.
Corcoran, Barbara. *Child of the Morning.* Atheneum, 1982. 6–9. A young girl working with a theatre company discovers she has epilepsy.
Dacquino, Vincent T. *Kiss the Candy Days Good-Bye.* Delacorte, 1982. 6–8. A young boy finds out he has diabetes.
Ferris, Jean. *Invincible Summer.* Farrar, Straus & Giroux, 1987. 7–12. Two teens who are hospitalized with leukemia fall in love.
Girion, Barbara. *A Handful of Stars.* Scribner's, 1981. 6–9. A young girl discovers she has epilepsy.
Gould, Marilyn. *Golden Daffodils.* Addison-Wesley, 1982. 5–7. A child adjusts to having cerebral palsy.
Hermes, Patricia. *What If They Knew?* Harcourt Brace Jovanovich, 1980. 7-up. A young girl dreads her new friends will not accept her because she has epilepsy.

Kenny, Kevin, and Krull, Helen. *Sometimes My Mom Drinks Too Much.* Illus. Helen Cogancherry. Raintree, 1980. 5–8. A child discovers she is not responsible for her mother's alcoholism.

Killilea, Marie. *Karen.* Prentice-Hall, 1962. 7-up. What parents can do for a child who suffers from spastic cerebral palsy.

Klein, Norma. *Going Backwards.* Scholastic, 1986. 7-up. A child copes with the pain of seeing his grandmother suffering from Alzheimer's disease.

Levy, Marilyn. *The Girl in the Plastic Cage.* Ballantine, 1982. 6-up. A child deals with having curvature of the spine.

Radley, Gail. *CF in His Corner.* Four Winds, 1984. 6–8. A boy discovers his younger brother has cystic fibrosis and learns to deal with it.

Schoor, Gene. *Babe Didrikson: The World's Greatest Woman Athlete.* Doubleday, 1978. 6-up. Chronicles the athletic triumphs of the woman as well as her fight against cancer.

Shilts, Randy. *And the Band Played On.* St. Martin's, 1987. 7-up. How early efforts to publicize and understand AIDS impeded the fight against it.

Skurzynski, Gloria. *Manwolf.* Clarion, 1981. 7-up. An "illegitimate" child in medieval Poland is afflicted with a rare disease and persecuted because of it.

Slepian, Jan. *Lester's Turn.* Macmillan, 1981. 5–8. Two disabled friends' relationship and how one must deal with a tragedy.

Strauss, Linda Leopold. *Coping When a Parent Has Cancer.* Rosen, 1988. 7-up. The added responsibilities children bear when parents are diagnosed as having cancer.

G. SAFETY AND FIRST AID

Grades K Through Three

Accident Prevention

Gobbell, Phyllis and Laster, Jim. *Safe Sally Seat Belt and the Magic Click.* Illus. Stephanie McFetridge Britt. Childrens Press, 1986. K–5. A child is saved from being hurt by her seat belt and tells her classmates about the experience.

Johnsen, Karen. *The Trouble with Secrets.* Parenting Press, 1986. K–3. Helps children distinguish between secrets that may harm people and those that do not.

Purves, Marjory. *Home Safety.* Illus. Carole Hughes; cartoon drawings by Keith Logan. Ladybird, 1981. Pres.–3. Identifies possible hazards and their prevention.

Seuling, Barbara. *Stay Safe, Play Safe.* Illus. Kathy Allert. Golden, 1985. Pres.–3. Factual information on safety for parents to share with their children.

Stanek, Muriel. *All Alone After School.* Illus. Ruth Rosner. Whitman, 1985. K–4. How to deal with feelings of loneliness and anxiety as a latchkey child.

Vandenburg, Mary Lou. *Help! Emergencies That Could Happen to You and How to Handle Them.* Illus. R. L. Markham. Lerner, 1980. K–5. Explains safety precautions and first-aid procedures.

Wachter, Oralee. *Close to Home.* Illus. Jane Aaron. Scholastic, 1986. Pres.–3. Common sense rules about safety discussed.

Safety at Play

Brown, Margaret Wise. *Red Light, Green Light.* Illus. Leonard Weisgard. Doubleday, 1944. 3–5. Explains traffic safety.

Chlad, Dorothy. *Stop, Look, and Listen for Trains.* Childrens Press, 1983. Pres.–2. Explains safety rules for being around trains.

————. *When I Cross the Street.* Childrens Press, 1982. K–3. Explains safety rules for crossing the street.

Cleary, Beverly. *Lucky Chuck.* Illus. J. Winslow Higginbottom. Morrow, 1984. K–3. Explains motorcycle safety rules.

Kaye, Marilyn. *Will You Cross Me?* Illus. Ned Delaney. Harper & Row, 1985. Pres.–3. Two friends across the street from each other rely on passers-by to help them cross the street to be together.

McLeod, Emilie Warren. *The Bear's Bicycle.* Little, Brown, 1975. Pres.–3. Explains bicycle safety rules.

Viorst, Judith. *Try It Again, Sam: Safety When You Walk.* Illus. Paul Galdone. Lothrop, Lee & Shepard, 1970. Pres.–2. Learning the safety rules for going somewhere alone.

Waddell, Martin. *The Park in the Dark.* Illus. Barbara Firth. Lothrop, Lee & Shepard, 1989. Pres.–1. Three stuffed animals sneak out in the dark and make their way to the playground by themselves.

Watson, Wendy. *Tales for a Winter's Eve.* Farrar, Straus & Giroux, 1988. Pres.–2. Tales are told to a fox by family and friends after the fox has a skiing accident.

Yamashita, Haruo. *Mice at the Beach.* Illus. Kazuo Iwamura. Morrow, 1987. Pres.–K. A mouse family practices safety at the beach.

Young, Miriam. *Beware the Polar Bear: Safety on the Ice.* Illus. Robert Quackenbush. Lothrop, Lee & Shepard, 1970. K–4. Two siblings learn rules of ice skating safety. Includes a section on safety.

People and Places That Can Provide Help

Aylesworth, Jim. *Siren in the Night.* Illus. Tom Centola. Whitman, 1983. Pres.–K. Explains the work of firefighters.

Bundt, Nancy. *The Fire Station Book.* Carolrhoda, 1981. K–4. An explanation of the work of firefighters.

Chlad, Dorothy. *When There Is a Fire, Go Outside.* Childrens Press, 1983. K–3. Explains fire safety rules for the home.

Keller, Irene. *Benjamin Rabbit and Fire Chief.* Illus. Dick Keller. Childrens Press, 1986. K–5. Explanation of fire safety rules.

Pelta, Kathy. *What Does a Lifeguard Do?* Dodd, Mead, 1977. 2–4. History of lifesaving and techniques currently used.

Rockwell, Anne. *The Emergency Room.* Illus. Harlow Rockwell. Macmillan, 1985. Pres.–2. Equipment and procedures used in an emergency room.

Sobol, Harriet Langsam. *Jeff's Hospital Book.* Illus. Patricia Agre. Walck, 1975. K–2. Photo-documentary account of a child's stay in the hospital for an operation.

•Udry, Janice May. *Mary Jo's Grandmother.* Illus. Eleanor Mill. Whitman, 1970. K–3. A child's grandmother has an accident while she is visiting; how they cope with the accident.

Weber, Altons. *Elizabeth Gets Well.* Illus. Jacqueline Blass. Crowell, 1970. 3–5. The story of one child's experiences in the hospital.

Grades Four Through Six

Safety Precautions

Baker, Eugene. *Fire.* Illus. Tom Dunnington. Creative Education, 1980. 3–5. Fire hazards existing at home, in stores, and at campsites.

———. *Home.* Illus. Tom Dunnington. Creative Education, 1980. 3–5. Safety in the home.

———. *School.* Illus. Tom Dunnington. Creative Education, 1980. 3–5. Safety at school.

Brink, Carol. *Baby Island.* Macmillan, 1973. 4–6. Two girls are shipwrecked with four babies on an island; safety with infants.

Chlad, Dorothy. *Poisons Make You Sick.* Illus. Lydia Halverson. Childrens Press, 1984. 3–5. A child explains the dangers of ingesting poisons.

———. *Strangers.* Illus. Lydia Halverson. Childrens Press, 1982. 3–5. Safe behavior around strangers.

Curtis, Robert H. *Medical Talk for Beginners.* Illus. William Jaber. Messner, 1976. 4–6. A simple medical dictionary for young people.

Gray, Genevieve. *Keep an Eye on Kevin.* Illus. Don Madden. Lothrop, Lee & Shepard, 1973. 2–6. Safety around the home is explained.

•Greenberg, Keith Elliot. *Out of the Gang.* Illustrated with photographs. Lerner, 1992. 4-up. The dangers of city gangs are explored through the experiences of a former gang member and a boy who has stayed out of gangs.

Mazer, Harry. *Cave Under the City.* Crowell, 1986. 6-up. Two brothers hide under New York City's streets to escape being sent to a
shelter.
Meyer, Linda B. *Safety Zone.* Illus. Marina Megale. Charles Franklin Press,
1984. 3–5. Safety around strangers.
Moeri, Louis. *Save Queen of Sheba.* Dutton, 1981. 4–6. Two pioneer
children search for their parents after a massacre.
Newman, Susan. *Never Say Yes to a Stranger: What Your Child Must Know
to Stay Safe.* Photographs by George Tiboni. Putnam, 1985. 5-up.
Stresses awareness of dangerous situations around strangers.
O'Dell, Scott. *Island of the Blue Dolphins.* Houghton Mifflin, 1960. 4–6. A
child learns to survive alone amidst life-threatening circumstances.

Being Safe at Play

Baker, Eugene. *Outdoors.* Illus. Tom Dunnington. Creative Education,
1980. 3–5. Being safe while playing.
———. *Water.* Illus. Tom Dunnington. Creative Education, 1980. 3–5.
Water safety.
Chlad, Dorothy. *Bicycles Are Fun to Ride.* Illus. Lydia Halverson. Childrens
Press, 1984. 3–5. Explains bicycle safety practices.
Haskins, Jim. *Break Dancing.* Lerner, 1985. 4-up. Explains break dancing
and safe practices for doing it.
Hopper, Nancy J. *The Truth or Dare Trap.* Dutton, 1985. 5-up. The
dangers of taking dares; fireworks safety practices.
Kessler, Leonard. *Who Tossed That Bat?* Lothrop, Lee & Shepard, 1973.
4–6. Sports safety practices.

Who Keeps Us Safe?

Arnold, Caroline. *Who Keeps Us Safe?* Photographs by Carole Bertole.
Watts, 1983. 4-up. Discusses police, fire, and other emergency person-
nel and how they aid their communities.
Berry, Joy Wilt. *What To Do When Your Mom or Dad Says Be Careful.*
Childrens Press, 1983. K–6. Illustrates safety procedures.
Kay, Eleanor. *The Emergency Room.* Watts, 1970. 4–6. An account of what
goes on in an emergency room.
———. *The First Book of the Clinic.* Watts, 1971. 4–6. Explains the
functions and purposes of a health clinic.
Rothkopf, Carol Z. *The First Book of the Red Cross.* Watts, 1971. 4–6.
Explains the history, organization, and activities of the Red Cross,
including the Junior Red Cross and its activities.

Grades Seven and Up

Safety Precautions

Berry, Joy. *Every Kid's Guide to Responding to Danger*. Childrens Press, 1987. 4–7. How to avoid dangerous situations.
Haines, Gil Kay. *Natural and Synthetic Poisons*. Morrow, 1978. 6–8. Animals, plants, and other substances that can harm people.
Haskins, James. *The Child Abuse Help Book*. Addison-Wesley, 1982. 6–9. Explanation of child abuse with straightforward, realistic advice on what to do.
Nourse, Alan E. *Fractures, Dislocations and Sprains*. Watts, 1978. 4–8. Explains these injuries and gives first-aid tips.

Stories of Risks, Accidents, and Survival

Bauer, Marion Dane. *On My Honor*. Clarion, 1986. 4–7. A boy drowns his friend and must live with his conscience and his grief.
Bennett, Jay. *The Haunted One*. Watts, 1987. 7-up. A lifeguard causes a girl's death because he was smoking marijuana and unable to save her from drowning.
Byars, Betsy. *The Not-Just-Anybody Family*. Illus. Jacqueline Rogers. Dell, 1986. 6–8. Explains how a family copes with accidents and embarrassment.
George, Jean Craighead. *Julie of the Wolves*. Harper & Row, 1982. 6-up. A young girl joins a wolf pack in order to survive on the Arctic tundra.
Hamilton, Dorothy. *Last One Chosen*. Illus. James L. Converse. Herald Press, 1982. 6-up. A farmer lives with the guilt of causing a farm accident that has disabled his son.
Hinton, S. E. *The Outsiders*. Viking Kestrel, 1967. 7-up. A tough, lower-class gang feuds with a middle-class gang.
Holman, Felice. *Slake's Limbo*. Macmillan, 1974. 6-up. A child survives in the subway, hoping to make a life for himself.
L'Engle, Madeleine. *An Acceptable Time*. Farrar, Straus & Giroux, 1989. 6-up. Polly O'Keefe is transported to prehistoric times and involved in a dangerous confrontation between freedom and oppression.
Lewis, Elizabeth Foreman. *To Beat a Tiger*. Illus. John Heuhnergarth. Holt, 1956. 7-up. A group of boys in ancient Shanghai attempt to survive grim circumstances of gang life in the streets.
Mathieson, David. *Trial by Wilderness*. Houghton Mifflin, 1985. 7-up. A girl must learn to survive in the wilderness after a plane wreck.
Mayhar, Ardath. *Medicine Walk*. Atheneum, 1985. 6-up. A child must survive alone in the desert after a plane crash.

Miklowitz, Gloria. *After the Bomb*. Scholastic, 1985. 6-up. Survival under a city in a shelter after a bomb dropped during a war.

Moore, Ruth Nulton. *Danger in the Pines*. Illus. James Converse. Herald Press, 1983. 6-up. A child must survive in the wilderness in New Jersey during a forest fire.

Morris, Judy K. *The Crazies and Sam*. Viking Kestrel, 1983. 5–7. A single parent's child must learn to recognize danger in a large city.

Naylor, Phyllis Reynolds. *The Dark of the Tunnel*. Atheneum, 1985. 7-up. Safety practices in case of a nuclear attack are explained.

O'Brien, Robert. *Z for Zachariah*. Macmillan, 1975. 6-up. A girl survives a nuclear war in a valley with an unstable companion.

Rickett, Frances, and McGraw, Steven. *Totaled*. Ballantine, 1983. 7-up. An eighteen-year-old's struggle to lead a normal life after an auto accident.

Schneider, Hansjorg. *Robinson and Friday*. Ken and Barbi Rugg, translators. Carol Korty, editor. Baker's Plays, 1980. 7-up. Play based on *Robinson Crusoe*, examining what we do to physically survive.

Skurzynski, Gloria. *Caught in the Moving Mountains*. Illus. Ellen Thompson. Lothrop, Lee & Shepard, 1984. 6-up. Two brothers survive an earthquake during a hiking trip.

Speare, Elizabeth George. *The Sign of the Beaver*. Houghton Mifflin, 1984. 6–8. A boy left alone in the Maine woods in the 1700s learns survival from a Native American whom he befriends.

H. CONSUMER HEALTH

Grades K Through Three

Berenstain, Stan, and Berenstain, Jan. *The Berenstain Bears Go to the Doctor*. Random House, 1981. 1–3. The bears go in for a check-up, from temperatures to getting booster shots.

Chalmers, Mary. *Come to the Doctor, Harry*. Harper & Row, 1981. 1–3. Harry the cat learns that a visit to the doctor can be a good experience.

Ciliotta, Claire, and Livingston, Carole. *Why Am I Going to the Hospital?* Illus. Dick Wilson. Lyle Stuart, 1981. K–2. Basic information about hospitals and hospital procedures.

DeSantis, Kenny. *A Doctor's Tools*. Photographs by Patricia A. Agre. Dodd, Mead, 1985. Pres.–2. Introduction to the doctor's office.

Goodsell, Jane. *The Mayo Brothers*. Illus. Louis Glanzman. Harper & Row, 1972. 2–4. The story of the Mayo brothers and their clinic.

Hutchins, Pat. *Don't Forget the Bacon!* Greenwillow, 1987. Pres.–3. A humorous trip to the grocery store.

Hyde, Margaret O. *Know About Alcohol*. Illus. Bill Morrison. McGraw-Hill, 1978. 3-up. Facts about alcohol, responsible drinking, dealing with alcoholic friends and relatives, coping with peer pressure; includes sources for assistance.

Linn, Margot. *A Trip to the Dentist.* Illus. Catherine Siracusa. Harper & Row, 1988. Pres.–2. Questions and answers about visiting the dentist.

———. *A Trip to the Doctor.* Illus. Catherine Siracusa. Harper & Row, 1988. Pres.–2. Questions and answers about visiting the doctor.

Marino, Barbara Pavis. *Eric Needs Stitches.* Photographs by Richard Rudinski. Addison-Wesley, 1979. K–3. Follows a child through the process of having stitches in the emergency room to getting ice cream afterward.

Martin, Charles E. *Summer Business.* Greenwillow, 1984. 1–4. Story about friends who undertake small businesses in order to make money over a summer.

Miller, J. P. *Little Rabbit Goes to the Doctor.* Random, 1987. Pres.–1. Information about visiting the doctor.

Moncure, Jane Belk. *The Healthkin Food Train.* Illus. Lois Axeman. Childrens Press, 1982. 2-up. Information about the food groups and a good diet.

Pearson, Tracey Campbell. *The Storekeeper.* Dial, 1988. K–3. The activities of a storekeeper, from opening to closing.

Rockwell, Anne, and Rockwell, Harlow. *Sick in Bed.* Macmillan, 1982. Pres.–3. Documents a small boy's illness from beginning to recovery.

Smith, Barry. *Tom and Annie Go Shopping.* Houghton Mifflin, 1989. K–3. Two children go on a shopping trip.

Steig, William. *Doctor De Soto.* Farrar, Straus & Giroux, 1982. Pres.–3. A mouse dentist may be at the mercy of his fox patient.

Grades Four Through Six

Arnold, Caroline. *Who Keeps Us Healthy?* Illus. Carole Bertole. Watts, 1982. 4-up. Introduces and explains the work of various health care professionals and examines programs for public health.

Baker, Rachel. *The First Woman Doctor.* Illus. Evelyn Copelman. Scholastic, 1987. 6-up. Details the life of the first woman to become a doctor.

Betancourt, Jeanne. *Smile! How to Cope with Braces.* Illus. Mimi Harrison. Knopf, 1982. 4-up. Information and advice for those having their teeth straightened.

Boylston, Helen Dore. *Clara Barton, Founder of the American Red Cross.* Illus. Paula Hutchison. Random, 1955. 4–7. Biography of Clara Barton, emphasizing her work during the Civil War.

Charren, Peggy, and Hulsizer, Carol. *The TV-Smart Book for Kids.* Illus. Marylin Hafner. Dutton Children's Books, n.d. 2–6. A way to help children manage their TV habits.

Crofford, Emily. *Healing Warrior: A Story about Sister Elizabeth Kenny.* Illus. Steve Michaels. Carolrhoda, 1989. 3–6. Biography of a nurse who found a way to fight polio.

Daniel, Anita. *The Story of Albert Schweitzer.* Random, 1957. 4–6. Explains Schweitzer's life and work.

De Angeli, Marguerite. *The Door in the Wall.* Doubleday, 1969. 4–6. Play that takes place during the bubonic plague.

Fekete, Irene, and Ward, Peter Dorrington. *Your Body.* Facts on File, 1984. 5-up. History of the study of the human body from ancient Greece to the present.

Gilbert, Sara. *You Are What You Eat; A Common-Sense Guide to the Modern American Diet.* Macmillan, 1977. 5-up. A skeptical look at the food industry and its impact on our eating habits.

Killen, Barbara. *Economics and the Consumer.* Lerner, 1989. 5-up. Who consumers are, how they make decisions, and how the decisions affect the economy.

Krantz, Hazel. *Daughter of My People: Henrietta Szold and Hadassah.* Dutton, 1988. 5–6. Biography of a woman who developed health services in Israel.

Lowry, Lois. *A Summer to Die.* Illus. Jenni Oliver. Houghton Mifflin, 1977. 5-up. Explains the medical treatment of leukemia through the story of a family coping with the death of a daughter.

McNeer, Mary, and Ward, Lynd. *Armed with Courage.* Illus. Lynd Ward. Abingdon, 1952. 4–7. Biographies of seven dedicated men and women.

Shiels, Barbara. *Winners, Women and the Nobel Prize.* Dillon, 1985. 5-up. Eight biographies of women who have won the Nobel Prize.

Grades Seven and Up

Aaseng, Nathan. *The Disease Fighters.* Lerner, 1987. 6-up. Biographies of people instrumental in fighting diseases.

•Bess, Clayton. *Story for a Black Night.* Houghton Mifflin, 1982. 6-up. Contrast between old African and modern Christian attitudes toward helping the sick.

Bowman, Kathleen. *New Women in Medicine.* Creative Education, 1976. 5–7. Seven biographies of successful women in medicine.

•Brown, Marion Marsh. *Homeward the Arrow's Flight.* Abingdon, 1980. 5–7. Fictionalized biography of the first woman Native American doctor.

Clapp, Patricia. *Doctor Elizabeth: The Story of the First Woman Doctor.* Lothrop, Lee & Shepard, 1974. 6-up. Obstacles to women in careers in the nineteenth century.

•Clifford, Eth. *The Wild One.* Illus. Arvis Stewart. Houghton Mifflin, 1974. 6–9. Biography of Santiago Ramon, who won the Nobel Prize for medicine in 1906.

Gordon, James S. *Holistic Medicine.* Chelsea House, 1988. 6–9. A comprehensive overview of the many ways of healing.

Matthew, Scott. *The First Woman of Medicine: The Story of Elizabeth Blackwell.* Illus. Wayne Atkinson. Contemporary Perspectives, 1978. 6–9. Biography of the first American woman doctor.

Morgan, Elizabeth. *The Making of a Woman Surgeon.* Putnam's, 1980. 6–9. Biography of the first woman surgeon.
•Patterson, Lillie. *Sure Hands, Strong Heart: The Life of Daniel Hale Williams.* Illus. David Scott Brown. Abingdon, 1981. 6–9. Biography of one of the first black men to become a physician.
Perl, Lila. *Junk Food, Fast Food, Health Food: What America Eats and Why.* Clarion, 1980. 6-up. Information on American eating habits and the various diets.
Ranahan, Demerris C. *Contributions of Women: Medicine.* Dillon Press, 1981. 6–9. Biographies of five women who made outstanding contributions to medicine.
Sullivan, George. *How Do They Package It?* Westminster, 1976. 5–7. Explains the history and functions of packaging.
Van Devanter, Lynda, and Morgan, Christopher. *Home Before Morning: The Story of an Army Nurse in Vietnam.* Beaufort, 1983. 6–9. Recounting of a woman's experiences as an army surgical nurse in Vietnam and stress experienced after coming home.
Walz, Michael K. and Killen, M. Barbara. *The Law and Economics: Your Rights as a Consumer.* Lerner, 1990. 6–9. Describes consumer laws, e.g., contracts and warranties that protect the consumer.
Weiner, Michael. *Bugs in the Peanut Butter: Dangers in Everyday Food.* Little, Brown, 1976. 5–8. Discusses the natural and artificial poisons found in our foods.

I. DRUG USE AND ABUSE

Grades Four Through Six

Alexander, Anne. *Connie.* Illus. Gail Owens. Atheneum, 1976. 6–8. A child adjusts to a new life when her father loses his job.
Buckvar, Felice. *Ten Miles High.* Morrow, 1981. 6-up. A teen finds love and understanding with a former drug addict.
Corcoran, Barbara. *The Woman in Your Life.* Atheneum, 1984. 6-up. Diary of a girl in prison who was transporting drugs across the border for a boyfriend.
Dorman, N. B. *Laughter in the Background.* Elsevier/Nelson, 1980. 6-up. An obese and slovenly teen learns to take control of her life after her alcoholic mother's boyfriend tries to rape her.
Gilmour, H. B. *Ask Me If I Care.* Fawcett, 1985. 6-up. A girl gets hooked on drugs after her move to her father's new home.
Hamilton, Dorothy. *Joel's Other Mother.* Illus. Esther Rose Graber. Herald, 1984. 6-up. The experience of having an alcoholic mother and finding out how to help.
Hawley, Richard A. *Think About Drugs and Society.* Walker, 1988. 6-up. Explores drugs and drug abuse in our culture.

Hinton, Susan Eloise. *Rumble Fish.* Delacorte, 1975. 5–8. Two brothers deal with having an alcoholic father and with belonging to street gangs.

Holland, Isabelle. *Alan and the Animal Kingdom.* Lippincott, 1977. 5–8. A child who has been in many foster homes learns to accept adults as caring individuals after many negative experiences.

Hyde, Margaret O. *Know About Drugs.* Illus. Bill Morrison. McGraw-Hill, 1979. 4-up. Information for young readers on drugs and their effects.

———. *Know About Smoking.* Illus. Dennis Kendrick. McGraw-Hill, 1983. 4-up. History of tobacco and cigarettes and their effects on the body.

•Lampman, Evelyn Sibley. *The Potlatch Family.* Atheneum, 1976. 4-up. A young girl is ashamed of her Native American family and her alcoholic father.

Miner, Jane Claypool. *A Day at a Time: Dealing with an Alcoholic.* Crestwood House, Inc., 1982. 6-up. A girl deals with having an alcoholic father.

Porterfield, Kay Marie. *Coping with an Alcoholic Parent.* Rosen, 1985. 5-up. The effects of alcoholism on a family and what to do.

Robinson, Mary. *Give It Up, Mom.* Houghton Mifflin, 1989. 5–9. One girl's attempts to stop her mother from smoking.

Rock, Gail. *A Dream for Addie.* Illus. Charles C. Gehm. Knopf, 1975. 4–7. An adolescent learns how to give and receive friendship and deal with an alcoholic friend.

Ryan, Elizabeth A. *Straight Talk about Drugs and Alcohol.* Facts on File, 1989. 6-up. The process of making decisions about using drugs and alcohol.

Seixas, Judith S. *Living with a Parent Who Drinks Too Much.* Greenwillow, 1979. 4–8. Describes alcoholism, alcoholic behavior, and resulting family problems.

Sonnett, Sherry. *Smoking.* Watts, 1988. 4-up. Informational book about the physiological effects of tobacco on the body.

Stwertka, Eve, and Stwertka, Albert. *Marijuana.* Watts, 1986. 5–8. History, appearance, and effects of smoking marijuana.

Woods, Geraldine. *Drug Use and Drug Abuse.* Watts, 1986. 4–6. Medicinal and recreational use of drugs explained.

Yost, Don. *The Case of the Blue Notes.* Bridgework Theater, 113½ East Lincoln Ave., Goshen, IN 46526. 4-up. Play providing information about substance abuse.

Grades Seven and Up

Bauer, Marion Dane. *Shelter from the Wind.* Seabury Press, 1976. 6-up. A story about parental alcoholism.

Berg, Jean Horton. *I Cry When the Sun Goes Down: The Story of Herman Wrice.* Westminster, 1975. 6–9. Biography of a community leader and drug counselor.

Black, Claudia. *It Will Never Happen to Me.* Ballantine, 1987. 6–9. Story of children of alcoholics.

Bottner, Barbara. *Let Me Tell You Everything: Memoirs of a Lovesick Intellectual.* Harper & Row, 1989. 6–9. A teen's problems with an alcoholic father and a crush on a new teacher.

Brancato, Robin Fidler. *Something Left to Lose.* Knopf, 1976. 7-up. A girl's friendship with a girl whose mother is an alcoholic.

Carlson, Dale Bick. *Triple Boy.* Atheneum, 1977. 7-up. A child deals with his mother's alcoholism.

•Childress, Alice. *A Hero Ain't Nothin' but a Sandwich.* Coward, McCann, 1973. 6-up. A young boy's life as a heroin addict.

Dodson, Susan. *Have You Seen This Girl?* Four Winds, 1982. 7-up. The life of a runaway in a big city; problems of drug and alcohol abuse.

•Glass, Frankcina. *Marvin & Tige.* St. Martin's, 1977. 7-up. A man and a boy come to respect and love each other, although unrelated by race or culture.

Godfrey, Martin. *Heroin.* Illus. Peter Harper. Watts, 1987. 6-up. Why people take heroin, its effect on the body, cost of addiction, its manufacture, and sources of help.

Goldreich, Gloria. *Lori.* Holt, 1979. 6-up. A child's experiences after being caught smoking marijuana.

Greene, Shep. *The Boy Who Drank Too Much.* Viking Kestrel, 1979. 7-up. The story of a high school hockey player who is an alcoholic.

Hanlon, Emily. *It's Too Late for Sorry.* Bradbury, 1978. 6-up. Story of marijuana smoking among teens and prejudice against handicapped.

Hawkes, Nigel. *The Heroin Trail.* Illus. Ron Hayward Associates. Gloucester, 1986. 7-up. Story of the manufacture, sale, and uses of heroin, and consequences for addicts.

Hinton, S. E. *That Was Then, This Is Now.* Viking Kestrel, 1971. 7-up. Two friends deal with one's problems as a drug pusher and the question of loyalty.

Kinter, Judith. *Cross-Country Caper.* Illus. Furan Illustrators. Crestwood House, Inc., 1981. 6–9. The courage of making a decision about drugs and drug pushing.

Mazer, Harry. *The War on Villa Street: A Novel.* Delacorte, 1978. 6–9. An only child deals with his father's alcoholism and finds independence.

Mazer, Norma Fox. *Dear Bill, Remember Me? And Other Stories.* Delacorte, 1976. 7-up. Eight short stories about teens' family problems, one dealing with parental alcoholism.

McFann, Jane. *Maybe by Then I'll Understand.* Avon, 1987. 6-up. A teen deals with her boyfriend's alcoholism.

Meyer, Carolyn. *The Center: From a Troubled Past to a New Life.* Atheneum, 1979. 7-up. A troubled teenager's two years of experiences in a place for those with problems like his.

Milgram, Gail Gleason. *Coping with Alcohol.* Rosen Press, 1980. 6-up. Questions and answers about alcoholism, with resources.

Neville, Emily Cheney. *Garden of Broken Glass.* Delacorte, 1975. 6-up. A child deals with his alcoholic mother and his own loneliness.

O'Dell, Scott. *Alexandra.* Houghton Mifflin, 1984. 6-up. A young girl deals with drug traffic coming in from the Caribbean to her southern Florida town.

O'Hanlon, Jacklyn. *Fair Game*. Dial, 1977. 6–9. Sisters deal with the sexual advances of their mother's alcoholic boyfriend and with their father's mental illness and drug problems.
Roos, Stephen. *You'll Miss Me Whan I'm Gone*. Delacorte, 1988. 7-up. A sixteen-year-old deals with his own alcoholism.
Scoppettone, Sandra. *The Late Great Me*. Putnam, 1976. 7-up. A seventeen-year-old girl deals with her own alcoholism.
Shyer, Marlene Fanta. *Me & Joey Pinstripe, the King of Rock*. Scribner's, 1987. 7-up. A teen deals with the effects of drugs in her school.
Snyder, Anne. *First Step*. Holt, 1975. 6–9. A senior high student copes with her divorced mother's drinking and the fear that her mother will abuse her little brother.
————. *My Name Is Davy: I'm an Alcoholic*. New American Library, 1978. 6-up. The nightmares of being a young alcoholic.
Tapp, Kathy Kennedy. *Smoke from the Chimney*. Atheneum, 1986. 6–8. A child creates a fantasy world to escape her father's alcoholism.
Terry, Megan. *Keggar*. Omaha Magic Theatre, 1417 Farnam St., Omaha, NE 68102. 6-up. Play about alcohol abuse among young people.
Windsor, Patricia. *Diving for Roses*. Harper & Row, 1976. 7-up. A teen deals with her mother's alcoholism and her own pregnancy.
Wrenn, C. Gilbert and Schwartzrock, Shirley. *Facts and Fantasies About Alcohol*. Illus. Carol Nelson. American Guidance Service, Inc., 1971. 6–9. Facts and fantasies presented about alcoholism.

J. COMMUNITY HEALTH MANAGEMENT

Grades K Through Three

Types of Pollution; Environmental Protection

Bartlett, Margaret F. *The Clean Brook*. Illus. Aldren A. Watson. Harper & Row, 1960. 1–3. How a brook purifies itself through the activities of plants and animals.
Bodeker, N. M. *The Mushroom Center Disaster*. Illus. Erik Blegvad. Atheneum, 1974. 2–4. Fantasy about insects living in a community being littered by humans and what they can do about it.
Breiter, Herta S. *Pollution*. Raintree, 1978. 2–4. An introduction to the problems of pollution.
Cowcher, Helen. *Rain Forest*. Farrar, Straus & Giroux, 1988. Pres.–2. The destruction of the rain forest by machines and its consequences.
Foord, Isabelle. *Junkyard*. Toronto, Ontario: Playwrights Co-op, 1971. 3-up. Three children plan to save their favorite playground, a junkyard, from conversion into a parking lot.

Parnall, Peter. *The Mountain.* Doubleday, 1971. Pres.–3. Picture storybook tracing the transformation of a mountainside into a treeless national park.

Seuss, Dr. *The Butter Battle Book.* Random House, 1984. All ages. Commentary on the absurdity of war.

Shanks, Anne Zane. *About Garbage and Stuff.* Viking Kestrel, 1973. K–2. Introduction to recycling waste materials and how children can help.

Showers, Paul. *Where Does the Garbage Go?* Illus. Loretta Lustig. Harper & Row, 1974. 2–4. The problems of sanitation, conservation, and recycling garbage from a child's point of view.

Tusa, Tricia. *Stay Away from the Junkyard!* Macmillan, 1988. 1–3. The story of turning a village junkyard into an object of delight.

Ecosystems

Cajacob, Thomas, and Burton, Teresa. *Water for Life.* Photographs by Thomas Cajacob. Carolrhoda, 1987. 2–5. Discusses the value of water in our lives.

Cortesi, W. W. *Explore a Spooky Swamp.* Photographs by J. H. Bailey. National Geographic Society, 1978. K–4. Two children explore the Okefenokee Swamp, identifying the plants and animals they see.

Lerner, Carol. *A Forest Year.* Morrow, 1987. All ages. Effects of the seasons in a forest on its plants and animals.

Levitin, Sonia. *The Fisherman and the Bird.* Ill. Frances Livingston. Houghton/Parnassus, 1982. K–4. A fisherman becomes the keeper of a nest of birds on the mast of his boat.

Milgram, H. *ABC of Ecology.* Illus. Donald Crews. Macmillan, 1972. K–3. Each letter of the alphabet introduces an example of urban pollution. Book gives suggestions for solving pollution problems.

Newton, James R. *A Forest Is Reborn.* Illus. Susan Bonners. Crowell, 1982. 2–4. Describes the part fire plays in forest ecology.

Nixon, Hershell H., and Nixon, Joan Lowery. *Land Under the Sea.* Dodd, Mead, 1985. All ages. Information about the land formations beneath the sea.

The Paper Bag Players. *Dandelion.* Baker's Plays, 1978. 3-up. Play about periods in evolution of the earth, lessons in conservation, and care of the environment are presented.

Tresselt, Alvin. *The Beaver Pond.* Illus. Roger Duvoisin. Lothrop, Lee & Shepard, 1970. K–2. Explores the ecosystem in which the beaver lives.

Environmental Awareness

Aliki. *The Story of Johnny Appleseed.* Prentice-Hall, 1963. K–3. Picture book about the man who wandered the Midwest spreading apple seeds and love.

Arnold, Caroline. *A Walk on the Great Barrier Reef.* Photographs by Arthur Arnold. Carolrhoda, 1989. 2–5. The plants and animals of Australia's Great Barrier Reef are described and illustrated.

———. *Saving the Peregrine Falcon.* Photographs by Richard R. Hewett. Carolrhoda, 1989. 2–5. A brief natural history of the peregrine falcon is described.

Baylor, Byrd. *I'm in Charge of Celebrations.* Illus. Peter Parnall. Scribner's, 1986. 3-up. A dweller in the wilderness celebrates natural phenomena.

•———. *The Desert Is Theirs.* Illus. Peter Parnall. Scribner's, 1975. 1–4. Poetic explanation of the Papago Indians' respect for the resources of the desert.

———. *The Way to Start a Day.* Illus. Peter Parnall. Aladdin, 1986. 1–4. Examples of those who have celebrated the dawn throughout history.

Blood-Patterson, Peter. *Rise Up Singing.* New Society Publishers, 1988. All ages. Twelve hundred songs, including those about ecology and nature.

Burns, Diane L. *Arbor Day.* Illus. Kathy Rogers. Carolrhoda, 1989. K–3. Explains the history of Arbor Day and some activities that take place on the day.

Caduto, Michael J., and Bruchac, Joseph. *Keepers of the Earth.* Illus. John Kahionhes Fadden and Carol Wood. Fulchrum, 1989. All ages. Native American tales accompanied by related hands-on environmental activities. The same format is used in *Animals of the Earth.*

Caveney, Sylvia, and Giesen, Rosemary. *Where Am I?* Lerner, 1980. K–3. A look at people's places in the world.

•dePaola, Tomie, reteller. *The Legend of the Bluebonnet: An Old Tale of Texas.* Putnam, 1983. K–3. An Indian girl sacrifices her dearest possession to bring rain to save her people.

de Papp Severo, Emöke, translator. *The Good-Hearted Youngest Brother: An Hungarian Folk Tale.* Illus. Diane Goode. Bradbury, 1981. K–4. The concern of a younger brother for all living things removes a princess from a spell and restores the countryside to life.

Elkington, John, and others. *Going Green: A Kid's Handbook to Saving the Planet.* Illus. Tony Ross. Puffin, 1990. 4–6. Introduces environmental issues and includes a checklist for environmental awareness.

Fischer-Nagel, Heiderose, and Fischer-Nagel, Andreas. *Fir Trees.* Carolrhoda, 1989. 2–5. Describes the ecosystem and the development of fir trees.

Hines, Anna Grossnickle. *Come to the Meadow.* Clarion, 1984. Pres.–3. A family goes on a picnic in the meadow in springtime.

Isadora, Rachel. *City Seen from A to Z.* Greenwillow, 1983. K–3. Urban environments from a to z described.

Lewis, J. Patrick. *A Hippopotamusn't and Other Animal Verses.* Illus. Victoria Chess. Dial, 1990. Pres.–3. Thirty-five humorous poems about animals, insects, and birds.

Mayer, Marianna. *The Unicorn and the Lake.* Illus. Michael Hague. Dial, 1982. K–3. The unicorn restores beauty to the earth, saving all other animals so they can communicate once again.

Norman, Charles. *The Hornbeam Tree and Other Poems*. Illus. Ted Rand. Holt, 1988. K–4. Poems about the beauty and power of nature.

Osborne, Mary Pope. *Favorite Greek Myths*. Illus. Troy Howell. Scholastic, 1989. 2–5. Nature is revealed through these tales.

Pearson, Susan. *My Favorite Time of Year*. Illus. John Wallner. Harper & Row, 1988. K–3. Celebrates the seasons with illustrations.

Powzyk, Joyce. *Tasmania: A Wildlife Journey*. Lothrop, Lee & Shepard, 1987. 1–4. A journey through the isolated island, highlighting its unusual animals in their natural settings.

Radin, Ruth Yaffe. *High in the Mountains*. Illus. Ed Young. Macmillan, 1989. K–4. The environment of the Colorado Rockies illustrated through a child's experiences there.

Russo, Susan, compiler. *The Ice Cream Ocean and Other Delectable Poems of the Sea*. Lothrop, Lee & Shepard, 1984. Pres.–2. Anthology of verses about the sea.

Selsam, Millicent, and Hunt, Joyce. *Keep Looking!* Illus. Normand Chartier. Macmillan, 1989. K–3. The wildlife present in the winter in the country.

Siebert, Diane. *Heartland*. Illus. Wendell Minor. Harper & Row, 1989. Pres.–3. Poetry about America's heartland.

A Song of Seasons. San Diego: Readers Theatre Script Service, P.O. Box 178333, San Diego, CA 92117. K–3. Play in which Mother Nature teaches the twelve months their jobs for the new year.

Van Allsburg, Chris. *Just a Dream*. Houghton Mifflin, 1990. K–6. A trip into the polluted world of the future awakens Walter to his responsibility to the environment.

Grades Four Through Six

Types of Pollution; Environmental Protection

Berger, Melvin. *Hazardous Substances: A Reference*. Enslow, 1986. 6-up. A dictionary of toxic and hazardous materials in our environment.

Briggs, Raymond. *When the Wind Blows*. Schocken, 1982. 6-up. An elderly British couple prepare for a nuclear attack by following the government's guidelines.

Brown, Joseph E. *Oil Spills: Danger in the Sea*. Dodd, Mead, 1978. 6–9. The sources and effects of oil spills on the environment.

Elliott, Sarah M. *Our Dirty Water*. Messner, 1973. 4–6. Causes and dangers of polluted water.

Gregor, Arthur S. *Man's Mark on the Land; The Changing Environment from the Stone Age to the Age of Smog, Sewage, and Tar on Your Feet*. Scribner's, 1974. 4–6. Explains the effects of the arrival of humans on our environment.

Hamilton, Virginia. *M. C. Higgins, the Great*. Macmillan, 1974. 5-up. A thirteen-year-old boy tries to save his family's Appalachian home from the slag heap that threatens to destroy it.

Hyde, Dayton O. *Thunder Down the Track.* Atheneum, 1986. 5–8. The fight against dumping toxic waste on a site near a railroad line.

Hyde, Margaret O., and Hyde, Bruce G. *Everyone's Trash Problem: Nuclear Wastes.* McGraw-Hill, 1979. 4-up. The effects of nuclear waste on our environment.

Larrick, Nancy. *I Heard a Scream in the Street: Poems by Young People.* Evans, 1970. 4–9. Several of the poems deal with pollution.

Lloyd, David. *Air.* Illus. Peter Visscher. Dial, 1982. 3–6. The effects of air as an element in the natural world.

Maguire, Gregory. *I Feel Like the Morning Star.* Harper & Row, 1989. 6-up. Three friends question their survival in an underground community built to save them from a nuclear war.

Marek, Margot. *Matt's Crusade.* Four Winds, 1988. 5–7. A boy deals with the decision to house nuclear missiles at an army base near his home.

Martin, Laurence. *Nuclear Warfare.* Lerner, 1989. 5-up. The history of the atomic bomb, development of weapons, and current hopes for disarmament.

•Maruki, Toshi. *Hiroshima No Pika.* Lothrop, Lee & Shepard, 1982. 4-up. A child's story as she and others try to flee the 1945 atomic holocaust.

•Mayo, Gretchen Will. *Earthmaker's Tales: North American Stories About Earth Happenings.* Walker, 1987. 4–7. Legends that engender respect for the earth.

McMahan, Ian. *Lake Fear.* Macmillan, 1985. 5-up. A pollutant in a city reservoir causes a mysterious rash on the town's children.

Miller, Christina G., and Berry, Louise A. *Wastes.* Watts, 1986. 5–8. Discussion of the problem of disposing of wastes in our time.

Moeri, Louise. *Downwind.* Dutton, 1984. 6-up. The problems that threaten one family after a nuclear power plant's disaster.

Murray, Marguerite. *A Peaceable Warrior.* Atheneum, 1985. 4–8. How to deal with someone transporting and storing dangerous wastes.

Orlowsky, W., and Perera, T. B. *Who Will Wash the River?* Illus. Richard Cuffari. Coward, 1970. 3–6. Causes and cure for water pollution discovered by two children.

Ostmann, Robert, Jr. *Acid Rain, A Plague upon the Waters.* Dillon Press, 1982. 6-up. The economic and political ramifications of acid rain.

Pringle, Laurence. *Lives at Stake: The Science and Politics of Environmental Health.* Macmillan, 1980. 4–8. Examines the effects of pollution on our environment.

————. *The Only Earth We Have.* Macmillan, 1969. 5–8. A discussion of how man has misused the Earth.

Ricciuti, Edward R. *They Work with Wildlife: Jobs for People Who Want to Work with Animals.* Harper & Row, 1983. 5-up. The work involved in managing wildlife.

Service, Pamela F. *Winter of Magic's Return.* Atheneum, 1985. 5-up. Two girls meet a boy with strange powers five hundred years after the nuclear devastation that almost destroyed their world.

Sootin, H. *Easy Experiments with Water Pollution.* Illus. L. Bittner. Four Winds, 1974. 5–7. Easy experiments about pollution and how we can alleviate the problem.

Sorensen, Candace, adaptor. *The Martian Chronicles.* Dramatic Publishing, 1985. 5-up. Play in which, in one episode, Earth has been destroyed by a nuclear war and decides to colonize Mars.

Stern, Cecily. *A Different Kind of Gold.* Illus. Ruth Sanderson. Harper & Row, 1981. 4–6. A child deals with the effects of a hotel wanting to purchase the wilderness around her Alaskan home.

Swindells, Robert. *A Serpent's Tooth.* Holiday House, 1989. 4–6. A child whose parents are activists deals with a possible nuclear waste-disposal site coming to her village.

Vigna, Judith. *Nobody Wants a Nuclear War.* Whitman, 1986. 1–4. Information and hopeful reassurance provided about the possibility of nuclear war.

Walsh, Jill Paton. *Torch.* Farrar, Straus & Giroux, 1988. 4–7. A boy and girl in Greece after a world disaster inherit a symbolic torch.

White, Florence Meiman. *Linus Pauling: Scientist and Crusader.* Walker, 1981. 5-up. Biography of the winner of two Nobel Prizes; his work for control of atomic energy.

Zipko, Stephen J. *Toxic Threat: How Hazardous Substances Poison Our Lives.* Messner, 1986. 6-up. A discussion of environmental issues such as air pollution, pesticides, and radioactive waste.

Ecosystems

Billington, E. *Understanding Ecology.* Illus. G. R. Glaster. Warne, 1971. 5–7. Food chains, ecosystems, and other concepts are explained and some projects are included.

British Museum. *Nature at Work; Introducing Ecology.* Cambridge, 1978. 4–6. Introduces the concept of an ecosystem.

Cook, David. *Environment.* Crown, 1985. 4–7. Describes several different ecological systems inhabited by plants and animals adapted to them.

Dines, Glen. *John Muir.* Putnam, 1974. 4–6. A biography of the conservationist.

Doughty, Bix L. *Noah and the Great Ark.* Anchorage, 1978. 6-up. Play set on Noah's Ark that highlights the ecological conditions on today's Earth.

Edwards, Joan. *Caring for Trees on City Streets.* Scribner's, 1975. 4-up. Describes the usefulness of city trees and how to select, plant, and care for them.

Ehrlich, Anne H., and Ehrlich, Paul R. *Earth.* Watts, 1987. 6-up. The origins, character, and extent of changes to our environment, thanks to human actions.

Fodor, R. V. *Chiseling the Earth: How Erosion Shapes the Land.* Enslow, 1983. 5-up. An account of the changing surface of the Earth by a geologist.

Fradin, Dennis B. *Fires.* Childrens Press, 1982. 4–6. The characteristics of disastrous fires and how to prevent them.

Freschet, Berniece. *Year on Muskrat Marsh.* Illus. Peter Parnall. Scribner's, 1974. 3–5. The marsh as an ecosystem described.

George, Jean Craighead. *One Day in the Prairie.* Illus. Bob Marstall. Crowell, 1986. 4–7. Describes a day on the prairie and what happens when a natural disaster approaches.

——. *One Day in the Woods.* Illus. Gary Allen. Crowell, 1988. 4–7. A child discovers the plant and animal life in the woods of Hudson Highlands, New York.

Hughey, Pat. *Scavengers and Decomposers: The Cleanup Crew.* Photographs by Bruce Hiscock. Atheneum, 1984. 5–8. The characteristics and habits of animals and plants that clean up waste materials in our environment.

Johnson, Rebecca L. *The Greenhouse Effect: Life on a Warmer Planet.* Lerner, 1990. 5-up. Explains the nature of the greenhouse effect and what we can do to reduce its impact on global warming.

Leslie, Robert Franklin. *Ringo, the Robber Raccoon: The True Story of a Northwoods Rogue.* Illus. Leigh Grant. Dodd, Mead, 1984. 4–6. Author describes his relationships with a raccoon and bear in British Columbia's wilds and their survival story.

Linden, Saphira Barbara, and Rosenberg, Ira. *Creation.* New Plays, 1970. 5-up. Play where audience helps actors construct an environment that is free of pollution.

McClung, Robert M. *Whitetail.* Illus. Irene Brady. Morrow, 1987. 3–7. The life cycle of a deer and pros and cons of hunting.

McLaughlin, Molly. *Earthworms, Dirt, and Rotten Leaves: An Exploration in Ecology.* Illus. Rogert Shetterly. Atheneum, 1986. 4–8. Simple introduction to ecology focusing on the earthworm.

Miles, Betty. *Save the Earth!* Illus. Claire Nivola. Knopf, 1974. 4-up. An introduction to the study of ecology.

Muller, Jorg. *The Changing City and the Changing Countryside.* Atheneum, 1977. 4–8. Wordless folios depicting the effects of industrialization on our environment.

Patent, Dorothy Hinshaw. *Yellowstone Fires: Flames and Rebirth.* Photographs by William Munoz and others. Holiday House, 1990. 4-up. Several years after a 1988 fire has devastated nearly one-third of Yellowstone National Park, the forest begins to renew itself. A Notable Children's Trade Book in the Field of Social Sciences.

Pringle, Laurence. *Chains, Webs, Pyramids: The Flow of Energy in Nature.* Illus. Jan Adkins. Crowell, 1975. 4–7. How the sun's energy is changed to food energy in plants.

——. *City and Suburb: Exploring an Ecosystem.* Macmillan, 1975. 4–7. Study of human, animal, and vegetable life in an urban environment.

——. *Death Is Natural.* Four Winds, 1977. 4–7. Explains how death in nature is essential and how it affects the ecosystem.

——. *Into the Woods: Exploring the Forest Ecosystem.* Macmillan, 1973. 3–6. Explains the forest's energy cycle.

————. *Natural Fire: Its Ecology in Forests.* Morrow, 1979. 4–7. The part fire plays in forest ecology.

Ryden, Hope. *The Little Deer of the Florida Keys.* Putnam, 1978. 4–6. The natural environment and threatened survival of a species of small deer in the Florida Keys.

Swift, Hildegarde Hoyt. *From the Eagle's Wing: A Biography of John Muir.* Illus. Lynd Ward. Morrow, 1962. 4–6. Biography of the man fascinated by natural beauty who found peace in nature.

Turner, Ann. *Heron Street.* Illus. Lisa Desimini. Harper & Row, 1989. 3–7. Exploration of a marsh near the sea that was home to many animals, now a noisy city.

Whipple, Jane B. *Forest Resources.* Watts, 1985. 5-up. History of forest use, protection, and abuse.

Environmental Awareness

Attenborough, David. *Discovering Life on Earth: A Natural History.* Little, Brown, 1982. 5–8. Plant and animal life on Earth today and how it has survived.

Burnie, David. *Tree.* Knopf, 1988. 3-up. Tree growth, seeds, leaves, dispersal, and distribution.

Calhoun, Mary. *Julie's Tree.* Harper & Row, 1988. 5–7. A child tries to save a beloved tree in a new town.

Conly, Jane Leslie. *Racso and the Rats of NIMH.* Illus. Leonard Lubin. Harper & Row, 1986. Focuses on the meaning of relationships and on conservation, mental health, and communication.

Cooper, Clare. *Earthchange.* Lerner, 1986. 4–8. A child and her grandmother try to survive the world of the future.

Gallant, Roy A. *101 Questions and Answers about the Universe.* Macmillan, 1984. 4-up. Questions and answers from children visiting a planetarium.

George, Jean Craighead. *On the Far Side of the Mountain.* Dutton, 1990. 4–7. A suspenseful novel with a strong message about the needs to preserve the beauty of the mountains. Sequel to *My Side of the Mountain.*

————. *The Talking Earth.* Harper & Row, 1983. 5–8. A thirteen-year-old Seminole Indian girl survives in the Everglades and finds her ancestors are alive in modern society.

Graczyk, Ed. *Appleseed.* Anchorage, 1971. 4-up. Play covering the life and times of Johnny Appleseed and his love for the environment.

Hopkins, Lee Bennett, compiler. *The Sky Is Full of Song.* Illus. Dirk Zimmer. Harper & Row, 1983. 3–7. Thirty-eight poems capturing the moods of the seasons.

Kudlinski, Kathleen V. *Rachel Carson: Pioneer of Ecology.* Illus. Ted Lewin. Viking Kestrel, 1988. 4–6. The life and struggles of this scientist who fought for our natural resources.

Lauber, Patricia. *Seeing Earth from Space.* Orchard Books, 1990. 5-up. The planet and the earth are celebrated in a well researched text and stunning color photographs.

Livingston, Myra Cohn. *A Circle of Seasons*. Illus. Leonard Everett Fisher. Holiday House, 1982. 4-up. Poems and abstract pictures about the seasons.

————. *Earth Songs*. Illus. Leonard Everett Fisher. Holiday House, 1986. 5-up. Poems and paintings celebrating the features of the Earth.

Mattingley, Christobel. *The Miracle Tree*. Illus. Marianne Yamaguchi. Gulliver, 1986. 5-up. A family separated by the bombing of Nagasaki are reunited; plea for peace and human survival.

McGrath, Susan. *Saving Our Animal Friends*. National Geographic Society, 1986. 3–8. How people help wildlife in need of our protection.

Milne, Lorus J., and Milne, Margery. *Dreams of a Perfect Earth*. Illus. Stephanie Fleischer. Atheneum, 1982. 5-up. Discussion of the ecological changes taking place on Earth and how to prevent further harm to the environment.

Nagel, Shirley. *Tree Boy*. Sierra Club, 1978. 4–6. Story of a boy who overcame administrative red tape and planted tens of thousands of trees.

Roach, Marilynne K. *Down to Earth at Walden*. Houghton Mifflin, 1980. 6–8. Recreation of Thoreau and his life at Walden.

Scarry, Huck. *Our Earth*. Messner, 1982. 3–7. Reference book about Earth, solar system, evolution of humans, and their dominance on Earth.

Schnieper, Claudia. *An Apple Tree Through the Year*. Photographs by Othmar Baumli. Carolrhoda, 1987. 2–5. The growth process of an apple tree through the four seasons.

Smalley, Webster. *The Boy Who Talked to Whales*. Anchorage Press, 1980. 4-up. Play about a boy who proves he can communicate with whales and tries to save them from destruction.

Thompson, V. L. *Hawaiian Myths of Earth, Sea, and Sky*. Illus. Leonard Weisgard. Holiday House, 1966. 3–8. Explanations in myth and legend for natural phenomena.

Wood, John Norris. *Nature Hide & Seek: Jungles*. Illus. Kevin Dean and John Norris Wood. Knopf, 1987. 5-up. The art of camouflage in nature.

Wrightson, Patricia. *An Older Kind of Magic*. Illus. Neola Young. Harcourt Brace Jovanovich, 1972. 5–7. The little people use magic to foil a plan to destroy a botanical garden where they play.

Grades Seven and Up

Types of Pollution; Environmental Protection

Black, Hallie. *Dirt Cheap: The Evolution of Renewable Resource Management*. Morrow, 1979. 6–8. Methods for conserving our natural resources.

Cox, John. *Overkill: Weapons of the Nuclear Age*. Crowell, 1978. 7-up. Information about the proliferation of nuclear weapons throughout the world.

Cullen, Brian. *What Niall Saw.* St. Martin's, 1987. 7-up. A boy's diary found after the Bomb offers a testament to the end of the world.

Feldbaum, Carl B., and Bee, Ronald J. *Looking the Tiger in the Eye.* Harper & Row, 1988. 7-up. How private citizens can influence nuclear weapons policy and secure a different future.

Forman, James D. *Doomsday Plus Twelve.* Scribner's, 1984. 7–9. A group of teenagers in Oregon try to prevent another nuclear war in the future.

Gay, Kathlyn. *Acid Rain.* Watts, 1983. 7-up. The causes, effects, costs, and politics of acid rain explained.

Hall, Lynn. *If Winter Comes.* Scribner's, n.d. 7-up. A family lives under the threat of possible nuclear annihilation for several days.

Hawkes, Nigel. *Toxic Waste and Recycling.* Illus. Ron Hayward. Gloucester, 1988. 6–8. An overview of the problem of toxic waste with details, photographs, and diagrams.

Hughes, Monica. *Beyond the Dark River.* Atheneum, 1981. 5–8. Two children who have survived a nuclear holocaust in the twenty-first century meet and try to save some Amish children who are ill.

Hyde, Dayton O. *Thunder Down the Track.* Atheneum, 1986. 6–9. Two former railroad engineers start a railroad for tourists until an industrial waste company decides to dump near their dream railroad.

Johnson, Annabel, and Johnson, Edgar. *Finders, Keepers.* Four Winds, 1981. 7-up. Two children survive radiation following a nuclear power plant explosion, and deal with mob violence and hunger.

———. *The Danger Quotient.* Harper & Row, 1984. 7-up. An eighteen-year-old survivor of a nuclear holocaust returns to the 1900s for help via a time machine.

Karl, Jean. *Strange Tomorrow.* Dutton, 1985. 7-up. A family, sole survivors of an alien space attack, struggle to renew life on earth.

Kavaler, Lucy. *Dangerous Air.* Illus. Carl Smith. Day, 1967. 7-up. Causes of air pollution throughout the world and what can be done to eliminate it.

Kiefer, Irene. *Nuclear Energy at the Crossroads.* Illus. Judith Fast. Atheneum, 1982. Information on the future of nuclear energy in the United States.

———. *Poisoned Land: The Problem of Hazardous Waste.* Atheneum, 1981. 6–9. Discusses toxic waste and disposal problems.

Lawrence, Louise. *Children of the Dust.* Harper & Row, 1985. 7-up. Survivors of a nuclear war need to make peace in order to have hope for a future.

McCormick, John. *Acid Rain.* Illus. Ron Hayward Associates. Gloucester, 1986. 7-up. Explains where acid rain comes from and its effects.

Miller, Christina G., and Berry, Louise A. *Wastes.* Watts, 1986. 6-up. What happens to our waste materials and the dilemmas they pose.

Navarra, John. *One Noisy World: The Problem of Noise Pollution.* Doubleday, 1969. 6–9. Explains the problems caused by noise.

Naylor, Phyllis R. *The Dark of the Tunnel.* Atheneum, 1985. 7-up. A young man acts against the government's plans for nuclear defenses.

Ostmann, Robert, Jr. *Acid Rain: A Plague upon the Waters.* Dillon, 1982. 6-up. Where pollutants come from and how they cause acid rain.

Pringle, Laurence. *Nuclear War: From Hiroshima to Nuclear Winter*. Enslow, 1985. 7-up. History of nuclear weapons and probable consequences of their use.

———. *Our Hungry Earth: The World Food Crisis*. Macmillan, 1976. 5–7. Discusses the factors that have caused the world's food crisis.

———. *Rain of Troubles*. Macmillan, 1988. 7-up. Study of how acid rain is formed and transported and how it affects the environment, as well as why it has not been reduced.

———. *The Only Earth We Have*. Macmillan, 1969. 5–8. The effects of biocides such as DDT on the food chain.

———. *Throwing Things Away*. Crowell, 1986. 7-up. The effects of human waste disposal on our history, culture, and environment.

———. *Water: The Next Great Resource Battle*. Macmillan, 1982. 7-up. Information on the water crisis in the United States.

Sampson, Fay. *The Watch on Patterick Fell*. Greenwillow, 1980. 7-up. The social and moral questions presented by nuclear waste disposal.

Swindells, Robert. *Brother in the Land*. Holiday House, 1985. 7-up. Portrays the aftermath of a nuclear war graphically.

Thompson, Julian F. *A Band of Angels*. Scholastic, 1986. 7-up. Five teens embark on a campaign against nuclear weapons.

Weiss, Ann E. *The Nuclear Arms Race—Can We Survive It?* Houghton Mifflin, 1983. 5–8. People and questions involved in the post-World War II arms race are discussed along with current questions about arms control.

———. *The Nuclear Question*. Harcourt Brace Jovanovich, 1981. 5–8. The promises of nuclear power versus its potential dangers are presented.

Weiss, Malcolm E. *One Sea, One Law?: The Fight for a Law of the Sea*. Harcourt Brace Jovanovich, 1982. 4–8. Relates the seven-year struggle among nations to write a treaty of the sea.

———. *Toxic Waste: Cleanup or Cover-Up?* Watts, 1984. 7-up. Discusses the composition of hazardous wastes, origin of the disposal problem, and techniques for eliminating wastes.

Ecosystems

Bond, Nancy. *The Voyage Begun*. Atheneum, 1981. 7-up. Story of two young people living in the future where depleting natural energy is a problem.

Cochrane, Jennifer. *Air Ecology*. Illus. Cecilia Fitzsimons. Bookwright Press, 1987. 5-up. How living things interact with their environment and the role air plays.

Gay, Kathlyn. *The Greenhouse Effect*. Watts, 1986. 7-up. Explains the greenhouse effect and how it will change the temperature of the Earth.

Gutnik, Martin J. *Ecology*. Watts, 1984. 7-up. Explanation of ecology and why we must work to conserve our environment.

Hirsch, S. Carl. *The Living Community: A Venture into Ecology*. Illus.

William Steinel. Viking, 1966. 6–9. Study of the interrelationships among plants and animals.

McClung, Robert M. *Hunted Mammals of the Sea.* Illus. William Downey. Morrow, 1978. 6–8. Explains current efforts to save various sea mammals.

McCoy, Joseph J. *A Sea of Troubles.* Illus. Richard Cuffari. Houghton Mifflin, 1975. 6–8. Explains how the oceans have become polluted.

Miller, Christina G., and Berry, Louise A. *Coastal Rescue.* Atheneum, 1987. 5–9. Examines how pollutants are destroying the shoreline and marine life and measures to stop the destruction.

Polking, Kirk. *Oceans of the World: Our Essential Resource.* Philomel, 1983. 6-up. Discussion of the formation, features, life forms, uses, and future of the world's oceans.

Silverberg, Robert. *The Auk, the Dodo and the Oryx: Vanished and Vanishing Creatures.* Illus. J. Hnizdovsky. Crowell, 1967. 5–8. Discussion of creatures now and soon to be extinct.

Simon, Noel. *Vanishing Habitats.* Gloucester, 1987. 7-up. The destruction of natural lands for human habitation is discussed.

Environmental Awareness

Aiken, Joan. *Street.* Illus. Arvis Stewart. Viking, 1978. 6-up. Play about the negative effects of profit and progress on the natural environment.

Arnosky, Jim. *Drawing from Nature.* Lothrop, Lee & Shepard, 1982. 5–9. Directions for how to draw the landscape and animals.

•Ashabranner, Brent. *Morning Star, Black Sun: The Northern Cheyenne Indians and America's Energy Crisis.* Photographs by Paul Conklin. Dodd, Mead, 1982. 6-up. Should the Northern Cheyenne continue to mine coal on their land for jobs, and how can they reconcile this with their own beliefs and culture?

Branscum, Robbie. *The Adventures of Johnny May.* Illus. Deborah Howland. Harper & Row, 1984. 5–8. An eleven-year-old tries to reconcile having to kill animals to survive.

Hunt, Mabel Leigh. *Better Known as Johnny Appleseed.* Illus. James Daugherty. Lippincott, 1950. 7-up. Biography of John Chapman, American pioneer, missionary, and apple lover.

Hyde, Dayton O. *Island of the Loons.* Atheneum, 1984. 7-up. A criminal holds a fourteen-year-old boy prisoner, but is himself rehabilitated by birds, beauty, and peace of the island they are on.

Marek, Margot. *Matt's Crusade.* Four Winds, 1988. 6-up. In spite of opposition from his friends and father, a boy decides to support an anti-nuclear demonstration.

Sterling, Philip. *Sea and Earth: The Life of Rachel Carson.* Crowell, 1970. 7-up. Portrait of Carson's respect for nature and efforts to preserve the balance of ecology.

Sutton, Larry. *Taildraggers High.* Farrar, Straus & Giroux, 1985. 6–8. A

512 Children's Literature for Health Awareness

twelve-year-old helps save oranges during a Florida freeze, and realizes her dream of flying.

K. CAREERS IN THE HEALTH FIELD

All Grades

Carey, Helen H., and Hanka, Deborah R. *How to Use Your Community as a Resource.* Watts, 1983. 5-up. How to use people and places in the local community as resources.

Cavallaro, Ann. *The Physician's Associate: A New Career in Health Care.* Nelson, 1978. 7-up. Explains the career of physician's associate.

Davis, Mary. *Careers in a Medical Center.* Photographs by Milton J. Blumenfeld. Lerner, 1973. 6-up. Describes the various careers available to those working in a medical center.

Englebardt, Stanley L. *Jobs in Health Care.* Lothrop, Lee & Shepard, 1973. 5–7. Describes more than sixty health care careers.

Fricke, Pam. *Careers in Dental Care.* Lerner, 1984. 3–6. Explains the profession of dentist.

Heyn, Leah. *Challenge to Become a Doctor: The Story of Elizabeth Blackwell.* Feminist Press, 1971. 4–7. Biography of a woman determined to become a doctor despite discrimination in the male-dominated profession.

Hirsch, S. Carl. *Guardians of Tomorrow.* Illus. William Steinel. Viking Kestrel, 1966. 5–9. Biographies of seven American men and women concerned with protection of natural resources.

Jacobs, Francine. *Cosmic Countdown: What Astronomers Have Learned about the Life of the Universe.* Evans, 1983. 6-up. Theories on the past, present, and future of the universe.

Kane, Betty. *Looking Forward to a Career: Dentistry.* Illus. Dick Stuphen. Dillon, 1972. 4–6. Discusses a variety of dental careers.

Kassem, Lou. *Listen for Rachel.* Atheneum, 1986. 7-up. Civil War story about a young woman who learns the art of healing in her Appalachian home.

Keller, Mollie. *Marie Curie.* Watts, 1982. 7-up. Biography of the discoverer of radium and first woman to win the Nobel Prize.

Mays, Lucinda. *The Candle and the Mirror.* Atheneum, 1982. 7-up. Novel about a nurse in turn-of-the-century United States.

Pelta, Kathy. *What Does a Paramedic Do?* Dodd, Mead, 1978. 4–6. Discusses the work of paramedics and their training.

Poynter, Margaret. *Wildland Fire Fighting.* Atheneum, 1982. 5-up. Causes of forest fires and the responsibilities of rangers and forest firefighters.

Ricciuti, Edward R. *They Work with Wildlife: Jobs for People Who Want to Work with Animals.* Harper & Row, 1983. 5-up. Introduction to careers in field biology, marine biology, and nature writing.

Silverstein, Alvin, and Silverstein, Virginia B. *Futurelife: The Biotechnology Revolution*. Illus. Marjorie Thier. Prentice-Hall, 1982. 7-up. Explains the moral and legal implications of the biotechnology revolution.

Skurzynski, Gloria. *Safeguarding the Land: Women at Work in Parks, Forests, and Rangelands*. Harcourt Brace Jovanovich, 1981. 6–9. The responsibilities involved in three forestry professions.

Vandivert, Rita. *To the Rescue: Seven Heroes of Conservation*. Warne, 1982. 6–9. Biographies of seven men who contributed to protecting our natural resources.

Weiss, Ann E. *Bioethics: Dilemmas in Modern Medicine*. Enslow, 1985. 6–9. Examines issues such as the right to die, abortion, life support systems, and cloning.

Witty, Margot. *A Day in the Life of an Emergency Room Nurse*. Troll, 1979. 3–5. Examines the various situations encountered by an emergency room nurse.

L. MISCELLANEOUS ISSUES: PERSONS WITH HANDICAPS

Grades K Through Three

Informational Books

•Ancona, George and Beth, Mary. *Handtalk Zoo*. Photographs by George Ancona. Four Winds, 1989. All ages. A deaf actress and a group of children visit the zoo and demonstrate the signs and finger spellings for various familiar animals.

Aseltine, Lorraine; Mueller; Evelyn; and Tait, Nancy. *I'm Deaf and It's Okay*. Illus. Helen Coganchery. 1–4. A book for hearing-impaired children, to help them understand their emotions and build self-esteem.

Brown, Tricia. *Someone Special, Just Like You*. Photographs by Fran Ortiz. Holt, 1984. K–4. Helps promote understanding of children with special problems.

Fassler, Joan. *Howie Helps Himself*. Illus. Joe Lasker. Whitman, 1975. 1–3. Promotes positive attitudes toward handicapped children.

Henriod, Lorraine. *Grandma's Wheelchair*. Illus. Christa Chevalier. Whitman, 1982. Pres.–3. A child helps his disabled grandmother.

Hirsch, Karen. *Becky*. Illus. Jo Esco. Carolrhoda, 1979. 1–4. Deaf people aren't that different from those who can hear.

———. *My Sister*. Illus. Nancy Inderieden. Carolrhoda, 1977. K–3. A boy describes his mixed feelings about his handicapped sister.

Kuklin, Susan. *Thinking Big: The Story of a Young Dwarf*. Lothrop, Lee & Shepard, 1986. 1–4. A child's experiences with the world as a dwarf.

Lasker, Joe. *He's My Brother*. Whitman, 1974. 1–3. A child discusses feelings about a learning disabled brother.

————. *Nick Joins In*. Whitman, 1980. 1–3. The needs and feelings of the disabled are explored.

Levine, Edna S. *Lisa and Her Soundless World*. Illus. Gloria Kamen. Human Sciences Press, 1974. 1–3. Focus on deaf child who was not diagnosed for years and how she learns to speak.

Litchfield, Ada B. *A Button in Her Ear*. Illus. Eleanor Mill. Whitman, 1976. 2–4. Information on deafness for children.

————. *A Cane in Her Hand*. Whitman, 1977. 1–3. Story of a visually impaired child and how she copes.

————. *Making Room for Uncle Joe*. Illus. Gail Owens. Whitman, 1984. 3–5. Childrens' reaction when a mentally retarded uncle comes to live with them.

————. *Words in Our Hands*. Illus. Helen Cogancherry. Whitman, 1980. 2–4. The life of a hearing-impaired person explored.

Muldoon, Kathleen. *Princess Pooh*. Illus. Linda Shute. Whitman, 1989. 2–5. A sister's reaction to her wheelchair-bound sibling and how she gains understanding and sympathy for her.

Payne, Sherry Neuwirth. *A Contest*. Illus. Jeff Kyle. Carolrhoda, 1989. 1–4. A child with cerebral palsy has his first year at a public school.

Peterson, Jeanne Whitehouse. *I Have a Sister. My Sister Is Deaf*. Illus. Deborah Ray. Harper & Row, 1977. K–3. An account of a deaf child's development as seen by her older sister.

Powers, Mary Ellen. *Our Teacher's in a Wheelchair*. Whitman, 1986. Pres.–3. Photoessay about a young man in a wheelchair who teaches in a day care center.

Rosenberg, Maxine B. *My Friend Leslie*. Photographs by George Ancona. Lothrop, Lee & Shepard, 1983. K–3. Photoessay about a child with multiple handicaps and how her fellow classmates relate to her.

Sobol, Harriet Langsam. *My Brother Steven Is Retarded*. Photographs by Patricia Agre. Macmillan, 1977. 2–5. A sister's impressions of her retarded brother and of other people's reactions to him.

Stanek, Muriel. *My Mom Can't Read*. Illus. Jacqueline Rogers. Whitman, 1986. 1–4. A first grader discovers that her mother is illiterate.

Walker, Lou Ann. *Amy, the Story of a Deaf Child*. Photographs by Michael Abramson. Lodestar, 1985. 1–4. Details of a deaf child's life with deaf parents and a hearing brother.

Wolf, Bernard. *Anna's Silent World*. Lippincott, 1977. 1–4. Story of the active life of a six-year-old deaf child.

————. *Don't Feel Sorry for Paul*. Lippincott, 1974. 3-up. Two weeks in the life of a handicapped child learning to live in a world not made for him.

Realistic Fiction

Christopher, Matt. *Glue Fingers*. Illus. Jim Venable. Little, Brown, 1975. 2–4. A stutterer's experiences as a football player.

•Clifton, Lucille. *My Friend Jacob*. Illus. Thomas DiGrazia. Dutton, 1980. K–3. A young boy's relationship with an older, retarded friend is described.

Cohen, Miriam. *See You Tomorrow, Charles*. Illus. Lillian Hoban. Greenwillow, 1983. K–2. A blind child is welcomed into a typical first-grade classroom.

Gillham, Bill. *My Brother Barry*. Illus. Laszlo Acs. André Deutsch, 1981. 2–4. A child's feelings for his older, mentally handicapped brother and how he copes with difficult situations.

Gold, Phyllis. *Please Don't Say Hello*. Photographs by Carl Baker. Human Sciences Press, 1975. 2–4. A nine-year-old autistic child comes out of his shell, thanks to the support of his family.

•Greenfield, Eloise. *Darlene*. Illus. George Ford. Methuen, 1980. K–3. A child confined to a wheelchair learns to get along with others besides her mother, who normally cares for her.

•Heide, Florence Parry. *Sound of Sunshine, Sound of Rain*. Photographs by Kenneth Longtemps. Parent's Magazine Press, 1970. 3–5. The experiences and sensations of a blind child as he maneuvers in his world.

Kaufman, Curt, and Kaufman, Gita. *Rajesh*. Photographs by Curt Kaufman. Atheneum, 1986. 1–3. A child without legs and one hand learns to adapt in his first year of school.

Kibbey, Marsha. *My Grammy*. Illus. Karen Ritz. Carolrhoda, 1989. 1–4. A child's confusion and lack of understanding turns to resentment when her grandmother who has Alzheimer's disease moves in with her.

Litchfield, Ada B. *Captain Hook, That's Me*. Illus. Sonia O. Lisker. Walker, 1982. 2–4. A child with a hook instead of a left hand must adjust to a new home and new classmates.

―――. *Making Room for Uncle Joe*. Whitman, 1984. 2–5. Reactions of three children when a mentally retarded uncle comes to live with them.

―――. *Words in Our Hands*. Whitman, 1980. 2–4. A child explains his life with deaf parents.

MacLachlan, Patricia. *Through Grandpa's Eyes*. Illus. Deborah Ray. Harper & Row, 1980. 2–5. A child tells of a day with his blind grandfather and how the grandfather "sees" the world.

•Martin, Bill, Jr. and Archambault, John. *Knots on a Counting Rope*. Illus. Ted Rand. Holt, 1987. Pres.–1. Story of a blind Indian boy which conveys love, hope, and courage.

Sargent, Susan, and Wirt, Donna Aaron. *My Favorite Place*. Illus. Allan Eitzen. Abingdon, 1983. K–3. A blind child describes what she feels on a day at the beach.

Biography

DeGering, Etta. *Seeing Fingers: The Story of Louis Braille*. Illus. Emil Weiss. McKay, 1962. 4–8. Biography of Louis Braille.

Donovan, Pete. *Carl Johnston: The One-Armed Gymnast*. Childrens Press, 1982. 3–5. Story of a handicapped person who excels at gymnastics.

Kudlinski, Kathleen V. *Helen Keller: A Light for the Blind.* Illus. Donna Diamond. Viking Kestrel, 1989. 2–6. Biography of Helen Keller.

Fantasy

Boujon, Claude. *The Cross-Eyed Rabbit.* McElderry, 1988. K–3. A cross-eyed rabbit saves his careless brothers from danger.

Jonson, Marian. *The Cricket on the Hearth.* Morton Grove, IL: Coach House Press, 1981. 3-up. Play about a toymaker and his blind daughter searching for the truth.

Luenn, Nancy. *The Ugly Princess.* Illus. David Wiesner. Little, Brown, 1981. 3–6. Made ugly by a curse, a princess discovers the true nature of beauty.

Pryor, Bonnie. *Seth of the Lion People.* Morrow, 1988. 3–6. A handicapped child threatens his prehistoric clan with his ideas and must flee to save himself.

Winthrop, Elizabeth. *Journey to the Bright Kingdom.* Illus. Charles Mikolaycak. Holiday House, 1979. K–3. A child takes her blind mother to a magical underground kingdom.

•Yolen, Jane. *The Seeing Stick.* Illus. Remy Charlip and Demetra Maraslis. Crowell, 1977. K–3. A blind princess and blind old wise man teach others to see with a seeing stick.

Grades Four Through Six

Realistic Fiction

Brighton, Catherine. *My Hands, My World.* Macmillan, 1985. 3–6. A blind child copes with her handicap with the help of an imaginative companion.

Butler, Beverly. *Gift of Gold.* Dodd, Mead, 1972. 6-up. A blind child is determined to prove she can succeed as a speech therapist.

Byars, Betsy. *The Summer of the Swans.* Illus. Ted CoConis. Viking Kestrel, 1970. 4–8. A child recognizes the responsibility involved in love while taking care of her mentally retarded brother.

Carrick, Carol. *Stay Away from Simon!* Illus. Donald Carrick. Clarion, 1985. 3–5. A feared retarded child rescues a girl and her brother and gains their understanding.

Christopher, Matt. *Long Shot for Paul.* Little, Brown, 1966. 3–6. A retarded boy learns to play basketball and helps win an important game.

Cleaver, Vera, and Cleaver, Bill. *Me Too.* Lippincott, 1973. 4–6. A twelve-year-old tries to teach her retarded twin.

Corcoran, Barbara. *Axe-Time, Sword Time.* Atheneum, 1976. 6-up. A reading disabled child copes with family problems and her future on the eve of World War II's beginning.

Cowley, Joy. *The Silent One.* Illus. Hermann Greissle. Knopf, 1981. 5-up. A deaf-mute child wants to be included in the hunting activities of the men in his village, but his handicaps make his life difficult.

Cunningham, Julia. *Burnish Me Bright.* Dell, 1980. 4–6. A mute child survives the prejudices of his French village.

DeClements, Barthe. *Sixth Grade Can Really Kill You.* Scholastic, 1986. 5–8. A dyslexic child finds help and begins to adjust to school life.

•Dyer, T. A. *A Way of His Own.* Houghton Mifflin, 1981. 4–6. A crippled Native American child is left to die because he cannot keep up with his family, but he survives despite the odds.

First, Julia. *The Absolute, Ultimate End.* Watts, 1985. 5–7. A girl tutoring a blind child reevaluates her priorities.

Fleischman, Paul. *The Half-a-Moon Inn.* Illus. Kathy Jacobi. Harper & Row, 1980. 5-up. A mute child accepts his need for independence.

Forbes, Esther. *Johnny Tremain.* Houghton Mifflin, 1943. 5-up. An apprentice to a silversmith mutilates his hand in an accident, which transforms his formerly arrogant personality.

Garrigue, Sheila. *Between Friends.* Bradbury Press, 1978. 5-up. A girl makes friends with a retarded child despite her mother's efforts to stop their relationship.

Greenwald, Sheila. *Will the Real Gertrude Hollings Please Stand Up?* Little, Brown, 1983. 4–6. A learning disabled child spends three weeks with her overachieving cousin.

Haar, Jaapter. *The World of Ben Lighthart.* Delacorte, 1977. 5–7. A blind child decides he will not avoid friends and family because of his blindness.

Hall, Lynn. *Just One Friend.* Scribner's, 1985. 6-up. A child tells what it is like to be in a special education class and how she longs for a friend.

•Hansen, Joyce. *Yellow Bird and Me.* Clarion, 1986. 4–7. A child helps a dyslexic schoolmate become confident.

Heide, Florence Parry. *Secret Dreamer, Secret Dreams.* Lippincott, 1978. 6-up. A mentally handicapped girl tells her story about trying to understand the world in which she lives.

Hermes, Patricia. *Who Will Take Care of Me?* Harcourt Brace Jovanovich, 1983. 4–6. Two brothers, one retarded, who run away from home learn that each must live his own life.

Hunt, Irene. *The Everlasting Hills.* Scribner's, 1985. 4–7. A retarded child runs away from home and finds a loving relationship in which he grows and learns.

Kerr, M. E. *Little Little.* Harper & Row, 1981. 4–7. The perils of a dwarf with interfering parents.

Knowles, Anne. *Under the Shadow.* Harper & Row, 1983. 5-up. A girl helps her friend who has muscular dystrophy realize a dream.

Lee, Mildred. *The Skating Rink.* Seabury Press, 1969. 5–8. A stuttering child makes friends with a skating rink owner who helps him come out of his silence.

Levinson, Marilyn. *And Don't Bring Jeremy.* Illus. Diane de Groat. Holt, 1985. 5–7. Two brothers, one learning disabled, adjust to a new neighborhood.

Little, Jean. *Listen for the Singing.* Dutton, 1977. 5–9. A young Canadian girl with impaired vision prepares to begin high school as World War II begins.

————. *Take Wing.* Little, Brown, 1968. 4–7. A girl learns she doesn't need to be the only one who helps her retarded brother.

Martin, Ann M. *Inside Out.* Holiday House, 1984. 4–6. The need for acceptance felt by an autistic child.

————. *Yours Turly, Shirley.* Holiday House, 1989. 4–6. A dyslexic child struggles with her feelings of inferiority.

•Mathis, Sharon Bell. *Listen for the Fig Tree.* Viking Kestrel, 1974. 6-up. A blind girl copes with her problems and with taking care of her mother.

Rodowsky, Colby. *What About Me?* Sunburst, 1989. 5–7. A child is resentful of her mentally retarded brother and the attention he gets and embarrassment he sometimes causes.

Rounds, Glenn. *The Blind Colt.* Holiday House, 1960. 4–7. A blind mustang uses its other senses in order to survive.

Sallis, Susan Diana. *Only Love.* Harper & Row, 1980. 6-up. The story of a paraplegic teen and her struggles to live with her disability.

Savitz, Harriet May. *Fly, Wheels, Fly.* John Day, 1970. 5-up. Two paraplegics train for wheelchair sports.

Shyer, Marlene Fanta. *Welcome Home Jellybean.* Scribner's, 1978. 4–6. Effects on a family of their retarded child's return to the home.

Smith, Doris Buchanan. *Kelly's Creek.* Illus. Alan Tiegreen. Crowell, 1975. 3–6. Story of a child's struggles to cope with a learning disability.

Smith, Gene. *The Hayburners.* Delacorte, 1974. 4–6. A family is influenced by the retarded man they hire to do chores for them.

•Smucker, Barbara. *Runaway to Freedom.* Harper & Row, 1977. 4–6. Account of two young women's escape from slavery, one of whom is disabled.

Talbert, Marc. *Toby.* Dial, 1988. 4-up. A child with disabled parents deals with the possibility that he may have to go to a foster home.

Teague, Sam. *The King of Hearts' Heart.* Little, Brown, 1987. 3–7. Story of a child's struggles to make it into the Special Olympics.

Voight, Cynthia. *Dicey's Song.* Atheneum, 1982. 4–8. The children of a mentally ill mother and their problems with the grandmother they must live with.

•Weik, Mary Hays. *The Jazz Man.* Illus. Ann Grifalconi. Atheneum, 1966. 4–6. A story of a disabled child whose only delight is watching a man in another apartment play jazz on his piano.

Informational Books

Adams, Barbara. *Like It Is: Facts and Feelings About Handicaps from Kids Who Know.* Photographs by James Stanfield. Walker, 1979. 4–7. Handicapped children explain their individual problems and how they cope with them.

Alexander, Sally Hobart. *Mom Can't See Me.* Photographs by George Ancona. Macmillan, 1990. 4–6. The author's nine-year-old daughter describes her mother's blindness. A Notable Children's Trade Book in the Field of Social Studies.

Anders, Rebecca. *A Look at Mental Retardation.* Lerner, 1976. 3–6. Problems faced by mentally handicapped individuals.

Charlip, Remy, and Beth, Mary. *Handtalk Birthday: A Number and Story Book in Sign Language.* Photographs by George Ancona. Four Winds, 1987. 4–6. Teaches sign language through an amusing birthday story.

Curtis, Patricia. *Cindy, a Hearing Ear Dog.* Photographs by David Cupp. Dutton, 1981. 4–6. Follows a dog through obedience school to her home with a deaf child in a photoessay.

Dunbar, Robert F. *Mental Retardation.* Watts, 1978. 4–7. An account of the causes of mental retardation and its effects.

Greenberg, Judith E. *What Is the Sign for Friend?* Photographs by Gayle Rothschild. Watts, 1985. 2–5. A deaf child's everyday interests and activities.

•Greenfield, Eloise, and Revis, Alesia. *Alesia.* Photographs by Sandra Turner Bond. Illus. George Ford. Philomel, 1981. 4–6. A child's struggle to make it as a handicapped person.

Haskins, James. *Who Are the Handicapped?* Doubleday, 1978. 4–6. Causes, therapies, cures, and mental problems associated with various handicaps.

Hermann, Helen, and Hermann, Bill. *Jenny's Magic Wand.* Photographs by Don Perdue. Watts, 1988. 4–7. A blind child adjusts to home and school.

Hyman, Jane. *Deafness.* Watts, 1980. 4-up. Discusses various types of hearing loss and their causes.

Kamien, Janet. *What If You Couldn't?* A *Book About Special Needs.* Illus. Signe Hanson. Scribner's, 1979. 5–7. Discusses various physical handicaps and their treatment.

Marek, Margot. *Different, Not Dumb.* Photographs by Barbara Kirk. Watts, 1985. 3–5. A dyslexic child's experiences in a special class.

Rosenberg, Maxine B. *Finding a Way: Living with Exceptional Brothers and Sisters.* Photographs by George Ancona. Lothrop, Lee & Shepard, 1988. 4–7. Problems of being the sibling of a disabled child.

Roy, Ron. *Move Over, Wheelchairs Coming Through! Seven Young People in Wheelchairs Talk about Their Lives.* Photographs by Rosmarie Hausherr. Clarion, 1985. 5-up. The daily activities of seven young people confined to wheelchairs.

Savitz, Harriet May. *Wheelchair Champions: A History of Wheelchair Sports.* Crowell, 1978. 4–6. Athletes and events that are part of wheelchair competitions.

Shapiro, Patricia Gottlieb. *Caring for the Mentally Ill.* Watts, 1982. 6-up. What emotional dysfunction is, how to treat it, and what legal rights the mentally ill have.

Sullivan, Mary Beth. *Feeling Free.* Addison-Wesley, 1979. 4–8. Explores physical disabilities through young people's perceptions.

Wolf, Bernard. *Connie's New Eyes*. Lippincott, 1976. 5-up. Story of the life
of a seeing eye dog and his new owner.
————. *Don't Feel Sorry for Paul*. Lippincott, 1974. 4-up. A disabled child
with self-confidence and his life.
Wright, Betty Ren. *My Sister Is Different*. Illus. Helen Cogancherry.
Raintree, 1981. 4–6. An older brother realizes how much he loves his
retarded sister when she gets lost.

Biography

Neimark, Ann E. *A Deaf Child Listened: Thomas Gallaudet, Pioneer in
American Education*. Morrow, 1983. 5-up. Biography of the pioneer in
education for the deaf.
•Nelson, Mary Carroll. *Michael Naranjo: The Story of an American Indian*.
Dillon, 1975. 4–7. The struggles of a blind American Indian and his life
as a sculptor.

Plays

Groff, Phyllis. *The Christmas Nightingale*. Anchorage Press, 1935. 4-up.
Play about a family who helps a mute child and receives a gift.
Kral, Brian. *Special Class*. Anchorage Press, 1981. 5-up. Play that explores
the dreams and disappointments of handicapped children in our society.
Kraus, Joanna Halpert. *Circus Home*. New Plays, 1979. 5-up. Play about a
disfigured child trying to find acceptance in normal family surroundings.

Grades Seven and Up

Realistic Fiction

Adler, C. S. *Kiss the Clown*. Clarion, 1986. 6-up. A Guatemalan immigrant
falls in love with a dyslexic. Explains the effects this disability can have on
one's self-esteem.
Albert, Louise. *But I'm Ready to Go*. Bradbury, 1976. 6–9. A girl makes a
successful career for herself despite a learning disability.
Baastad, Bobbie Friss. *Don't Take Teddy*. Scribner's, 1967. 6–8. Two
brothers run away after the mentally retarded brother accidentally
injures a boy.
Bates, Betty. *Love Is Like Peanuts*. Holiday House, 1980. 7-up. A girl
matures while babysitting for a brain-damaged child over a summer.
•Blos, Joan W. *Brothers of the Heart*. Scribner's, 1985. 7-up. A crippled boy

survives and matures in Michigan wilderness, thanks to an old Indian woman.

Blume, Judy. *Deenie.* Bradbury, 1973. 6-up. A child deals with the fact that she has scoliosis, thanks to supportive friends.

Canada, Lena. *To Elvis, with Love.* Everest House Publishers, 1978. 7-up. A child dying of cerebral palsy finds strength, thanks to correspondence from a caring star.

Clark, Margaret Goff. *Who Stole Kathy Young?* Dodd, Mead, 1980. 7-up. A deaf girl is kidnapped, and her friends try to find her.

Denzel, Justin. *Boy of the Painted Cave.* Philomel, 1988. 5–8. Story of a crippled boy trying to live independently in prehistoric times.

Evernden, Margery. *The Kite Song.* Illus. Cindy Wheeler. Lothrop, Lee & Shepard, 1984. 5–7. A special school helps a troubled child find his way back to life.

Farish, Terry. *Why I'm Already Blue.* Greenwillow, 1989. 7-up. Neighbors whose lives are brought together, one of whom has muscular dystrophy.

Garfield, James B. *Follow My Leader.* Illus. Robert Greiner. Viking, 1957. 4–8. Story of a child's rehabilitation after a firecracker accident damages his eyes.

Greenberg, Joanne. *In This Sign.* Holt, 1970. 7-up. Story of deaf parents raising a hearing daughter.

Hall, Lynn. *Half the Battle.* Scribner's, 1982. 7-up. A blind boy trains for a hundred-mile endurance horseback ride, causing resentment in his sighted brother.

•Hamilton, Virginia. *The Planet of Junior Brown.* Macmillan, 1971. 6-up. With the help of his friend, an obese, unhappy young man learns to feel wanted and find his place in the world.

Hanlon, Emily. *It's Too Late for Sorry.* Bradbury, 1978. 7-up. A mentally retarded teen moves from an institution to his family home and must cope with reactions of neighbors and friends.

———. *The Swing.* Bradbury, 1979. 7-up. A deaf child must share a swing she considers hers and makes friends in the process.

Hartling, Peter. *Crutches.* Lothrop, Lee & Shepard, 1988. 6–9. A homeless disabled veteran helps a German child search for his mother after World War II.

Heide, Florence Parry. *Secret Dreamer, Secret Dreams.* Harper & Row, 1978. 6–8. The hopes and fears of a mentally handicapped girl are revealed.

Kent, Deborah. *Belonging.* Illus. Gary Watson. Dial, 1978. 6–8. A blind teenager discovers her self-worth.

Knowles, Anne. *Under the Shadow.* Harper & Row, 1983. 6–8. A friendship develops between a young girl and handicapped boy.

L'Engle, Madeleine. *The Young Unicorns.* Farrar, Straus & Giroux, 1968. 6-up. Several characters, among them a blind twelve-year-old musician, are involved in a scheme relying on the ability of a loser to gain complete power over people's minds.

•Likhanov, Albert. *Shadows Across the Sun.* Richard Lourie, translator. Harper & Row, 1983. 7-up. A handicapped child and her friend raise pigeons in their housing complex in urban Russia.

•Mathis, Sharon Bell. *Listen for the Fig Tree.* Viking Kestrel, 1974. 7-up. A gifted blind girl deals with having an alcoholic mother.

Pevsner, Stella. *Keep Stompin' Till the Music Stops.* Houghton Mifflin, 1977. 5–7. Some experiences of a dyslexic child.

Phipson, Joan. *A Tide Flowing.* Atheneum, 1981. 5–9. A lonely motherless child makes friends with a quadriplegic girl.

Radley, Gail. *CF in His Corner.* Four Winds, 1984. 7-up. A brother deals with his younger brother's cystic fibrosis, despite his mother's denial.

Richmond, Sandra. *Wheels for Walking.* Atlantic, 1985. 7-up. Explains the experiences of a quadriplegic after a spinal cord injury strikes her at the age of eighteen.

Riskind, Mary. *Apple Is My Sign.* Houghton Mifflin, 1981. 5–9. A deaf child's experiences of the world and how it changes his life.

Rodowsky, Colby F. *P.S. Write Soon.* Watts, 1978. 5–8. A child with a paralyzed leg deals with feelings of inferiority and anger.

Sallis, Susan. *Only Love.* Harper & Row, 1980. 7-up. A sixteen-year-old girl in a wheelchair determines to experience life to the fullest.

Voigt, Cynthia. *Tree by Leaf.* Atheneum, 1988. 4–8. A child deals with her father's disfigurement after World War I and her friend's misfortunes because of an alcoholic father.

Wolff, Virginia Euwer. *Probably Still Nick Swansen.* Holt, 1988. 6–9. The experiences and feelings of a learning disabled child.

Informational Books

Berger, Gilda. *Physical Disabilities.* Watts, 1979. 6–8. Characteristics, causes, and consequences of common physical handicaps.

Butler, Beverly. *Maggie by My Side.* Dodd, Mead, 1987. 6-up. Account of a blind person and her seeing eye dog.

Drimmer, Frederick. *Born Different.* Atheneum, 1988. 7-up. Histories of some of the world's famous disabled people.

Gill, Derek L. T. *Tom Sullivan's Adventures in Darkness.* McKay, 1978. 5–9. Biography of the singer and entertainer who has been blind from birth.

Hayman, Leroy. *Triumph!: Conquering Your Physical Disability.* Messner, 1982. 7-up. Author discusses his disability and how it affected him physically and emotionally.

Hilbok, Bruce. *Silent Dancer.* Photographs by Liz Glasgow. Messner, 1981. 7-up. Experiences of a ten-year-old deaf girl studying ballet at the Joffrey School.

Hocken, Sheila. *Emma and I.* Thomas Congdon Books, 1978. 7-up. Experiences of a blind child and her seeing eye dog.

Marcus, Rebecca B. *Being Blind.* Hastings, 1981. 5–8. Informative book about the lives of blind people and how they are assisted.

Sullivan, Tom, and Gill, Derek. *If You Could See What I Hear.* Signet Books, 1976. 7-up. A child deprived of sight excels and tells his story as an adult, including his hopes and fears.

Biography

Haskins, James. *The Story of Stevie Wonder.* Lothrop, Lee & Shepard, 1976. Biography of the blind musician.

Hunter, Edith Fisher. *Child of the Silent Night.* Dell, 1983. 6-up. Biography of a girl who lost sight and hearing from scarlet fever and learned to read and communicate with others.

Little, Jean. *Little by Little: A Writer's Education.* Viking Kestrel, 1988. 5–8. Autobiography of a blind author who found success, thanks to her family.

Fantasy

Wilder, Cherry. *Yorath the Wolf.* Atheneum, 1984. 6–9. Magic helps Yorath overcome his physical disability and eventually become a peace-loving individual.

DEATH AND DYING

Grades K Through Three

Realistic Fiction

Carrick, Nancy. *The Accident.* Illus. Donald Carrick. Houghton Mifflin, 1976. K–3. A family learns to grieve after the death of its pet dog.

•Clifton, Lucille. *Everett Anderson's Goodbye.* Illus. Ann Grifalconi. Holt, 1983. Pres.–3. A child works through his grief after his father's death.

Cohen, Miriam. *Jim's Dog Muffins.* Illus. Lillian Hoban. Greenwillow, 1984. Pres.–3. A boy's best friend helps him grieve after his dog dies.

•Coutant, Helen. *First Snow.* Illus. Vo-Dinh. Knopf, 1974. 2–4. A Vietnamese family's first New England winter brings sadness at the grandmother's death.

Dabcovich, Lydia. *Mrs. Huggins and Her Hen Hannah.* Dutton, 1985. K–3. An old woman grieves after the death of her hen, but finds new friendship with the hen's offspring.

Gould, Deborah. *Grandpa's Slide Show.* Illus. Cheryl Harness. Lothrop, Lee & Shepard, 1987. Pres.–1. A slide show including shots of his grandparents helps a child mourn his grandfather's death.

Hoopes, Lyn Littlefield. *Nana.* Illus. Arieh Zeldich. Harper & Row, 1981.

K–3. A child's remembrances of her grandmother just after the grandmother's death.

Jewell, Nancy. *Time for Uncle Joe.* Illus. Joan Sandin. Harper & Row, 1981. Pres.–1. A child finds in everyday things memories of her uncle who has died.

Joosse, Barbara M. *Better with Two.* Illus. Catherine Stock. Harper & Row, 1988. Pres.–2. A child helps a neighbor to grieve for her dog.

Jukes, Mavis. *Blackberries in the Dark.* Illus. Thomas B. Allen. Knopf, 1985. 3–5. A child and his grandmother grieve together over the grandfather's death.

Keller, Holly. *Goodbye, Max.* Greenwillow, 1987. Pres.–3. A child grieves for his dog who has died and finds reassurance in the sharing of his grief.

Levitin, Sonia. *All the Cats in the World.* Illus. Charles Robinson. Harcourt Brace Jovanovich. Pres.–3. A friendship forms over caring for a number of wild cats near a lighthouse.

Little, Jean. *Home from Far.* Illus. Jerry Lazare. Little, Brown, 1965. 3–6. Jenny grieves for her twin brother who is killed in an auto accident.

•Miles, Miska. *Annie and the Old One.* Illus. Peter Parnall. Little, Brown, 1971. Pres.–3. A story of Navajo traditions and the bravery of a child.

Newman, Nanette. *That Dog!* Illus. Marylin Hafner. Crowell, 1983. 1–4. A child grieves for his dead dog with help from family and friends.

Porte, Barbara Ann. *Harry's Mom.* Illus. Yossi Abolafia. Greenwillow, 1985. K–3. A child grieves for his deceased mother with help from family.

Powell, E. Sandy. *Geranium Morning.* Illus. Renee Graef. Carolrhoda, 1990. 1–4. A child finds strength to cope with his father's death from a friend whose mother is dying.

Simon, Norma. *We Remember Philip.* Illus. Ruth Sanderson. Whitman, 1979. 2–4. A realistic story about death.

Skorpen, Liesel M. *Old Arthur.* Illus. Wallace Tripp. Harper & Row, 1972. K–5. An aging dog finds a new home.

Thomas, Ianthe. *Hi, Mrs. Mallory!* Illus. Ann Toulmin-Rothe. Harper & Row, 1979. K–3. A child deals with the death of an older woman who had become her friend by remembering their times together.

Thomas, Jane Resh. *Saying Good-bye to Grandma.* Illus. Marcia Sewall. Clarion, 1988. 1–4. A child follows the family's rituals at grandma's funeral.

Townsend, Maryann, and Stern, Ronnie. *Pop's Secret.* Addison-Wesley, 1980. Pres.–1. A book assembled by a child in order to come to terms with his grandfather's death.

Varley, Susan. *Badger's Parting Gifts.* Lothrop, Lee & Shepard, 1984. Pres. Badger's friends remember him and the thoughtful things he did for them in life.

Viorst, Judith. *The Tenth Good Thing About Barney.* Illus. Erik Blegvad. Atheneum, 1971. K–4. A child deals with the death of a pet.

Zolotow, Charlotte. *My Grandson Lew.* Illus. William Pène du Bois. Harper & Row, 1974. K–4. Celebration of memory, which enables one to heal in times of death of a loved one.

Informational Books

Bernstein, Joanne E., and Gullo, Stephen V. *When People Die.* Illus. Rosmarie Hausherr. Dutton, 1977. K–3. A comprehensive discussion of death.

Cohn, Janice. *I Had a Friend Named Peter: Talking to Children about the Death of a Friend.* Illus. Gail Owens. Morrow, 1987. Pres. A child talks with parents and classmates about death when a friend dies.

Osborn, Lois. *My Dad Is Really Something.* Illus. Rodney Pate. Whitman, 1983. K–3. A child invents a father to cope with his own loss.

Rogers, Fred. *When a Pet Dies.* Photographs by Jim Judkis. Putnam, 1988. Pres.–2. Study of how to cope with the loss of a pet.

Simon, Norma. *The Saddest Time.* Whitman, 1986. 1–4. Three stories of the emotions children feel when death touches their lives. Whitman, 1986. 1–4.

Fantasy

•DeArmond, Dale. *The Seal Oil Lamp.* Sierra Club Books, 1988. K–4. A child left to die because of blindness is saved by mouse people.

•Goble, Paul. *Beyond the Ridge.* Bradbury, 1989. All ages. The path of a grandmother's spirit during her death and her vision of heaven.

Sendak, Maurice. *Higglety, Pigglety, Pop! or There Must Be More to Life.* Harper & Row, 1967. 2–4. A dog leaves home in search of experiences, and her final letter home is written after her death.

White, E. B. *Charlotte's Web.* Illus. Garth Williams. Harper & Row, 1952. K–3. Wilbur the pig copes with the death of the spider who saved his own life.

Grades Four Through Six

Realistic Fiction

Bauer, Marion Dane. *On My Honor.* Clarion, 1986. 4–7. A child deals with guilt after his friend dies of drowning because of his dare.

Blue, Rose. *Grandma Didn't Wave Back.* Watts, 1972. 4–6. A child realizes her grandmother may have to go to a nursing home and deals with their parting.

Boyd, Candy Dawson. *Circle of Gold.* Apple, 1984. 4–6. A child tries to deal with the death of her father amidst problems at home and school.

Bunting, Eve. *The Empty Window.* Illus. Judy Clifford. Warne, 1980. 4–6. A young boy deals with guilt and sadness as his friend dies.

————. *The Ghost Children.* Clarion, 1989. 4–7. Siblings cope with living with an aunt after their mother's death.

•————. *The Happy Funeral.* Illus. Vo-Dinh Mai. Harper & Row, 1982. A child deals with the death, funeral, and burial of her grandfather.

Byars, Betsy. *Good-Bye, Chicken Little.* Harper & Row, 1979. 4–6. A child deals with death, guilt, and feelings of abandonment after his uncle's death.

•Cave, Hugh B. *Conquering Kilmarnie.* Macmillan, 1989. 3–7. A child copes with his father, who can't get over the deaths of his wife and other son.

Colman, Hila. *Suddenly.* Morrow, 1987. 6-up. A young girl deals with the death of her friend and guilt feelings.

Davis, Jenny. *Good-Bye and Keep Cold.* Orchard Books, 1987. 4–6. A child reflects about life after her father's death in a mining accident.

•Ellis, Sarah. *A Family Project.* McElderry, 1988. 4–7. A family deals with the new baby's death.

Graeber, Charlottte. *Mustard.* Illus. Donna Diamond. Macmillan, 1982. 2–5. A child faces the death of his aging pet cat and grieves after the death with his family's help.

Green, Connie Jordan. *The War at Home.* McElderry, 1989. 4–6. A child helps her friend grieve when his mother is killed in an accident during World War II.

Greenberg, Jan. *A Season In-Between.* Farrar, Straus & Giroux, 1979. 6-up. A child deals with emotions when her father is stricken with cancer and dies.

Greene, Constance C. *Beat the Turtle Drum.* Illus. Donna Diamond. Viking Press, 1976. 3–7. A sister learns to cope after her sibling dies suddenly.

Griffiths, Helen. *Rafa's Dog.* Holiday House, 1983. 3–6. A child befriends a stray dog and deals with his mother's death.

Hermes, Patricia. *Nobody's Fault.* Harcourt Brace Jovanovich, 1981. 5–7. A child describes her feelings after her younger brother's death.

————. *You Shouldn't Have to Say Good-Bye.* Harcourt Brace Jovanovich, 1982. 4–6. A child accepts the fact that her mother is dying of cancer.

Hest, Amy. *Pete and Lily.* Clarion, 1986. 4–7. A girl deals with the death of her father and her mother's new husband.

Holl, Kristi D. *The Rose Beyond the Wall.* Atheneum, 1985. 4–6. A child copes with the knowledge that her grandmother has come home to die and her best friend is going his own way.

Howker, Janni. *Isaac Campion.* Greenwillow, 1987. 5-up. A child is forced to leave school and work for his father after his brother's tragic death.

Joosse, Barbara. *Pieces of the Picture.* Harper & Row, 1989. 4–6. A child deals with her father's death and a move to a new town.

•Lasky, Kathryn. *Beyond the Divide.* Macmillan, 1983. 4–7. A child's father dies, and a girl struggles for survival during the Gold Rush.

Levy, Elizabeth, adapter. *The Shuttered Window.* Yearling Books, 1981. 4–7. A child deals with her uncle's death with a friend's assistance.

Little, Jean. *Home from Far.* Illus. Jerry Lazare. Little, Brown, 1965. 4–6. A child deals with the death of her twin.

————. *Mama's Going to Buy You a Mockingbird.* Viking Kestrel, 1985. 4–6. A young boy deals with his father's death by helping others.

Lorentzen, Karin. *Lanky Longlegs.* Joan Tate, translator. Illus. Jan Ormerod. McElderry, 1983. 3–6. A child's dog has puppies while her brother grows sicker and dies.

Lowry, Lois. *A Summer to Die.* Illus. Jenni Oliver. Houghton Mifflin, 1977. 5–7. A child's older sister dies from leukemia, and she must deal with her jealous feelings and grief.

Mann, Peggy. *There Are Two Kinds of Terrible.* Doubleday, 1977. 4–7. A child's mother dies of cancer, and he must learn to love his father while they cope with the death.

Payne, Bernal C., Jr. *The Late Great Dick Hart.* Houghton Mifflin, 1986. 5-up. A child deals with his best friend's death and the fact that he seems to be calling to him from the grave.

•Phipson, Joan. *A Tide Flowing.* McElderry, 1981. 6-up. A child is haunted by his mother's mysterious death and his rejection by his father and finds strength in friendship with a quadriplegic girl.

Ruckman, Ivy. *This Is Your Captain Speaking.* Walker, 1987. 4–6. A child learns about living and dying through his friendship with a nursing home patient.

Rylant, Cynthia. *Missing May.* Orchard Books, 1992. 5–7. Summer grieves the death of the aunt who has raised her, and, with her beloved uncle, leaves her West Virginia trailer home in search of the strength to go on living.

•Sachs, Marilyn. *Call Me Ruth.* Doubleday, 1982. 4–6. A Russian immigrant deals with her father's death and mother's involvement in the labor movement.

Smith, Doris B. *A Taste of Blackberries.* Illus. Charles Robinson. Crowell, 1973. 2–5. Death of a best friend from the child's point of view.

————. *The First Hard Times.* Viking Kestrel, 1983. 5–7. A child struggles to accept her father's death in Vietnam.

Wallace-Brodeur, Ruth. *The Kenton Year.* Atheneum, 1980. 5-up. A child deals with her father's death in an accident.

Whelan, Gloria. *A Time to Keep Silent.* Putnam, 1979. 4–6. A child makes a friend and manages to cope with her mother's death.

Plays

Harris, Aurand. *The Arkansaw Bear.* Anchorage Press, 1980. 4-up. An old bear teaches a young girl the meaning of life and death, helping her to cope with her grandfather's approaching death.

————. *The Magician's Nephew.* Dramatic Publishing Co., 1984. 4-up. Two friends travel to a distant land to acquire a healing apple for one friend's dying mother.

Miller, Kathryn Schultz. *You Don't See Me.* Coach House Press, 1984. 5-up.

A child whose brother has died copes by creating a fantasy world in which her brother appears.
Wiles, Julian. *The Boy Who Stole the Stars.* Dramatic Publishing Co. 1985. 4-up. A child and his grandfather cope together with the grandfather's imminent death.

Folktales

Yolen, Jane. "The Boy Who Sang for Death." In *Dream Weaver.* Collins, 1979. 4-up. A child attempts to bring his mother back from the land of the dead.
————, ed. "Youth Without Age and Life Without Death." In *Favorite Folktales from Around the World.* Pantheon, 1986. 5-up. A youth seeks to overcome age and death.
•————, ed. "Woman Chooses Death." In *Favorite Folktales from Around the World.* Pantheon, 1986. 3–6. A Blackfoot tale about the origin of death.

Fantasy

Babbitt, Natalie. *Tuck Everlasting.* Farrar, Straus & Giroux, 1975. 4–6. A child is befriended by a family that has everlasting life and must choose between eternal life and mortality.
•Hamilton, Virginia. *Sweet Whispers, Brother Rush.* Philomel, 1981. 6-up. A girl learns the startling facts about her family from the ghost of her uncle. She must cope with the death of her older brother from a rare inherited illness, and grows to accept herself.

Informational Books

Krementz, Jill. *How It Feels When a Parent Dies.* Knopf, 1981. 5–9. Eighteen children give their own accounts of feelings when their parents died.
LeShan, Eda. *Learning to Say Good-By: When a Parent Dies.* Illus. Paul Giovanopoulos. Macmillan, 1976. 5–7. Testimonies of children's reactions to death.
Pringle, Laurence. *Death Is Natural.* Four Winds, 1977. 4–6. Explanation of death related to nature.
•Rofes, Eric E., ed. *The Kids' Book about Death and Dying.* Little, Brown, 1985. 4-up. Fourteen children share their ideas about death, after the death of a pet, parent, or friend.
Zim, Herbert S., and Bleeker, Sonia. *Life and Death.* Illus. René Martin. Morrow, 1970. 4–7. Comprehensive account of aspects of aging, death, and dying.

Grades Seven and Up

Realistic Fiction

Amoss, Berthe. *Secret Lives*. Atlantic-Little, Brown, 1979. 7-up. A child tries to find out the facts about her mother's death.

Asher, Sandy. *Missing Pieces*. Delacorte, 1984. 7-up. Story of a girl facing her father's death and her first romance.

Bacon, Katharine Jay. *Shadow and Light*. Macmillan, 1987. 7-up. A girl copes with the fact that her grandmother is dying.

•Bosse, Malcolm J. *Ganesh*. Crowell, 1981. 7-up. After his father dies, an Indian child comes to America and discovers the culture.

Boyd, Candy Dawson. *Breadsticks and Blessing Places*. Macmillan, 1985. 6–8. A child grieves after the death of her best friend, with help from family and other friends.

Carter, Alden R. *Sheila's Dying*. Putnam, 1987. 7-up. A basketball star can't break up with his girlfriend once he finds out she is dying of cancer.

Christiansen, C. B. *A Small Pleasure*. Atheneum, 1988. 7-up. A girl must come to terms with her father's death and find meaning in her own life.

Colman, Hila. *Suddenly*. Morrow, 1987. 7-up. A child deals with guilt after an accident that kills a friend.

Crutcher, Chris. *Running Loose*. Greenwillow, 1983. 7-up. A boy loses his girlfriend in a fatal accident.

Deaver, Julie Reece. *Say Goodnight, Gracie*. Harper & Row, 1988. 7-up. A girl learns to come to grips with the death of her best friend by savoring memories of him.

Evernden, Margery. *The Kite Song*. Lothrop, Lee & Shepard, 1984. 5–8. A child blames himself for his parents' deaths and must face his past in order to move on.

•Fenton, Edward. *The Morning of the Gods*. Delacorte, 1987. 7-up. A child deals with the death of her mother in an accident while spending a spring and summer in Greece, her mother's home.

Grant, Cynthia D. *Phoenix Rising: Or How to Survive Your Life*. Atheneum, 1989. 7-up. A younger sister can't move on with life after her sister's death from cancer.

Holland, Isabelle. *Alan and the Animal Kingdom*. Lippincott, 1977. 5–8. A child who is orphaned attempts to live alone with his animals rather than face another foster home.

Hopkins, Lee Bennett. *Wonder Wheels*. Knopf, 1979. 6-up. Relationships among teens in a roller rink are strained when one of them dies.

Hunter, Mollie. *A Sound of Chariots*. Harper & Row, 1972. 5–9. A child closest to her father deals with his death.

Jukes, Mavis. *Blackberries in the Dark*. Illus. Thomas B. Allen. Knopf, 1985. 7-up. A child and his grandmother grieve together for the grandfather who has died.

Klass, David. *The Atami Dragons*. Scribner's, 1984. 5–6. A boy and his sister and father work through their grief over the mother's death during a summer in Japan.

Little, Jean. *Mama's Going to Buy You a Mockingbird*. Viking Kestrel, 1986. 5–7. A child comes to terms with his father's death, thanks to a friend and memories of his father.

Martin, Ann M. *With You and Without You*. Holiday House, 1986. 6–8. A family has a last Christmas with the father, who is dying.

Mazer, Harry. *When the Phone Rang*. Scholastic, 1985. 7-up. Three siblings deal with grief after the death of both parents.

Mazer, Norma Fox. *After the Rain*. Morrow, 1987. 7-up. A child cares for her dying grandfather.

McLean, Susan. *Pennies for the Piper*. Farrar, Straus & Giroux, 1981. 5–9. A child must deal with her mother's death alone.

Miller, Sandy. *Two Loves for Jenny*. New American Library, 1982. 7-up. A child whose father recently died adjusts to life in a new town.

Mills, Claudia. *All the Living*. Macmillan, 1983. 5–8. A girl must learn to live in the present instead of focusing on death.

Naughton, Jim. *My Brother Stealing Second*. Harper & Row, 1989. 6-up. A child's emotional recovery from his older brother's death, thanks to fond memories.

Naylor, Phyllis Reynolds. *A String of Chances*. Atheneum, 1983. 7-up. A child faces birth, love, and death during a summer with her cousin.

———. *The Dark of the Tunnel*. Atheneum, 1985. 7-up. A boy faces the death of his mother and decisions about his future.

Olsen, Violet. *Never Brought to Mind*. Atheneum, 1985. 7-up. Friends are still depressed and guilty four months after the death of two other friends, and must seek understanding and acceptance from others.

Oneal, Zibby. *A Formal Feeling*. Viking Kestrel, 1982. 7-up. A girl is detached and isolated after her mother's death and must learn to grieve.

Paulsen, Gary. *The Voyage of the Frog*. Orchard Books, 1989. 6–8. An uncle who has died of cancer bequeaths a sailboat to his nephew which he must sail alone to scatter the ashes at sea.

———. *Tracker*. Bradbury, 1984. 6-up. A boy who loves hunting comes to realization of its evil while accepting his grandfather's imminent death.

Peck, Robert Newton. *A Day No Pigs Would Die*. Knopf, 1972. 6-up. A boy comes of age in the 1920s, facing life, fears, triumphs, and death.

Rinaldi, Ann. *Term Paper*. Walker, 1980. 6-up. A child must do a special term paper in order to release her guilt over her father's death during an argument with her.

•Sullivan, Mary Ann. *Child of War*. Holiday House, 1984. 5–8. A child loses her mother and little brother in the political struggles in Northern Ireland, retreating into a world of fantasy.

Talbert, Marc. *Dead Birds Singing*. Little, Brown, 1985. 7-up. A teen rebuilds his life when a car accident kills his mother and critically injures his sister.

Voigt, Cynthia. *Dicey's Song*. Atheneum, 1982. 7-up. A child learns from her grandmother how to reach out and let go when her mother dies.

Zindel, Paul. *A Begonia for Miss Applebaum*. Harper & Row, 1989. 6-up. Friends deal with the terminal illness of a beloved former teacher.

Plays

Benet, Stephen Vincent. *Johnny Pye and the Footkiller*. Readers Theatre Script Service, n.d. 6-up. Johnny Pye from boyhood to old age, as he tries to cope with death.

Informational Books

Llewellyn, Chris. *Fragments from the Fire: The Triangle Shirtwaist Company Fire of March 25, 1911.* Viking Kestrel, 1987. 7-up. Poetry about the women and children who died in this factory fire.

McHugh, Mary. *Young People Talk About Death*. Watts, 1980. 7-up. Teenagers, psychologists, doctors, and social workers discuss their feelings about death, euthanasia, legislation on aging and dying, funerals, and grief.

Palmer, Laura. *Shrapnel in the Heart: Letters and Remembrances from the Vietnam Memorial*. Random House, 1987. 7-up. About the families and friends who have left remembrances at the Vietnam Memorial.

ABUSE

Grades K Through Three

Informational Books

Baker, Amy C. *It's OK to Say No*. Illus. Frederick Bennett Green. Grosset & Dunlap, 1986. K–3. It's all right to refuse adults you are uncomfortable around.

Buschman, Janis, and Hunley, Debbie. *Strangers Don't Look Like the Big Bad Wolf!* Franklin, 1985. K–3. Teaches how to avoid being abducted by strangers.

Davis, Diane. *Something Is Wrong at My House*. Parenting Press, 1985. K–3. Discusses adults who fight, domestic violence, and provides list of state coalitions against domestic violence.

Dayee, Frances S. *Private Zone*. Illus. Marina Megale Horosko. Charles Franklin Press, 1982. K–4. What a child needs to know to prevent or report sexual assault.

Freeman, Lory. *It's My Body & Mi Cuerpo es Mio*. Parenting Press, 1985. K–3. How to resist uncomfortable touches by others. Presents hypothetical situations to help children tell the difference between good and bad touching.

————. *Loving Touches.* Parenting Press, 1985. K–3. A book that helps identify the positive, caring kinds of touching and teaches respect for the bodies of others.

Girard, Linda Walvoord. *My Body Is Private.* Illus. Rodney Pate. Whitman, 1984. Pres.–3. Explains one's right to privacy and how important it is to tell someone if you are being abused.

————. *Who Is a Stranger and What Should I Do?* Illus. Helen Cogancherry. Whitman, 1985. 2–6. Warns parents and children of possible dangerous situations and presents actions to take.

Hyde, Margaret O. *Sexual Abuse: Let's Talk about It.* Westminster, 1984. 2–6. Information about how to help children protect themselves from sexual abuse. Includes bibliography and resources.

Jance, Judith A. *Dial Zero for Help.* Franklin, 1985. K–4. Teaches abduction prevention skills for when a custodian tries to take a child.

————. *It's Not Your Fault.* Franklin, 1985. K–4. Reassures that molestation is not the fault of children and encourages them to speak out if they are being molested.

Meyer, Linda D. *Safety Zone: A Book Teaching Child Abduction Prevention Skills.* Franklin, 1984. K–4. Teaches stranger abduction prevention skills.

Stanek, Muriel. *Don't Hurt Me, Mama.* Illus. Helen Cogancherry. Whitman, 1983. 1–3. Offers an understated introduction to parental abuse.

Fantasy and Other Types of Stories

Berenstain, Stan, and Berenstain, Jan. *The Berenstain Bears Learn about Strangers.* Random, 1985. Pres.–2. Rules to follow in dealing with strangers in order to avoid danger.

Huck, Charlotte, reteller. *Princess Furball.* Illus. Anita Lobel. Greenwillow, 1989. K–4. A princess rebels against her abusive father in a folktale that hints of incest.

Keller, Irene. *Benjamin Rabbit and the Stranger Danger.* Illus. Dick Keller. Dodd, Mead, 1985. 1–3. Advice about helping children deal with strangers.

Steig, William. *The Amazing Bone.* Farrar, Straus & Giroux, 1976. K–3. Vulnerable Pearl, a romantic pig, is captured by a fox who prepares to eat her, but she is saved from danger through the help of a magical talking bone. Teaches alertness to danger.

Grades Four Through Six

Realistic Fiction

Banks, Lynne Reid. *Melusine: A Mystery.* Harper & Row, 1989. 6-up. A teen is caught up in a mystery involving incest and death.

Bawden, Nina. *Squib.* Illus. Hank Blaustein. Lothrop, Lee & Shepard, 1982. 4–6. Explains the trials of one abused child.

Byars, Betsy. *Cracker Jackson.* Viking Kestrel, 1985. 4–6. Domestic violence threatens the world of a boy's babysitter.

———. *The Pinballs.* Harper & Row, 1977. 4–7. Three foster children attempt to cope with their problems.

Christopher, Matt. *The Hockey Machine.* Little, Brown, 1986. 4–6. An athlete held captive by a fan must play hockey in order to survive and plan his escape.

Duffy, James. *Missing.* Scribner's, 1988. 4–6. Portrays family support and strength in the case of a kidnapped child.

Geller, Mark. *Raymond.* Harper & Row, 1988. 5–8. An abused child tries to escape his dangerous home situation.

Hall, Lynn. *The Boy in the Off-White Hat.* Scribner's, 1985. 4–6. Story of the damaging effects on a child of a man's sexual abuse. Gives clues to behavior for parents and older children.

Howard, Ellen. *Gillyflower.* Atheneum, 1986. 4–6. Story of a child being sexually abused by her father who finds the bravery to report it.

Hunt, Irene. *The Lottery Rose.* Ace Tempo Books, 1978. 4–6. A victim of child abuse overcomes his fears when placed in a home with other boys.

Irwin, Hadley. *Abby, My Love.* McElderry, 1985. 5-up. A young man discovers his girlfriend is a victim of incest.

Magorian, Michelle. *Good Night, Mr. Tom.* Harper & Row, 1981. 6-up. An abused child heals when sent to live with a lonely older man in the English countryside during World War II.

McLean, Susan. *Pennies for the Piper.* Farrar, Straus & Giroux, 1981. 5-up. A child and her mother plan for the mother's death from heart disease.

Nathanson, Laura. *The Trouble with Wednesdays.* Putnam, 1986. 4–6. A child is sexually abused by her dentist and manages to speak out.

Newton, Suzanne. *An End to Perfect.* Viking Kestrel, 1984. 4–6. A child's friend is the victim of an abusive mother.

Roberts, Willo Davis. *Don't Hurt Laurie!* Illus. Ruth Sanderson. Aladdin, 1988. 4–6. A child deals with her abusive mother to save herself.

Shreve, Susan. *Lucy Forever & Miss Rosetree, Shrinks.* Knopf, 1988. 4–6. Two sixth graders uncover a case of child abuse.

Whitley, Mary Ann. *A Sheltering Tree.* Walker, 1985. 5–6. A young girl struggles to escape an abusive stepfather.

Informational Books

Dolan, Jr., Edward F. *Child Abuse.* Watts, 1980. 4–6. Nature, history, and causes of child abuse, including pertinent legislation and community action programs.

Hyde, Margaret O. *Cry Softly! The Story of Child Abuse.* Westminster Press, 1980. 5–8. Explains that child abuse is present at all socioeconomic levels and provides list of organizations that help abusive parents as well as abused children.

Terkel, Susan Neiburg, and Rench, Janice E. *Feeling Safe, Feeling Strong: How to Avoid Sexual Abuse and What to Do If It Happens to You.* Lerner, 1984. 4–8. Six persons tell their encounters with sexual abuse, and each gives factual information and advice.

Wachter, Oralee. *No More Secrets for Me.* Illus. Jane Aaron. Little, Brown, 1983. 4–6. Four short stories illustrate possible adult-child sexual encounters, suggesting ways for children to cope with them and to seek help.

Fantasy

Walsh, Jill Paton. *A Chance Child.* Farrar, Straus & Giroux, 1978. 5-up. An abused child takes a journey back in time to where children were treated as harshly as he is in the present.

Plays

Out of the Trap. Bridgework Theater, 113½ Lincoln Ave., Goshen, IN 46526. 4-up. Play providing information and skills for prevention of sexual abuse.

Yost, Don, and Plummer, Carol. *Little Bear.* Bridgework Theater, 1981. 3–5. Play designed to teach children information and skills to make them less vulnerable to sexual abuse. Includes a curriculum guide.

Grades Seven and Up

Fiction

Adler, C. S. *Fly Free.* Coward, McCann, 1984. 7-up. A verbally and physically abused child finds solace in her relationship with her frequently absent father and her younger brother.

Arrick, Fran. *Chernowitz.* Bradbury, 1981. 6-up. A child deals with an anti-Semitic bully who is himself abused.

Cole, Brock. *The Goats.* Farrar, Straus & Giroux, 1987. Two teens are victims of a cruel prank by fellow campers.

Conrad, Pam. *Holding Me Here.* Harper & Row, 1986. 6–9. A child learns about the effects of divorce when a battered woman rents a room from her mother.

Dizenzo, Patricia. *Why Me? The Story of Jenny.* Avon, n.d. 7-up. A teen tells about her rape, its aftermath, and how people around her reacted.

Hermes, Patricia. *A Solitary Secret.* Harcourt Brace Jovanovich, 1985. 7-up. A first-person story of a girl's sexual abuse by her father.

Hunt, Irene. *Lottery Rose.* Scribner's, 1976. 6–8. A child is victimized by his mother, until the authorities step in.

Lasky, Kathryn. *Prank*. Dell, 1984. 7–9. A girl from a troubled family looks forward to a better life for herself.

Lee, Kingman. *The Refiner's Fire*. Houghton Mifflin, 1981. 7-up. A girl goes to live with her father and meets his unconventional housemates, one of whom is physically abused.

MacLean, John. *Mac*. Houghton Mifflin, 1987. 7-up. A teen's world crumbles when he is molested by a physician and he tries to ignore the experience.

Miklowitz, Gloria D. *Did You Hear What Happened to Andrea?* Delacorte, 1979. 6-up. Story of a girl's rape, and the counselor, therapist, and boyfriend who help her.

————. *Secrets Not Meant to be Kept*. Delacorte, 1987. 7-up. Story of sexual abuse at a preschool.

Moeri, Louise. *The Girl Who Lived on the Ferris Wheel*. Dutton, 1979. 7-up. How one girl deals with child abuse.

Peck, Richard. *Are You in the House Alone?* Viking Kestrel, 1976. 7-up. A girl is raped by a rich, popular boy from school, and no one believes her.

Sebestyen, Ouida. *The Girl in the Box*. Little, Brown, 1988. 7-up. A girl forced to live in an underground room by an unknown captor finds a way to survive.

Informational Books

Benedict, Helen. *Safe, Strong, and Streetwise*. Little, Brown, 1987. 7-up. A rape-crisis specialist explains how young adults can prepare for and protect against sexual assault.

Bode, Janet. *Rape: Preventing It; Coping with the Legal, Medical, and Emotional Aftermath*. Watts, 1979. 7-up. Case histories and interviews with rape victims discuss rape as a social problem.

Kosof, Anna. *Incest: Families in Crisis*. Watts, 1985. 7-up. Explores family situations where incest occurs and how important it is to report it.

Parrot, Andrea. *Coping with Date Rape & Acquaintance Rape*. Rosen, 1988. 7-up. Explanation of date and acquaintance rape and what to do for help and support.

SUICIDE

Grades Four Through Six

Realistic Fiction

Byars, Betsy. *The Burning Questions of Bingo Brown*. Viking Kestrel, 1988. 4–7. A child deals with a bully and the attempted suicide of his teacher.

Clifford, Eth. *Killer Swan.* Houghton Mifflin, 1980. 5–8. A child's involvement with a family of swans helps him work through the problems he has because of his father's suicide.

Eyerly, Jeannette. *See Dave Run.* Harper & Row, 1978. 7–9. A runaway boy and his suicide as seen through the eyes of those around him.

Killien, Christi. *Artie's Brief: The Whole Truth and Nothing But.* Houghton Mifflin, 1989. 3–7. A child deals with his older brother's suicide.

Peck, Richard. *Remembering the Good Times.* Delacorte, 1985. 6-up. Two teens cope with the suicide of their best friend.

Pevsner, Stella. *How Could You Do It, Diane?* Clarion, 1989. 5–9. A stepsister tries to cope with her sibling's suicide.

Radley, Gail. *The World Turned Inside Out.* Crown, 1982. 7-up. A child and his family adjust to the suicide of his brother.

Shreve, Susan. *Family Secrets: Five Very Important Stories.* Illus. Richard Cuffari. Knopf, 1979. 7-up. A child learns to cope with death, divorce, suicide, old age, and cheating at school.

Steele, Mary Q. *The Life (and Death) of Sara Elizabeth Harwood.* Greenwillow, 1980. 5–8. A girl becomes disgusted with herself and considers suicide.

Informational Books

•Krementz, Jill. *How It Feels When a Parent Dies.* Knopf, 1988. 7-up. Two children report how they coped with the suicide of a parent.

Madison, Arnold. *Suicide and Young People.* Houghton Mifflin, 1981. 6-up. Talks about the epidemic of teen suicides and discusses prevention.

Plays

Kral, Brian. *Apologies.* Anchorage Press, 1988. 6-up. A child leaves a note and takes her life, and family and friends are left wondering why.

Fantasy

Arkin, Alan. *The Lemming Condition.* Harper & Row, 1976. 4-up. One lemming finds the courage to fight instinct and resists joining the mass suicide.

Grades Seven and Up

Realistic Fiction

Adler, Carole S. *The Shell Lady's Daughter.* Putnam, 1983. 6–9. A child deals with her mother's nervous breakdown and attempted suicide.

Arrick, Fran. *Tunnel Vision*. Bradbury, 1980. 6-up. Story of a fifteen-year-old and why he committed suicide.

Bridgers, Sue Ellen. *Notes for Another Life*. Knopf, 1981. 7-up. A boy attempts suicide when his life begins to fall apart.

Faucher, Elizabeth. *Surviving*. Scholastic, 1985. 7-up. An overachiever and a problem teen decide life isn't worth the effort.

Ferris, Jean. *Amen, Moses Gardenia*. Farrar, Straus & Giroux, 1985. 7-up. A teen needing a family and friends considers suicide.

Hughes, Dean. *Switching Tracks*. Atheneum, 1982. A story of a boy tormented by his father's suicide for which he feels responsible.

Irwin, Hadley. *So Long at the Fair*. McElderry, 1987. 7-up. A friend deals with his best friend's suicide by trying to lose himself at a county fair.

Korschunow, Irina. *Who Killed Christopher?* Eva Mayer, translator. Philomel, 1980. 7-up. Two young people try to understand the possible suicide of their friend.

Landis, J. D. *The Band Never Dances*. Harper & Row, 1989. 6-up. A girl deals with her older brother's suicide by immersing herself in music.

Menlus, Opal. *No Escape*. Elsevier/Nelson, 1979. 6-up. A teen deals with his father's last message before he committed suicide.

Miklowitz, Gloria D. *Close to the Edge*. Dell, 1984. 7-up. A child finds help from senior citizens in understanding her friend's suicide.

Oneal, Zibby. *The Language of Goldfish*. Viking Kestrel, 1980. 7-up. An adolescent having difficulty growing up considers suicide.

Pfeffer, Susan Beth. *About David*. Delacorte, 1980. 7-up. A girl deals with shock and guilt, feeling she could have stopped a friend's murder of his parents and his suicide.

Tapp, Kathy Kennedy. *The Sacred Circle of the Hula Hoop*. McElderry, 1989. 5–9. A sister tries to help when her older sibling tries suicide.

Van Leeuwen, Jean. *Seems Like This Road Goes on Forever*. Dial, 1979. 7-up. A child who feels unloved by her stern, preoccupied parents attempts suicide and gets help from a therapist.

Informational Books

Giovacchini, Peter. *The Urge to Die*. Viking Kestrel, 1983. 7-up. Author suggests love and understanding as the treatment for teens struggling with life.

Harrison, William. *In a Wild Sanctuary*. Morrow, 1969. 7-up. Four friends make a suicide pact, and a father tries to understand it before they carry it out.

Hermes, Patricia. *A Time to Listen: Preventing Youth Suicide*. Harcourt Brace Jovanovich, 1987. 6-up. Interviews reveal pain and suffering of suicidal young people and those who survive them.

Hyde, Margaret O., and Forsyth, E. H. *Suicide: The Hidden Epidemic*. Discusses misconceptions, patterns, and theories behind suicides.

Klagsbrun, Francine. *Too Young to Die: Youth and Suicide*. Houghton

Mifflin, 1976. 7-up. Author examines issues likely to cause suicide, and book lists crisis treatment centers.

Kolehmainen, Janet, and Handwerk, Sandra. *Teen Suicide: A Book for Friends, Family, and Classmates*. Lerner, 1986. 7-up. Dispels myths surrounding suicide, describes potential victims, and lists eight classic warning signs. Also presents six histories describing situations that typically lead to suicide.

Langone, John. *Dead End: A Book About Suicide*. Little, Brown, 1986. 7-up. Offers facts and insights into suicide for teens, parents, and teachers.

Leder, Jane M. *Dead Serious: A Book About Teenagers and Teenage Suicide*. Atheneum, 1987. 7-up. What to do and not do for friends and parents of those considering suicide.

Mack, John E. *Vivienne: The Life and Suicide of an Adolescent Girl*. New American Library, 1982. 7-up. Case study of suicidal behavior which includes a bibliography for further reading.

Plays

The Living Stage Theatre. *Suicide*. Living Stage Theatre Company, 6th and Maine Ave. S.W., Washington, DC 20024. 6-up. The surviving member of a suicide pact struggles with family and the ghost of his girlfriend, who is urging him to commit suicide.

Appendix I: Health-Related Material and Resources

Source information is given for the materials and resources listed below. Some sources are listed only after the last item in the series when consecutive items are from the same source. The following symbols identify the type of resource:

> * = audiovisual material
> ** = posters
> # = material in print

A. GROWTH AND DEVELOPMENT

Development

*Infancy Through Adolescence: School-Age Child. grades 1–6. Subjects: motor skill refinement, socialization activities, drive to learn and cognitive development, effect of entering school, and importance of family influence.
    American Journal of Nursing Company
    Educational Services Division
    555 West 57th Street
    New York, NY 10019-2961

Exercise

*Exercise Is Wise. grades K–2.
    American Heart Association
    7320 Greenville Avenue
    Dallas, TX 75231

General

*Early Start to Good Health. grades K–3. Stresses how the body works, importance of a positive self-image, good health habits, and making choices.

American Cancer Society, Inc.
National Headquarters
1599 Clifton Road
Atlanta, GA 30329
(404) 320-3333

Heart and Circulatory System

*Adventure of a Man in Search of a Heart. grades K–2. Introduces four major heart health risk factors and urges adoption of appropriate habits for a healthier heart.

*Circulation of the Blood. grades 3–5. Animated diagrams explain how the blood circulates through the heart to the lungs and the rest of the body.
    American Heart Association
    7320 Greenville Avenue
    Dallas, TX 75231

**Curriculum on Blood: Primary Level. Identifies and explains the main blood components; vocabulary cards for word pronunciation; wall posters use cartoon characters to show functions of components; three lessons and optional follow-up activities.
    University of Washington
    Distribution Coordinator
    HSCER, T-281, SB-56
    Seattle, WA 98195

*Dr. Truso's Jet Powered Pedaller. grades 3–5. Dr. Truso's adventures emphasize the importance of cardiovascular fitness and healthy snacks.
    American Heart Association
    7320 Greenville Avenue
    Dallas, TX 75231

*Heart Medley. grades 3–5. Five entertaining computer games: Heart-works, Heart Attack Risk, Tic-Tac Heart, Heart Jeopardy, and the Healthy Heart Food game.

Heartbeat Journal. grades 4–6. Series of heart health education publications:

*It's a Heart. grades K–2. The Tin Woodman, the Scarecrow, and the Lion introduce the physiology of the heart and circulatory system.

#Putting Your Heart into the Curriculum. grades 3–5. Activities: Cardiovascular Terms Word Find; Scrambled Words; Vein and Artery Flow; Heart

Sounds; Pulse Rate Variation; Animal Heart Dissection; Discussion Topic, Cardiovascular Disease Statistics; and Magic Square.

**Songs from the Heart. grades K–2. Music for piano and guitar on individual record or audiocassette, and coloring pages. Songs include: "The Heart Is the Part That Goes Thump, Kee-Thump," "It's a Heart," "The Circulatory System and Your Heart," and "Around and Round the Circulatory System."

Take Care of Your Heart. grades K–2. Four risk factors from the film "Adventures of a Man in Search of a Heart" help students make decisions about the risk factors.

**Your Heart and How It Works. grades 3–5.

**Your Heart Is Just About the Strongest Part of Your Body. grades K–2. On a dot-to-dot format, boys and girls can trace the circulation of the blood through the heart.
>   American Heart Association
>   7320 Greenville Avenue
>   Dallas, TX 75231

Vision

*The Eyes Have It. grades K–3. Eye safety at home and school demonstrated using marionettes. Supplemental teacher's packet.

*The Magic of Sight. grades 5–6. Filmstrip audiocassette presentation for teaching about vision, eye health, and safety; teacher's guide, chart of the eye, folder with illustration of the eye and how it works, first-aid sticker, three quiz testing sheets, and a crossword puzzle sheet.
>   National Society to Prevent Blindness
>   500 East Remington Road
>   Schaumburg, IL 60173

Organizational Resources

American Dental Association
211 E. Chicago Avenue
Chicago, IL 60611

American Foundation for the
    Blind
15 W. 16th Street
New York, NY 10011
(212) 620-2000

American Heart Association
7320 Greenville Avenue
Dallas, TX 75231
(214) 750-5300

American Kidney Fund
7315 Wisconsin Avenue
Suite 203E
Bethesda, MD 20814
(800) 638-8299
(301) 986-1444 in MD

American Liver Foundation
998 Pompton Avenue
Cedar Grove, NJ 07009
(800) 223-0179
(201) 857-2626 in NJ

Better Hearing Institute
(800) 424-8576

Brain Research Foundation
134 S. La Salle Street
Chicago, IL 60603

Council on Stroke
American Heart Association
7320 Greenville Avenue
Dallas, TX 75231

Heart Information Center
National Heart Institute
U.S. Public Health Service
Bethesda, MD 20014

National Federation of the Blind
1800 Johnson Street
Baltimore, MD 21230
(301) 659-9314

National Heart, Lung, and Blood
    Institute
9000 Rockville Pike
Bethesda, MD 20205
(301) 496-4236

National Institute of Dental
    Research
9000 Rockville Pike
Bethesda, MD 20205

National Kidney Foundation
Two Park Avenue
New York, NY 10016
(212) 889-2210

B. MENTAL/EMOTIONAL HEALTH

Discipline

Loving Your Child Is Not Enough: Positive Discipline That Works. Nancy Samalin with Martha Moraghan Jablow. Using dialogues between parent and child, this book provides an accessible approach to nonpunitive discipline. New York: Viking/Penguin Books, 1988.

Emotions

First Feelings: Milestones in the Emotional Development of Your Baby and Child from Birth to Age 4. Stanley Greenspan, M.D., and Nancy Thorndike

Greenspan. Offers parents and professionals a new approach in dealing with the emotions of small children. New York: Viking/Penguin Books, 1989.

Growing Up

*Summer's End. The story of a tomboy's struggle with her mother's image of how a girl growing into womanhood should look and act, and how the mother and daughter reach understanding.
> Direct Cinema, Ltd.
> P.O. Box 69589
> Los Angeles, CA 90069

*How to Be a Perfect Person in Just Three Days. A dramatization of Stephen Manes' book; introduces 12-year-old Milo, weighted with troubles, and Dr. K. Pinkerton Silverfish, who, while apparently teaching Milo how to be "perfect," in reality teaches him a great deal more about self-esteem and confidence.
> Learning Corp. of America
> 108 Wilmot Road
> Deerfield, IL 60015-9990

Mental Illness

*After the Tears: Teens Talk About Mental Illness in Their Families. Videotape of teens with relatives suffering from mental illness; they discuss their anger, guilt, fear, resentment, and confusion, and the effects of mental illness upon their lives.
> United Mental Health, Inc.
> 1945 Fifth Avenue
> Pittsburgh, PA 15219

The Children at Santa Clara. Elizabeth Marek. A young teacher reveals her experiences in teaching and learning from the disturbed adolescents in a special school in the Southwest. New York: Viking/Penguin Children's Books, 1987.

Prejudice

*Family Issues: Differences. grades 3–8. A dramatic film showing how a 12-year-old white boy and a 9-year-old Native American girl overcome prejudice and become friends.

AIMS Media
6901 Woodley Avenue
Van Nuys, CA 91406-4878
(800) 367-2467
(818) 785-4111 in CA and AK

Self-Esteem

About Self-Esteem. Explores self-esteem and explains that different talents and abilities make everyone special.
    Channing L. Bete Co., Inc.
    200 State Road
    S. Deerfield, MA 01373

Acting You. grades 6-up. A series of teaching guides on the use of improvisational theater activities and theater games for developing skills of trust, group awareness, self-expression, self-esteem, and a nonjudgmental environment. Includes *Results Don't Count, Not Sex But SEX,* and *First Kiss.*
    Girls Clubs of America, Inc.
    205 Lexington Avenue
    New York, NY 10016

Everyone Is Special. Helps children develop positive feelings for those who are different.
    Channing L. Bete Co., Inc.
    200 State Road
    S. Deerfield, MA 01373

Joyful Child: New Age Activities to Enhance Children's Joy. Peggy D. Jenkins. A New Thought guide geared to aid children in becoming more positive, this book emphasizes self-esteem through the use of directed activities based on affirmations and positive self-programming. New York: Dodd, Mead, 1988.

Organizational Resources

American Mental Health Fund
(800) 433-5959
(800) 826-2336 in IL

American Psychiatric Association
1400 K Street, N.W.
Washington, DC 20005

American Psychological
   Association
1200 17th Street, N.W.
Washington, DC 20036

Bethany Lifeline
(800) 238-4269

Depressives Anonymous
P.O. Box 1777
Grand Central Station
New York, NY 10017
(212) 942-6540

National Clearinghouse for
    Mental Health Information
Public Inquiries Section
5600 Fishers Lane
Room 11A-21
Rockville, MD 20857
(301) 443-4513

National Institute of Mental
    Health
Science Communications Branch
Public Inquiries Section
5600 Fishers Lane

Room 15C-17
Rockville, MD 20857
(301) 443-4513

National Mental Health
    Association
1021 Prince Street
Arlington VA 22314
(703) 684-7722

Northern Light Productions
169 Newbury Street
Boston, MA 02116

Phobia Society of America
6110 Executive Boulevard
Rockville, MD 20852
(301) 321-9350

C. PERSONAL HEALTH

Dental Health

Casper's Dental Health Activity Book. Uses secret codes, crossword puzzles, and color-by-code, to present brief instructive dental care messages.

Casper Presents Space-Age Dentistry. Features Casper, the Friendly Ghost, fighting against plaque.

Dental Health Activity Book. grades 3–4. Includes dozens of dot-to-dot, coloring, and cutout activities.
    American Dental Association
    211 E. Chicago Avenue
    Chicago, IL 60611

**Do You?* grades K–2. Shows the importance of regular toothbrushing, visiting the dentist, and proper foods for dental health.
    National Dairy Council
    Order Department
    6300 North River Road
    Rosemont, IL 60018-4233

**Elementary School Posters Set. Four separate dental health messages.
   American Dental Association
   211 East Chicago Avenue
   Chicago, IL 60611

*Fantastic Fluoride. Animation presents the process of tooth decay, how fluoride works, why it is needed, and various methods of using fluoride.
   Science Transfer and Research Analysis Branch
   National Institutes of Health
   5333 Westbard Avenue
   Bethesda, MD 20892

*Flash That Smile. Uses contemporary music and dancing to present information on preventive dentistry.

*The Haunted Mouth. Features invisible B. Plaque (the voice of Caesar Romero) who takes the viewer through the dental health message.
   American Dental Association
   211 E. Chicago Avenue
   Chicago, IL 60611

**Have a Healthy, Happy Smile. grades 2–4. Shows healthy smiles.
   General Mills, Inc.
   Nutrition Department (45)
   P.O. Box 1112
   Minneapolis, MN 55427

I'm Going to the Dentist. Helps children to know what to expect when they visit a dentist.

*It's Dental Flossophy, Charlie Brown. Lucy teaches Charlie Brown and Snoopy to floss, and Woodstock makes his own use of the floss to build a nest.

Learning About Your Oral Health. grades K–3 and 4–6. Teaches about plaque control, fluoride, the teeth, and dental personnel. Each packet includes teacher's guide, lesson plans, duplication master, activity sheets, and overhead transparencies.

*Merlin's Magical Message. Animated characters Merlin and King Arthur demonstrate the importance of home dental care.

*Portrait of the Enemy. Basketball strategy is an analogy for a message on periodontal disease.

*Protect Your Smile. Tabletop exhibit. Stresses the importance of sealants and systemic and topical fluorides for oral health.

So Many Things to See. pres. What happens when two children visit a dental office.

Spiderman Comic Book. With a dentist's help Spiderman defeats a villain.
American Dental Association
211 E. Chicago Avenue
Chicago, IL 60611

*Supervised School-Based, Self-Applied Fluoride Programs to Protect Children's Teeth (tabletop exhibit). Promotes the use of self-applied, fluoride tablet and mouth-rinsing procedures in school settings.
Science Transfer and Research Analysis Branch
National Institutes of Health
5333 Westbard Avenue
Bethesda, MD 20892

Tommy and Toni Teeth. Teaches that to be healthy, children must eat the proper foods and brush their teeth.
General Mills, Inc.
Nutrition Department (Department 45)
P.O. Box 1112
Minneapolis, MN 55427

*Toothbrushing with Charlie Brown. Charlie Brown teaches Linus and Snoopy how to brush.

Tooth Survival Book. grades 3–4. On plaque, fluoride, braces, endodontics, and related subjects.

A Visit from the Dentist. grade 2. A dentist presents a show-and-tell message about dental care.
American Dental Association
211 E. Chicago Avenue
Chicago, IL 60611

**Wanted: Tooth Rustlers. grades pres.–2. Demonstrates how plaque, bacteria, and sugar produce tooth decay and brushing teeth thoroughly, eating OK snacks, and regular dental checkups controls cavities.
General Mills, Inc.
Nutrition Department
P.O. Box 1112
Minneapolis, MN 55427

Decision Making

*Health Network. grades 4–6. Helps children to learn to make decisions about their own health.

American Cancer Society, Inc.
National Headquarters
1599 Clifton Road
Atlanta, GA 30329
(404) 320-3333

About Good Health. Emphasizes eating right, cleanliness, brushing the teeth, exercising, practicing safety, getting enough sleep, and eating healthy foods.
    Channing L. Bete Co., Inc.
    200 State Road
    S. Deerfield, MA 01373

Emotions

*Feelings Grow, Too. grades 5–9. The emotional ups and downs accompanying puberty. Part I: "You and Yourself," the unfamiliar feelings with the physical changes of puberty; Part II: "You and Others," puberty's effect on male-female relationships.

*Looking Great, Feeling Great. grades 5–9. Develops awareness of the new personal hygiene demands accompanying puberty; discusses hormonal and physical changes of puberty and approaches to health and hygiene.

*Liking Me: Building Self-Esteem. grades 5–9. Self-esteem and its importance in school performance, resisting peer pressure, and coping generally. Part I: "Your Self-Image"; and Part II: "Step By Step," correlation between high self-esteem and success.
    Sunburst Communications
    Rm. MV9
    39 Washington Avenue
    Pleasantville, NY 10570

General

**Well Kid Posters. Lessons on safety, nutrition, and dental health using Humpty Dumpty, Nellie Needle, Wilbur Wackeroo, and Curly-Headed Keith.
    Great Performance, Inc.
    700 N. Green Street, Suite 302
    Chicago, IL 60622

Hi! I'm Jeepers. Personal hygiene messages in simple verses.
    ABI Arts, Inc.

312 Griffit Street
P.O. Box 108
Hopkins, MN 55343

*Healthy Decisions. grades 4–6. Uses a computer program adventure game to examine environmental cues that influence making choices. Apple II series.
American Cancer Society, Inc.
National Headquarters
1599 Clifton Road
Atlanta, GA 30329
(404) 320-3333

Sexual Abuse

*Sexual Abuse Prevention: A Middle School Primer. Live-action video helps middle and junior high students deal with sexual abuse.
Human Relations Media
175 Tompkins Ave.
Pleasantville, NY 10570

Vision

Having an Eye Test. A child has vision test, wears a patch, and has eye surgery.
Pediatrics Projects, Inc.
P.O. Box 1880
Santa Monica, CA 90406-1880

Organizational Resources

Acne Helpline
(800) 235-ACNE
(800) 225-ACNE in California

Adoptees' Liberty Movement
Association (ALMA) Society
P.O. Box 154
Washington Bridge Station
New York, NY 10033
(212) 581-1568

Aerobics International Research
Society
1200 Preston Road
Dallas, TX 75230

American Association of Retired
Persons
1909 K Street, N.W.
Washington, DC 20049
(202) 872-4700

American Chiropractic
Association
1916 Wilson Boulevard
Arlington, VA 22201

American Holistic Medical
Association
Route 2 Welsh Coulee
La Crosse, WI 54601

American Kidney Fund
(800) 638-8299
(800) 492-8361 in MD

American Running and Fitness
Association
2420 K Street, N.W.
Washington, DC 20037

Better Sleep Council Committee
National Association of Bedding
Manufacturers
One Crystal Gateway
1235 Jefferson Davis Highway
Suite 601
Arlington, VA 22202

Gray Panthers
3635 Chestnut Street
Philadelphia, PA 19104
(215) 382-3300

Medic Alert Foundation
2323 Colorado
Turlock, CA 95380
(209) 668-3333

Medic Alert Organ Donor
Program
P.O. Box 1009
Turlock, CA 95381
(209) 668-3333

National Clearinghouse on Aging
330 Independence Avenue, S.W.
Washington, DC 20201
(202) 245-2158

National Council on the Aging
600 Maryland Avenue
Washington, DC 20024

National Council of Senior
Citizens
925 15th Street, N. W.
Washington, DC 20005
(202) 347-8800

National Eye Care Project
Helpline
(800) 222-EYES

National Gay Health Education
Foundation
P.O. Box 784
New York, NY 10036
(212) 563-6313

National Gay Task Force
80 Fifth Avenue
New York, NY 10011
(212) 741-1010

National Gay Youth Network
P.O. Box 14412
San Francisco, CA 94114
(415) 554-6025

National Institute of Dental
Research
Science Transfer and Research
Analysis Branch
National Institutes of Health
5333 Westbard Avenue
Bethesda, MA 20892

National Institute on Aging
National Institutes of Health
Bethesda, MD 20014

National Maternal and Child
Health Clearinghouse
3520 Prospect Street, N.W.
Washington, DC 20057

National Self-Help Clearinghouse
33 West 42nd Street
City University of New York
New York, NY 10036
(212) 840-1259

Office of Health Information,
   Health Promotion, Physical
   Fitness and Sports Medicine
Department of Health and
   Human Services
200 Independence Avenue, S. W.
Washington, DC 20201

Parents and Friends of Lesbians
   and Gays (Parents FLAG)
P.O. Box 24565
Los Angeles, CA 90024

PMS Access
(800) 222-4767
(608) 833-4767 in WI

Project Focus
Department P, FAS, Room 9438
60 Hudson Street
New York, NY 10013

Resources for Children in
   Hospitals
P.O. Box 10
Belmont, MA 02178

Shriners Hospital Referral Line
(800) 237-5055
(800) 282-9161 in FL

Women's Sports Foundation
(800) 227-3988
(415) 563-6266 in CA
(212) 972-9170 in AK, HI, and
   NYC

D. FAMILY LIFE

Adoption

*The Importance of Being Ernesto. A film about building a family through
adoption.
   Northern Light Productions
   169 Newbury Street
   Boston, MA 02116

Aging

The Aging Adult in Children's Books & Nonprint Media: An Annotated
Bibliography. Catherine Townsend Horner. Comprehensive list of fiction
and nonprint materials about the aging adult.
   Scarecrow Press
   P.O. Box 4167
   52 Liberty Street
   Metuchen, NJ 08840

Blended Families

*Stepdancing: Portrait of a Remarried Family. A candid and encouraging portrait of blended family life—the trials, tribulations, and joys of living with two families and in two homes.
>   Kensington Communications, Inc.
>   800-421-2304

Death/Dying

When a Parent Is Very Sick. Eda Le Shan. Advice for how to respond to an ill parent. Boston: Little, Brown, 1987.

Family Stress

Dennis the Menace Comic Book: Coping with Family Stress. Real-life situations producing stress in the family with possible solutions for each situation.
>   National Mental Health Association
>   1021 Prince Street
>   Alexandria, VA 22314-2971

Until Daddy Comes Home Again. Deals with young children's fears or anxieties when father is away.
>   Channing L. Bete Co., Inc.
>   200 State Road
>   S. Deerfield, MA 01373

Motherhood

Remaking Motherhood: How Working Mothers Are Shaping Our Children's Future. Anita Shreve. Assessment of the risks and rewards for working mothers and their families. New York: Viking/ Penguin Books, 1987.

Parent/Child Relationships

*My Parents and I Series. grades 5–9:

*My Mother and Father Are Getting a Divorce. Addresses the anger, depression, fear, or confusion children experience during divorce. Part I: "When Parents Separate," and Part II: "Finding Help."

*You and Your Parents: Making It Through the Tough Years. Vignettes on tensions in parent-child relationships during the "growing up" years from ages 11–14. Part I: "Why the Problem," and Part II: "Learning to Cope."
Sunburst Communications
Rm. MV9
39 Washington Avenue
Pleasantville, NY 10570

Reproduction

As You Grow Up. Introduces the basic facts about human reproduction and the physical changes that young people encounter during puberty.
Channing L. Bete Co., Inc.
200 State Road
S. Deerfield, MA 01373

Did the Sun Shine Before You Were Born? grades pres.–2. Helps parents communicate facts about sex, reproduction, and the family to their children.

Girls Are Girls and Boys Are Boys, So What's the Difference? grades 1–4. Presents nonsexist sex education.
Ed-U-Press
7174 Mott Road
Fayetteville, NY 13066

Sex Talk for a Safe Child. grades 1–3. To be read to children. Details body structure and functions, human reproduction, types of relationships and feelings and discusses sexual abuse and what children should do if someone attempts to abuse them.
American Medical Association
Order Department
P.O. Box 10946
Chicago, IL 60610-0946

Sexuality

*Another Half. grades 6–12. Focuses on helping teenagers become conscious of gender role pressures and how these pressures affect their sexual behavior.
Wadsworth Productions
1913 W. 37th St.
Austin, TX 78731

Children and Sex: The Parents Speak. Such topics as reproduction, parental double standards, nudity, masturbation, sexual information, and sexual innuendo in the media are discussed.

The Study Group of New York
Facts on File
460 Park Ave., So.
New York, NY 10016

Date Rape. Christina Dye. Defines date rape and discusses possible means of prevention.
Do It Now (DIN) Publications
P.O. Box 21126
2050 East University Drive
Phoenix, AZ 85036

The Family Book About Sexuality. Mary Calderone, M.D., and Eric W. Johnson. Presents answers to questions about sex in direct and specific terms. New York: Bantam, 1983.

Healthy Sex and Keeping It That Way. Richard Lumiere and Stephani Cook. Sections for expectant mothers, gay men, and teenagers, plus information on herpes and AIDS, help the reader to be a sensitive and responsible sexual partner. New York: Simon & Schuster, 1983.

*How Not to Make a Baby. Discusses making conscious decisions about whether to engage in sexual intercourse, saying no and waiting, and using birth control. "Part 1: Making Choices"; "Part 2: Taking Charge."
Human Relations Media
175 Tompkins Ave.
Pleasantville, NY 10570

The Parent's Guide to Teenage Sex and Pregnancy. Howard Lewis and Martha Lewis. Has a special section explaining how to respond to teenagers' questions about sexuality and how to encourage them to accept responsibility for their sexual decisions. New York: St. Martin's Press, 1980.

Putting the Boys in the Picture. Joy G. Dryfoos. Focuses on the role of boys in the teenage pregnancy crisis.
Network Publications
P.O. Box 1830
Santa Cruz, CA 95061-1830

Raising a Child Conservatively in a Sexually Permissive World. Judith Gordon and Sol Gordon. Provides advice and good sense for parents who are raising children in the modern world. New York: Simon & Schuster, 1986.

*Sex and the American Teenager. grades 6–12. Confirms the number of youngsters who, unprepared emotionally and without taking precautions, engage in sex. Provocative discussion material for teens and adults.

Pyramid Film and Video
P.O. Box 1048
Santa Monica, CA 90406

*Sex Myths and Facts. The most common misconceptions concerning sex are honestly and explicitly clarified in a question-and-answer quiz format. Alfred Higgins Productions, Inc.
9100 Sunset Blvd.
Los Angeles, CA 90069

*Sexual Responsibility: A Two-Way Street. Carl Anthony Payne, who plays Cockroach on the Cosby Show, narrates; emphasizes that communication is the most important part of girl-boy relationships, especially where sex is concerned.
Human Relations Media
175 Tompkins Ave.
Pleasantville, NY 10570

Straight Talk: Sexuality Education for Parents and Kids 4–7. grades pres.–2. Susan Chamlin and Marilyn Ratner. A handbook that clearly, sensibly, and sensitively shows how to become a confident, comfortable, "askable" parent. New York: Viking/Penguin Books, 1987.

Siblings

Another Look at the Rainbow: Straight from the Siblings. grades K–3. Sisters and brothers of children with catastrophic diseases draw and tell brief stories about the effects on them.

I Have a Sister, My Sister Is Deaf. Judith A. Jance. grades K–6. A child describes her deaf sister who laughs, plays, and rocks her doll to sleep without a song.

Living with a Brother or Sister with Special Needs: A Book for Siblings. Explores information and feelings about chronic illnesses and disabilities.

Losing Someone You Love: When a Brother or Sister Dies. grades 3–6. Children and teens talk about loss of their siblings from various conditions.
Pediatric Projects, Inc.
P.O. Box 1880
Santa Monica, CA 90406-1880

Women

Action Agenda for Equalizing Girls' Options. Practical steps to remove barriers keeping girls from realizing their true potential.

*Guide to Developing Sports Programs for Girls; Ten Principles for Girls' Sport Participation. A sports resource kit for planning effective sports programs for girls ages 6–18.
    Girls Clubs of America
    Resource Center
    441 West Michigan Street
    Indianapolis, IN 46202

I Wish My Parents Understood: A Report on the Teenage Female. Lesley Jane Nonkin. Presents complex attitudes and concerns of today's teenaged girls. New York: Viking/Penguin Books, 1987.

Sports Resource Kit. Comprehensive set of materials for planning effective sports programs for girls, ages 6–18. Includes *Sports Resource Guide; On Your Mark: A Complete Guide to Developing Sports Programs for Girls; Ten Principles of Girls' Sports Participation;* "Sports Beyond Winning," a video promoting women's sports involvement; and other materials. Books are available separately. Others available from:
    Girls Clubs of America
    Resource Center
    441 West Michigan Street
    Indianapolis, IN 46202

Organizational Resources

Adam Walsh Child Resource
    Center
1876 N. University Drive
Suite 306
Fort Lauderdale, FL 33322
(303) 475-4847

American Association of
    Marriage and Family
    Counselors
225 Yale Avenue
Claremont, CA 91711
Center for Population
    Options
2031 Florida Avenue, N.W.
Suite 301
Washington, DC 20008

Childfind
P.O. Box 277
New Paltz, NY 12561
(800) 431-5005

Equal Rights for Fathers
P.O. Box 6327
Albany, CA 94706

The Edna Gladney Home
(800) 433-2922
(800) 772-2740 in TX

Family Communications, Inc.
4802 Fifth Avenue
Pittsburgh, PA 15213

Family Service Association of
    America
44 E. 23rd Street
New York, NY 10010
(212) 674-6100

International Childbirth
    Education Association
P.O. Box 20048
Minneapolis, MN 55420

National Center for Education in
Maternal and Child Health
38th and R Streets N.W.
Washington, DC 20057

National Clearinghouse for
Family Planning Information
P.O. Box 2225
Rockville, MD 20852
(301) 251-5153

National Gay Task Force
Crisisline
(800) 221-7044
(212) 529-1604 in NY, AK, and
HI

National Hotline for Missing
Children
(800) 843-5678
(202) 644-9836 in DC

National Organization of Mothers
of Twins Clubs
5402 Amberwood Lane
Rockville, MD 20853

National Pregnancy Hotline
(800) 852-5683
(800) 831-5881 in CA
(213) 380-8750 in Los
Angeles

National Runaway Switchboard
(800) 621-4000

Planned Parenthood Federation
of America
810 Seventh Avenue
New York, NY 10019

Runaway Hotline
(800) 231-6946
(800) 392-3352 in TX

Sibling Information Network
3429 Glenbrook Road
Box U-64
University of Connecticut
Storrs, CT 06268
(203) 486-4034

E. NUTRITIONAL HEALTH

Cardiovascular Fitness

Children's Help Your Heart Cookbook. grades K–2. Emphasizes healthy
heart habits as kids learn to make unusual treats.

Dr. Truso's Jet Powered Pedaller. grades 3–5. Emphasizes the importance
of cardiovascular fitness and healthy snacks; includes activity sheet.
American Heart Association
7320 Greenville Avenue
Dallas, TX 75231

Dairy

**Milk From Cow to You. grades 2–4. Highlights the important steps in
producing, processing, and delivering to protect the high-quality, safety,
and good flavor of milk.

*Milk . . . in the Computer Age. grades 4–7. A sixth-grade class tours a modern dairy farm and a milk processing plant; emphasizes protecting safety, quality, and good flavor of milk.
National Dairy Council
Order Department
6300 N. River Road
Rosemont, IL 60018-4233

Dental

**OK Snacks Shop. grades pres.–2. Animated teeth enjoy safe snacks (cheese, fresh fruits and vegetables, popcorn, tacos, and sugarless gum); explain the relationship between foods, toothbrushing, flossing, and tooth decay.
General Mills, Inc.
Nutrition Department (Dept. 45)
P.O. Box 1112
Minneapolis, MN 55427

The Tooth Chicken. pres.–2. Detective Tooth Chicken investigates a serious snacking problem and talks about good nutrition.
American Dental Association
211 E. Chicago Avenue
Chicago, IL 60611

**Which of These Foods Cause Cavities? Answers the question and suggests ways to prevent cavities.
General Mills, Inc.
Nutrition Department (Department 45)
P.O. Box 1112
Minneapolis, MN 55427

Diet Problems

Food Additives and Their Impact on Health. Mary Ellen Huls and David A. Tyckoson, compilers. Provides the researcher with 251 fully annotated references on the subject of food additives; references generally available in most libraries. Phoenix, AZ: Oryx Press, 1988.

How Schools Can Help Combat Eating Disorders: Anorexia Nervosa and Bulimia. Michael P. Levine. A very readable and comprehensive research review on anorexia nervosa and bulimia; helps distinguish normal dieting from abnormal behavior; appendices include bibliographies, filmographies, organizations, etc. Washington, DC: National Education Association, 1987.

 # Special Diets and Kids: How to Keep Your Child on Any Prescribed Diet. John F. Taylor and R. Sharon Latta. Experienced child psychologist and a mother with children on special diets present a helpful, comprehensive program for motivating a child to stay on a prescribed diet; offers clear, easy-to-follow advice on coping with the psychological ramifications of raising a child who must eat differently from peers and other family members.
  National Education Association
  1201 16th St., N.W.
  Washington, DC 20036

Food Groups

#About Good Nutrition. Uses pictures and puzzles to teach the four basic food groups and the importance of eating three meals a day without eating too much sugar.
  Channing L. Bete Co., Inc.
  200 State Road
  South Deerfield, MA 01373

Every Day Eat the 3-2-4-4 Way! grades pres.–2. Illustrates four food groups, explaining the kinds and amounts of foods needed each day.
  National Dairy Council
  Order Department
  6300 N. River Road
  Rosemont, IL 60018-4233

Food Encounters. grades 3–6. Computer program provides information needed to understand four food groups; has students deliver nutritious foods to space stations. Computer courseware is programmed in color, with optional sound. For use with the Apple II plus, IIc, IIe, or IIe enhanced computer.
  National Dairy Council
  Order Department
  6300 N. River Road
  Rosemont, IL 60018-4233

#Good to Eat Coloring Book. Reviews four food groups.
  General Mills, Inc.
  Nutrition Department (Department 45)
  P.O. Box 1112
  Minneapolis, MN 55427

#Let's Explore Nutrition. grades 3–6. Teaches children the basics of good nutrition and to eat right to stay healthy.
  Channing L. Bete Co., Inc.
  200 State Road
  South Deerfield, MA 01373

*Nutrition for Everyone's Needs. Promotes positive approach to good eating.
> American Journal of Nursing Company
> Educational Services Division
> 555 W. 57th Street
> New York, NY 10019-2961

**The Starting Line Up. grades K–12. Photographs show that nutritious food tastes good; provides recommended servings and nutritional information about the five food groups for planning a balanced diet.
> Modern Talking Picture Service
> 5000 Park Street North
> St. Petersburg, FL 33709-9989

#*The Thing the Professor Forgot.* grades pres.–3. Professor Oonoose Q. Eckwoose teaches about five food groups.
> General Mills, Inc.
> Nutrition Department (Department 45)
> P.O. Box 1112
> Minneapolis, MN 55427

Food Relationships

#*Mudluscious.* Jan Irving and Robin Currie. Stories and activities featuring food for preschool children.
> Libraries Unlimited
> P.O. Box 263
> Littleton, CO 80160

General

**Big Muscles. grades K–12. Shows a strong young boy and the type of breakfast needed to build his muscles; shows the cause-and-effect syndrome of good nutrition habits.
> Modern Talking Picture Service
> 5000 Park Street North
> St. Petersburg, FL 33709-9989

#*Creative Food Experiences for Children.* Introduces children to cooking; offers dozens of recipes, games, and activities designed to develop good eating habits.
> Center for Science in the Public Interest
> 1501 16th Street, NW
> Washington, DC 20036

#Foods . . . Your Choice. grades 1–6. Comprehensive program: overview, learning activities, nutrition primer, duplicating masters for student handouts and work sheets, and resource materials specific to each grade level.
National Dairy Council
Order Department
6300 N. River Road
Rosemont, IL 60018-4233

*Good Food Puppets. grades pres.–2. Puppets Annie Apple, Charlie Carrot, and Super Bean used to teach basics of good food and good health and create play activities; stories, lessons, scripts, and songs available.
Yummy Designs
P.O. Box 14243
Portland, OR 97214

**Growth Record. grades pres.–2. Shows growth patterns using bar graphs to chart changes in height and weight; discusses foods needed for growth and health.

**What Did You Have for Breakfast This Morning? grades 2–5. Shows children from different ethnic groups to help children recognize that food habits can be different but still good. Teacher's guide available.

*Wholly Cow! grades 3–12. Animated presentation of how a cow's food is digested and how the nutrients are absorbed and used to make milk.
National Dairy Council
Order Department
6300 N. River Road
Rosemont, IL 60018-4233

Snacking

*The Barnyard Snacker. Features detective Tooth Chicken who discovers a serious snacking problem and teaches Hungry Hog and other animals a lesson in nutrition.
American Dental Association
211 E. Chicago Avenue
Chicago, IL 60611

**Meals and Snacks for You. grades pres.–2. Shows children eating nutritious meal; encourages discussions of good food selection. Teacher's guide available.
National Dairy Council
Order Department
6300 N. River Road
Rosemont, IL 60018-4233

**Snack Light, Snack Right. For the classroom or cafeteria, to remind students that nutritious snacks matter.
    Modern Talking Picture Service
    5000 Park Street North
    St. Petersburg, FL 33709-9989

Vitamins

\# Vitamins: An Alphabet Soup for Good Health. Quick introduction to specific aspects of nutrition.
    Abbott Labs
    Department 792V
    North Chicago, IL 60064

Organizational Resources

American Anorexia Nervosa/
    Bulimia Association, Inc.
133 Cedar Lane
Teaneck, NJ 07666
(201) 836-1800

American Institute of
    Nutrition
9650 Rockville Pike
Bethesda, MD 20814

American Society for Clinical
    Nutrition (Same as American
    Institute of Nutrition)

Anorexia Bulimia Treatment and
    Education Center
(800) 33-ABTEC
(301) 332-9800 in MD

Bulimia Anorexia Self-Help
(800) 227-4785

Dairy and Nutrition Council,
    Mideast
5811 Canal Road

Cleveland, OH 44125
(216) 447-1012

Food and Nutrition Board
National Research Council
2101 Constitution Avenue, NW
Washington, DC 20418

Food and Nutrition Information
    Center
National Agricultural Library
    Building
Room 304
Beltsville, MD 20705
(301) 344-3719

National Anorexic Aid Society,
    Inc.
P.O. Box 29461
Columbus, OH 43229
(614) 895-2009

National Dairy Council
Order Department
6300 N. River Road
Rosemont, IL 60018-4233

National Nutrition Education
  Clearinghouse
Society for Nutrition
  Education
2140 Shattuck Avenue
Suite 1110
Berkeley, CA 94704

Overeaters Anonymous
2190 W. 190th Street
Torrance, CA 90504
(213) 320-7941

TOPS (Take Off Pounds
  Sensibly)
P.O. Box 07489
4575 S. Fifth Street
Milwaukee, WI 53207
(414) 482-4620

Weight Watchers International,
  Inc.
800 Community Drive
Manhasset, NY 11030
(516) 627-9200

F. PREVENTION AND CONTROL OF DISEASES
AND DISORDERS

AIDS

AIDS. William A. Check. Presents a concise history of the disease, as well as research efforts and ways to avoid transmission.
  Chelsea House Publishers
  Dept. WP4
  P.O. Box 914
  1974 Sproul Road, Suite 400
  Broomall, PA 19008-0914

AIDS: Ending an Epidemic. Jim Parker. A clear overview of the disease; what it is, how it is transmitted, the symptoms and prognosis, how to reduce the risk of contracting the disease, etc.

The AIDS Crisis. Christina Dye. A slightly older but in-depth look at AIDS; also includes two useful charts.

Drugs & AIDS. Danielle Hain. A question-and-answer format and a matter-of-fact style pamphlet.
  Do It Now (DIN) Publications
  P.O. Box 21126
  2050 East University Drive
  Phoenix, AZ 85036

Into Adolescence: Learning About AIDS. grades 5–8. First in Contemporary Health Series; targets middle grades; emphasis on AIDS education as part of comprehensive health education program. Santa Cruz, CA: Network Publications, 1988.

Talking with Children about AIDS. A subfile in Center for Disease Control's computer file; contains programs, curricula, guidelines, policies, regulations, and materials.
> BRS Information Technologies
> 800-345-4277
> 1200 Route 7
> Latham, NY 12110

Cancer

*Coping with Cancer: The Early School Years. An 8-year-old boy and 9-year-old girl in play therapy explore their fears, anxieties, and understanding of the ways of coping with their cancer experiences. Demonstrates use of puppets and modified hospital equipment in play techniques.

*Coping with Cancer: The Sibling Perspective. The story of four children, aged 6 to 16, with siblings with cancer as they deal with changes in their families, school lives, and friendships, while still believing in life.
> American Journal of Nursing Company
> Educational Services Division
> 555 W. 57th St.
> New York, NY 10019-2916

Diabetes

Educational Materials For and About Young People with Diabetes: Selected Annotations.
> National Institute of Arthritis, Diabetes, and Digestive and Kidney
> Diseases
> Building 31, Room 9A-04
> 9000 Rockville Pike
> Bethesda, MD 20205

Skin

Your Skin and the Sun. grades 4–6. Increases children's awareness of the sun and its effect on the skin. Includes activity sheets, a teacher's guide, wall poster, fifty take-home booklets, and a reply card.
> Johnson and Johnson Baby Products Company
> Grandview Road
> Skillman, NJ 08558

Organizational Resources

AIDS Information Hotline
Public Health Service
(800) 342-AIDS

AIDS Medical Foundation
10 East 13th Street, Suite LD
New York, NY 10003
(212) 206-0670

Alzheimer's Disease and Related
  Disorders Association
360 N. Michigan Avenue
Suite 601
Chicago, IL 60601
(800) 621-0379
(800) 572-6037 in IL
(312) 853-3060

AMC Cancer Information
(800) 525-3777

American Diabetes Association
2 Park Avenue
New York, NY 10016
(212) 683-7444
(800) 232-3472
(703) 549-1500 in VA and DC
  metro area

American Leprosy Missions
(Hansen's Disease)
(800) 543-3131
(201) 794-8650 in NJ

Arthritis Foundation
1314 Spring Street, N.W.
Atlanta, GA 30309
(404) 872-7100

Arthritis Information
  Clearinghouse
P.O. Box 9782
Arlington, VA 22209
(703) 558-8250

Association of Heart Patients
P.O. Box 54305
Atlanta, GA 30308
(800) 241-6993
(404) 523-0826 in GA

Asthma and Allergy Foundation
  of America
1302 18th Street, N.W.
Suite 303
Washington, DC 20036
(202) 293-2950

Cancer Connection
4410 Main
Kansas City, MO 64111

Cancer Information Service
  (CIS)
National Cancer Institute
9000 Rockville Pike
Bethesda, MD 20205
(800) 4-CANCER
(808) 524-1234 in Oahu, HI
  (Neighbor Islands call collect)
(800) 628-6070 in AK

The Candlelighters Childhood
  Cancer Foundation
1901 Pennsylvania Avenue, N.W.
Suite 1001
Washington, DC 20006

Center for Disease Control
BRS 1200 Route 7
Latham, NY 12110
(800) 345-4277

Center for Prevention Services
Centers for Disease Control
1600 Clifton Road, N.E.
Atlanta, GA 30333
(404) 329-1819

Center for Sickle Cell Disease
2121 Georgia Avenue N.W.
Washington, DC 26059
(202) 636-7930

Cooley's Anemia Foundation
(800) 221-3571
(212) 598-0911 in New York City

Cystic Fibrosis Foundation
6000 Executive Boulevard
Suite 309
Rockville, MD 20852
(800) 344-4823
(301) 951-4422 in MD

Down's Syndrome Congress
P.O. Box 1527
Brownwood, TX 76801

Heartlife
(800) 241-6993
(404) 523-0826 in GA

Herpes Resource Center
Box 100
Palo Alto, CA 94302
(415) 321-5134

High Blood Pressure Information
Center
120/80 National Institutes of
Health
Bethesda, MD 20205
(301) 496-1809

Huntington's Disease Society of
America
(800) 345-4372
(212) 242-1968 in NY

Institute of Arthritis, Diabetes,
and Digestive and Kidney
Diseases
Building 31, Room 9A-04
9000 Rockville Pike
Bethesda, MD 20205

Juvenile Diabetes Foundation
International Hotline
(800) 223-1138
(212) 889-7575 in NY

Leukemia Society of America,
Inc.
733 Third Avenue
New York, NY 10017
(212) 573-8484

Lung Line National Asthma
Center
(800) 222-5864
(303) 355-LUNG in Denver

Lupus Foundation of America
11921A Olive Boulevard
St. Louis, MO 63141

Mended Hearts
7320 Greenville Avenue
Dallas, TX 75231
(214) 750-5442

National Association for Sickle
Cell Disease
(800) 421-8453
(213) 936-7205 in CA

National Association of Patients
on Hemodialysis and
Transplantation
156 William Street
New York, NY 10038
(212) 619-2727

National Asthma Center
(800) 222-LUNG

National Clearinghouse for
Human Genetic Disease
1776 East Jefferson Street
Rockville, MD 20852
(301) 279-4642

National Diabetes Information
Clearinghouse
Box NDIC
Bethesda, MD 20205
(301) 468-2162

National Digestive Diseases and
Education and Information
Clearinghouse
1555 Wilson Boulevard
Suite 600
Rosslyn, VA 22209
(301) 496-9707

National Down Syndrome
Congress
(800) 232-6372
(309) 452-3264 in IL

National Down Syndrome
Society Hotline
(800) 221-4602
(212) 460-9330 in NY

National Genetics Foundation
9 West 57th Street
New York, NY 10019

National Headache Foundation
(800) 843-2256
(800) 523-8858 in IL

National Institute of Neurological
and Communicative Disorders
and Stroke
National Institutes of Health
Bethesda, MD 20205

National Jewish Hospital/
National Asthma Center
(800) 222-LUNG

National Psoriasis Foundation
6415 S.W. Canyon Court
Suite 200
Portland, OR 97221

National Retinitis Pigmentosa
Foundation
(800) 638-2300
(301) 225-9400 in MD

National Reye's Syndrome
Foundation
(800) 233-7393
(800) 231-7393 in OH

National SIDS Foundation
(800) 221-SIDS
(301) 459-3388 or 3389 in MD

National Tuberous Sclerosis
Association
(800) 225-6872
(312) 668-0787 in IL

NIDA Helpline
(800) 662-HELP

Patients' Aid Society
521 Fifth Avenue
17th Floor
New York, NY 10017
(212) 687-0890

Rosewell Park Memorial Institute
(800) 462-1884

Shanti Project
890 Hayes Street
San Francisco, CA 94117
(415) 558-9644

Spina Bifida Information and
Referral
(800) 621-3141
(301) 770-7222 in MD

Sudden Infant Death Syndrome
Clearinghouse
1555 Wilson Boulevard
Suite 600
Rosslyn, VA 22209
(703) 528-8480

VD Hotline (Operation
Venus)
(800) 227-8922

V.D. National Hotline
(800) 227-8922 in California
(800) 982-5883

G. SAFETY AND ACCIDENT PREVENTION

Babysitting

*Liz Sits the Schlegels. ages 9-13. Reinforces important babysitting rules, bicycle safety points, and such courtesies as family members calling home when late.
Beacon Films
P.O. Box 575
Norwood, MA 02062

First Aid

*First Aid: Newest Techniques. grades 5–12. Presents true-to-life first-aid emergencies in vignette form in two separate series. Series A includes artificial respiration, bleeding, poison, shock, burns, fractures, rescue and transfer, and a first-aid review. Series B includes frostbite/hypothermia, excessive heat, choking, sudden illness, bites, snakebite, head injuries, and multiple injuries.
Sunburst Communications
Rm. MV9
39 Washington Avenue
Pleasantville, NY 10570

I Take Good Care of Me! Teaches basic first aid and rescue techniques; fire, water, street, and electrical safety; as well as abduction and sexual assault prevention.
Chas. Franklin Press
7821 175th Street, S.W.
P.O. Box 108
Edmonds, WA 98026

Prevention

Help Yourself to Safety: A Guide to Avoiding Dangerous Situations with Strangers and Friends. Kate Hubbard and Evelyn Berlin. ages 6–11. Teaches prevention of sexual assault and abduction and gives common-sense tips.
Chas. Franklin Press
7821 175th Street, S.W.
Edmonds, WA 98026

**42nd Annual AAA School Traffic Safety Poster Program. K–3. Be Extra Alert in Bad Weather; Be Seen After Dark; Bicyclist STOP! Before Entering Traffic; Buckle, Buckle, Buckle Your Safety Belt; Help Your Safety Patrol; I Cross at Corners; Keep From Between Parked Cars; Look All Ways; Play Away From Traffic; Walk Facing Traffic
> American Automobile Association
> Public Relations
> 8111 Gatehouse Road
> Falls Church, VA 22047

*I'm No Fool Series. grades K–6. Walt Disney safety film series featuring safety instructor Jiminy Cricket teaching important safety lessons: I'm No Fool as a Pedestrian; I'm No Fool Having Fun; I'm No Fool in Water; I'm No Fool with a Bicycle; I'm No Fool with Electricity; I'm No Fool with Fire (Revised)
> Coronet/MTI Film and Video
> 108 Wilmot Road
> Deerfield, IL 60015

Safety

Series on various safety topics: About After-School Safety; Buckle Up for Safety; Car Safety; Drive Your Bicycle Safely; Fire Prevention; Fire Safety; Holiday Safety; Join the Bus Safety Team; School Bus Safety; Telephone for Help; Traffic Safety. ages 9–13.
> Channing L. Bete Co., Inc.
> 200 State Road
> S. Deerfield, MA 01373

Safety Belts

A Safer Way for Everyday. grades K–3. Stresses the importance of using safety belts, encourages students to promote safety belt use.

3 Seconds to Safety. grades 3–6. Examines the need for seat belts and analyzes common tales about them. Helps students develop critical reading skills and teaches them about sequencing and drawing conclusions.
> Mazer Corporation
> Seat Belt Safety
> P.O. Box 1400-K
> Dayton, OH 45414

**Get Home Safely
> National PTA
> 700 North Rush Street
> Chicago, IL 60611-2571

Vision

Seymour Safely Materials. Seymour Safely, a space alien puppet, and his puppet friends teach children about the need or benefit of thorough vision care: Happy Boo Day to You Booklet—Halloween Safety Tips; Meet Seymour Safely Activity Kit; Reflections of Bike Basics Booklet; Seymour Safely Bag Puppet; Seymour Safely Flyer (can be sent home with children after a presentation or be stuffed into statements going to parents); Seymour Safely Library Booklet (tells how fun it is to read and provides reading and vision tips); Seymour Safely Meets Op-Tic Booklet; Seymour Safely Poster ("Protect Your Eyes. Take Care of Your Vision"); Seymour Safely Self-Adhesive Stickers

American Optometric Association
243 N. Lindberg Blvd
St. Louis, MO 63141

Organizational Resources

American Automobile
  Association
8111 Gatehouse Road
Falls Church, VA 22047
(703) 222-6000

American Paralysis Association
(800) 225-0292
(201) 379-2690 in NJ

American Trauma Society
(800) 556-7890
(301) 328-6304

Auto Safety Hotline
(800) 424-9393
(202) 426-0123 in Washington,
  DC

Clearinghouse for Occupational
  Safety and Health
  Information
Technical Information Branch
4676 Columbia Parkway
Cincinnati, OH 45226
(513) 684-8326

HUD User
P.O. Box 280
Germantown, MD 20874
(301) 251-5154

Insurance Institute for Highway
  Safety
Watergate Six Hundred
Washington, DC 20037
(202) 333-0770

National Association for Crime
  Victims' Rights
P.O. Box 16161
Portland, OR 97216
(503) 252-9012

National Burn Victim
  Foundation
308 Main Street
Orange, NJ 07050
(201) 731-3112

National Child Safety Council
  Childwatch
(800) 222-1464

National Highway Traffic Safety
Administration
U.S. Department of
Transportation
400 7th Street, S.W.
Room 5130
Washington, DC 20590
(800) 424-9393
(202) 426-9294

National Safety Council
425 North Michigan Avenue
Chicago, IL 60611

(800) 621-7619 for placing orders
(312) 527-4800 in IL

National Victims of Crime
715 8th Street, S.E.
Washington, DC 20003
(202) 543-5379

Phoenix Society
National Organization for Burn
Victims
11 Rust Hill Road
Levittown, PA 19056
(215) 946-4788

H. CONSUMER HEALTH

Consumer Information Center
(CIC)
Pueblo, CO 81009 or
18th and E Streets, N.W.
Washington, DC 20405
(202) 566-1794

Consumer Product Safety
Commission
Washington, DC 20207
(800) 638-CPSC
(800) 638-8270 TDD
(800) 492-8104 TDD in MD

Consumers Union
256 Washington Street
Mount Vernon, NY 10550

Council of Better Business
Bureaus

1515 Wilson Boulevard
Arlington, VA 22209
(703) 276-0100

Food and Drug
Administration
5600 Fishers Lane
Room 188-31
Rockville, MD 20857
(301) 443-6260

Hill-Burton Hospital Free
Care
(800) 638-0742
(800) 492-0359 in MD

National Second Surgical
Opinion Program Hotline
(800) 638-6833
(800) 492-6603 in MD

I. SUBSTANCE USE AND ABUSE

Alcohol

About Alcohol and Drugs. Teaches kids about the dangers of substance abuse and discusses reasons why people drink, the effects of alcohol and drugs, and alternatives to substance abuse.

Channing L. Bete Co., Inc.
200 State Road
South Deerfield, MA 01373

Alcohol: How It Can Affect Your Health & Nutrition. Christina Dye.
Aimed at social drinkers, rather than alcohol abusers, describes the effects
of minimal amounts of alcohol consumption in the body, and emphasizes
moderate use at all times.

All About Series. grades 5-8. The following illustrated foldouts give facts
about effects and other aspects of substance use and abuse: All About
Alcohol; All About Downers; All About Marijuana; All About Saying No;
All About Sniffing; All About Speed

Amyl/Butyl Nitrite & Nitrous Oxide: The Sour Smell of Excess. Christina
Dye. Although legal, these chemicals can be as powerful as street
drugs.
Do It Now (DIN) Publications
P.O. Box 21126
2050 East University Drive
Phoenix, AZ 85036

Are You a Drug Quiz Whiz? Multiple-choice questions for young people
to test their knowledge about drugs and drug abuse; detailed answers.

Be Smart, Don't Start. Stories and activities on the "Be Smart, Don't
Start! Just Say NO!" theme regarding alcohol use. Includes tips from TV
stars (Tony Danza), rock stars (the Jets), and athletes (Mary Lou Retton and
Dave Winfield).

Buzzy's Rebound. Fat Albert and the Cosby Kids in a story about Buzzy,
a basketball player with a drinking problem. Discusses effects and
consequences of alcohol abuse.
National Clearinghouse for Alcohol and Drug Information
P.O. Box 2345
Rockville, MD 20852

COA Review: The Newsletter About Children of Alcoholics. For teachers
interested in helping COAs. Contains reviews of current fiction and
nonfiction on alcoholism and its effects.
Thomas W. Perrin, Inc.
P.O. Box 423
Rutherford, NJ 07070

*Broken Bottles, Broken Dreams: Understanding and Helping the Children of
Alcoholics.* Charles Deutsch. New York: Teacher's College Press,
1982.

Elementary School Children and Alcohol Education: Update. Lists audiovisuals, program descriptions, and professional and organizational resources to assist educators of young children.
> National Clearinghouse for Alcohol and Drug Information
> P.O. Box 2345
> Rockville, MD 20852

An Elephant in the Living Room: The Children's Workbook. Marion Hyppo and Jill M. Hastings. Helps children from alcoholic homes understand that alcoholism is a disease and that they are not alone. Enables them to express feelings, improve self-esteem and family relationships, and seek support from appropriate groups.
> Compcare Publications
> P.O. Box 27777
> Minneapolis, MN 55427

Facts and Reflections on Girls and Substance Abuse. Booklet providing a review of current research on the prevalence, patterns, and causes of girls' substance abuse, health risks, and intervention strategies.
> Girls Clubs of America
> Resource Center
> 441 West Michigan Street
> Indianapolis, IN 46202

Feeling Better Together. Presents a simple story about a mother who drinks too much, how her problem affects the family, and how she finally goes to the hospital for help. Emphasizes the feelings of the two young children in the family.
> Pathway Center Memorial Hospital
> 615 North Michigan
> South Bend, IN 46601

*Glug. Film/videotape features a group of 12-year-olds who meet weekly to experiment with alcohol. One becomes dependent, and his experiences teach him the need for serious help.
> Churchill Films
> 662 North Robertson Blvd.
> Los Angeles, CA 90069

*Is It Time to Stop Pretending? grade 6. Film/videotaped dramatization of Nancy talking with a school health officer about a "friend" who is having a family problem involving alcohol abuse.
> American Automobile Association
> Public Relations
> 8111 Gatehouse Road
> Falls Church, VA 22047

*It's Your Choice Series.* Discourages use of alcohol, tobacco, and marijuana, provides peer models, presents realistic situations and choices, builds decision-making skills, encourages "smart" choices, and makes reading fun! Includes: Saying No to Alcohol: A Teacher's Guide (Nancy Abbey and Ellen Wagman); Serena's Secret (Christine DeVault and Bryan Strong); Alcohol: The Real Story (David R. Stronck).
>Network Publications
>Department JSH
>P.O. Box 1830
>Santa Cruz, CA 95061-1830
>(408) 438-4060

*Kids and Drinking.* Anne Snyder. Short stories based on real experiences of children who develop drinking problems during elementary school. Includes short questions and answers about alcohol and a short parent/teacher's guide.
>Channing L. Bete Co., Inc.
>200 State Road
>South Deerfield, MA 01373

*Kootch Talks About Alcoholism.* Mary Kay Schwant. Kootch the worm helps young children understand three basic principles about alcoholism and alcoholics.
>Serenity Work
>1455 North University Drive
>Fargo, ND 58102

*Let's Learn About Alcohol.* ages 9–13. Motivates kids to learn the facts about alcohol and alcohol abuse. Describes the effects of alcohol on young people.
>Compcare Publications
>P.O. Box 27777
>Minneapolis, MN 55427

*****A Little About Alcohol. Uses the cartoon character "Al" to present basic alcohol facts.

*Little Al's Coloring Book.* Presents basic facts about alcohol using a cartoon character named "Al."
>Alcohol Research Information Service
>1120 East Oakland Avenue
>Lansing, MI 48906

*****Lots of Kids Like Me. Film/videotape emphasizes that children of alcoholics are not alone and not to blame for their parents' drinking. Includes suggestions for coping with problems that arise from parental alcohol abuse.

MTI Teleprograms
Divisions of Simon & Schuster Communications
108 Wilmot Road
Deerfield, IL 60015

*Should He Tell? grade 6. Film/videotape about a boy's decision to tell his mother about his father's problem drinking.
American Automobile Association
Public Relations
8111 Gatehouse Road
Falls Church, VA 22047

What Every Kid Should Know About Alcohol. Tells the facts about the dangers of alcoholism and problems faced by young people who drink in order to prepare youngsters to make sensible choices.

What Kids Should Know About Parents and Drinking. Helps children cope with a parent's drinking problem, explains how a parent's drinking may affect their own feelings and behavior. Suggests ways children can help themselves and find outside support.
Compcare Publications
P.O. Box 27777
Minneapolis, MN 55427

You're Not Alone: Kids' Book on Alcoholism and Child Abuse. older elementary. Presents a short story about a child and an alcoholic grandmother. The child grows up to be an alcoholic, too. Discusses many myths about alcohol and alcoholism.
National Committee for the Prevention of Child Abuse
332 S. Michigan Avenue
Chicago, IL 60604

Alcohol and Driving

*MTV: It's Your Right To Say No! Tells children it's all right to say "no" to alcohol. Urges children to resist peer pressure and not to ride with drivers who have been drinking.

*Mr. Punch versus the Drug Alcohol. Punch and Judy show the effects of drugs and alcohol on drivers.
American Automobile Association
Public Relations
8111 Gatehouse Road
Falls Church, VA 22047

Drugs

"Adam" & "Eve" & "Ecstasy": Facts About MDMA XTX, MDMA. Christina Dye. "Adam" and its spinoff "Eve" are comeback hallucinogenics from the 1970s that find a new market with upscale users. Presents the history of the drug, known for its high and its miserable hangover.

Angel Dust: Facts About PCP. Christina Dye. Uses powerful language to warn against PCP—an erratic, explosive substance that ranks fifth among the causes of drug-related emergencies at U.S. hospitals.
   Do It Now (DIN) Publications
   P.O. Box 21126
   2050 East University Drive
   Phoenix, AZ 85036

Be Fantastic. ages 8–11. Vocabulary facts about marijuana with quiz, essay sheet, and sticker for each child.
   National Parents' Resource Institute for Drug Education (PRIDE)
   100 Edgewood Avenue
   Suite 1002
   Atlanta, GA 30303

*Cocaine and Crack: Formula for Failure. Narrated by Graham Beckel, with interviews with former cocaine users such as jazz guitarist Larry Coryell, the film explains cocaine's addictive effects and how initial pleasant effects turn to depression and need. Useful for health and social studies classes.
   Human Relations Media
   175 Tompkins Ave.
   Pleasantville, NY 10570-9973

Cocaine: Waking Up to a Nightmare. Christina Dye. Presents the complex, deadly impact of cocaine on physical and psychological health, emphasizing impact on the human heart.
   Do It Now (DIN) Publications
   P.O. Box 21126
   2050 East University Drive
   Phoenix, AZ 85036

Drug Abuse. Raymond J. Reitz. A collection of recently published papers on various aspects of the drug problem, including graphs and lengthy bibliographies. Bloomington, IN: Phi Delta Kappa, 1987.

Drugs: A Multimedia Sourcebook for Young Adults. Sharon Ashenbrenner and Charles and Sari Feldman. Annotations for fiction, nonfiction, and nonprint materials on all kinds of drugs, as well as an appendix containing

professional reading, a list of publishers, and an author, title, and subject index. Santa Barbara, CA: ABC-Clio/Neal-Schuman, 1980.

Drugs and Alcohol: Simple Facts About Alcohol/Drug Combinations. Christina Dye. Stresses the simplicity of staying healthy by staying away from dangerous combinations of liquor and drugs, both prescription and street varieties.
Do It Now (DIN) Publications
P.O. Box 21126
2050 East University Drive
Phoenix, AZ 85036

*The Drug Knot. The dramatization of a community with a drug problem centering on one particular family. The real-life David Tome is shown and highlighted as he presents his anti-drug, pro-family message of love and involvement to change peoples' lives.
Walt Disney Educational Media Co.
500 S. Buena Vista St.
Burbank, CA 91521

DrugSmart: Test Your Chemical I.Q. Jennifer James. Multiple choice questions covering PCP to tobacco.
Do It Now (DIN) Publications
P.O. Box 21126
2050 East University Drive
Phoenix, AZ 85036

** The Head of the Class. Shows a boy asleep at his desk with the message that there are two kinds of heads: the ones that do well in school and the ones that smoke pot and do drugs.
National Clearinghouse for Alcohol and Drug Information
P.O. Box 2345
Rockville, MD 20852

Help Your Children Say No to Drugs. John Q. Baucom. Information for parents on the extent of drug abuse problems among young people, helping identify teen users, helping drug abusers, and helping teens avoid drug use. Includes a glossary and a chart helping to identify potential abusers. Grand Rapids, MI: Pyranee/Zondervan, 1987.

How to Keep the Children You Love Off Drugs. Ken Barun and Philip Bashe. Facts about signs of use of particular drugs, the appearance of drugs, physical effects, paraphernalia, and immediate and long-term effects. Includes a list of drug treatment programs and addresses to write for free information, as well as other important sources. New York: Atlantic Monthly Press, 1988.

*Learning Drug Facts Series. grades 5–9. Making Decisions: You Can Learn How; Learning to Say NO; Marijuana: What Do You Know?; Drugs and You: How Will You Decide?; Alcohol: What Do You Know?
  Sunburst Communications
  Rm MV9
  39 Washington Avenue
  Pleasantville, NY 10570

Marijuana: Health Effects. Christina Dye. History of the "truths" of marijuana based on scientific research.

Marijuana: Personality and Behavior. Christina Dye. Presents research into marijuana use and its effect on the senses.
  Do It Now (DIN) Publications
  P.O. Box 21126
  2050 East University Drive
  Phoenix, AZ 85036

*Mr. Finlay's Pharmacy. Film/videotape of puppet production that advises children how to use drugs properly.
  Kinetic, Inc.
  255 Delaware Avenue
  Suite 340
  Buffalo, NY 14202

*Say NO! to Drugs. Presents a practical, easy-to-follow approach to improve family communication concerning drug use. Combines interviews with dramatic vignettes.
  National Federation of Parents for Drug-Free Youth
  8730 Georgia Avenue
  Suite 200
  Silver Spring, MD 20910

Saying No to Drugs. grades 4–6. Presents successful ways for rejecting alcohol and drugs.
  Weekly Reader Skills Books
  4343 Equity Drive
  P.O. Box 16618
  Columbus, OH 43216

**School Daze. Shows the face of a dazed boy with the message: School is tough enough without having to learn through a mind softened with drugs. Urges kids to say NO to drugs.
  National Clearinghouse for Alcohol and Drug Information
  P.O. Box 2345
  Rockville, MD 20852

*Schoolyard. Shows that drug-free kids can be successful and accepted. A 13-year-old is offered drugs and when he hesitates, an older student tells him to "Just Say No!"
Modern Talking Picture Service
5000 Park Street North
St. Petersburg, FL 33709-9989

Soozie and Katy. young children. Presents the purpose of medicine, its appropriate use, the legal distribution of drugs, and the dangers that can accompany misuse.
National Clearinghouse for Alcohol and Drug Information
P.O. Box 2345
Rockville, MD 20852

*Stand up for Yourself: Peer Pressure and Drugs. A discussion format presents drug situations and strategies for just saying no.
Churchill Films
662 North Robertson Blvd.
Los Angeles, CA 90069

Steering Clear: Helping Your Child Through the High Risk Drug Years. Dorothy Cretcher. Covers such areas as "Prevention, Dealing with the Drug Use of Your Child and the Who, What, and Why of Adolescent Drug Use."
Winston Press, Inc.
430 Oak Grove
Minneapolis, MN 55403

*Where's Shelly? Helps children understand some factors that can affect their decisions about using drugs.
Kinetic, Inc.
255 Delaware Avenue
Suite 340
Buffalo, NY 14202

*Why Say No to Drugs? Deals with drug issues young people confront every day in social situations. Offers decision-making guidelines that will help kids say no to drugs.
National Federation of Parents for Drug-Free Youth
8730 Georgia Avenue
Suite 200
Silver Spring, MD 20910

General

Everyday Detox: A Guide to Living Without Chemicals. Jim Parker. young adults. A self-help guide to recognizing chemical dependency on drugs, alcohol, caffeine, sugar, and junk food, and how to detoxify and change.

Do It Now (DIN) Publications
P.O. Box 21126
2050 East University Drive
Phoenix, AZ 85036

Facts and Reflections on Girls and Substance Abuse. Reviews current research on the prevalence, patterns, and causes of girls' substance abuse, health risks, and intervention strategies.
Girls Clubs of America
Resource Center
441 West Michigan Street
Indianapolis, IN 46202

*How Do You Tell? A combination of live interviews and animation encourages children to say no to marijuana, tobacco, and alcohol use.
MTI Teleprograms
Divisions of Simon and Schuster Communications
108 Wilmot Road
Deerfield, IL 60015

*A Story About Feelings. ages 5–8. Shows the role of feelings in people's lives and that some people change the way they feel by using drugs and alcohol.
Kinetic, Inc.
255 Delaware Avenue, Suite 340
Buffalo, NY 14202

Substance Abuse Materials for School Libraries: An Annotated Bibliography. Theodora Andrews. Contains 496 entries including reference works, general discussions, fiction, personal narratives, and materials on various aspects of substance abuse with appropriate age levels.
Libraries Unlimited
P.O. Box 263
Littleton, CO 80160

Smoking

All About Smoking. grades 5–8. Reviews how tobacco affects the body, noting its cancerous effects on the heart and lungs, lips, mouth, and throat. Discusses nicotine addiction, smoking as a habit, and snuff and "clove" cigarettes.
Do It Now (DIN) Publications
P.O. Box 21126
2050 East University Drive
Phoenix, AZ 85036

*Be a Winner. grades 6–8. Uses a sports perspective to discuss peer pressure and the health hazards of smokeless tobacco. Can integrate puppets with a slide presentation.
Dougherty County Health Department
P.O. Box 3048
Albany, GA 31708

Best Tip Yet: Don't Start. Presents a strong, graphic antismoking message: If You've Got Your Health, You've Got It All; Smoking Pollutes You and Everything Else; 12 Things to Do Instead of Smoking Cigarettes; What's Wrong with This Picture?
American Cancer Society
90 Park Avenue
New York, NY 10016

*The Chews Blues. grades 5–12 and college. Portrays socially unacceptable aspects of use, marketing, and advertising strategies; health consequences of use; and conflict of nicotine dependency with students' needs and desires. Compares fiscal interests of tobacco industry with motives of health educators.
BALANCE Productions
27 Wellstone Drive
Portland, ME 04103

**Chew Tobacco? ages 6–17.
Idaho Department of Health and Welfare
Dental Health Section
Statehouse
Boise, ID 83720

* A Conversation with Dr. Elbert Glover on Smokeless Tobacco. grades 7–12 and adults. Dr. Glover, one of the first health scientists in the country to recognize the problems of smokeless tobacco, speaks informally on the history of smokeless tobacco, today's users, and the health consequences of use and dependency.
BALANCE Productions
27 Wellstone Drive
Portland, ME 04103

**Don't Get Hooked! Shows a fish smoking a cigarette caught by a fishing hook.
Office of Smoking and Health
Technical Information Center
5600 Fishers Lane
Park Bldg., Room 1-10
Rockville, MD 20857

*Don't Take the Risk. ages 9–18. Presents the health risks of smokeless tobacco.

California Dental Association
P.O. Box 13749
Sacramento, CA 95853-4749

Facts About Smokeless Tobacco. grades 4–8. Presents 10 crucial questions as part of the "Healthy Me Tobacco Free" project.
Bowling Green State University
School of Health, Physical Education, and Recreation
Bowling Green, OH 43403

*Goldy and the Four Smokey Bears. Describes the social and health hazards of smoking and smokeless tobacco.
Muskingum County Health Department
421 Main Street
Zanesville, OH 43701

*The Heart That Changed Color. grades 3–5. The adventures of the Tin Woodman and Scarecrow traveling through Nicotina.
American Heart Association
7320 Greenville Avenue
Dallas, TX 75231

*The Huffless, Puffless Dragon. grades 5–9. Introduces antismoking subject with lots of energy and satire.

Huff 'n Puff. grades K–3. Tells an antismoking story that parodies the "Three Little Pigs."
American Cancer Society
90 Park Avenue
New York, NY 10016

* Mr. Gross Mouth. This model displays the oral effects of using smokeless tobacco.
Health Ed Co., Inc.
P.O. Box 21207
Waco, TX 76702-1207

The No Smoking Coloring and Activities Book. Explains what a cigarette is, why people smoke, the effects of smoking on the body and the environment, and the fact that one can say "no" to smoking.
Channing L. Bete Co., Inc.
200 State Rd.
S. Deerfield, MA 01373

* The Smokeless Showdown. grades 2–4. Uses puppets to get its message across.

West Virginia University
Extension Service
616 Knapp Hall
Morgantown, WV 26506

Smokeless Tobacco: A Pinch Is Not Safer Than a Puff. Discusses the hazards
of chewing tobacco.
Dental Health Section
Statehouse
Boise, Idaho 83720

Smokeless Tobacco: No Way. elementary, junior high, and high school.
Illustrates the fact that whether chewed or smoked, tobacco is hazardous to
health.
American Lung Association
1740 Broadway
New York, NY 10019

Smokeless Tobacco. Part 1: Historical and Current Information. Provides the
most current and accurate information about smokeless tobacco, its use,
and the profiles of its users. *Part 2: Teaching Unit and Discussion Guide.*
BALANCE Productions
27 Wellstone Drive
Portland, ME 04103

*Smokeless Tobacco: The Whole Truth. Addresses the idea that these
products are less harmful than cigarettes. Former Boston Red Sox star Jim
Longborg discusses smokeless tobacco dangers: gum disease, tooth loss,
and mouth and gum cancer.
Sunburst Communications
Rm. MV9
39 Washington Avenue
Pleasantville, NY 10570

** This Is a Dumb Bunny. Pictures a rabbit smoking a cigarette.
Office of Smoking and Health
Technical Information Center
5600 Fishers Lane
Park Bldg., Room 1-10
Rockville, MD 20857

Steroids

Anabolic Steroids. Christina Dye. Defines steroids, tells how they work
(or don't), and discusses their dangers.

*Benny and the 'Roids. grades 7–12. The story of a teenaged high school football player, Benny Zimmer, who has worked hard to be on this year's team. When practice begins, Benny desperately turns to anabolic steroids.

Do It Now (DIN) Publications
P.O. Box 21126
2050 East University Drive
Phoenix, AZ 85036

Organizational Resources

Action on Smoking and Health
  (ASH)
2013 H Street, N.W.
Washington, DC 20006
(202) 659-4310

Al-Anon and Alateen
One Park Avenue
New York, NY 10016
(212) 683-1771

Al-Anon Family Group
  Headquarters
(800) 356-9996
(212) 245-3151 in NY and
  Canada

Alcohol, Drug Abuse, and Mental
  Health Administration
5600 Fishers Lane
Rockville, MD 20857
(301) 443-4883

Alcoholics Anonymous
P.O. Box 459
Grand Central Station
New York, NY 10017
(212) 686-1100

Alcoholism and Drug Addiction
  Treatment Center
(800) 382-4357

American Cancer Society
90 Park Avenue

New York, NY 10016
(212) 599-8200

American Heart Association
7320 Greenville Avenue
Dallas, TX 75231
(214) 750-5300

American Lung Association
1740 Broadway
New York, NY 10019
(212) 315-8700

Cocaine Anonymous
CokEnders (215) 735-2525

Drug Abuse Prevention
(800) 638-2045
(800) 492-6605 in MD

Emphysema Anonymous
P.O. Box 66
Ft. Myers, FL 33902

Five-Day Plan To Stop Smoking
6830 Laurel Street, N.W.
Washington, DC 20012
(202) 723-0800

Just Say No Kids Club
(800) 258-2766

Mothers Against Drunk Driving
(MADD)
669 Airport Freeway
Suite 310
Hurst, TX 76053
(817) 268-6233

Narcotics Anonymous
16155 Wyandotte Street
Van Nuys, CA 91406
(818) 780-3951

National Clearinghouse for
Alcohol Information
P.O. Box 2345
Rockville, MD 20852
(301) 468-2600

National Clearinghouse for Drug
Abuse Information
P.O. Box 416
Dept. DQ
Kensington, MD 20795
(301) 443-6500

National Cocaine Hotline
(800) COC-AINE

National Coordinating Council on
Drug Education, Inc.
1830 Connecticut Avenue, N.W.
Washington, DC 20009

National Council on Alcoholism
(800) NCA-CALL

National Federation of Parents
for Drug-Free Youth
(301) 585-5437 in MD

National Information Center for
Orphan Drugs and Rare
Diseases
(800) 336-4797
(202) 429-9091 in DC

National Institute on Alcohol
Abuse and Alcoholism

5600 Fishers Lane
Rockville, MD 20857

National Institute on Drug Abuse
11400 Rockville Pike, Room 110
Rockville, MD 20852
(800) 638-2045
(301) 492-2948 in MD

National Interagency Council on
Smoking and Health
c/o American Cancer Society
90 Park Avenue
New York, NY 10016

National Parents' Resource Institute for Drug Education
(PRIDE)
100 Edgewood Avenue
Suite 1002
Atlanta, GA 30303
(800) 241-7946
(404) 658-2548 in GA

Office of Smoking and Health
Technical Information Center
5600 Fishers Lane
Park Bldg., Room 1-10
Rockville, MD 20857
(301) 443-1690

Office of Substance Abuse
Prevention
(301) 443-6500 in MD

Pyramid East
7101 Wisconsin Avenue
Suite 1006
Bethesda, MD 20814
(301) 654-1194

Pyramid West
8746 Mt. Diablo Boulevard
Suite 200
Lafayette, CA 94549
(415) 284-5300 or 939-6666

Students Against Drunk Driving
(SADD)
10812 Ashfield Road
Adelphi, MD 20783
(301) 937-7936

Women For Sobriety, Inc.
P.O. Box 618
Quakertown, PA 18951
(215) 536-8026

J. COMMUNITY HEALTH

Nuclear Holocaust

*The Big Snit. junior high, senior high, adults. Award-winning animated film in which an oddball domestic couple's quarrel is portrayed in relation to a worldwide "snit" (nuclear holocaust).
Phoenix Films
468 Park Avenue So.
New York, NY 10016

Population Growth

*What Is the Limit? A global issues video that explores the damaging effects of population growth, using discussion-provoking examples from around the world.
Northern Light Productions
169 Newbury Street
Boston, MA 02116

Organizational Resources

Americans for Nuclear Energy
P.O. Box 28371
Washington, D.C. 20005
(703) 528-4430

Asbestos Hotline
(800) 334-8571

Black Lung Association
1222 Washington Street East
Charleston, WV 25301

Center for Environmental Health
Centers for Disease Control

1600 Clifton Road, N.E.
Atlanta, GA 30333

Council for a Livable World
100 Maryland Avenue, N.E.
(202) 543-4100

Environmental Protection Agency
(EPA)
Public Information Center
Room PM 211-B

401 M Street, S.W.
Washington, DC 20460
(202) 382-7550
(800) 424-9346 Hazardous Waste
  Hotline

Friends of the Earth
124 Spear Street
San Francisco, CA 94105
(415) 495-4770

National Audubon Society
950 Third Avenue
New York, NY 10022
(212) 832-3200

National Institute of
  Environmental Sciences
P.O. Box 12233
Research Triangle Park, NC
  27709
(919) 541-3345

National Institute of
  Environmental Health Services
P.O. Box 12233
Research Triangle Park, NC
  27709
(919) 541-3345

National Pesticide Information
  Clearinghouse
(800) 531-7790 in Texas
(800) 292-7664

SANE: Committee for a Sane
  Nuclear Policy
711 G Street, S.E.
Washington, DC 20003
(202) 546-7100

Sierra Club
530 Bush Street
San Francisco, CA 94108
(415) 981-8634

K. GENERAL RESOURCES FOR HEALTH EDUCATORS

Child Abuse

Child Abuse and Neglect: The NEA Training Program. Presents an in-depth analysis of detecting and reporting abuse and neglect, as well as legal advice to protect both the teacher and the student.
  National Education Association
  1201 16th St., N.W.
  Washington, DC 20036

General Health

Bibliography of Books Concerned with Death

Bibliography of Books Concerned with Mental Retardation

Bibliography of Books Concerned with Physical Handicaps
  National Society of Genetic Counselors
  Genetic Counseling Program
  710 O'Neil Building
  Binghamton, NY 13901
  (607) 723-9692

 # The Encyclopedia of Health. Dale C. Garrell, M.D., and Salomon H. Snyder, M.D., general editors. Up-to-date information covering a wide range of topics, from basic anatomy to ethical and legal issues.
 Chelsea House Publishers
 Dept. WP4
 P.O. Box 914
 1974 Sproul Road, Suite 400
 Broomall, PA 19008-0914

 # Health Resource Builder: Free and Inexpensive Materials for Librarians and Teachers. Carol Smallwood. Health hints on many topics, as well as addresses and phone numbers for services or available materials. Jefferson, NC: McFarland and Co., 1988.

General Skills

 # Say It With Puppets Program. grades 3–5. Helps students build reading, study, and group participation skills. Includes a kit with 32 puppet outlines to create puppet characters; six plays that cover family relationships, drug prevention, environment, thoughtfulness, death, and caring; teacher's guide.
 Say It With Puppets, Inc.
 2212 Main Street
 P.O. Box 693
 Glastonbury, CT 06033

Parenting

 # Parenting and Child Development. Offers selected books under the following topics: Parenting, Child Development, Family & Crisis Counseling, Health & Sexuality, Pregnancy, and Educational Resources.
 Harper & Row Publishers, Inc.
 10 East 53rd Street
 New York, NY 10022-5299

Self Help

 # The Directory of National Self-Help and Mutual-Aid Resources. Lists information packets available by mail from each group.
 AHA Services
 4444 W. Ferdinand
 Chicago, IL 60624
 (800) AHA-2626

Organizational Resources

American Academy of Pediatrics
141 Northwest Point Boulevard
P.O. Box 927
Elk Grove Village, IL 60009

American Association of Sex
  Educators, Counselors, and
  Therapists
5010 Wisconsin Avenue, N.W.
Suite 304
Washington, DC 20016
(202) 686-2523

American Cancer Society
90 Park Avenue
New York, NY 10016
(212) 599-8200

American Guidance Services
Publishers' Building
P.O. Box 99
Circle Pines, MN 55014

American Medical Association
535 North Dearborn Street
Chicago, IL 60610

American Medical Radio News
(800) 621-8094

American Nurses Association
2420 Pershing Road
Kansas City, MO 64108

American Osteopathic
  Association
212 East Ohio Street
Chicago, IL 60611
(312) 280-5800

American Red Cross
17th and D Streets, N.W.
Washington, DC 20006
(202) 737-8300

Association for the Care of
  Children's Health
3615 Wisconsin Avenue, N.W.
Washington, DC 20016

Boston Women's Health Book
  Collective
240 A Elm St.
Somerville, MA 02144

Center for Health Promotion and
  Education
Centers for Disease Control
Building 1 South, Room SSB249
1600 Clifton Road, N.E.
Atlanta, GA 30333
(404) 329-3492 or 329-3698

Center for Prevention Services
Centers for Disease Control
1600 Clifton Road, N.E.
Atlanta, GA 30333
(404) 329-1819

Centers for Disease Control
1600 Clifton Road, N.E.
Atlanta, GA 30333
(404) 329-3286

Chelsea House Publishers
Dept. WP4
P.O. Box 914
1974 Sproul Road, Suite 400
Broomall, PA 19008-0914

Children's Defense Fund
122 C Street, N.W.
Washington, DC 20001

Churchill Films
662 N. Robertson Boulevard
Los Angeles, CA 90069-5089

Communicating With Dolls
Migima Designs
P.O. Box 70064
Eugene, OR 97401

Consumer Information
Center
Pueblo, CO 81009
(202) 566-2794

Department of Health and
Human Services
3700 East-West Highway
Room 1-57
Hyattsville, MD 20782
(301) 436-8500

Educational Materials Center
School of Health
Loma Linda University
Loma Linda, CA 92350

Educational Resources
Information Center (ERIC)
Clearinghouse on Teacher
Education
Department of Education
One Dupont Circle,
Suite 810
Washington, DC 20036
(202) 293-2450

Films For the Humanities &
Sciences, Inc.
P.O. Box 2053
Princeton, NJ 08543

Genetic Counseling Program
(National Society of Genetic
Counselors, Inc.)
168 Water St.
Binghamton, NY 13901

Greenhaven Press
P.O. Box 289009
San Diego, CA 92128-9009

Health Data Centers (Online
Computer Services)
Bibliographic Retrieval Services
1200 Route 7
Lantham, NY 12110
(800) 833-4707
(518) 583-1161 in New York

Journal of School Health
American School Health
Association
7263 S.R. #43
Kent, OH 44240

Library of Congress National
Referral Service
(202) 287-5670

Living Bank
(800) 528-2971
(713) 528-2971 in Texas

Medical Self-Care Magazine
P.O. Box 717
Inverness, CA 94937

MTI Teleprograms
3710 Commercial Avenue
Northbrook, IL 60062

National Center for Education in
Maternal and Child Health
3520 Prospect Street, N.W.
Suite 1
Washington, DC 20057
(202) 625-8400

National Education Association
1201 16th St., N.W.
Washington, DC 20036

National Health Information
Clearinghouse
P.O. Box 1133
Washington, DC 20013-1133
(800) 336-4797
(703) 522-2590 in VA

National Heart, Lung, and Blood
Institute
9000 Rockville Pike
Bethesda, MD 20205

National Injury Information
Clearinghouse
5401 Westbard Avenue, Room
625
Washington, DC 20207
(301) 492-6424

National Institutes of Health
(NIH)
9000 Rockville Pike
Bethesda, MD 20205
(301) 496-4000

National Library of Medicine
MEDLARS Management Section
Building 38A, Room 4N-421
8600 Rockville Pike
Bethesda, MD 20209
(800) 638-8480
(301) 496-6193

National Maternal and Child
Health Clearinghouse &
National Center for Education
in Maternal and Child Health
38th and R Streets, N.W.
Washington, DC 20057

National Technical Information
Service (NTIS)
Department of Commerce
5285 Port Royal Road
Springfield, VA 22161

National Women's Health
Network
224 Seventh Street, S.E.
Washington, DC 20003

Network Publications
ETR Associates
P.O. Box 1830
Santa Cruz, CA 95061-1830

ODN Productions, Inc.
74 Varick Street, Rm. 304
New York, NY 10013

ODPHP National Health
Information Center
(800) 336-4797
(202) 429-9091 in DC

Pediatric Projects, Inc.
P.O. Box 1880
Santa Monica, CA 90406-9920

Public Health Service
200 Independence Avenue, SW
Washington, DC 20201

Research Press
P.O. Box 3177
Dept. K
Champaign, IL 61821-9988

Sex Information and Education
Council of the U.S. (SIECUS)
137-155 N. Franklin Street
Hempstead, NY 11550
(516) 483-3033

Sick Kids Need Involved People,
Inc. (SKIP)
216 Newport Drive
Severna Park, MD 21146
(301) 647-0164

Sunburst Communications
101 Castleton Street
Pleasantville, NY 10570-3498

U.S Department of Health,
Education, and Welfare
Public Health Service
Health Services Administration
Bureau of Community Health
Services
5600 Fishers Lane
Rockville, MD 20857

L. MISCELLANEOUS ISSUES

Abduction Prevention

Safety Zone. Linda D. Meyer. ages 4–9. Teaches stranger abduction prevention skills, which are different from those children must know to prevent noncustodial parental abduction (in case of divorce).
  Chas. Franklin Press
  7821 175th Street, S.W.
  Edmonds, WA 98026

Stay Safe Around People You Don't Know Well. Helps children distinguish between those they feel they can trust and people they don't know well and teaches them to recognize unsafe situations, how to get away, and to report incidents to parents and police.
  Channing L. Bete Co., Inc.
  200 State Road
  S. Deerfield, MA 01373

Strangers Don't Look Like the Big Bad Wolf. Janis Buschman and Debbie Hunley. ages 2–6. Teaches stranger abduction prevention skills to preschoolers.
  Chas. Franklin Press
  7821 175th Street, S.W.
  Edmonds, WA 98026

Coping With Death

Children and Death. Hannelore Wass and Charlene A. Corr, eds. Information and guidelines on dying children and their families with special focus on helping siblings, bereaved children and families, suicidal behavior, etc. Includes chapters on death education, books for children. New York: Hemisphere Publishing Corp., 1985.

*Griff Gets a Hand. Griff, whose parents were killed in an accident, can't find a sense of order or purpose to his life after his friend Danny dies. An older brother and his classmates help show him that there are still people who care for him.
  Beacon Films
  1250 Washington St.
  P.O. Box 575
  Norwood, MA 02062

Helping Children Cope with Death. 2nd edition. Hannelore Wass and Charlene A. Corr, eds. Presents effective guidelines for creative and

practical counseling to apply when helping children cope with death. Contains a section on books for children. New York: Hemisphere Publishing Corp., 1985.

Helping Children to Understand Death: A Selected Bibliography.
Bureau of Community Health Services
Rm. 7-16, Parklawn Building
5600 Fishers Lane
Rockville, MD 20857
(301) 443-1650

Thumpy Series: Thumpy's Story, Sharing with Thumpy, El Cuento de Thumpy.
Children's Hospice International
1101 King Street, Suite 131
Alexandria, VA 22314

* When Children Grieve. Offers a way to help children through the death of a parent. Families with a terminally ill parent, as well as doctors and social workers, are interviewed.
Churchill Films
662 N. Robertson Blvd.
Los Angeles, CA 90069

Disabilities

* Griff Makes a Date. Unpopular Griff makes a new friend, Lisa. However, their friendship is endangered by Griff's callous attitude towards a mentally retarded man.
Beacon Films
1250 Washington St.
P.O. Box 575
Norwood, MA 02062

* Growing Up Proud: A Parent's Guide to the Psychological Care of Children with Disabilities. A helpful guide to aid parents in raising a handicapped child. New York: Warner, 1983.

Mental Retardation: An Issue in Literature for Children. Bibliography.
Association for Retarded Citizens
2501 Avenue J
Arlington, TX 76011

A Reader's Guide For Parents of Children with Mental, Physical, Emotional Disabilities.

Maryland State Planning Council on Developmental Disabilities
201 W. Preston Street
Baltimore, MD 21201

Hospitalization

At the Hospital. Tells what to take to the hospital, about tests, hospital personnel, equipment, hospital clothing, and about the body.
Channing L. Bete Co., Inc.
200 State Road
S. Deerfield, MA 01373

Books That Help Children Deal with a Hospital Experience. preschool and elementary. Presents a comprehensive bibliography of books suitable to the needs of the specific child.
U.S. Department of Health, Education, and Welfare
Public Health Service
Bureau of Community Health Services
5600 Fishers Lane
Rockville, MD 20857

The Child and Health Care: A Bibliography.
Association for the Care of Children's Health
3615 Wisconsin Avenue, N.W.
Washington, DC 20016

Emergency Room: An ABC Tour. Explains the emergency room with photos and sensitive, brief stories.
Pediatric Projects, Inc.
P.O. Box 1880
Santa Monica, CA 90406-1880

Going to the Doctor. Why children visit the doctor, medical instruments, and things to do to stay healthy.
Channing L. Bete Co., Inc.
200 State Road
S. Deerfield, MA 01373

Little Doctor. An Asian girl plays doctor with her doll and a rocking horse.

Mr. Rogers: Going to the Hospital; Having an Operation; Wearing a Cast. Fred Rogers explains (in a series of three books) about health care and how to cope with unfamiliar medical and surgical events.
Pediatric Projects, Inc.
P.O. Box 1880
Santa Monica, CA 90406-1880

Using Media to Make Kids Feel Good: Resources and Activities for Successful Programs in Hospitals. Maureen Gaffney. Hands-on guide to over fifty films, videos, and closed-circuit TV programs and related projects and activities that effectively alleviate children's fears and feelings of isolation during hospitalization.

> Oryx Press
> 4041 N. Central, Suite 700
> Phoenix, AZ 85012-3330

Sexual Abuse

*Child Abuse: The Untold Story. Videotaped portrayal of a victim as she discloses her experiences, feelings, and struggle to regain a normal life. Assists school nurses in helping child abuse victims.

> American Journal of Nursing Company
> Educational Services Division
> 555 W. 57th Street
> New York, NY 10019-2961

Child Sexual Abuse Prevention Education Program Kit. Attempt to assist victims of assault and prevent assault through education. Includes: an activity guide, discussion guide, booklets for teens, parents, and youth workers.

> Child Sexual Abuse Prevention Education Program
> King County Rape Relief Center
> 1025 South Third
> Renton, WA 98055

*Coping Strategies for Sexual Abuse. grades 5–9. Assists teachers in introducing the topic of child abuse, illustrating ways children might be abused, and profiling a typical abuser; teacher assertiveness techniques to ward off abusers.

> Sunburst Communications
> 101 Castleton Street
> Pleasantville, NY 10570-3498

Hi! My Name Is Sissy. I Am Six Years Old. Ruth Amerson. elementary and preschool. Teaches children what to do if someone touches them in a sexual manner.

> Lee County Department of Social Services
> P.O. Box 1066
> Sandford, NC 27330

I Take Good Care of Me! I Take Good Care of Us! Linda D. Meyer and Denelle Peaker, illustrator. Covers sexual assault and abduction prevention, as well as fire, water, and electrical safety.

Chas. Franklin Press
7821 175th Street, S.W.
Edmonds, WA 98026

It's Not Your Fault. Judith A. Janice. ages 4–10. Reassures children that they are not to blame when they are molested and encourages children to tell.
American Medical Association
Order Department
P.O Box 10946
Chicago, IL 60610-0946

It's OK to Say NO! Educates young people about body safety and discusses dangers of child molestation and abduction.
Creative Child Press
Playmore, Inc.
Publisher & Waldman Publishing Corp.
200 Fifth Avenue
New York, NY 10010

A Little Bird Told Me About . . . My Feelings. Marcia K. Morgan. Teaches children to trust their feelings and say "no" to inappropriate touching and conveys the difference between good and bad touching and what the child can do in response to a bad touch. Includes parents' guide.
Migima Designs
P.O. Box 70064
Eugene, OR 97401

The New Child Protection Team Handbook. Donald C. Bross, Richard D. Krugman, Marilyn R. Lanherr, Donna Andrea Rosenberg, and Barton D. Schmitt. A reference source that offers practical information on evaluating, treating, and managing abused and neglected children. New York: Garland, 1989.

No More Secrets. Caren Adams and Jennifer Fay. A guide to help parents talk to their children about sexual assault. San Luis Obispo, CA: Impact Publishers, 1981.

No More Secrets for Me. Oralee Wachter. Tells four realistic stories on lack of respect for children's right to privacy and criminal child abuse. The stories portray children handling the circumstances successfully and teach children that there are adults they can tell who can help and protect them.
Little, Brown, and Co.
34 Beacon Street
Boston, MA 02106

Private Zone. Frances S. Dayee. ages 3–9. Teaches sexual assault prevention skills, covering privacy of body parts, who can touch them when, and who kids can tell if they have been molested.

Chas. Franklin Press
7821 175th Street, S.W.
Edmonds, WA 98026

The Silent Children: A Parent's Guide to Prevention of Sexual Abuse. Linda Tschirhart Sanford. Prevention approaches for parents to use including chapters on special populations such as physically disabled, mentally handicapped, and deaf victims. Garden City, NY: Anchor, 1980.

*The Sixth Sense. Film/videotape gives children common-sense ideas on how to determine whether or not they are in danger of being molested. Also tells children what to do when confronting such a danger.
    Kinetic, Inc.
    255 Delaware Avenue, Suite 340
    Buffalo, NY 14202

Spider Man and Power Pack. elementary or preschool. Features two stories dealing with sexual abuse, emphasizing to children that they should not feel guilty or "bad" if this happens to them. Stresses that children should tell parents or other authority figures.
    National Committee for the Prevention of Child Abuse
    332 S. Michigan Avenue
    Suite 950
    Chicago, IL 60604

*Strong Kids, Safe Kids. Videotape using music, humor, and straight talk from television personalities and cartoon characters to teach children basic skills which can help prevent sexual abuse and abduction.
    Ed-U-Press
    7174 Mott Road
    Fayetteville, NY 13066

Take Care of Yourself: A Young Person's Guide to Understanding, Preventing and Healing from the Hurts of Child Abuse. Laurie White and Steven Spencer. elementary or preschool. Informs the child that he or she is not to blame in the case of abuse and discusses different types of abuse and various solutions.
    DayStar Press
    915 Maxime
    Flint, MI 48503

A Teaching Guide to Preventing Adolescent Sexual Abuse. Joan Krebill and Julie Taylor. A manual presenting activities and strategies to prevent adolescent sexual abuse. Santa Cruz, CA: Network Publications, 1988.

What Every Kid Should Know About Sexual Abuse. Helps children to understand what sexual abuse is and how to protect themselves from it.
    Channing L. Bete Co., Inc.
    200 State Road
    S. Deerfield, MA 01373

You Belong to You. elementary and preschool. Tells children what they
should do if someone attempts to abuse them, stressing the message that
"It's not your fault" when adults act this way.
   YWCA Sexual Assault Crisis Center
   Domestic Violence/Sexual Assault Services
   310 East Third Street
   Flint, MI 48502

You're in Charge! preschool. Presents a positive message to preschoolers
through pictures and puzzles that their bodies are special, and to say "NO"
to a "bad" touch.
   Channing L. Bete Co., Inc.
   200 State Road
   S. Deerfield, MA 01373

Suicide

*Before It's Too Late. Teaches students how to spot suicidal behavior in
friends and peers, and ways to prevent suicide. Students are urged to take
suicide threats seriously and direct a friend to a trusted adult.
   Walt Disney Educational Media
   500 S. Buena Vista St.
   Burbank, CA 91521

*Suicide: Call for Help. Discussion at a teen center on typical situations
that can trigger suicidal feelings.
   AIMS Media
   6901 Woodley Avenue
   Van Nuys, CA 91406-4878
   (800) 367-2467 in CA, AK, and HI call collect

Teen Suicide. Nancy Merritt. Information on potentially suicidal teens,
reasons they commit it, warning signs, and how others can help.
   Do It Now (DIN) Publications
   P.O. Box 21126
   2050 East University Drive
   Phoenix, AZ 85036

*Understanding Suicide. grades 5–9. Helps students understand about
peer suicide, recognize warning signals in classmates, and learn what they
can do to prevent it.
   Sunburst Communications
   Rm. MV9
   39 Washington Avenue
   Pleasantville, NY 10570

Organizational Resources

AIMS Media
6901 Woodley Avenue
Van Nuys, CA 91406-4878
(800) 367-2467 in CA, AK and
   HI call collect

American Association of
   Suicidology
2459 S. Ash
Denver, CO 80222
(303) 692-0985

American Cleft Palate
   Association
(800) 24-CLEFT
(800) 23-CLEFT in PA

American Council of the Blind
(800) 424-8666
(202) 393-3666 in DC

American Foundation for the
   Blind (AFB)
(800) 232-5463
(212) 620-2147.

Association for Children and
   Adults with Learning Disorders
4156 Library Road
Pittsburgh, PA 15234
(412) 341-1515

Association for Retarded
   Citizens
P.O. Box 6109
Arlington, TX 76006

Batterers Anonymous
1295 N.E. Street
San Bernardino, CA 92405
(714) 383-2972
Self-help group for men who are
   abusive toward women.

Child Abuse Prevention Project:
   An Educational Program for
   Children
Cordelia Kent. Sexual Assault
   Services
Hennepin County Attorney's
   Office
C-2000 Government Center
Minneapolis, MN 55487

Child Assault Prevention (CAP)
   Project
Women Against Rape
P.O. Box 02084
Columbus, OH 43202

Children's Hospice
   International
1101 King St., Suite 131
Alexandria, VA 22314

Clearinghouse on Child Abuse
   and Neglect
P.O. Box 1182
Washington, DC 20013
(301) 251-5157

Clearinghouse on the
   Handicapped
Switzer Bldg.
330 C St., S.W.
Washington, DC 20201
(202) 245-0196

Coordinating Council for
   Handicapped Children
Parent Information Center
407 South Dearborn Street
Chicago, IL 60605

Dial a Hearing Test
(800) 222-EARS
(800) 345-EARS in PA

Epilepsy Foundation of America
1828 L Street N.W.
Washington, DC 20036

Epilepsy Information Line
(800) 426-0660
(206) 323-8174 in Washington
state

Euthanasia—Concern for Dying
250 W. 57th Street
New York, NY 10107
(212) 246-6962

The Federation for Children with
Special Needs
312 Stuart Street, 2nd Floor
Boston, MA 02116
(617) 482-2915, Toll free within
MA (800) 331-0688

Grapevine
(800) 352-8888
(800) 346-8888 in CA

Hearing Helpline
(800) 424-8576
(703) 642-0580 in VA

HEATH Resource Center
(800) 544-3284
(202) 939-9320 in DC

Hospice Education Institute
Hospicelink
(800) 331-1620
(203) 767-1620 in CT

Incest Survivors Anonymous
Box 5613, Dept P
Long Beach, CA 90805-0613

Job Accommodation Network
(800) 526-7234
(800) 526-4698 in WV

The John F. Kennedy Institute for
Handicapped Children

707 North Broadway
Baltimore, MD 21205

Library of Congress
National Library Services for the
Blind and Physically
Handicapped
Washington, DC 20542
(800) 424-8567
(202) 287-5100 in DC

Make Today Count
P.O. Box 303
Burlington, IA 52601

March of Dimes Birth Defects
Foundation
Public Health Education
Foundation
1275 Mamaroneck Avenue
White Plains, NY 10605
(914) 428-7100

National Association for Hearing
and Speech Action Line
(800) 638-8255
(301) 897-0039 in HI, AK, and
MD call collect

National Association for
Retarded Citizens
2709 Avenue E
East Arlington TX 76011

National Association of the Deaf
814 Thayer Avenue
Silver Springs, MD 20910

National Center for Stuttering
(800) 221-2483
(212) 532-1460 in NY

National Center for the
Prevention and Control of Rape
5600 Fishers Lane
Room 6C-12
Rockville, MD 20857

National Center on Child Abuse
Office of Child Development
P.O. Box 1182
Washington, DC 20013

National Child Abuse Hotline
(800) 422-4453

National Committee for the
 Prevention of Child Abuse
332 S. Michigan Avenue
Chicago, IL 60604

National Down's Syndrome
 Hotline
(800) 221-4602
(212) 764-3070 in New York

National Easter Seal Society
2023 West Ogden Avenue
Chicago, IL 60612
(312) 243-8400 (voice)
(312) 243-8800 (TDD)

National Federation of the Blind
1800 Johnson Street
Baltimore, MD 21230

National Hearing Aid Helpline
(800) 521-5247
(313) 478-2610 in MI

National Hearing Aid Society
20361 Middlebelt Road
Livonia, MI 48152

National Hospice Organization
1901 N. Fort Meyer Drive
Suite 402
Arlington, VA 22209

National Information Center for
 Handicapped Children and
 Youth
1555 Wilson Blvd.
Rosslyn, VA 22209
(703) 522-3332

National Information System for
 Health Related Services (NIS)
(800) 922-9234
(800) 922-1108 in SC

National Rehabilitation Center
(800) 34-NARIC
(202) 635-5822 in DC

National Rehabilitation
 Information Center
4407 Eighth Street, N.E.
Washington, DC 20017-2299

National Society for Crippled
 Children and Adults
2023 West Ogden Avenue
Chicago, IL 60612

National Spinal Cord Injury
 Association
(800) 962-9629
(617) 964-0521 in MA

Office for Handicapped
 Individuals
200 Independence Avenue, S.W.
Washington DC 20201

The Orton Dyslexia Society
(800)ABCD-123

Parents Anonymous
2810 Artesia Boulevard
Redondo Beach, CA 90278
Hotline (800) 421-0353, in CA
 (800) 352-0386

Parent's Campaign for
 Handicapped Children and
 Youth/Closer Look
1201 Sixteenth Street, N.W.
Washington, DC 20036

Parents United
P.O. Box 952, Dept. P
San Jose, CA 95108

President's Committee on Mental
  Retardation
Office of Human Development
200 Independence Avenue, S.W.
Washington, DC 20201

Prevent Sexual Abuse
Box 2866
Chicago, IL 60690

Special Olympics
1701 K Street, N.W.
Washington, DC 20006
(202) 331-1346

Spinal Cord Injury Hotline
(800) 526-3456
(800) 638-1733 in MD

TAPP Project
Federation for Children with
  Special Needs
312 Stuart Street
Boston, MA 02116

Victims Anonymous
9514-9 Reseda Boulevard, #607
Northridge, CA 91324
(213) 993-1139

Appendix II: Children's Literature Resources

BOOKLISTS AND BIBLIOGRAPHIES

A to Zoo, Subject Access to Children's Picture Books. 3rd ed. Carolyn Lima. New York: R.R. Bowker, 1989. List (not annotated) of over 4,400 titles and authors for preschool to grade 2 arranged by subject headings, subject guide, bibliographic guide, title index, and illustrator index.

Accept Me as I Am: Best Books of Juvenile Nonfiction on Impairments and Disabilities. Joan Brest Friedberg, June B. Mullins, and Adelaide Weir Sukiennik. New York: R.R. Bowker, 1985. A listing of over 300 titles.

Adventuring with Books: A Booklist for Pre-K–Grade 6. Mary Jett-Simpson, ed. Urbana, IL: National Council of Teachers of English, 1989. Published about every two years. Contains annotations for various types of books arranged by type, subject, and theme.

The Aging Adult in Children's Books & Nonprint Media: An Annotated Bibliography. Catherine Townsend Horner. Metuchen, NJ: Scarecrow Press, 1982. Describes fiction and nonprint materials about relationships, illness, death, and other topics on the aging adult.

Anatomy of Wonder: A Critical Guide to Science Fiction. 3rd edition. Neil Barron, ed. New York: R.R. Bowker, 1987. Provides evaluative summaries of 2,000 adult and juvenile science fiction stories.

Best Books for Children. 4th edition. John T. Gillespie and Corinne J. Naden, eds. New York: R.R. Bowker, 1990. 11,000 annotated entries "to provide a list of books . . . that are highly recommended to satisfy both a child's recreational reading needs and the demands of a special school curriculum."

The Best in Children's Books: The University of Chicago Guide to Children's Literature, 1979–1984. Zena Sutherland, ed. Chicago, IL: University of Chicago Press, 1986. Reviews of over 1,000 books arranged by author, title, subject, curricular area, reading level, and developmental values.

The Best Science Books and A-V Materials for Children: Selected and Annotated. Kathryn Wolff et al., eds. American Association for the Advancement of Science, 1333 H Street, NW, 8th Floor, Washington, DC 20005. 1983. An annotated list of outstanding literature and media in the various sciences.

The Black Experience in Children's Books. Rev. ed. Barbara Rollock, comp. New York: New York Public Library, 1984. Annotated listing of books about the experiences of blacks in America and other parts of the world.

Books for the Gifted Child. Barbara H. Baskin and Karen H. Harris. New York: R.R. Bowker, 1990. Annotated list of books for gifted children.

Books to Help Children Cope with Separation and Loss. 2nd ed. Joanne E. Bernstein. New York: R.R. Bowker, 1983. Discusses such topics as death, divorce, adoption, and handicaps. Selections are for children from age three through sixteen.

Children's Books of the Year. Child Study Children's Book Committee at Bank Street College, 610 West 112th St., New York, NY 10025. An annual annotated list of over 500 books published in the current year. Books are chosen for artistic quality, child appeal, presentation of positive role models, and lack of stereotypes.

Choices: A Core Collection for Young Reluctant Readers. Carolyn Fleming and Donna Schatt, eds. Evanston, IL: John Gordon Burke, 1984. Annotated list of over 300 books for reluctant readers in grades two through six.

Choosing Books for Young People, Volume 2: A Guide to Criticism and Bibliography, 1976–1984. John R.T. Ettlinger and Diana L. Spirt. Phoenix, AZ: Oryx Press, 1987. Annotated bibliography evaluating more than 400 books on children's literature published in the above years.

The Community Bibliographer. 129 Felix St., Apt. 8, Santa Cruz, CA 95060. Distributes bibliographies to meet community needs, advocates for libraries, and addresses community organizations and leadership conferences.

Drugs: A Multimedia Sourcebook for Young Adults. Sharon Charles and Sari Feldman. Available from ABC-Clio/Neal-Schuman, Riviera Campus, Box 4397, Santa Barbara, CA 93103. 1980. An annotated list of fiction, nonfiction, and nonprint materials. Includes information on professional reading, and an author, title, and subject index.

The Elementary School Paperback Collection. John Thomas Gillespie. Chicago, IL: American Library Association, 1985. Annotated list of recommended paperbacks.

Fantasy for Children: An Annotated Checklist and Reference Guide. 2nd ed. Ruth Nadelman Lynn. New York: R.R. Bowker, 1983. Each annotated entry of more than 2,000 titles includes reading level, summary, review citations, and awards won.

Girls Are People Too! A Bibliography of Nontraditional Female Roles in Children's Books. Joan E. Newman. Metuchen, NJ: Scarecrow Press, 1982. A listing of fiction and nonfiction books for readers in preschool through grade nine. Focuses on minority groups and disabled characters.

Health, Illness, and Disability: A Guide to Books for Children and Young Adults. Pat Azarnoff. New York: R.R. Bowker, 1983. Describes over 1,000 books on health concerns and issues.

Helping Children Through Books. Rev. ed. Helen Ott, 1979. Church and Synagogue Library Association, P.O. Box 1130, Bryn Mawr, PA 19010. 1987. An annotated list of books about contemporary concerns including living with oneself and others, friendship, and personal problems.

High-Interest Books for Teens: A Guide to Book Reviews and Biographical Sources. 2nd ed. Adele Sarkissian, ed. Detroit, MI: Gale Research Co., 1988.

A Hispanic Heritage, Series IV: A Guide to Juvenile Books about Hispanic People and Cultures. Isabel Schon. Metuchen, NJ: Scarecrow Press, 1991. A list of books that provide students in kindergarten through grade twelve with an understanding and appreciation of the people, history, art, and political, social, and economic problems of Hispanic people. Author, subject, and title indexes. Previous series cover earlier children's books.

Indian Children's Books. Hap Gilliland. Bozeman, MT: Montana Council for Indian Education, 1980. Annotated list of over 1,500 books about Native American life.

Mexico and Its Literature for Children and Adolescents. Isabel Schon, comp. Tempe, AZ: Arizona State University Press, 1977. Annotated list of Mexican children's books.

More Notes from a Different Drummer: A Guide to Juvenile Fiction Portraying the Disabled. Barbara Baskin and Karen Harris. New York: R.R. Bowker, 1984. In addition to an annotated list of books portraying the disabled, this resource also contains essays on the history of the portrayal of disabled persons in children's literature and selection criteria.

Museum of Science and Industry Basic List of Children's Science Books. Bernice Richter, ed. Chicago, IL: Museum of Science and Industry, 1985. A list of trade books from the Museum's library and annual book fair. The books are evaluated.

Notable Children's Books, 1976–1980. Chicago, IL: *American Library Association, 1986. Annotated list of quality books chosen by the American Library Association.*

Notes from a Different Drummer: A Guide to Juvenile Fiction Portraying the Handicapped. Barbara Baskin and Karen Harris. New York: R.R. Bowker, 1977. In addition to reviews of more than 400 books with disabled characters, this book discusses criteria for the selection of books about disabled people.

Paperbound Books for Young People, Kindergarten through Grade 12. 2nd ed. New York: R.R. Bowker, 1980. Non-annotated list of 15,000 paperback books for ages preschool through grade 12. Title, author, subject, and illustration indexes.

Science Books for Children; Selections from Booklist, 1976–1983. Denise Murcko Wilms. Chicago, IL: American Library Association, 1985. Reviews of outstanding science trade books in a variety of genres. Includes author, title, and subject indexes.

Selected Jewish Children's Books. Marcia Posner, comp. New York: Jewish Book Council, 1984. A topical guide to books with Jewish themes.

The Single-Parent Family in Children's Books: An Annotated Bibliography. 2nd ed. Catherine Townsend Horner. Metuchen, NJ: Scarecrow Press, 1988. An annotated bibliography of 600 books published between 1965 and 1986 concerning the single-parent family. Includes grade level and a rating system.

INDEXES

Children's Books in Print. New York: R.R. Bowker. An annual listing of children's books still in print, grades K-12.

Children's Catalog. 4th ed. Isaacson, Richard, H., and Gary L. Bogard, eds. New York: H.W. Wilson, 1981. Analytical author, title, subject index with brief excerpts from reviews. Published periodically.

Index to Fairy Tales, 1978–1986: Including Folklore, Legends, and Myths in Collections, fifth supplement. Norma O. Ireland and Joseph W. Sprug, comps. Metuchen, NJ: Scarecrow Press, 1989. An author, compiler, subject, and title index. Part of a series that covers tales published from the 1920s to recent years.

Index to Poetry for Children and Young People, 1976–1981. John E. Brewton et al. Bronx, NY: H.W. Wilson Co., 1984. Poems on various topics are indexed according to subject, author, title, and first line. Previous editions date from the 1940s.

Storyteller's Sourcebook. Margaret Read MacDonald, ed. Detroit, MI: Gale Research, 1982. A subject, motif, variant, and title index of folktales in 700 collections.

Subject Guide to Children's Books in Print. New York: R.R. Bowker. An annual guide which categorizes all children's books currently in print under various subject headings.

Subject Index to Poetry for Children and Young People. Dorothy B. Frozzell Smith and Eva L. Andrews. Chicago, IL: American Library Association, 1977.

RESOURCES ON SPECIAL TOPICS

Beyond Fact: Nonfiction for Children and Young People. Jo Carr, comp. Chicago, IL: American Library Association, 1982. An overview of nonfiction, with many suggested titles.

Bilingual Books in Spanish and English for Children. Doris Cruger Dale. Littleton, CO: Libraries Unlimited, 1985. Reviews of bilingual books for preschool and elementary school children.

The Bookfinder, Volume 3: When Kids Need Books: Annotations of Books Published 1979–1982. Sharon Spredemann Dreyer. American Guidance Service, Circle Pines, MN 55014. 1985. Subject, author, title index and reviews of books, fiction and nonfiction, on problems children may experience as well as feelings and relationships.

Books by African-American Authors and Illustrators for Children and Young Adults. Helen E. Williams. Chicago, IL: American Library Association, 1991.

Books to Help Children Cope with Separation and Loss. 3rd ed. Joanne E. Bernstein. New York: R.R. Bowker, 1989. Information about bibliotherapy, and annotative lists of books on such topics as death, divorce, adoption, and foster children.

Children's Books of International Interest. 3rd ed. Barbara Elleman, ed. Chicago, IL: American Library Association, 1984. An annotated list of books that depict the American way of life and contain universal themes of interest to children.

Children's Literature: An Issues Approach. Masha Kabakow Rudman. 2nd ed. New York: Longman, 1984. Essays and annotated lists about literature on such issues as sibling relationships, divorce, adoption, sexuality, gender roles, multicultural experiences, the disabled, old age, and death. Contains teaching ideas.

Creative Uses of Children's Literature. Mary Ann Paulin. Hamden, CT: Library Professional Publications, 1982. Tips for teaching and sharing literature with preschool and elementary school children.

For Reading Outloud! Margaret Mary Kimmel and Elizabeth Segel. New York: Delacorte, 1983. A guidebook to selecting good read-aloud books and ways to share them. Contains a subject, title, and author index.

Information Sources in Children's Literature: A Practical Reference Guide for Children's Librarians, Elementary School Teachers, and Students of Children's Literature. Mary Meacham. Westport, CT: Greenwood Press, 1978. A guide to reviews and periodicals.

A Multimedia Approach to Children's Literature: A Selective List of Films, Filmstrips, and Recordings Based on Children's Books. Mary Alice Hunt. 3rd ed. Chicago, IL: American Library Association, 1983. Reviews media on children's literature.

Poetry Alive! P.O. Box 9643, Asheville, NC 28815, (704) 298–4927. Combines theatrical techniques with memorized poetry to entertain as well as stimulate creativity.

The Read-Aloud Handbook. Jim Trelease. Rev. ed. New York: Penguin Books, 1985. Contains ideas for reading aloud and an annotated list of good books to read aloud.

Readers Theatre Script Service. P.O. Box 178333, San Diego, CA 92117. Describes readers-theatre–style scripts and materials about using readers theatre in the classroom.

Reading Ladders for Human Relations. Eileen Tway, ed. 6th ed. Washington, DC: American Council on Education, 1981. An annotated listing of titles for ages preschool to high school arranged according to five themes.

Reference Books for Children. Carolyn Peterson and Ann Fenton. 4th ed. Metuchen, NJ: Scarecrow Press, 1992. Describes over 1,000 reference books.

Substance Abuse Materials for School Libraries: An Annotated Bibliography. Theodora Andrews. Littleton, CO: Libraries Unlimited, 1984. A listing of fiction, reference works, personal stories and various materials.

This Way to Books. Caroline Fuller Bauer. Bronx, New York: H.W. Wilson Co., 1983. Literature activities.

PERIODICALS

Appraisal: Children's Science Books. Children's Science Book Review Committee, 36 Cummington Street, Boston, MA 02215. A quarterly that features outstanding science trade books in various genres of literature.

Book Review Digest. Bronx, NY: H.W. Wilson. Published ten times a year, this periodical evaluates more than 3,000 adult and children's books and provides quotations from reviews of the books.

Bulletin of the Center for Children's Books. Chicago, IL: The University of Chicago Press. Published eleven times yearly, contains reviews of recommended books and indexes on curricular use and developmental values.

CBC Features. Available from Children's Book Council, 67 Irving Place, New York, NY 10003. A semi-annual newsletter about various authors, illustrators, and subjects related to children's books. Contains information about free and inexpensive materials such as posters and bookmarks.

Childhood Education. Association for Childhood Education International, 3615 Wisconsin Avenue N.W., Washington, DC 20016. A regular column contains annotated reviews of new children's books.

The Children's Literature Association Quarterly. Available from Children's Literature Association, P.O. Box 138, Battle Creek, MI 49016. Contains book reviews, articles on children's literature, with special sections on poetry, plays, censorship, teaching children's literature, and other topics of interest. Membership in Children's Literature Association required.

Children's Literature in Education. A quarterly that contains articles on children's literature, book reviews, authors and illustrators of children's books, and teaching. Available from Human Services Press, Inc., 233 Spring Street, New York, NY 10013–1578.

The Five Owls. Available from The Five Owls, Inc., 2004 Sheridan Avenue South, Minneapolis, MN 55405. A bi-monthly intended for libraries, educators, parents, authors, illustrators, and other readers who are personally and professionally involved in children's literature.

The Horn Book Magazine. Horn Book, Inc., Park Square Building, 31 St. James Ave., Boston, MA 02116. A bi-monthly which includes book reviews, articles about children's literature, interviews, information about children's literature conferences, and other related items.

Interracial Books for Children Bulletin. Council on Interracial Books for Children, 1841 Broadway, New York, NY 10023. Contains articles and reviews of books that depict ethnic, religious, and gender experiences. Also featured are books about people with handicaps.

Journal of Youth Services in Libraries. Chicago, IL: American Library Association, 50 E. Huron St., Chicago, IL 60611. Contains articles on children's and young adult literature, Newbery and Caldecott Award acceptance speeches, and current issues in teaching and library work. Published quarterly.

The Lion and the Unicorn. Department of English, Brooklyn College, Brooklyn, NY 11210. Articles about children's literature.

The New Advocate. Christopher-Gordon Publishers, Inc., P.O. Box 809, Needham Heights, MA 02194–0006. A quarterly journal that includes book and media reviews, articles about illustrators and authors, and teaching methods.

Plays Magazine. Plays, Inc., 120 Boylston Street, Boston, MA 02116. A monthly publication (Oct.-May) which contains short plays, skits, monologues, and dramatized classics.

School Library Journal. New York: R.R. Bowker & Co. A monthly journal that contains book reviews and articles. Annual December issue includes "Best Books" of the current year.

Science Books and Films. American Association for the Advancement of Science. 1515 Massachusetts Ave., N.W., Washington, DC 20005. Reviews of literature and reference materials.

Science and Children. National Science Teachers Association, 1201 16th Street N.W., Washington, DC. Contains a monthly column which reviews children's books and non-print media.

VOYA (Voice of Youth Advocates). Metuchen, NJ: Scarecrow Press. Bi-monthly journal of book reviews and articles aimed at librarians serving young adults.

The Web: Wonderfully Exciting Books. The Ohio State University, The Reading Center, 200 Ramseyer Hall, Columbus, OH 43210. Reviews books and offers ideas for teaching literature that are centered around specific topics.

Subject Index

Abuse. *See* Child abuse; Drug abuse; Health behavior
Adolescence. *See* Health behavior; Human sexuality; Personality and individuality; Self
Aging and the elderly. *See* Family life and health
AIDS, 25–26, 167–171, 257, 275, 282, 284, 297, 355–356, 486–487
Alcoholism and teenage drinking:
   coping with alcoholic parents, 103, 190, 284, 294–297, 497–500
   teenage drinking, 33–34, 244, 258, 289, 295–297, 498–500
Annotated bibliography: organization of, by Growing Healthy Curriculum subject area:
   by major curricular categories (*see under*: Growing Healthy Curriculum)
   detailed subject listing (*see* Annotated Bibliography Indexed by Growing Healthy Curriculum Subject Area, pp. 620–622)
Appearance. *See* Grooming; Personality and individuality; Self; Weight control
Appendixes to this book: descriptions of information contained in, 175, 317, 348

Basal reading program: description and evaluation of, 304–310
Biographies for children, 183–192 (*See also* Children's literature: discussions and evaluations of)
Birth and fetal development. *See under* Growth and development
Body parts and systems. *See under* Growth and development

Child abuse, 104, 167, 171, 172, 224, 258, 288, 531–535
Child care/working parent(s), 32, 178, 221, 275, 288
"Children's Choices": recommendations of, for health-oriented literature, 217–226, 318
Children's cookbooks, 109, 125–126, 155, 177–178, 182, 278–279, 472–473, 475, 480
Children's literature: creative use of illustrations/layouts to enhance, 65–66, 72–74, 139–141, 146, 148, 154, 169, 179–181, 195–196, 199
Children's literature: discussions and evaluations of, by literature category:
   broad discussions of: biographies, 183–192; fantasy and science fiction, 78–97; folktales, 68–78; historical fiction, 115–129; informational

611

books, 162–182; plays, 192–210; poetry, 129–161; realistic fiction, 97–115

characteristics of good children's literature: biographies, 186–188; fantasy and science fiction, 80–84; folktales, 70–73; historical fiction, 80–84; informational books, 164–172; plays, 200–205; poetry, 137–147; realistic fiction, 98–101

checklists for evaluating: biographies, 188–189; fantasy and science fiction, 96–97; folktales, 75; historical fiction, 148; informational books, 172–173; plays, 205; poetry, 147; realistic fiction, 100

"something to do" projects to enhance children's skills in evaluating: biographies, 191; fantasy literature, 84; historical fiction, 122–123; informational books, 175; plays, 209; poetry, 152–153; realistic fiction, 107

Children's literature: uses of, in classroom teaching highlighted:

by teaching design: creating appropriate groupings/thematic units, 314, 333–338; creating meaningful activities, 19, 344–345; creating a reading environment, 317–318; creating "whole group" experiences, 320, 338–342; forming a classroom lending library, 318–320; linking literature to writing, 346–352; promoting independent reading, 342–343; structuring read-aloud sessions with open-ended follow up, 321–322, 324–326; teachers as facilitators/meaning makers, 323–331

classroom teachers cited for excellent instructional approaches: Bolton, Dona, 318–320, 330–331; Doan, Beth, 341; Dye, Melanie, 326; Fulks, Mary Beth, 341; Gambrill, Noreen, 350; Goddard, Carrie, 121–122, 351; McGill, Geri, 327, 341; Miller, Donna, 342; Parks, LaCheryl, 335; Smith, Peg, 336, 350; Steward, Barbara, 335, 342

Children's literature selection, xvi,63–68, 134–137, 152–153, 173–175, 193–200, 210–217, 226–227, 305, 317, 318 (See also "Children's Choices")

Cleanliness. See Grooming

Conformity/individuality, 112, 197, 198, 222, 225, 243, 265, 389–394 (See also Self)

Conservation. See Environment

Consumer rights, 291–293, 300–301

Cookbooks. See Children's cookbooks

Coping strategies and behaviors, 245, 266, 329, 372–376

Culture and cultural differences. See under Eating and food preparation; Food; Social Issues

Day care/working parent(s), 32, 178, 221, 275, 288

Death and dying, 25, 158, 196–197, 209, 224, 258, 274, 275, 288, 339, 523–531

death of a family member, 66, 102–103, 208, 273, 326, 342, 350 (see also Disease)

death of a pet, 223, 275, 339

teenage deaths: statistics on, 7, 24–25, 29 (see also Suicide)

unhealthy lifestyles, effects of, 6–7, 25–27

unsettling events seen on TV, 121–122

Dental health/visits, 55, 133, 248, 256, 260, 269, 290, 292, 351, 411
Depression (emotional), 111, 133, 166, 223–224, 272, 276, 340 (*See also* Mental illness)
Diet. *See* Food; Nutrition; Weight control
Disabilities and handicaps, 222, 225, 258, 284, 289, 339–340, 362, 513–523
Disease: (*See also* AIDS; Family life and health; Health behavior; Mental illness)
    communicable/infectious disease, 11, 25, 56, 200, 257, 271
    coping with, 482, 484–486, 488–489 (*see also* Physical handicaps and disabilities)
    disease fighters, biographies of, 188, 271, 283, 291
    germs/bacteria/viruses, 11, 282–284
    prevention and control of, 25–27, 55–56, 190, 256, 257, 281–285, 481–489
    sexually transmitted, 7, 166, 172, 244, 257, 276
    specific diseases, 27, 257, 276, 282–285, 481–482, 483, 486–487
Divorce. *See under* Family composition: changing circumstances
Doctor and hospital visits, 248, 249, 269, 282, 286, 290, 411–412, 414
Drinking. *See* Alcoholism and teenage drinking
Drug abuse, 56, 171, 224, 252, 258, 271, 272, 275, 276, 285, 293–297, 418, 497–500

Eating and food preparation: (*See also* Food; Nutrition; Weight control)
    campfire meals/cookouts, 116, 155
    customs in other lands/cultures, 77, 107–109, 123,-124, 177–178, 278, 280
    eating disorders, 179, 272, 480
    festive meals, 105, 123, 155, 278
    food preparation, 76, 105, 160, 178, 180, 199, 219, 278–280 (*see also* Children's cookbooks)
    overeating (*see* Weight control)
    pleasure taken in, 140–141, 154 , 155, 160–161, 278–280, 350
    table manners, 123–124, 156, 159, 182, 280
    utensils, 108–109, 124, 182
Emotional problems/disorders. *See* Health behavior; Mental illness; Personality and individuality
Environment, 297–301, 500–512
    ecosystems, 225, 298, 301, 501, 505–507, 510–511
    environmental awareness, 95, 335, 501–503, 507–508, 511–512
    environmental conservation, 19, 87, 95, 190–191, 204 , 255, 298–301, 335, 500–512
    how progress has adversely affected, 85, 87, 199, 299–300, 335
    nuclear accidents (*see* Nuclear war/accident)
    poems about, where to find, 158, 236
    pollution/waste disposal, 25, 94, 299–301, 503–505, 508–510
    workplace hazards, 300–301

Esteem, self. *See* Self
Evaluating:
children's literature (*see* Children's literature: discussions and evaluations of; Illustrations)
health education models, 28–36
reading instruction programs, 211–212, 303–304, 305–313
Exercise, 250, 269, 270–272, 412–413, 415–419 (*See also* Physical fitness and sports)

Facts of life. *See under* Human sexuality
Family composition: changing circumstances:
adoption, 207, 274, 351, 428–430, 441, 442
birth of a new sibling, 102, 172, 222, 442
divorce, separation, and single-parent families, 66, 198, 207, 224, 248, 273, 326, 428–430, 440–442
estranged parents, communication with 114, 171, 441
foster families, 429, 441
grandparents as child rearers, 114, 190, 429, 441
stepparents, 197, 248, 273, 429, 441, 442
Family life and health, 272–277, 420–466 (*See also* Family composition; Human sexuality)
birth (*see under* Growth and development)
cultures, life in other (*see under* Eating and food preparation; Food; Social issues)
cycle of life, 24, 449–450
gender issues, 436–439
grandparents, communication with, 114, 190, 209, 273, 274, 275, 350, 351, 425–428
illness among family members, 254, 282, 350, 351
relationships with siblings, 207, 221, 222, 421–425, 452–454
various kinds of families, 430–435, 442–449
working parent(s)/child care issues, 32, 221, 275, 288
Fantasy literature, 78–97 (*See also* Children's literature: discussions and evaluations of)
Fear: coping with. *See* Mental illness; Personality and individuality; Stress, coping with
Fetal development and birth. *See under* Growth and development
First aid and safety, 489–494 (*See also under* Annotated Bibliography Indexed by Growing Healthy Curriculum Subject Area, pp. 620–622)
Folktales, 68–78 (*See also* Children's literature: discussions and evaluations of; Food; Nutrition)
use of, in teaching language/writing/health skills, 69, 71–73, 195, 206, 327, 341, 352
Food: (*See also* Eating and food preparation; Nutrition; Weight control)
as a cause of conflict, 69–70, 157–158
attraction/aversion to specific foods, 71, 89, 90, 155, 156
cookbooks/recipes for children (*see* Children's cookbooks)

cultural differences in food customs: 77, 107–109, 177–178, 278, 280, 466–467, 473, 475–476, 479–480

food customs: past and changing, 123, 181–182

harvesting/planting/farm life, 124–125, 180–182, 280, 467–469

hunger/famine/drought, 74, 123, 125–128, 136 (*see also under* Social issues)

hunting/foraging for, 88, 109, 160

in survival situations, 69, 123–125, 155

junk food, 90, 93–94, 278, 280, 336

sharing of, 92, 104–105, 125, 154, 160, 199, 278, 472–473, 475, 480

workings of, in body, 177, 179, 280

Food stories: themes and activities in early grades, 69–70, 74–77, 91, 159, 466–473

nutrition: role of, in teaching (*see* Nutrition: role of children's literature in teaching)

pots: cooking, magic, and escape of food from, 76–77, 160, 327, 341

use of, to reveal attitudes and feelings, 23, 156, 158, 177, 181

Friends and friendships, 220–221, 248–249, 265, 275, 384–388, 398–400, 409–411

peer acceptance/influence, 223, 248, 256

responsibility/commitment to, 56, 209, 220

separation/loss, 220, 254, 288

Gender issues, 308, 436–439 (*See also* Human sexuality; Women's achievements)

Grooming, 219, 220, 269, 271, 412, 415–416, 418–419

Growing Healthy Curriculum, xv–xvii, 38–57, 214, 246, 255–259

"Curricular Progression Chart," 39–54

"Curricular Progression Chart" summarized, 55–57

Growing Healthy Curriculum: literature recommendations by curricular component:

Careers in the Health Field, 512–513

Community Health Management, 297–301, 500–512

Consumer Health, 289–293, 494–497

Disease Prevention and Control, 281–285, 481–489

Drug Use and Abuse, 293–297

Family Life and Health, 272–277, 420–466

Growth and Development, 247–255, 259–263, 365–372

Mental and Emotional Health, 264–268, 372–411

Miscellaneous Issues, 513–538

Nutrition, 277–281, 466–480

Personal Health, 268–272, 411–419

Safety and First Aid, 285–289, 489–494

Growth and development, 247–255, 259–263, 365–372

birthing process, 169, 275, 276, 420–421

body parts and systems 55–56, 66, 261–263, 365–372

chart of, depicting students' characteristics and needs (by grade levels), 247–255

facts of life/reproduction (*see under* Human sexuality)
fetal development, 164, 168–170, 275

Handicaps. *See* Mental illness; Physical handicaps and disabilities
Health advisors. *See* Dental health/visits; Doctor and hospital visits
Health awareness promotion, xvi, 7, 13–14, 25–26, 30, 57, 217–226, 242–246
Health behavior: (*See also* Disease; Human sexuality; Nutrition; Weight control)
    inconsistency between school curricula and community activities, 23–24, 30, 176, 244
    social/cultural forces influencing, 256, 281, 345, 464–466
    teenage behavior, 7, 33–34, 166, 168, 244, 258, 450–452, 454–456, 462–464
    unhealthy lifestyles, health risks of, 6–7, 25–27
Health education: (*See also* Growing Healthy Curriculum)
    consistency between school curricula and community activities, 23–24, 30, 176, 244, 358
    goals of/traditional approaches to teaching, described, 27–30, 316
    models for (components of/criteria for evaluating), 28–29, 36, 255–259, 311–313
    role of children's literature in teaching (*see* Children's literature: discussions and evaluations of)
    standard health textbooks: inadequacies of, 9–17
    statistics on existing programs of, and teacher preparation for, 36–38
    successful ideas/projects, 325–331, 335–337, 339–342, 345, 350–352, 355–356
    using the "Kolbe" model, 30–31, 35
Health statistics, 7, 24–25, 32, 33–34, 244, 258
Historical fiction, 115–129 (*See also* Children's literature: discussions and evaluations of)
Holistic view of health, 8, 9, 226
Homelessness. *See* Social issues
Homosexuality. *See under* Human sexuality
Honesty. *See* Friends and friendships; Personality and individuality
Human sexuality, 275–276, 439–440, 454–456
    AIDS, 25, 26, 167–171, 275, 282, 284, 355–356
    birthing process (*see* Growth and development)
    facts of life/reproduction, 165, 169, 254, 274–276, 370, 439–440, 454–456
    homosexuality, 64, 168, 272, 276, 455–456
    pregnancy/teen pregnancy, 166, 168, 171, 454–456
    sexual abuse, 167, 171–172, 205 (*see also* Child abuse)
    sexual maturation, 197, 254, 263, 275, 276
    sexuality/sexual identity, 164–170, 197, 225, 254, 276
    sexually transmitted diseases, 7, 166, 172, 244, 276
    teenage behavior (*see under* Health behavior)

Hunger. *See* Food; Nutrition; Social issues
Hygiene. *See* Grooming

Illness and medical care. *See* Disease; Doctor and hospital visits; Mental illness
Illustrations/unusual layouts: creative use of, to enhance children's literature, 65–66, 72–74, 139–141, 146, 148, 154, 169, 179–181, 195–196, 199
Image (self). *See* Self
Individuality and conformity, 112, 197, 198, 222, 225, 243, 265, 389–394 (*See also* Self)
Informational books for children, 162–182 (*See also* Children's literature: discussions and evaluations of)

Junk food, 90, 93–94, 278, 280, 336 (*See also* Nutrition)

Librarians: role of, in sparking interest in reading/health reading, xiv, 317–318, 322, 347
Lifestyle, fostering a healthy/consequences of an unhealthy. *See* Health behavior; Nutrition
Literacy training: reading/writing/interpretative skills, 19, 61–64, 132–137, 311–352
Literature: discussions of, by type. *See* Children's literature: discussions and evaluations of
Literature: use of, to develop problem solving/writing skill, 18–19, 313, 329–331, 346–352
Literature selection. *See* Children's literature selection

Manners/table manners. *See* Eating and food preparation; Grooming; Individuality and conformity
Maturation. *See* Growth and development; Human sexuality; Personality and individuality
Mental illness, 224, 244, 264–268, 272, 276, 278
  depression, 111, 133, 166, 223–224, 272, 276, 340
  eating disorders/obsessions with specific foods (*see* Weight control)
  stress (*see* Stress, coping with)

Nuclear war/accident, 64, 94, 96, 113, 187, 257, 289, 299–301, 350, 504–505, 508–510 (*See also* Environment)
Nutrition, 277–281, 466–480 (*See also* Eating and food preparation; Food; Weight control)
  changing views/attitudes/customs, 123, 158, 181–182
  consistency between school curricula and community activities, 23–24, 30, 176, 244, 358

cooking nutritious meals 125–126, 176–178

effects of poor diet on school performance, 35, 244

effects of TV promotion of junk food on decision making, 281, 345

healthy foods and diets, 26, 27, 56, 69, 88, 104, 157–159, 176–179, 182, 223, 270, 278–280, 336–337, 467–470, 477–478, 479

nutrients, 56, 477, 478–479

obsessions with eating/eating specific foods, 155, 159, 272

overeating/overweight (*see under* Weight control)

promoting an interest in, 159, 177–178, 278

role of children's literature in teaching (discussed by literature type): 69, 77, 78, 88–94, 104–114, 123–128, 153–161, 175–182

starvation/hunger, 74, 123–128, 240, 280 (*see also under* Social issues)

unhealthy foods and consequences of eating, 24, 27, 93–94, 153, 220, 280, 336, 470

vitamins, 176, 290, 345, 363

Parental separation/divorce. *See under* Family composition: changing circumstances

Personal appearance/hygiene. *See* Grooming; Individuality and conformity; Weight control

Personality and individuality, 219–224 (*See also* Human sexuality; Self)

appearance, 223, 265 (*see also* Grooming; Self; Weight control)

conformity/individuality, 112, 197, 198, 222, 225, 243, 265, 389–394

depression, 111, 133, 166, 223–224, 272, 276, 340 (*see also* Mental illness)

endurance/survival skills, 134, 243, 265, 289, 350

fear/bravery, 219, 221–223, 329, 379–384

gender issues, 308, 436–439 (*see also* Human sexuality; Women's achievements)

honor/integrity/truthfulness/trust, 219, 224, 243, 275 (*see also* Friends and friendships)

possibilities for change, 178, 224, 243

Persons with handicaps. *See* Mental illness; Physical handicaps and disabilities

Physical fitness and sports, 223, 250, 253, 269–272, 412–419

Physical handicaps and disabilities, 222, 225, 258, 284, 289, 339–340, 362, 513–523

Plays for children, 192–210 (*See also* Children's literature: discussions and evaluations of)

finding good plays, 193–200

use of in teaching health issues, 206–209

Poetry for children, 129–161 (*See also* Children's literature: discussions and evaluations of)

children's poetry interests, 147–152

making it enjoyable, 132–137, 312, 351

use of appearance (layout) to enhance, 139–141, 146, 148, 154

Pregnancy/teen pregnancy. *See* Growth and development; Health behavior; Human sexuality
Prejudice. *See* Social issues
Puberty. *See* Family life and health; Health behavior; Human sexuality; Personality and individuality; Self

Reading instruction:
  basal reading program, description of, 304–307
  evaluation of traditional reading programs, 211–212, 303–304, 305–310
  use of naturalistic research to assess, 311–313
Realistic fiction for children, 97–115 (*See also* Children's literature: discussions and evaluations of)
Recipes. *See* Children's cookbooks
Reproduction. *See* Growth and development; Human sexuality

Safety and first aid, 285–289, 489–494 (*See also under* Annotated Bibliography Indexed by Growing Healthy Curriculum Subject Area, pp. 620–622)
Science fiction. *See* Fantasy literature
Selecting children's literature. *See* "Children's Choices"; Children's literature selection
Self: (*See also* Human sexuality; Personality and individuality)
  self vs. need to belong, 221, 223, 224 , 403 (*see also* Family and health)
  self-acceptance, 18, 220–223, 243, 336, 378, 389–394
  self-awareness, 18, 219, 223, 376–379, 398, 403
  self-image/esteem, 184, 189, 209, 219, 222, 223, 243, 267, 376–379, 407–409
  self-reliance and survival skills, 178, 289, 350
Separation and loss. *See* Death and dying; Family composition; Friends and friendships
Sexual abuse, 167, 171–172, 205 (*see also* Child abuse)
Sexual discrimination, *See* Gender issues; Social issues; Women's achievements
Sexually transmitted diseases. *See* Human sexuality
Sibling relationships, 207, 221, 222, 421–425, 452–454
Smoking and tobacco use, 7, 17, 31, 33–34, 133, 171, 295, 372
Social issues: (*See also* Environment)
  conflicting human values, 204, 223
  consumer rights, 291–293
  hunger/homelessness, 176, 280, 479–480 (*see also under* Food)
  sexual discrimination, 436–439 (*see also* Women's achievements)
  social awareness/other cultures, 225, 388–389
  social injustice, 126–129, 199, 225, 276, 293, 340, 388–389, 394–397
Sports and physical fitness, 223, 250, 253, 269–272, 412–419
  women's achievements (in sports and science), 185, 187–190, 263

Starvation. *See* Food; Nutrition; Social issues
Statistics on:
  health/student health education, 7, 24–25, 32, 33–34, 244, 258
  reading, as a classroom activity, 212, 307–308
  teacher training/preparation in health-related areas, 36–38, 356–357
Stress, coping with, 184, 198, 223, 335, 400–404, 405–407
Suicide/teenage suicide, 7, 133, 208–209, 244, 258, 275, 535–538
Survival:
  of the individual (*see* Food; Personality and individuality; Self; Working parent(s)/child care issues)
  of the world (*see* Environment; Social issues)

Teacher training/preparation in health-related areas, 36–38, 356–357
Teenage behavior. *See* Health behavior; Human sexuality; Personality and individuality
Teenage pregnancy. *See* Growth and development; Health behavior; Human sexuality
Tobacco use, 7, 17, 31, 33–34, 133, 171, 295, 372

Vision and hearing. *See* Growth and development; Physical handicaps and disabilities
Vitamins, 176, 290, 345, 363

Waste disposal. *See* Environment
Weight control: (*See also* Eating and food preparation; Food; Junk food; Nutrition)
  eating disorders, 179, 272, 480
  obsessions with eating/eating specific foods, 89, 90, 111, 155, 159, 272
  overeating, 90, 111, 155–156, 159, 253, 279, 480
  overeating, consequences of, 111, 138, 155, 160, 270, 281, 476–477, 480
  overweight/obesity, 110–113, 179, 271, 280, 470–471, 476–477, 480
Women's achievements (in science and sports), 185, 187–190, 263
Working parent(s)/child care issues, 32, 178, 221, 275, 288
Workplace health/hazards, 300–301
Writing: using literature to develop skills in, 313, 346–352

ANNOTATED BIBLIOGRAPHY INDEXED BY
GROWING HEALTHY CURRICULUM SUBJECT AREA

Community Health Management: 500–512; ecosystems, 501, 505–507, 510–511; environmental awareness, 501–503, 507–508, 511–512;

types of pollution/environmental protection, 500–501, 503–505, 508–510
Consumer Health: 494–497

Disease Prevention and Control: 481–489; coping with disease, 482; coping with disease/lifestyle choices, 484–486, 488–489; disease prevention, 482, 483, 487–488; types of diseases, 481–482, 483, 486–487
Drug Use and Abuse: 497–500

Family Life and Health: 420–466; adolescence, 450–452, 462–464; all kinds of families, 430–435, 442–449; cycle of life, 449–450; divorce, single-parent families, foster families, 428–430, 440–442; families the world over, 435–436; family life, 456–462; gender issues, 436–439; grandparents, 425–428; relationships with siblings, 421–425, 452–454; reproduction and birth, 420–421; reproduction and human sexuality, 439–440, 454–456; social and cultural forces that influence health behavior, 464–466

Growth and Development: 365–372; body parts, 365–368; body systems, 368–370; the human body, 371–372

Mental and Emotional Health: 372–411; coping strategies and behaviors, 372–376; coping with stress, 400–404, 405–407; developing a personal identity, 407–409; emotions and feelings, 379–384; friendships, all kinds of, 398–400; human differences and similarities, 388–389; relationships, 384–388, 394–397; relationships between physical well-being and, 389–394, 409–411; responsibility to self/others, 376–379
Miscellaneous Issues: 513–538; abuse, 531–535; careers in the health field, 512–513; death and dying, 523–531; persons with handicaps, 513–523; suicide, 535–538

Nutrition: 466–480; effects of a poor diet, 476–477; fanciful food stories, 471–472, 476; food choice/types of foods, 477–478, 479; food identification, nutrition and health, 469–470; food sources, 467–469; food sources/food customs, 473–475; food sources/world health problems, 479–480; nutrition and health, nutrients, 477, 478–479; personal and ethnic variations in foods, 466–467, 476; preparing and sharing foods, cookbooks, 472–473, 475, 480; snacks, 471; unhealthy eating habits, 470–471; weight control/eating disorders, 480

Personal Health: 411–419; health advisors, 411, 414; health care practices, 411–412, 414–415; improving personal health care, 418; personal health care habits, 419; physical fitness, 412–413, 415–418

Safety and First Aid: 489–494; accident prevention, 489–490; people and places that can provide help, 490–491; safety at play, 490, 492; safety precautions, 491–492 493; stories of risks, accidents, and survival, 493, 494; who keeps us safe, 492

Author and Illustrator Index

Notes: Bold type indicates that the author's poetry has been recited on this page. This index does not include authors whose work is referenced solely in the Annotated Bibliography; neither does it include authors (of research studies) cited only in chapter notes, unless their work is directly quoted in the text. References to illustrators are limited to citations appearing in the text.

Aaron, C., 127, 234
Aaseng, N., 189, 190, 238, 252,
 283, 389, 415–416, 484, 496
Ackerman, K., 273
Adams, A., 262
Adler, C. S., 249, 384, 389, 405,
 437, 440, 452, 456, 484,
 520, 534, 536
Adoff, A., **140–141**, 153, **154**,
 235, 250, 279, 335, 340,
 361, 394, 416, 436, 443,
 473
Agree, R. H., **155–156**, 235, 476
Aho, J. S., 172, 236, 454
Aiken, J., 172, 199, 239, 443, 511
Aldis, D., **142**, **154–155**, 159,
 235, 400
Alexander, M., 102, 233, 379,
 421
Alexander, S., 103, 233, 430
Aliki, 123, 124, 181, 185, 191,
 234, 236, 238, 260, 347,
 352, 362, 365, 372, 379,
 425, 452, 469, 502
Allensworth, D. D., 30, 58, 59, 60
Amadeo, D. M., 282
American Medical Association, 8,
 23, 36

American Public Health Associa-
 tion, 26–27
Amon, A., 300, 335, 362
Ancona, G., 169, 187, 236, 238,
 420, 421, 437, 456, 478, 513
Andersen, H. C., 84, 232, 350,
 362, 376
Anderson, G., 178, 236, 475
Anderson, M. K., 300
Andrews, E. L., 152
Andrews, J., 109, 233, 376, 379
Angell, J., 292, 389, 456
Anspaugh, D., 33, 59, 78
Apy, D., 70, 231
Arbuthnot, M. H., 65, 98, 99–
 100, 186, 227
Archambault, J., 219, 222
Armstrong, D., 172
Arnold, C., 179, 236, 286, 291,
 414, 484, 492, 495, 502
Aruego, J., 221
Asbjornsen, P. C., 231, 352, 362,
 437, 471
Asch, F., 248, 372, 412, 430
Asch, J., 248, 411, 412
Aseltine, L., 340, 362, 372, 513
Ashe, F., 221, 240
Atwell, N., 312, 352, 360

623

Babbitt, N., 249, 436, 528
Bach, A., 285
Baeher, P., 225, 390, 409
Baggett, N., 271
Baker, E., 287, 491, 492
Baldwin, A., 282, 390, 482
Baldwin, D., 262, 368
Balestrino, P., 260
Banks, A., 288
Barr, J., 209, 239, 376
Bates, B., 283, 443, 450, 520
Bateson, I., 110, 238
Bauer, M. D., 288, 493, 498, 525
Bedard, R. L., 196, 240
Behrens, R., 30
Bell, R., 276, 354, 462
Benet, S. V., 208, 240, 531
Benjamin, C. L., 280, 390, 416
Berenstain, J., 248, 372, 380,
    384, 411, 421, 426, 436,
    470, 494, 532
Berenstain, S., 248, 372, 380,
    384, 411, 421, 426, 436,
    470, 494, 532
Berger, G., 176–177, 236, 295,
    297, 450, 522
Berger, M., 176–177, 236, 292,
    365, 368, 414, 477, 478,
    484, 487, 503
Berghammer, G., 197, 240
Bergman, T., 266
Berlin, E., 288
Bernick, D., 178–179, 236, 270
Berry, J., 267, 390, 493
Bershad, C., 178–179, 236, 270
Bertol, R., 352, 362
Bettelheim, B., 4, 21, 72, 92–93,
    227
Bierhorst, J., 69, 231
Bisignano, A., 178, 236
Blackburn, L., 152
Blegvad, L., 222, 372, 380
Blume, J., 221, 316, 342, 362,
    400, 409, 414, 421, 440,
    443, 452, 454, 462, 484, 521
Bolton, D., 318, 320, 330–331,
    360

Bond, M., 200–203, 204, 232,
    240, 471
Bond, N., 94–95, 232, 510
Bonderoff, J., 190, 238, 409
Bosma, B., 327, 361
Boston Hospital Children's Hos-
    pital Staff, 276
Boujon, C., 223, 466, 516
Boundy, D., 296
Bowe-Gutman, S., 168, 171, 236,
    454
Boylston, H. D., 352, 362, 495
Braden, V., 270
Bradley, A., 200–203, 204, 240
Brandenberg, F., 160, 235, 421
Branley, F. M., 335, 362, 368
Branscum, R., 224, 255, 279,
    408, 464, 511
Bratter, T. E., 272
Brenner, B., 255, 371, 421, 436
Brewton, J., 152
Bridwell, N., 316
Brinckloe, J., 222
Brooks, B., 297
Brown, F. G., 276, 284
Brown, L. K., 248, 273, 372
Brown, M. (Marc), 248, 273, 286,
    355, 372, 376, 380, 412,
    421, 430, 467
Brown, M. (Marcia), 70, 77, 231,
    330, 365, 467
Brown, M. M., 185, 238, 496
Brown, M. W., 339, 362, 490
Browne, A., 222, 376, 380, 388,
    430
Browne, D., 271
Brunner, J., 12, 21
Bruun, B., 250, 263, 371
Bruun, R. D., 250, 263, 371
Bryan, A., 327, 362, 370
Bunting, E., 251, 273, 384, 400,
    426, 525–526
Burgess, G., 156
Burnett, F. H., 196, 225, 252,
    372
Burningham, J., 181, 236, 421,
    426, 467, 469

Burns, M., 177, 236, 390, 479
Burton, V. L., 84, 232
Bush, M., 206, 240, 267, 450
Butler, D., 312, 360
Byars, B., 111, 233, 251, 291,
  390, 394, 398, 400, 437,
  443, 450, 456, 493, 516,
  526, 533, 535

Califano, J., 28, 59
Calkins, L., 352
Cameron, A., 266, 372, 376, 384
Carlsen, R., 316, 360
Carlson, J., 351, 362
Carlson, N., 221, 223, 373, 376,
  380, 384, 388, 412, 430
Carr, J., 183, 229
Carroll, L., 157, 342
Cassedy, S., 223, 390, 409, 443
Cavallaro, A., 271, 512
Cesarani, G. P., 186, 239
Chaback, E., 288
Chan, J. M. T., 12, 21
Charlip, R., 153, 160, 235, 286,
  519
Chase, R., 352, 362
Children's Defense Fund, 32
Childress, A., 199, 240, 267, 336,
  362, 409, 414
Chlad, D., 286, 288, 490, 491,
  492
Chorao, K., 351, 362, 373, 422
Christopher, M., 294, 390, 395,
  400–401, 416, 514, 516, 533
Clark, E., 279
Claypool, J., 295, 419
Cleary, B., 101–102, 224, 233,
  251, 294, 376, 398, 401,
  437, 443, 490
Cleaver, B., 336, 362, 438, 450,
  516
Cleaver, V., 224, 336, 362, 401,
  438, 444, 450, 516
Clifford, E., 337, 362, 384, 444,
  496, 536
Coats, L. J., 274

Cobb, V., 248, 269, 414, 467,
  468, 473, 477
Cochran-Smith, M., 322, 360
Coerr, E., 187, 239, 257, 438, 484
Cohen, B., 225, 401, 409
Cohen, L. B., 279
Cohen, M., 336, 362, 515, 523
Cole, J., 170, 172, 219, 220, 236,
  260, 262, 286, 371, 373,
  420, 422, 439
Cole, W., 153, 156, 235, 454, 476
Coleridge, S., 335, 362
Collier, C., 117–118, 234
Collier, J. L., 117–118, 234
Commission on Reading, 210,
  304, 306
Conford, E., 223, 390, 401
Conly, J. L., 325, 362, 507
Conrad, P., 119, 234, 370, 380,
  401, 405, 430, 457, 534
Cooney, B., 124, 234, 298, 430
Corey, D., 282
Cormier, R., 336, 362
Cosgrove, S., 221, 377
Cox, D., 219
Crago, H., 312, 360
Crago, M., 312, 360
Crofford, E., 291, 484, 495
Crutcher, C., 254, 405, 529
Cunningham, J., 249, 384, 385,
  519
Curtis, R. H., 267, 491
Cutchins, J., 222, 298
Cuyler, M., 220, 385, 408, 422,
  478
Cwiklik, R., 280, 367

Danzinger, P., 268, 395, 401, 457
Davis, J., 271, 398, 408, 450, 526
Davis, K., 276
Davis, O., 199, 240, 409
De Angeli, M., 199, 240, 481,
  485, 496
DeClements, B., 111, 223, 224,
  233, 297, 391, 401, 410,
  444, 517

Degen, B., 153, 160, 235, 260, 472
de Jenkins, L. B., 276
Denson, W., 254, 408
dePaola, T., 76, 109, 180, 231, 233, 237, 341, 362, 377, 426, 469, 471, 472, 502
de Regniers, B. S., 197, 240, 265, 381
Dewey, A., 221, 476
Diamond, D., 69, 232
Dickmeyer, L. A., 250, 412
Dines, G., 191, 239, 505
Dobrin, A., 178, 237, 472
Donovan, J., 64, 230
Dragonwagon, C., 165, 237, 278, 381, 420, 422, 429
Drescher, J., 269, 373, 430
Drimmer, F., 255, 522
Drucker, M., 275, 476
Duncan, L., 224, 336, 362
Dunning, S., 133, 235, 454

Eagan, A. B., 272, 462
Edwards, G., 297
Egoff, S., 80, 227
Ehlert, L., 180, 237, 469
Elliott, D., 9, 219
Elting, M., 265
Engdahl, S. L., 87, 232, 449
Ennis, H., 322, 360
Erickson, R. E., 91, 232
Erlanger, E., 179, 237, 479, 480
Esbensen, B., 136, 351, 388
Evans, I., 262
Evernden, M., 298, 521, 529
Ezell, G., 33, 59

Farjeon, E., 145
Faucher, E., 224, 537
Ferris, H., 144, 235
Field, R., 144, 159, 290, 345, 362
Fine, J., 284
Fine, J. C., 280, 477
Finney, S., 300
Fisher, A., 143–144, 235

Fisher, C., 151, 229
Fisher, L. E., 292, 414
Flandermeyer, K. L., 270
Fleishman, P., 292, 414, 449, 457, 517
Flournoy, V., 221, 273, 426, 449
Fodor, R. V., 253, 279, 419, 477, 505
Fontana, V. J., 172
Forbes, E., 118, 234, 517
Forsyth, E. H., 171, 237
Fortunato, P., 288
Fox, M., 351, 362, 373
Fox, P., 126, 234, 295, 362, 395, 398, 444, 457, 462
Francis, C. B., 157
Frank, M., 352
Freedman, R., 186, 239, 366, 420
Freeman, L., 288, 531, 532
Friedman, I. R., 108, 233, 467
Fritz, J., 185, 186–187, 239, 414, 450, 476
Froelich, M. W., 103, 233, 457
Froman, R., 147, 235
Fry, D., 321–322, 323, 360

Gackenbach, D., 198, 240, 377, 385
Gaes, J., 282
Galdone, P., 76, 231, 232, 352, 471, 472
Gammell, S., 105, 234
Gaskin, J., 280
Gates, R., 298
Gay, K., 300
George, J. C., 237, 349, 362, 493, 506, 507
Gerbino, M., 253, 281, 418
Gertz, S., 290
Giblin, J. C., 123, 182, 237, 280, 474
Gilbert, A., 156
Gilbert, C. B., 174
Gilbert, S., 179, 237, 266, 391, 444, 454, 477, 480, 496
Gillespie, J. T., 174
Ginsburg, M., 70, 231, 468

Goble, P., 316
Goodland, J., 211, 229
Goodman, K. N., 33, 59
Gordon, N., 352
Gore, H. M., 287
Gould, D., 248, 372, 373, 523
Grahame, K., 84, 92, 232, 436
Gravelle, K., 285
Gray, N., 265
Green, M., 247, 302
Greenberg, H. R., 276
Greenberg, J., 224, 395, 398,
    450, 463, 465, 485, 521, 526
Greene, G., 16
Greenfeld, H., 347, 362
Greenfield, E., 102, **138**, 139,
    140, 189, 233, 235, 239,
    342, 389, 426, 445, 457–
    458, 515, 519
Greimes, C., 224
Grimm Brothers (J. & W.), 231,
    232, 373, 422, 452
Gunther, J., 326, 362
Guy, R., 251, 297, 405

Haffner, D. W., 356
Hall, D., 124, 234, 431, 468
Hall, K., 157
Hall, L., 103, 233, 255, 391, 405,
    408, 451, 463, 509, 517,
    521, 533
Hamilton, V., 113, 233, 252, 268,
    316, 381, 395, 402, 445,
    503, 521, 528
Hammid, H., 170, 236
Harder, E., 272, 395
Harder, R., 272, 395
Harris, A., 196, 197, 208, 209,
    240, 391, 395, 399, 527
Harris, L., 33, 59
Harris, R., 352, 362, 439
Harvey, B., 119, 120, 125, 234,
    431, 445
Haskins, J., 237, 289, 293, 492,
    493, 519, 523
Hausherr, R., 282
Hautzig, D., 220, 480

Hawkins, C., 219, 381
Hawkins, J., 219, 381
Hayes, B., 225
Hayes, G., 220, 385
Hayes, S., 278, 395
Hazard, P., 62, 227
Hearn, M. P., 157, 235, 471, 474
Hearne, B., 61, 68, 227
Heide, F. P., 290, 345, 362, 377,
    391, 517, 521
Helbig, A., 130, 228
Helgerson, J., 301
Henderson, N., 198, 240, 410
Henkes, K., 221, 250, 373, 422,
    427
Hepler, S., 115, 228
Hermes, P., 223, 224, 326, 362,
    396, 399, 402, 485, 488,
    517, 526, 534, 537
Hest, A., 221, 252, 374, 385,
    427, 431, 445, 452, 471, 526
Hickman, J., 115, 228
Hill, E., 248, 374
Himler, R., 165, 187, 237, 239,
    257
Hines, A. G., 221, 248, 374, 377,
    422, 427, 431, 502
Hinton, S. E., 266, 399, 405, 458,
    493, 498, 499
Hiser, C., 278
Hoban, L., 155, 351, 362, 363,
    366, 385
Hoban, R., 89, 155, 156, 232,
    235, 422, 467
Hoberman, M. A., 158, 159, 470
Holden, J., 336
Holl, K. D., 266, 391, 402, 441,
    451, 526
Holland, I., 295, 415, 455, 465,
    477, 498, 529
Holloran, P., 350–351
Holman, F., 136, 147, **148**, 235,
    289, 336, 363, 402, 405, 493
Hoover, H. M., 87, 232, 300
Hopkins, L. B., 134, 136, 156,
    220, 228, 235, 265, 386,
    507, 529
Hotze, S., 268, 402, 405

Howe, J., 250, 291, 381, 402, 414
Hubbard, K., 288
Huck, C. S., 6, 21, 115, 228, 532
Hughes, B., 285
Hughes, L., 133, 134, 142, 143, 235, 251, 402
Hughes, M., 285, 478, 509
Hughes, T., 134
Hunt, E. T., 134
Hunt, M. A., 135
Hunt, M. L., 191, 239, 511
Hurwitz, J., 222, 377, 396, 402, 441, 458
Hutchins, P., 250, 363, 370, 423, 471, 494
Hutton, W., 223, 352, 363, 396
Hyde, M. O., 167, 171, 237, 297, 391, 458, 486, 494, 498, 504, 532, 533, 537
Hyland, B., 224, 485
Hyman, T. S., 73, 232
Hymes, J. L., 158
Hymes, L., 158

Irwin, H., 224, 533, 537
Isenberg, B., 269, 413

Jackson, L. A., 351, 363, 487, 512
Jacobs, F., 156, 484, 487, 512
Jacobs, H. H., 253, 419
Jacobs, J., 158, 232
Jaffe, M., 269
Jance, J. A., 294, 532
Janeczko, P. B., 276, 280, 336, 363, 391, 406, 455
Jarrell, R., 70, 232
Jennings, C. A., 197, 240, 449
John, B. A., 285
Johnson, E. W., 165–166, 170, 237, 254, 276, 439–440, 486
Johnson, P., Jr., 156
Johnston, G., 222, 298, 391
Jones, J. L., 225

Kalina, S., 263
Keller, H. (Helen), ix

Keller, H. (Holly), 223, 423, 427, 524
Kelley, A., 291, 488
Kellogg, S., 298, 377
Kennedy, X. J., 156
Kenny, K., 294, 489
Kent, J., 221, 316, 413, 432
Kerr, M. E., 112, 233, 406, 465, 517
Kerrod, R., 301
Kessler, L., 269, 492
Kettelkamp, L., 263, 488
Khalsa, D. K., 337, 363, 449
Kheridian, D., 190, 239, 445
Kibbey, M., 282, 427, 517
Kitzinger, S., 164–165, 168, 237, 420
Klass, D., 253, 418, 529
Kleeberg, I. C., 275, 374
Knudson, R. R., 187, 239, 250, 253, 270, 402, 413, 417, 419
Kolbe, L. J., 8, 20, 29–31, 35, 59
Kolodny, N. J., 255, 272, 406, 480
Kolodny, R. C., 255, 272, 405
Konigsburg, E. L., 252, 402, 408, 458
Korschunow, I., 222, 396, 537
Kosof, A., 254, 458, 535
Kozuszek, J. E., 271
Kral, B., 204, 206, 208, 240, 451, 520, 536
Kramer, S., 262
Kraus, J. H., 196, 207, 240, 396, 410, 411, 520
Kraus, R., 222, 336, 363, 382, 423
Krementz, J., 66, 230, 237, 411, 417, 429, 441, 458, 475, 528, 536
Krensky, S., 182, 237, 286
Kroeber, T., 254, 408
Krull, H., 294
Kuklin, S., 248, 269, 290, 411, 441, 465, 487, 513
Kumin, M. W., 157
Kuskin, K., 133, 136, 145, **146**, 159, 235, 451
Kyte, K. S., 251, 289, 292, 402, 438

629

Lambert, M., 285, 300, 301
Landau, E., 172, 237, 482, 483
Lang, A., 352, 363
Langone, J., 237, 406, 455, 465, 538
Langton, J., 265
Lasker, J., 124, 234, 432, 514
Lasky, K., 166, 237, 374, 420, 423, 427, 474, 526, 535
Lattimore, D., 278, 377
Lauber, P., 237, 366, 371, 507
Laurie, R., 196, 240, 432
Leaf, M., 287
Leder, J. M., 417, 538
Leiner, K., 296
L'Engle, M., 252, 485, 493, 521
Lenski, L., 157
Lerner, E. A., 167, 237, 483
LeShan, E., 237, 266, 374, 392, 402, 441, 446, 528
LeSieg, T., 260, 366
Lesser, R., 231
Lester, H., 220, 382, 386
Lester, J., 327, 363
Leuders, E., 133, 235
Levine, S., 272
Levy, E., 293, 455, 526
Lewis, N., 271
Lewis, R., 271, 378, 389
Lexau, J., 337, 363, 382
Lindberg, J., 285
Lindgren, A., 64, 231, 378, 396, 423
Lindon, J. A., 157
Lionni, L., 350, 363, 374, 378, 386
Lipsyte, R., 111, 233
Liss, H., 224, 465
Lister, C., 262
Little, L. J., 189, 239
Littledale, F., 221
Living Stage Theatre Company, 208, 240, 538
Livingston, M. C., 134, 156, 159, 232, 235, 236, 250, 316, 432, 474, 508
Lloyd, D., 221, 504
Lobel, A., 90–91, 149, 157–158,
232, 235, 249, 329, 341, 363
Lopshire, R., 220, 378
Lowry, L., 102, 103, 223, 225, 234, 396, 408, 423, 446, 451, 494, 527
Lukens, R., 83, 137, 227
Lukes, B. L., 179, 237, 281
Lysander, P., 207, 240, 459
Lyttle, R. B., 272, 419

McCaslin, N., 197, 378, 432, 449
McClure, A. A., 136, 152, 228, 312, 360
McCoy, J. J., 190, 239, 488, 511
McCoy, K., 276
McCullers, C., 156
McCully, E. A., 88, 232, 423, 427
McDonnell, C., 252, 386
McFann, J., 225, 499
McGinley, P., 133
McGinnis, J. M., vii, 35, 59
McKissack, P., 327, 363, 382
McKoy, K., 276, 465
MacLachlan, P., 248, 351, 363, 374, 427, 429, 432, 436, 451, 455, 481, 515
McLoughlin, J. C., 271
McMillan, B., 180, 237, 470, 474
McPhail, O., 248, 370, 423, 433
McPhee, J., 164
Madaras, L., 272, 275, 285, 463
Madison, A., 296, 392, 536
Mails, T. E., 293
Mandry, K., 155, 235
Manes, S., 225, 374, 477
Manna, A. L., 10, 21, 38, 60
Marek, M., 225, 504, 511
Margolis, R. J., 220, 423
Marino, B. P., 290, 495
Marshall, J., 89–90, 232, 386
Martin, A. M., 224, 382, 396, 402, 432, 446, 453, 459, 518, 530
Martin, B., Jr., 219, 222, 366, 382, 423, 437, 515

Martin, C. E., 287, 495
Martin, J., 197, 378, 446, 449
Martin, L., 177, 237, 473, 504
Martin, P. M., 197–198, 240,
    396, 482
Martin, R., 248, 374
Martin, T., 297
Martinez, M., 323–324, 360
Maruki, T., 64, 231, 504
Mathis, S. B., 341, 363, 446, 465,
    518, 522
Matthews, D., 253, 418
Mayer, M., 341, 363, 503
Mayle, P., 275, 420
Mazer, N. F., 223, 392, 399, 403,
    459, 499, 530
Meltzer, M., 118, 237
Meredith, G., 152
Merriam, E., 130, 131, 133, 159,
    235
Merrill, J., 86, 233
Metropolitan Life Foundation, 19,
    33–34
Middleton, K., 27, 59
Miklowitz, G. D., 257, 285, 494,
    535, 537
Miles, B., 263, 406, 506
Millay, E., 326
Miller, J., 168, 237, 262, 275,
    370
Miller, K. S., 208, 240, 392, 406,
    449, 527
Miller, M., 223, 403
Miller, R., 224
Minarik, E., 91, 386, 423, 437
Moe, J. E., 231, 352, 362
Moeri, L., 289, 446, 492, 504,
    535
Monjo, F. N., 185, 187, 188, 239,
    433
Morimoto, J., 250, 370
Morris, W., 223, 392, 408, 392,
    408
Morrison, L., 139, 235, 417
Mosel, A., 231, 337
Moss, J. F., 327, 340, 361
Mueller, E., 340
Musil, R. G., 207, 240, 433

Myers, W. D., 251, 296, 403, 429,
    459, 466

Nash, B., 253, 418
Nash, O., 157, 158
Natarella, M., 151, 229
Nathan, J., 278
National Center for Health Edu-
    cation, 39, 255
National Center for Health Statis-
    tics, 258
National Committee for the Pre-
    vention of Child Abuse, 258
National Education Association,
    35–36
Naylor, P. R., 225, 392–393, 406,
    424, 447, 451, 453, 459,
    494, 509, 530
Neff, F., 269
Negri, R., 185, 239
Newman, S., 297, 492
Newsome, M. E. L., 156
Nilsson, L., 164–165, 168, 237,
    275, 285, 424
Noble, I., 263, 447, 494
Noble, T. K., 336, 363
Nolan, P. T., 195, 240
Norman, J., 268
Nourse, A. E., 237, 263, 292,
    440, 464, 466, 479, 483,
    484, 487, 488, 493

O'Brien, R. C., 81, 85, 95–96,
    233, 494
Older, J., 287
Oliver, M., 336
Olsen, J. T., 293, 417
Oneal, Z., 254, 407
Ontario Science Centre, 177, 237,
    278, 336, 363
Orlev, U., 127–128, 234, 363,
    447
Osten, S., 207, 240
Ostrow, V., 284
Ostrow, W., 284
Oxenbury, H., 260, 290

Park, B., 223, 393, 399, 403, 407, 408, 442, 451, 453
Parks, L.-C., 335
Patent, D., 284, 370, 468, 483, 506
Patterson, L., 188, 239, 271, 497
Patz, N., 155, 236
Paulsen, G., 252, 289, 350, 363, 393, 460, 530
Payne, S. N., 282, 481, 514
Pearson-Davis, S., 198, 240, 375, 387, 427, 503
Peavy, L., 188, 239, 397
Peet, B., 222, 298, 382
Pelham, D., 168, 237, 262, 275, 370
Perl, L., 181–182, 237, 281, 466, 479, 497
Perrine, L., 129, 137, 142, 228
Perry, N., 12–13
Petersen, P. J., 289, 408
Petras, J. W., 172, 236
Philips, L., 156
Phillips, L., 270
Phipson, J., 289, 407, 522, 527
Pinkwater, D. M., 93–94, 219, 233, 378, 407, 474
Pogo, vii
Pollock, M., 27, 59
Pomerantz, C., 160, 236, 273, 427
Potter, B., 84, 88, 178, 196, 233, 240
Powledge, F., 254, 407
Prelutsky, J., 133, 142, 158–159, 220, 236, 336, 340, 363, 375, 382
Pringle, L., 238, 300, 301, 478, 479, 504, 506, 507, 510, 528
Proddow, P., 280
Pryor, B., 219, 378, 399, 516

Quackenbush, M., 356
Quackenbush, R., 220

Rabe, B., 282, 485
Radley, G., 103, 234, 486, 489, 522, 536

Ranahan, D. C., 190, 239, 497
Ray, D. K., 119, 234, 433
Readers Theatre Script Service, 278, 336, 363
Reit, S., 269, 290, 378
Rench, J. E., 171, 238, 440, 466
Rich, A., 336
Richmond, S., 289, 522
Rickman, I., 289
Riddell, C., 219
Rinkoff, B., 287
Robbins, R., 101
Roberts, W. D., 266, 375, 460, 533
Robinette, J., 209, 240, 397
Rockwell, A., 238, 468, 475, 491, 495
Rockwell, H., 238, 411
Rockwell, T., 196, 240, 399
Rodgers, M., 86, 233
Rogasky, B., 73, 232, 440
Rogers, A., 232
Roos, A., 352, 363
Rosenberg, E., 275
Roser, N., 323–324, 360
Ross, M. L., 207, 240, 453
Rothman, J., 260
Rousseau, J.-J., 242, 302
Routman, R., 312–313, 360
Roy, R., 105, 234, 284, 399, 407, 429, 482, 486, 519
Ryan, E. A., 252, 498
Rylant, C., 10, 21, 190, 225, 234, 239, 250, 251, 252, 268, 337, 351, 363, 387, 397, 408, 428, 433, 434, 440, 442, 448, 451, 464, 527

Sabin, F., 282
Sachar, L., 225, 393, 397, 404
Sacks, M., 225, 393, 451, 460, 464, 480, 527
Sadler, M., 222, 223, 378
Saltzberg, B., 221, 382, 393
Sanchez, G. J., 253, 281, 418
Sandberg, I., 17, 22
Sandberg, L., 17, 22

Sanders, S., 335, 363
Sargent, B., 223
Sawyer, R., 232
Schlesinger, A., 228
Schmitt, L., 293
Schneider, H., 252, 494
Schneider, T., 271
Schoor, G., 190, 239, 489
Schwarzrock, S., 17, 22
Sebesta, S. L., 216, 218, 230
Seixas, J. S., 176, 238, 280, 284,
    290, 294, 296, 345, 363,
    470, 498
Selden, G., 84, 233
Selsam, M., 169, 180, 181, 238,
    421, 468, 471, 478, 484,
    488, 503
Sendak, M., 5, 64, 81, 91, 161,
    231, 233, 236, 350, 363,
    382, 424, 470, 525
Settel, J., 271
Seuling, B., 263, 489
Seuss, Dr., 85–86, 231, 233, 299,
    472, 501
Seward, B., 335
Seward, S. A., 331
Shannon, P., 305, 308, 359
Sharmat, M., 248, 278, 379, 382,
    383, 387, 434, 467
Shaw, C. G., 336, 363
Shaw, D., 268, 466
Shiels, B., 190, 239, 496
Shorto, R., 252, 280
Showers, P., 11, 22, 238, 260,
    261, 283, 367, 369, 412,
    421, 424, 434, 501
Shreve, N., 275
Shulevitz, U., 66, 231
Silverstein, A., 66, 170, 171, 231,
    238, 250, 262, 270, 336,
    367, 369, 412, 419, 460,
    466, 481, 483, 484, 487,
    488, 513
Silverstein, S., 136, 158, 159,
    236, 316, 336, 363, 387, 393
Silverstein, V. B., 66, 170, 171,
    231, 238, 250, 262, 270,
    336, 367, 369, 412, 419,

460, 466, 481, 483, 484,
    487, 488, 513
Simon, N. (Nissa), 250, 272, 464
Simon, N. (Norma), 265, 274,
    383, 389, 429, 434, 524, 525
Simon, S., 250, 262, 368, 369,
    371, 415, 477
Siska, H. S., 110, 238
Smalley, W., 204, 240, 508
Smaridge, N., 157, 278, 336, 363
Smith, D. B., 66, 231, 252, 393,
    397, 404, 442, 448, 460,
    518, 527
Smith, H., 133, 235
Smith, J., 220, 387
Smith, L., 65, 227
Smith, U., 188, 239
Smith, W. J., 236
Sneve, V. D. H., 265
Snyder, C., 224, 393, 407
Snyder, Z. K., 249, 297, 375,
    404, 448
Sobol, H. L., 181, 238, 274, 429,
    442, 470, 478, 491, 514
Spier, P., 265
Springer, N., 224, 393, 397, 399,
    404
Stanek, L. W., 225, 410
Starbird, K., 156, 342
Steel, F. A., 232
Steig, W., 265, 375, 434, 495
Steinbeck, J., 326, 363
Steptoe, J., 223, 252, 387, 424,
    453
Stevens, J., 225, 410
Stevenson, J., 222, 375, 383, 387,
    424, 428, 434
Still, J., 209, 231, 240, 387
Stine, J., 267
Stine, J. B., 267
Stock, C., 248, 470
Stock, G., 251, 404
Stott, J., 327
Strasser, T., 253, 285, 400, 409,
    418
Strete, C. K., 274
Strieber, W., 301, 350
Sullivan, G., 189

Supree, B., 153, 160, 235, 286
Sutherland, Z., 65, 98, 99–100,
134, 159, 186, 227, 232,
236
Swenson, M., 270
Swift, H. H., 190–191, 239, 507
Symons, C. W., 38, 60. *See also*
Wolford, C. A.

Tashjian, V., 231, 232
Taylor, G. J., 253, 419
Taylor, P., 292, 294
Tchudi, S., 281, 301, 415, 479
Terkel, S. N., 171, 238, 413, 456,
534
Terry, A., 151, 229
Terry, M., 207, 240, 448, 500
Thayer, J., 223
Titherington, J., 181, 221, 238,
274, 425, 428, 469
Toto, J., 155, 235
Towle, F., 77, 231
Trait, N., 340
Trease, G., 116, 234
Trelease, J., 63, 162, 227, 229,
303
Trier, C. S., 248, 413
Turner, A., 236, 299, 448, 507
Turner, D., 278, 467, 469
Turner, G. T., 267
Tyler, L. W., 219, 383, 434, 481

UNICEF, 267

Vandenberg, M. L., 288, 490
Vandivert, R., 191, 239, 255,
300, 513
Ventura, P., 186, 239
Vestfals, J., 121–122
Vigna, J., 294, 299, 375, 425,
429, 482, 505
Villarreal, S., 356
Viorst, J., 99, 234, 339, 340, 350,
364, 383, 425, 434, 490, 524
Vogel, I.-M., 103, 234

Voigt, C., 254, 289, 394, 397,
407, 409, 449, 461, 464,
518, 522, 530

Waber, B., 248, 250, 375, 437
Wachter, O., 171, 238, 490, 534
Wahl, J., 223, 375
Walker, B. M., 125, 238, 480
Walker, L. A., 222, 514
Walker, M., 178, 238
Wallner, A., 155, 236
Ward, B. R., 250, 288, 296, 415,
418, 419, 440, 477
Warren, C., 284, 385, 487
Washton, A. W., 296
Watson, C., 137, **138–139**, 236
Watson, W., 137, **138–139**, 159–
160, 236, 379, 490
Waxman, S., 274, 437
Weiss, N., 221, 388, 425, 434
Wells, R., 222, 375, 383, 409,
425
Wersba, B., 99, 112, 234, 400,
461, 464, 480
Wexler, J., 180, 238
White, E. B., 81, 233, 388
White, E. E., 254, 407
Whitley, M. A., 224, 533
Wiesel, E., 127, 228
Wilbur, R., 156
Wilcox, C., 299
Wilcox, K., 272
Wilder, L. I., 120, 125, 234
Wildsmith, B., 350, 364
Wiles, J., 284, 528
Williams, G. B., 300
Williams, M., 85, 233
Williams, V. B., 105, 234, 379,
428, 434
Williams, W. C., 158
Winkel, L., 174
Winther, B., 195, 206, 240, 397,
400, 452
Wise, W., 158, 412
Wisema, B., 219
Wolf, B., 288, 290, 449, 482,
514, 520

Wolfe, B., 292, 411
Wolfe, D., 292, 411
Wolford, C. A., 30, 58, 59
Wolford, M. R., 30
Woods, W., 161
Wrenn, C. G., 17, 22, 500
Wright, B., 325, 364, 449, 486,
    520
Wrightson, P., 87, 233, 479,
    508
Wyndham, R., 70, 231

Yagawa, S., 231
Yolen, J., 82, 87, 98, 231, 327,
    440, 452, 476, 516, 528

Yost, D., 204, 240–241, 498, 534
Young, R., 199, 241, 473

Zeder, S., 197, 198, 209, 241,
    254, 339, 364, 397, 404,
    407, 442, 462
Zemach, M., 76, 232, 250, 376,
    469
Ziefert, H., 219, 220, 376, 425,
    428, 435, 470, 473
Zindel, P., 277, 326, 364, 407, 530
Zolotow, C., 101, 234, 249, 250,
    265, 371, 379, 384, 388,
    397, 425, 435, 437, 524
Zullo, A., 253, 418

Title Index

CONTENTS:

Section A: Children's Literature   635
Section B: Poetry   657
Section C: Book Series   658
Section D: Book Selection Guides   658
Section E: Literacy Training: Reading, Writing, Evaluating   658
Section F: Research Reports and Surveys   659

Notes: Titles cited only in the Annotated Bibliography are not included. Research reports are included only when directly quoted or named in the text.

Section A: Children's Literature

A, My Name Is Ami,   223
Aaron's Shirt,   248, 373
Abby, My Love,   224
About the Foods You Eat,   262
About Your Lungs,   262
Adventures in Babysitting,   224
Afraid to Ask: A Book for Families to Share About Cancer,   284
After Covering the Continent,   154
After the Goat Man,   111, 233
The Agony of Alice,   225
AIDS: Deadly Threat,   170, 171, 238
AIDS: What Does It Mean to You?   171, 237
Alan Alda: An Unauthorized Biography,   190, 238
Albert the Running Bear's Exercise Book,   269
Alcohol—What It Is, What It Does,   294
Alcohol and You,   295
Alexander and the Terrible, Horrible, No Good, Very Bad Day,   99, 234, 350, 364

Alexander's Midnight Snack,   248, 470
All About Asthma,   284
All About Eggs,   169, 238
All Kinds of Families,   274
All Together,   142
Almost Fifteen,   225
Alone at Home: A Kid's Guide to Being in Charge,   288
Altogether, One at a Time,   252, 402
Always and Forever Friends,   249, 384
Always Faithful,   225
The American Revolutionaries,   118, 237
American Sports Poems,   253, 270, 419
Amy: The Story of a Deaf Child,   222
Anansi and the Old Hag,   327
Anansi's Hat-Shaking Dance,   327
Anastasia, Ask Your Analyst,   223
Anastasia Krupnik,   102, 234
And I Heard a Bird Sing,   254, 405
And Then What Happened, Paul Revere?   121, 239
Androcles and the Lion,   196, 209, 240
Andy Bear: A Polar Bear Cub Grows Up at the Zoo,   222
Angel Dust Blues,   253, 418
Anna Banana and Me,   222
Anthony Burns: The Defeat and Triumph of a Fugitive Slave,   268
Apologies,   208, 240
The Apple and Other Fruits,   180, 239
Apples, How They Grow,   180, 237
The Arkansaw Bear,   208, 240
Arthur's Loose Tooth,   351, 362
Arthur's Pen Pal,   351, 363
The Artichoke,   157
Artichokes,   156
The Ash Lad Who Had an Eating Match With the Troll,   70, 231
At the Top of My Voice and Other Poems,   147–148, 235
Attila the Pun,   93, 233
Aunt Roberta,   138–139

Babe Didrikson: The World's Greatest Woman Athlete,   190, 239
A Baby for Max,   166–167, 237
A Baby Sitter for Frances,   89, 232
Back to School,   143–144
The Baker's Boy,   156
Barber Bear,   219
A Bargain for Frances,   89, 232
Basic for Better Living,   133
Beanpole,   223
A Bear Called Paddington,   200–203, 204, 232

Bear in There, 159
Bear's Picture, 219
Beauty and the Beast. (Apy, D.), 70, 231
Beauty and the Beast. (Harris, R.), 327, 352, 362
Beauty and the Beast. (Hutton, W.), 223
Beaver Moon—The Suicide of a Friend, 336
Bedtime for Frances, 89, 232
Behind the Attic Wall, 223
Being Born, 164–165, 168, 237
Being Greedy Chokes Anansi, 70, 231
Benjie, 337, 363
The Berenstain Bears Visit the Dentist, 248, 411
Best Friends, 220, 265
Better Known as Johnny Appleseed, 191, 239
Better Physical Fitness for Girls, 253, 419
Betty Botter Bought Some Butter, 150, 158
Bicycles, 287
The Big Mile Race, 269
The Big Red Barn, 273
Biology, 262
Bird's New Shoes, 219
The Birds of Summer, 297
A Birthday for Frances, 89, 232
The Birthday of the Infanta, 196
Black Out Loud: An Anthology of Modern Poems by Black Americans, 340, 361
Blimp, 271
Blow Wind Blow! and Go Mill Go! 150
A Blue-Eyed Daisy, 225
Body Maintenance, 250, 419
Body Sense, Body Nonsense, 250, 371
The Body Victorious, 285
Bodyworks, 178–179, 236
Bodyworks: The Kids' Guide to Food and Physical Fitness, 270
Bon Appetit, Mr. Rabbit! 223
A Book of Vegetables, 181, 238
Books, 331
Books from Writer to Reader, 347, 362
Born Different, 255, 522
Bossyboots, 219
The Boy from Over There, 266
The Boy Who Stole the Stars, 284
The Boy Who Talked to Whales, 204, 240
The Brain—What It Is, What It Does, 263
Bread, 278
Bread and Jam for Frances, 89, 232
Breakfast, Books, and Dreams, 157, 235
Breakfast With My Father, 105–106, 234

Bummer Summer,   224, 396
The Bun: A Tale from Russia,   70, 77, 231
The Burg-O-Rama Man,   281
But I'll Be Back Again,   190, 239, 252
The Butter Battle Book,   86, 231
By the Shores of Silver Lake,   125, 234

Can You Sue Your Parents for Malpractice?   268
The Cancer Lady: Maud Slye and Her Heredity Studies,   190, 239
Carrots and Kings,   280
The Cat Strikes Back,   347
Celebrating Life: Jewish Rites of Passage,   275
A Celebration of Bees,   351
Celery,   158
CF in His Corner,   103, 234
The Chalk Doll,   273
The Challenger,   121–122
Changing Bodies, Changing Lives,   276
Charles Drew,   352, 362
Charlotte's Web,   81, 209, 233, 240
The Checkup,   290
Chicken Soup with Rice,   161, 236, 350, 363
Child of the Silent Night,   190
Children and the AIDS Virus,   282
Children, Children Everywhere,   158
Children of Morrow,   300
Children Talk about Books,   321
The Children's Jewish Holiday Kitchen,   278
Children's Plays from Beatrix Potter,   196, 240
A Child's Chorus,   267
Childtimes: A Three-Generation Memoir,   189–190, 239
Chocolate,   140–141
Chocolate Cake,   199
Chocolate Dreams,   279
The Chocolate War,   336, 362
Christopher Columbus,   186, 239
A Circle Unbroken,   268
Clara Barton, Founder of the American Red Cross,   352, 362
Class Clown,   222
Clear Skin: A Step-by-Step Program to Stop Pimples, Blackheads,
    Acne,   270
Close to Home,   171, 238
Cocaine and Crack,   296
Come On, Patsy,   249
Conservation,   298
The Consumer Movement,   293
Consumer Protection Labs,   292

Contemporary Women Scientists of America, 263
A Contest, 282
Contributions of Women: Medicine, 190, 239
Cookies, 90–91
Cooking the Italian Way, 178, 236
Cookout Night, 155
Coping with Drug Abuse, 297
The Corn in the Rock, 69, 231
Corn is Maize, 181, 236
A Country Far Away, 265
Crack: The New Drug Epidemic, 297
Crack and Cocaine, 271
The Crack-of-Dawn Walkers, 221
The Crane Wife, 70, 231
The Crazy Horse Electric Game, 254, 405
The Cricket in Times Square, 84, 233
The Crocodile and the Crane, 298
Crunch and Lick, 159
Cry Softly! The Story of Child Abuse, 171, 237
Cuts, Breaks, Bruises, and Burns, 286

Daddy Makes the Best Spaghetti, 221
Dancer in the Mirror, 223
The Dancing Granny, 327, 362
Dancing Tepees: Poems of American Indian Youth, 265
Dandelion, 197
The Dark Bright Water, 87, 233
Dawn, 66, 231
The Day, 346
The Day Jimmy's Boa Ate the Wash, 336, 363
The Day Our TV Broke Down, 325, 364
The Dead Bird, 339, 362
Dead End: A Book About Suicide, 237
Dear Doctor, 272
Dear Mr. Henshaw, 251, 401
Death Be Not Proud, 326, 362
Death Is Natural, 238
Deep River Run, 190, 239
Delmore's Brainstorm, 252, 367
Demeter and Persephone, 280
Different, Not Dumb, 225
A Different Season, 253, 418
Dinky Hocker Shoots Smack, 112, 233
Dinosaurs, Beware! A Safety Guide, 286
Dinosaurs Divorce, 248, 273, 372
Dirge Without Music, 326
The Disappearance, 297

The Disease Fighters,   238, 283
Do Not Weep Little One,   134
Dogs & Dragons, Trees & Dreams,   146
Don't Panic! A Book about Handling Emergencies,   287
Don't Worry, You're Normal,   272
The Door in the Wall,   199–200, 240
The Doorbell Rang,   363
Doors,   198, 339, 364
Double Trouble,   224
Downwind,   289
Dramatic Literature for Children: A Century in Review,   196, 240
The Dream Keeper and Other Poems,   251, 402
Dreams into Deeds: Nine Women Who Dared,   239
Drug Abuse: The Impact on Society,   297
Drug-Related Diseases,   285
Drugs and Drug Abuse,   296
Drugs and You,   296

The Earth Is Sore: Native Americans on Nature,   300, 335, 362
The Earth Then and Now,   335
East of the Sun and West of the Moon. (Kral, B.),   206, 240
East of the Sun and West of the Moon, and Other Tales,   231, 352, 362
Eat Up, Gemma,   278
Eating,   280
Eating Disorders,   179, 237
Eat-It-All Elaine,   156, 342
Eats,   140–141, 153, 154, 235
The Effects of Gamma Rays on Man-in-the-Moon Marigolds,   277
Egg Thoughts and Other Frances Songs,   155, 235
Eggs,   278
Eleanor Farjeon's Poems for Children,   145
Emergency Room,   292
Emotional Illness in Your Family,   276
English Fairy Tales,   232
The Enormous Genie,   70, 231
Environmental Diseases,   300
Eric Needs Stitches,   290
Ernie's Little Lie,   219
Escape to Freedom,   199, 240
Escape to King Alfred,   234
Evan's Corner,   248, 374
Everybody's a Winner: A Kid's Guide to New Sports and Fitness,   271
The Excretory System: How Animals Get Rid of Waste,   262
Exercise: What It Is, What It Does,   248, 413

Facts and Fantasies About Smoking, 17, 22
The Facts of Life, 169, 237, 275, 370
Family Secrets: Five Very Important Stories, 275
Family Talk, 207, 240
The Far Side of Evil, 87, 232
The Farmer in the Soup, 221
Fat, A Love Story, 113, 234
Fat Free: Common Sense Guide for Young Weight Worriers, 179, 237
Fat Men from Space, 93, 233
Father Fox's Pennyrhymes, 137–138, 159–160, 236
Father Loses Weight, 156
Father William, 342
Favorite Folktales From Around the World, 231, 440
Favorite Poems Old and New, 144, 235
Feeling Safe, Feeling Strong, 171–172, 238
Finding a Poem, 133, 235
Firehouse, 288
First Aid, 288
The First Four Years, 125, 234
First Kiss, 336
First Snow, 89, 232
Fish is Fish, 350, 363
The Five Hundred Hats of Bartholomew Cubbins, 86, 233
Five Little Peppers, 207, 240
Flossie and the Fox, 327, 363
Folk Tale Plays Round the World, 195, 240
Foodworks, 177, 237, 278, 336–337, 363
Foolish Ones, 198
Foolish Rabbit's Big Mistake, 248, 374
Fool's Crow, 293
The Foundling Fox, 222
Fourth Floor Twins. (series), 316
Freaky Friday, 86, 233
Freckles and Willy: A Valentine's Day Story, 220
Fresh Cider and Pie, 160, 235
The Friendly Cinnamon Bun, 156
Friends Are Like That, 223
Friends Till the End, 285
Frog and Toad Are Friends, 249
Frog and Toad Together, 90, 232, 329, 341, 363
The Frog Prince, 327
From Hand to Mouth: Or, How We Invented Knives, Forks, Spoons, & Chopsticks, & the Table Manners to Go with Them, 123–124, 182, 237, 280
From Soup to Nuts, 156
From the Eagle's Wing: A Biography of Jon Muir, 190–191, 239, 507

Frontier Surgeons: A Story About the Mayo Brothers, 291
The Funny Little Woman, 70, 77, 231
The Future for the Environment, 300
Future Sources of Energy, 301

General Store, 290, 345, 362
Germs! 284
Germy Blew It, 225
Get Help: Solving the Problems of Your Life, 266
Get Well, Clown Arounds! 220
Getting Oxygen, 262
The Ghost-Eye Tree, 222
The Gingerbread Boy, 77, 231
The Girl With the Crazy Brother, 224
Going for the Big One, 289
Going Over to Your Place, 336, 363
The Good Food Book, 176–177, 236
Good for Me! 176, 236
Good-bye, Chicken Little, 251, 400
Goodbye House, 221, 372
Goodbye, Max, 223
Good-Bye Tomorrow, 257, 285
Grand Papa and Ellen Aroon, Being an Account of Some of the Happy
    Times Spent Together by Thomas Jefferson and His Favorite Grand-
    daughter, 187–188, 239
Grandma Ida's Cookie Dough for Apple Pie Crust, 154
Grandpa Bear, 219
Grandpa Had a Windmill, Grandma Had a Churn, 351, 363
The Great Giant Watermelon Birthday, 105, 234
The Great Mom Swap, 225
The Green Machine and the Frog Crusade, 301
Gregory, the Terrible Eater, 248, 278
Grover and the New Kid, 220
Growing Older, 187, 238
Growing Strong, 253, 419
Growing Up Feeling Good, 275
Growing Vegetable Soup, 180–181, 237
The Growth of the Potato, 181, 238

Hannah Bantry, 158
Hans in Luck, 70, 231
Hansel and Gretel, 69, 74, 231, 249, 373
Happy Birthday, Sam, 250, 370
Happy Birthday To Me, 238
Harriet Tubman, 342
Harry Takes a Bath, 220

Hat, 221
Hatchet, 252, 289
Hattie, Tom, and the Chicken Witch, 198–199, 240
Hear the Wind Blow, 335, 363
Heartbeats: Your Body, Your Heart, 66, 262
The Hedgehog Boy, 265
Help: Emergencies That Could Happen to You and How to Handle Them, 288
Help Yourself to Safety, 288
Henry and Mudge and the Forever Sea, 250, 433
Here Are My Hands, 219
Here We Go Round the Mulberry Bush, 150
Hereditary Disease, 284
A Hero Ain't Nothin' But a Sandwich, 335–336, 362
Heron Street, 299
Hiroshima No Pika, 64, 231
History in Poetry, 121
Hit and Run, 289
Holy Secrets, 271
Homeward the Arrow's Flight, 185, 238
Honey, I Love, 138–140, 235
The Honorable Prison, 276
Hormones, 263
A Horse to Love, 224
The Hospital Book, 250, 291
The Hospitals, 292
The Hot Pizza Serenade, 156
How a Book Is Made, 347, 362
How Do You Lose Those Ninth Grade Blues? 111, 223, 233
How It Feels When a Parent Dies, 66, 230
How It Feels When Parents Divorce, 66, 230, 237
How Many Teeth? 260
How My Parents Learned to Eat, 108–109, 233
How the Peasant Helped His Horse, 70, 231
How to Be a Reasonably Thin Teenage Girl, 179, 237, 281
How to Eat a Poem, 130–131
How to Eat a Poem and Other Morsels, 130–131, 155–156, 235
How to Eat Fried Worms, 196, 240
How to Live with Your Parents Without Losing Your Mind, 276
How to Make Elephant Bread, 155, 235
How You Were Born, 170, 236
The Human Body, 262, 370
The Human Body: How We Evolved, 262
The Human Body: Your Body and How It Works, 250, 263, 371
The Hundred Penny Box, 341, 342, 363
The Hunger Road, 280
Hungry Mungry, 159
Hunter in the Dark, 285

Hunter's Stew and Hangtown Fry: What Pioneer America Ate and
    Why,   182, 238
Hurricane Watch,   335, 362
Hygiene,   271

I Am the Running Girl,   250, 416
I Ate a Ton of Sugar,   156
I Can, I See, and I Hear,   260
I Do Not Like Thee, Doctor Fell,   150
I Eat My Peas with Honey,   158
I Must Remember,   159
I Raised a Great Hulabaloo,   158
I Saw a Ship A-Sailing,   149
I Touch,   260
I Want to Be Big,   248
I Want to Be Somebody New,   220
I Wish Daddy Didn't Drink So Much,   294
I Woke Up This Morning,   133, 145–146
I Wouldn't Be Afraid,   340
The Ice Is Coming,   87, 233
The Ice Wolf,   196
If All the World Was Paper,   156
If This Is Love, I'll Take Spaghetti,   223
I'll Get There, It Better Be Worth the Trip,   64, 230
I'm Deaf and It's Okay,   339–340, 362
I'm Hungry,   158
I'm in a Rotten Mood!   133
Immigrant Girl,   119, 234
In a Room Somewhere,   254, 407
In Charge: A Complete Handbook for Kids with Working Parents,   251,
    402
The Inch Boy,   250, 370
The Inventors: Nobel Prizes in Chemistry, Physics and Medicine,   190,
    238, 252, 484
An Invitation to Supper,   197–198
Ira Says Goodbye,   250, 375
Ira Sleeps Over,   248, 375, 437
Is Anybody Hungry?   154–155, 235
Is Anybody There?   251, 400
Ishi: Last of His Tribe,   254, 408
The Island on Bird Street,   127–128, 234, 340, 363
Island Rescue,   287
It Ain't All for Nothin',   251, 296
It Could Always Be Worse,   250, 376
It Doesn't Always Have to Rhyme,   235
It Looked Like Spilt Milk,   336, 363
It's a Baby,   169, 236

It's Not Easy Being a Bunny, 222
It's Raining, It's Pouring, the Old Man Is Snoring, 150
Izzy, Willy-Nilly, 254, 289

Jack and Jill Went Up the Hill, 150
Jack and the Beanstalk, 70. *See also* Jack and the Wonder Beans
Jack and the Northwest Wind, 352, 362
Jack and the Wonder Beans, 231
Jack Sprat, 158
The Jack Tales, 362
Jamberry, 153, 160, 235
Jamboree: Rhymes for All Times, 130
January Brings the Snow, 335, 362
Jenny's in the Hospital, 269
Jimmy's Boa Bounces Back, 336
Jingle Jangle Jingle, 278, 336, 363
Joey Runs Away, 221
John Muir, 191, 239
Johnny Appleseed, 298
Johnny Cash, 294
Johnny May Grows Up, 224, 255, 279
Johnny Pye and the Footkiller, 208, 240
Johnny Tremain, 118, 234
Journey Behind the Wind, 87, 233
Journey Cake Ho! 232
Julie of the Wolves, 349, 362
Junk Food—What It Is, What It Does, 280
Junk Food, Fast Food, Health Food: What America Eats and Why, 237,
    281

Keeping Clean, 248, 269, 407
Keeping in Shape, 271
Keepsake, 138
Kevin Corbett Eats Flies, 224
The Kids' Book of Questions, 251, 404
The Kids' Complete Guide to Money, 292
A Kid's Guide to First Aid, 288
The Kids' Whole Future Catalog, 292
Killing Mr. Griffin, 336, 362
Kimchi Kid, 207, 240
A Kindness, 268
The King of Ireland's Son, 70, 231
The King of the Golden River, 298
The King Who Loved Lollipops, 279
Know About Smoking, 171, 237

Lackawanna, 127, 234
The Lad Who Went to the North Wind, 70, 231
The Language of Goldfish, 254, 407
Latchkey Kid, 275
Laughing Time, 236
The Lawrence Taylor Story, 224
Lawyers for the People: A New Breed of Defenders and Their
  Work, 293
Learning About Sexual Abuse, 172, 236
The Leaving, 255, 408
The Leftover Kid, 224
Lemonade, 199
Lenses, Spectacles, Eyeglasses, and Contacts, 291
Leo the Late Bloomer, 336, 363
Life Is Not Fair, 225
Life Without Friends, 254, 407
A Light in the Attic, 159, 236
Lincoln: A Photobiography, 239
Listen to the Mustn'ts, 336
Little Bear, 205, 240
Little Chef Series, 177–178, 237
Little Hoo, 198
The Little House, 84, 232
Little House Cookbook, 125–126, 178, 238
Little House in the Big Woods, 125, 234
Little House on the Prairie, 125, 234
A Little Love, 113–114, 233
Little Miss Muffet, 150
The Little Princess, 196
Little Red Riding Hood, 69, 70, 231
A Little Time, 282
Little Town on the Prairie, 125, 234
The Little Wood Duck, 350, 364
Lives at Stake, 301
The Living Cell, 262
Living in a Risky World, 300
Living with a Parent Who Drinks Too Much, 284
Living with a Parent Who Takes Drugs, 296
Locked in Time, 224
Look At Your Eyes, 261
The Lorax, 299
The Louisa May Alcott Cookbook, 178, 236
Love and Sex in Plain Language, 165–166, 170, 237, 254, 276
Love Is the Crooked Thing, 113, 234
Lucky Charms & Birthday Wishes, 252, 386
Lunch, 157
Lynda Madaras' Growing Up Guide for Girls, 272
Lynda Madaras Talks to Teens about AIDS, 285

M. C. Higgins, the Great, 252, 503
Ma and the Kids, 197
The Macmillan Book of the Human Body, 265
The Magic Cooking Pot, 77, 231
The Magic Moscow, 93–94, 233
The Magic Pear Tree, 70, 231
The Magic Porridge Pot, 77, 231
The Magic School Bus Inside the Human Body, 260
The Magic Spell, 197
Make the Most of a Good Thing, 268
Making the Team, 223
Mama Is a Sunrise, 134
Mama One, Mama Two, 248, 374, 429
A Man for All Seasonings, 156
Man of Molokai: The Life of Father Damien, 352, 363
Martina Navratilova, 187, 239, 413
The Marvelous Pear Seed, 70, 231
Matches, Lighters, and Firecrackers Are Not Toys, 288
Maude and Sally, 221
Maybe by Then I'll Understand. 225
Me and Willie and Pa, 187, 239
The Meal, 159
Meat, 279
Medea's Children, 207, 240
Medicine in the Future, 285
A Medieval Feast, 123, 234
Megan's Beat, 225
Megan's Island, 266
Meg's Egg, 158
Menstruation: Just Plain Talk, 237
Merry Ever After, 124, 234
Michael and the Dentist, 290
Microbes and Bacteria, 282
The Midnight Ride of Paul Revere, 121, 239
Milk. (Giblin, J. C.), 182, 237
Milk. (Turner, D.), 278
Mind and Mood, 267
Mind Drugs, 171, 237, 297
Mind Your Manners, 156
Miss Rumphius, 298
Mist Over Altheney, 116, 234
The Mock Revolt, 336, 362
Molly's Pilgrim, 225
The Monkey's Haircut and Other Stories Told by the Maya, 231
Moonlight Moon, 295
More Stories Julian Tells, 266
More Tales of Uncle Remus, 327, 363
Mother Hicks, 198

Mother Mother I Feel Sick Send for the Doctor Quick Quick Quick, 153, 160, 235, 286
Mother to Son, 134, 142–143
A Mouse Named Junction, 249, 384
Move Over, Wheelchairs Coming Through, 284
Mr. East's Feast, 156
Mr. Jordan in the Park, 274
Mrs. Frisby and the Rats of NIMH, 85, 233, 325
Mufaro's Beautiful Daughters: An African Tale, 223, 252, 424
Munch, 155, 236
Munching, 156–157, 235
My Book for Kids with Cancer: A Child's Autobiography of Hope, 282
My Brother Sam Is Dead, 117–118, 234
My Five Senses, 260
My Grammy, 282
My Little Sister, 158
My Parents Think I'm Sleeping, 340
My Prairie Year, 120, 124–125, 234
My Sister Jane, 134
My Twin Sister Erika, 103, 234
My Uncle Dan, 134
The Mystery of Sleep, 270

Nadia the Willful, 103, 233
Nature Is . . . 158
Never Trust a Smiling Cat, 346–347
The New Baby at Your House, 172, 236
The New Kid on the Block, 133, 236
The New Physical Fitness: Something for Everyone, 272
Night of the Twisters, 289
No Bean Sprouts, Please! 278
No Kidding, 297
No Measles, No Mumps for Me, 11, 22, 283
No More Secrets for Me, 171, 238
No Place for Me, 297
No Pushing, No Dunking: Safety in the Water, 287
Nobody Asked Me If I Wanted a Baby Sister, 102, 233
Nobody Wants a Nuclear War, 299
Nobody's Baby Now, 280
Noise Pollution, 300
Norma Jean, Jumping Bean, 219
The Nose Tree, 352, 363
Nothing's Fair in Fifth Grade, 111, 233
Now Is Not Too Late, 295
Nuclear Accidents, 301
Nuclear Energy, 301
Nuclear War, Nuclear Winter, 300

O Sliver of Liver,   156
The Official Kids' Survival Kit: How to Do Things on Your Own,   288
Oh My Goodness, Oh My Dear,   138
Old Mother Hubbard,   158
On Eating Porridge Made of Peas,   156
On My Honor,   288
On the Banks of Plum Creek,   125, 235
Once There Was and Was Not: Armenian Tales Retold,   232
The One Bad Thing About Father,   185, 239
One Day in the Alpine Tundra,   237
One Fat Summer,   111–112, 233
One, Two, Buckle My Shoe,   150
Oodles of Noodles,   158
Oscar Mouse Finds a House,   223
Other Doors,   198
Out in the Dark and Daylight,   143–144, 235
Out of the Trap,   205, 241
Outside Over There,   64, 231
Overeating: Let's Talk About It,   253, 281
The Ox-Cart Man,   124, 234
Ozma of Oz,   209, 241

P. J. the Spotted Bunny,   223
Paddington on Stage,   200–203, 204, 240
The Pain and the Great One,   221
Pamela Camel,   222
Pancake?   159
The Pancake,   70, 77, 232
Pat a Cake, Pat a Cake, Baker's Man,   150
The Patchwork Quilt,   221, 273
Path of the Pale Horse,   292
Patrick and Ted,   220
Peabody,   222
Peanut Butter and Jelly,   199
Peanut Butter Batter Bread,   154
Peanut Butter Sandwich,   159
People,   265
People Like Us,   225
People of the Ice,   110, 238
The Perfect Family,   221, 351, 362
Perfect or Not, Here I Come,   266
Peter Rabbit's Natural Foods Cookbook,   178, 237
Phoebe's Revolt,   249, 436
A Photographic Story of Reproduction and Birth for Children,   275
Picnic,   88–89, 232
The Picnic,   159
Picnic Day,   159

Picture Book Theatre,   197, 240
Pie Problem,   158
Piggy,   156
The Pigman,   326, 364
Pippi Longstocking,   64, 231
The Pizza,   157
A Place for Ben,   221, 274
Play It Safe: The Kids Guide to Personal Safety and Crime Prevention,   289
Plays Children Love,   197, 239, 240
Plays from Folktales of Africa and Asia,   195, 240
A Pocketguide to Health and Health Problems in School Physical Activities,   247
Poem Stew,   153, 156, 235
Poems for Fathers,   250, 432
Poetry,   145
Point of View,   336
Polly, Put the Kettle On,   150
Pookins Gets Her Way,   220
Popcorn,   180, 238
The Popcorn Book,   180, 237
Popsicles,   157
Potatoes,   278
Prairie Songs,   119–120, 234
The Princess Who Was Hidden from the World,   206
Private High,   297
The Private Life of the American Teenager,   268
The Problem with Pulcifer,   290, 345, 362
Pumpernickel Tickle and Mean Green Cheese,   155, 236
Pumpkin Pumpkin,   181, 238
Punch and Judy Fought for a Pie,   150
The Puppy Who Wanted a Boy,   223
The Pushcart War,   86, 233

The Quiet Mother and the Noisy Little Boy,   265

Rabble Starkey,   225
Racso and the Rats of NIMH,   225, 325, 362
Rainbow Jordan,   267
Ralph Nader, Voice of the People,   293
Ramona and Her Father,   294
Ramona and Her Mother,   101, 233
Ramona Forever,   224
The Random House Book of Mother Goose,   149–150, 157–158, 235
The Random House Book of Poetry for Children,   142, 158, 220, 236, 336, 363

Rapunzel, 69, 70, 71–73, 232
Read-Aloud Rhymes for the Very Young, 158–159, 236
Reasons to Stay, 103–104, 233
The Red Fairy Book, 363
Red Is My Favorite Color, 350–351
The Red Pony, 326, 363
Reflections Dental, 133
Reflections on a Gift of Watermelon Pickle and Other Modern
    Verses, 133, 235
The Relatives Came, 105, 234
The Remembering Box, 337, 362
Restoring Our Earth, 301
Return to Bitter Creek, 66, 231, 252, 404
A Ring of Endless Light, 252, 485
Robinson and Friday, 252, 494
Robyn's Book, 224
Rope Rhyme, 139–140
The Rose on My Cake, 133, 145–146, 235
Rumble Fish, 266
Rumpelstiltskin, 69, 232
Running Is For Me, 269
Running with Rachel, 248, 412

Sad Sweet Story, 157
Sadako and the Thousand Paper Cranes, 187, 239, 257
Safety Can Be Fun, 287
Sarah Cynthia Sylvia Stout Who Would Not Take the Garbage Out, 136
Scoop After Scoop, 182, 237
The Scott, Foresman Anthology of Children's Literature, 134, 136, 159,
    232, 236
The Secret Garden, 225, 252, 372
Secrets of a Small World, 220
Seeing Things, 147
Selected Poems of Langston Hughes, 142, 235
729 Curious Creatures, 260
Sexual Abuse: Let's Talk About It, 167, 237
Sexually Transmitted Diseases, 172, 237
She Come Bringing Me That Little Baby Girl, 102, 233
A Sheltering Tree, 224
The Shopping Basket, 181, 236
A Shot for Baby Bear, 282
The Sick of Being Sick Book, 267
The Sidewalk Racer and Other Poems of Sports and Motion, 139, 235
The Sidewalk Racer or On the Skateboard, 139
Silent Killers: Radon and Other Hazards, 300
Sing For Your Supper, 145
The Skeletal System: Framework for Life, 238

The Skeleton Inside You, 260
Sky Seasoning, 159
Slake's Limbo, 336, 363
The Slave Dancer, 126–127, 234, 340, 362
Slaves of Spiegel, 93, 233
Sleep and Dreams, 250
Sleeping Beauty, 327
Slumber Party, 156
Slumps, Grunts, and Snickerdoodles: What Colonial America Ate and
    Why, 181, 238
Smart Choices, 255, 272
Smart Spending, 293
Smoking Not Allowed: The Debate, 295
Snack, 157
Snacks, 156
Snap! Snap! 219, 381
Snow White and the Seven Dwarfs, 70, 232
So Hungry, 219
So Many Raccoons, 223
So What? 336, 362
So What If I'm a Sore Loser, 249
The Solitary, 104, 233
Solomon Grundy, 150
Some Busy Hospital, 290
Some People, 144
Some People I Know, 158
Someone New, 250, 371
Something's Wrong in My House, 296
Sometimes My Mother Drinks Too Much, 294
Song and Dance Man, 273
Spaghetti, 159
Special Class, 204, 240
Spider's First Day at School, 222
Spinky Sulks, 265
A Spooky Sort of Shadow, 340
Sportsathon: Puzzles, Jokes, Facts & Games, 270
Starring Francine and Dave, 199, 241
The Steadfast Tin Soldier, 350, 362
Step on a Crack, 197
The Stepping Stone Series. (series), 316
A Stitch in Time for the Brothers Rhyme, 222
Storm Warnings, 336
The Story of Johnny Appleseed, 185, 238, 352,
    362
The Story of Poppyseed, 223
Straight Talk about Drugs and Alcohol, 252, 498
Straight Talk about Love and Sex for Teenagers, 254
Street, 199, 239

Street Gangs, Yesterday and Today, 289
Street Poems, 147, 235
Street Talk, 236
Strega Nona, 76, 341, 362
Strings: A Gathering of Family Poems, 276
Suicide, 208–209, 240
Sulk, 336
Summer Switch, 86, 233
A Summer to Die, 103, 234
Sunday Morning Toast, 154
Sunny Side Up, 155
Supermarket, 136, 147–148
Sure Hands, Strong Heart: The Life of Daniel Hale Williams, 239, 271
Sweet Dreams Body Book, 271
Sweetly Sings the Donkey, 224

Table Manners, 156
The Table, the Donkey, and the Stick, 352
Tackle Without a Team, 294
Take a Walk in Their Shoes, 267
Take Back the Moment, 225
The Tale of Peter Rabbit, 84, 88, 233
Tales of a Gambling Grandma, 337, 363
The Tales of Uncle Remus, 327, 363
Tales the People Tell in China, 231
The Talking Fish, 69, 232
A Taste of Purple, 158
Taught Me Purple, 134
Teddy Bears Go Shopping, 290
Tee-Tee, 221
Teen Guide to Childbirth, 276
Teen Pregnancy, 168, 171, 236
Teenage Body Book Guide to Sexuality, 276
Teenagers Face to Face with Cancer, 285
Tennis Is For Me, 250, 412
The Tenth Good Thing About Barney, 339, 364
Theatre for Youth: Twelve Plays with Mature Themes, 197, 240
The Theft of Fire, 327
There's a Boy in the Girl's Bathroom, 225
There's a Little Bit of Me in James, 282
There's a Nightmare in My Closet, 341–342, 363
They Really Like Me, 248, 374
A Thief in the Village (and Other Stories), 267
This Can Lick a Lollipop: Body Riddles for Kids, 260
This Delicious Day, 280
This Is Just to Say, 158
This Is the Bread I Baked for Ned, 278

This Time of Darkness, 87, 232
Those Happy Golden Years, 125, 235
Three Apples Fell from Heaven: Armenian Tales Retold, 70, 231
The Three Billy Goats Gruff, 330, 362
The Three Brothers, 352, 363
The Three Little Kittens, 209, 239
The Three Little Pigs, 70, 232
The Three Princesses of Whiteland, 352, 363
Three Rolls and One Doughnut: Fables from Russia, 231
The Three Wishes. (Galdone), 70, 75, 76, 232
The Three Wishes. (Zemach), 76, 232
Through Grandpa's Eyes, 351, 363
Throwing Shadows, 255, 408
Tiger Eyes, 342, 362
Timothy Too! 101, 234
Tinker Autumn, 254
To the Rescue: Seven Heroes of Conservation, 191, 239, 255, 300
Toaster Time, 159
Tobacco—What It Is, What It Does, 294
Tom Tit Tot, 69, 232
Too Blue, 133
Too Fat? Too Thin? Do You Have a Choice? 179, 236
Too Many Lollipops, 220
Too Much Garbage, 237
The Tooth Book, 260, 292
Tornado! 335
Tough Beans, 283
Tracker, 350, 363
Trash, 299
Trouble at Dinner, 157
The Trouble with Derek, 272
The Trouble with Thirteen, 263
Turtle Soup, 157
Tutti-Frutti, 156
The TV Kid, 291
Two Plays About Foolish People, 197–198, 240
Two Under Par, 250, 373

The Ugly Duckling, 84, 232, 350, 362, 376
Understanding AIDS, 167–168, 237
Understanding and Preventing AIDS, 284
Ups and Downs with Oink and Pearl, 351, 362

The Velveteen Rabbit, 85, 209, 233, 240
Very Last First Time, 109–110, 233
Vitamins—What They Are, What They Do, 176, 238, 290, 345,
  363

The Voyage Begun,   94–95, 232
The Voyage of the Dragonfly,   206–207, 240, 267

Waiting for Johnny Miracle,   285
Waiting for Mom,   219
Waiting to Waltz,   251, 464
Walk Together,   198, 240
Warton and the Castaways,   91, 232
Watch Out for the Chicken Feet in Your Soup,   109, 233
The Way I Feel. . .Sometimes,   265, 381
The Way Things Are and Other Poems,   235
The Ways of Living Things,   158
We Don't Look Like Our Mom and Dad,   274
The Wee Bannock,   70, 77, 232
A Weed Is a Flower: The Life of George Washington Carver,   185, 238
A Weekend with Wendell,   221
Welcome Home,   294
What a Teacher Needs,   353
What Does It Mean to You?   237
What Is a Girl? What Is a Boy?   274
What Is the Sign for Friend?   224
What Shall We Do With the Land? Choices for America,   301
What Teenagers Want to Know About Sex—Questions and Answers,   276
What to Do When There's No One But You,   287
What to Eat and Why,   279
What to Say to Clara,   221
What Will We Buy?   291
What's Happening to Me?   275
The What's Happening to My Body? Book for Boys,   272, 275
The What's Happening to My Body? Book for Girls,   272, 275
What's On Your Plate?   278, 336, 363
What's the Big Idea, Ben Franklin?   239
What's Under My Bed?   222
Wheels for Walking,   289
When a Parent Is Very Sick,   237
When Grandfather Journeys into Winter,   274
When Grownups Drive You Crazy,   266
When I Ride in a Car,   286
When I See My Dentist. . .   269
When I See My Doctor. . .   248, 290, 411
When I Was Lost,   142
When I Was Young in the Mountains,   337, 351, 363
When the New Baby Comes, I'm Moving Out,   102, 233
When the Rattlesnake Sounds,   199, 240, 409
When Your Kids Drive You Crazy,   266

Where Are You Going, Little Mouse? 221
Where Do You Think You're Going, Christopher Columbus? 186–187,
  239
Where Does All That Smoke Come From? 17, 22
Where in the World Is the Perfect Family? 252, 445
Where Is Nicky's Valentine? 219
Where the Sidewalk Ends, 159, 236, 336, 363
Where the Wild Things Are, 81, 233
Where's Chimpy? 282
Whiff, Sniff, Nibble and Chew: The Gingerbread Boy Retold, 160, 236
Who Are the Handicapped? 237
Who Ever Sausage a Thing? 156
Who Keeps Us Safe? 286
Who Killed Cock Robin? 150
Who Laughs Last? 197
Why Am I Different? 265
Why Am I So Miserable If These Are the Best Years of My Life? 272
Why Are You So Mean To Me? 220
Why Does My Nose Run? 271
Why I Cough, Sneeze, Shiver, Hiccup, and Yawn, 236
Why Me? Coping With Family Illness, 254, 458
Why There Is No Arguing in Heaven, 278
Wiggly Giggles, 336
The Wild Children, 289
Wild Strawberries, 159
Wiley and the Hairy Man, 198, 209, 241
Wilfrid Gordon McDonald Partridge, 351, 362
William's Doll, 249, 437
Willy the Wimp, 222
Wilma's Revenge, 207, 240
The Wind in the Willows, 84, 92, 232
Wind Rose, 165, 237
Winners: Women and the Nobel Prize, 190, 239
Winners Never Quit: Athletes Who Beat the Odds, 189, 238
Wish in One Hand, Spit in the Other, A Collection of Plays by Susan
  Zeder, 198, 240
With His Mouth Full of Food, 159
The Wolf and the Seven Little Kids, 70, 232
Wolf of Shadows, 301, 350
Women of Our Time. (series), 185
A Word From Our Sponsor or My Friend Alfred, 292
The World of Tomorrow, 301
The Wump World, 298

A Year in the Life of Rosie Bernard, 255, 436
Yellow Butter, 159

The Yellow Fairy Book,   363
The You Can Do It! Kids Diet,   253, 418
You Can Say No to a Drink or a Drug,   297
You Can't Make a Move Without Your Muscles,   238, 261
You Can't Sneeze With Your Eyes Open & Other Freaky Facts About the
    Human Body,   263
You Don't See Me,   208, 240
You Shouldn't Have to Say Goodbye,   326, 362
You'll Survive,   254, 407
Your Body Fuel,   262
Your Body, Your Heart,   231
Your Doctor, My Doctor,   269
Your Marvelous Mind,   263
Your Nerves and Their Messages,   263
Yummers!   89, 232
Yummers Too,   89–90, 232

Z for Zachariah,   81, 82, 95–96, 233
Zanballer,   250, 417

Section B: Poetry

After Covering the Continent,   154
Aunt Roberta,   139
Back to School,   143–144
Books,   331
The Challenger,   121–122
Chocolate,   140–141
Hannah Bantry,   158
How to Eat a Poem,   130
I Saw a Ship A-Sailing,   149
I Woke Up This Morning,   146
If All the World Was Paper,   156
Keepsake,   138
Mother to Son,   143
Oh My Goodness, Oh My Dear,   138
Poetry,   145
Rope Rhyme,   140
The Sidewalk Racer or On the Skateboard,   139
Supermarket,   148
What a Teacher Needs,   353
When I Was Lost,   142

Section C: Book Series

Brown Paper School Books,   177
Coping With,   17
Fourth Floor Twins,   316
Little Chef,   177
Magic Moscow Trilogy,   93
Stepping Stone,   316
Women of Our Time,   185

Section D: Book Selection Guides

Best Books for Children,   174
Children and Books,   65
Children's Choices,   216–226, 318
Choosing Books for Children,   68
The Elementary School Library Collection,   174
Index to Children's Plays in Collections,   194
Index to Poetry for Children and Young People: 1976–1981,   152
Pass the Poetry Please,   134, 136
Plays Magazine,   195
Subject Index to Poetry for Children and Young People,   152

Section E: Literacy Training: Reading, Writing, Evaluating

The Art of Teaching Writing,   352
The Basal Reading Program,   304–310
A Celebration of Bess: Helping Children Write Poetry,   136, 351
The Child as Critic   327
Children Talk About Books,   321–322
Children's Responses to Poetry in a Supportive Literacy Context,   312
Classroom Experiences,   352
Cushla and Her Books,   312
Drop Everything and Read (D. E. A. R.),   342–343
Fairy Tales, Fables, Legends, and Myths,   327
The Family of Stories,   327
Focus Units in Literature,   340–342

Growing Healthy, xv,   38–57, 214, 255–301
If You're Trying to Teach Kids How to Write, You've Gotta Have This
   Book,   352
In the Middle,   312, 352
Moving from the Basal into Literature,   311
A Prelude to Literacy,   312
The Read-Aloud Handbook,   21, 63, 162, 344
Sustained Silent Reading (S. S. R.),   342–343
Transitions,   312–313

Section F: Research Reports and Surveys

Becoming a Nation of Readers: The Report of the Commission on
   Reading,   210, 304, 306
Carnegie Corporation's Task Force on the Education of Young Adoles-
   cents,   244
Children's Poetry Preferences: A National Survey of the Upper Ele-
   mentary Grades,   151
Health Education and Youth: A Review of Research and Development,   8
Healthy People: The Surgeon General's Report on Health Promotion and
   Disease Prevention,   24, 25, 26
The National Adolescent Student Health Survey,   57
National Assessment of Educational Progress,   212, 315
1985 School Health Education Survey,   xiii, 8, 21
Primary Grades Health Curriculum Project,   xv, 39
School Health Curriculum Project. (grades 4–7),   xv, 39
School Health Education Evaluation study, (SHEE),   viii, 33–34
School Health in America,   36–38
Young Children's Preferences in Poetry: A National Survey of First,
   Second, and Third Graders,   151

About the Authors

Anthony L. Manna (B.A., Seton Hall University; M.A.T., Fairleigh Dickinson University; Ph.D., The University of Iowa) is an Associate Professor of literature, educational drama, and English education at Kent State University. Dr. Manna has taught at every level of education, from preschool to graduate school, both in the U.S.A. and overseas. He has been awarded research fellowships by the Shakespeare Institute, Stratford-upon-Avon, England; the Alden B. Dow Creativity Center, Midland, Michigan; and the Institute for Humanities and Medicine at the Northeast Ohio Universities College of Medicine, where he has served as an adjunct instructor. Dr. Manna is currently a visiting lecturer at Aristotle University, Thessaloniki, Greece. He is the recipient of a Distinguished Teaching Award from Kent State University. In addition to serving as director of publications for the international Children's Literature Association, Dr. Manna is the editor of the visual arts column of the *Children's Literature Association Quarterly*. He has published numerous articles and chapters on literature and drama.

Cynthia Wolford Symons is an Associate Professor of Health Education at Kent State University. She holds a B.S. degree from Lock Haven University, and an M.Ed. and D.Ed. in Health Education from The Pennsylvania State University. Prior to her work in higher education, Dr. Wolford Symons taught public school health education for seven years. She has been honored both as a distinguished teacher at Penn State and for her work with school- and community-based health promotion professionals by the College and Graduate School of Education at Kent State University. Her publication record indicates particular expertise in child and adolescent health issues in context of school-based health promotion initiatives.